Management Engineering for Effective Healthcare Delivery:

Principles and Applications

Alexander Kolker
Children's Hospital and Health System, Wisconsin, USA

Pierce Story
GE Healthcare, USA

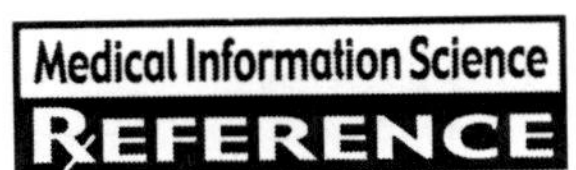

Senior Editorial Director:	Kristin Klinger
Director of Book Publications:	Julia Mosemann
Editorial Director:	Lindsay Johnston
Acquisitions Editor:	Erika Carter
Development Editor:	Michael Killian
Production Editor:	Sean Woznicki
Typesetters:	Keith Glazewski, Natalie Pronio, Milan Vracarich, Jr.
Print Coordinator:	Jamie Snavely
Cover Design:	Nick Newcomer

Published in the United States of America by

Medical Information Science Reference (an imprint of IGI Global)
701 E. Chocolate Avenue
Hershey PA 17033
Tel: 717-533-8845
Fax: 717-533-8661
E-mail: cust@igi-global.com
Web site: http://www.igi-global.com

Library of Congress Cataloging-in-Publication Data

Management engineering for effective healthcare delivery : principles and applications / Alexander Kolker and Pierce Story, editors.

p. ; cm.

Includes bibliographical references and index.

Summary: "This book illustrates the power of management engineering for quantitative managerial decision-making in healthcare settings, that assists in predicting performance and/or real resource requirements and allowing decision-makers to be truly proactive rather than reactive"-- Provided by publisher.

ISBN 978-1-60960-872-9 (hardcover) -- ISBN 978-1-60960-873-6 (ebook) -- ISBN 978-1-60960-874-3 (print & perpetual access) 1. Health services administration--Decision making. 2. Medical care. I. Kolker, Alexander, 1952- II. Story, Pierce.

[DNLM: 1. Delivery of Health Care--organization & administration. 2. Decision Making. 3. Health Services Administration. 4. Leadership. 5. Models, Organizational. 6. Practice Management--organization & administration. W 84.1]

RA971.M34237 2012

362.1068--dc23

2011022228

British Cataloguing in Publication Data

A Cataloguing in Publication record for this book is available from the British Library.

Editorial Advisory Board

Table of Contents

Chapter 12
Reducing Patient Waiting Time at an Ambulatory Surgical Center 246
David Ben-Arieh, Kansas State University, USA
Chih-Hang Wu, Kansas State University, USA

Chapter 13
Scheduling Healthcare Systems: Theory and Applications 261
Arben Asllani, The University of Tennessee - Chattanooga, USA

Chapter 14
Appointment Order Outpatient Scheduling System with Consideration of Ancillary Services and Overbooking Policy to Improve Outpatient Experience 287
Yu-Li Huang, New Mexico State University, USA

Section 3
Electronic Health Records

Chapter 15
Electronic Health Record: Adoption, Considerations and Future Direction...................................... 309
Janine R. A. Kamath, Mayo Clinic, USA
Amerett L. Donahoe-Anshus, Mayo Clinic, USA

Chapter 16
Electronic Medical Records (EMR): Issues and Implementation Perspectives.................................. 333
Dean E. Johnson, Wellspan Health, USA

Chapter 17
Health Information Exchange for Improving the Efficiency and Quality of Healthcare Delivery 352
Jing Shi, North Dakota State University, USA
Sudhindra Upadhyaya, North Dakota State University, USA
Ergin Erdem, North Dakota State University, USA

Section 4
Patient Flow

Chapter 18
Evaluating Patient Flow Based on Waiting Time and Travel Distance for Outpatient Clinic Visits.......376
S. Reza Sajjadi, North Dakota State University, USA
Jing Shi, North Dakota State University, USA
Kambiz Farahmand, North Dakota State University, USA

Detailed Table of Contents

Section 1
Efficient Managerial Decision-Making and Management of Operations

This chapter illustrates the predictive and analytical decision-making power of healthcare management engineering compared to traditional management reasoning. An overview of the domain of healthcare management engineering is provided, including capacity management, staffing, scheduling, the entire hospital patient flow, probabilistic resource allocation, patient volume forecasting, principal components analysis for a large patient demographic data base. Four types of problems are illustrated in details: (i) dynamic supply and demand balance using discrete event simulation, (ii) the probabilistic resource optimization, (iii) principal component analysis for identifying a few significant independent contributing variables (factors), and (iv) recursive forecasting of a time series using its auto-correlation function to identify the strongly correlated past data-points. Traditional managerial decision-making and management engineering methodology are discussed and applied side by side to analyze the same problems in order to illustrate and explain their differences. Some fundamental management engineering principles are summarized in conclusion.

Hospitals are dynamic systems and must be analyzed and managed as such. Therefore, we need dynamic analytical tools and thinking to fix hospitals' most pressing issues. This is the premise of the chapter on Dynamic Capacity Management (DCAMM). Concepts such as "Dynamic Standardization" and "Outlier Management" can augment the existing, static process improvement systems such as Lean and Six Sigma. This chapter will provide an overview of the concepts and structures necessary to profoundly change the way our hospitals, and health systems, are managed.

Healthcare has delivered incredible improvements in diagnosis and treatment of diseases but faces challenges to improve the delivery of services. This chapter reviews the current challenges and methods including the use of simulation modeling. Analysis of emergency patient flows through a major hospital shows the capability of simulation modeling to enable improvement of the healthcare delivery system. This chapter enables healthcare managers to understand the power simulation modeling brings to the improvement of healthcare delivery.

The chapter will broaden the engineer's perception in regards to the gamut of simulation implements. This ranges from paper-and-pencil and board-game reproductions of situations to complex computer-aided interactive systems. Some of the problem-solving models discussed include labor and delivery room utilization, neonatal intensive care unit expansion, emergency department staffing and process improvement, radiology process improvement, patient transport, operating room elective case surgery optimization, partial pediatric unit conversion to Intermediate Medical Care unit, family practice, and women's health clinics.

Biomedical technology is a valuable asset of healthcare facilities. It is now universally accepted that, to assure patient safety, medical devices must be correctly managed and used, and that the quality of healthcare delivery is related to the suitability of the available technology. The activities that guarantee a proper management are carried on by the people working on a Clinical Engineering (CE) Department. In the chapter we describe a model to estimate the number of clinical engineers and biomedical equipment technicians (BMET) that will constitute the clinical engineering department staff. It was used by managers of Regione Piemonte to start a regional network of clinical engineering departments.

Chapter 6
Intensive Care Unit Operational Modeling and Analysis 132
Yue Dong, Mayo Clinic, USA
Huitian Lu, South Dakota State University, USA
Ognjen Gajic, Mayo Clinic, USA
Brian Pickering, Mayo Clinic, USA

The outcome of critical illness depends not only on life threatening disturbances, but also on several complex "system" dimensions. Systems engineering tools offers a novel approach which can enable the emergence of a "systems understanding" of patient-environment interactions facilitating advances in the science of healthcare delivery. Patient variation and uncertainties present an additional challenge to investigators wishing to model and improve healthcare delivery processes. In this chapter authors present a systems engineering approach to modeling critical care delivery using sepsis resuscitation as an example.

Chapter 7
Human-Centered Systems Engineering: Managing Stakeholder Dissonance
in Healthcare Delivery 148
GM Samaras, Samaras & Associates, Inc., USA

Deploying new tools and technologies often results in creating new problems while solving existing problems. A root cause is the interaction between tool design and organizational deployment. One undesirable result is the creation of stakeholder dissonance (SD). SD is a term for the conflict between the needs, wants, and desires (NWDs) of different stakeholders. In healthcare delivery systems, it is evidenced by errors, workarounds, and threats to patient safety and organizational profitability. Human-Centered Systems Engineering (HCSE) is the foundational paradigm for managing SD. HCSE emphasizes the criticality of the interfaces between humans, their tools, and their organizations, offering methods to recognize, measure, and control SD. It is complimentary to Lean, Six Sigma, Balanced Scorecard, and Quality Function Deployment approaches.

Chapter 8
Enabling Real-Time Management and Visibility with RFID 172
Peter J. Hawrylak, The University of Tulsa, USA
Ajay Ogirala, University of Pittsburgh, USA
Bryan A. Norman, University of Pittsburgh, USA
Jayant Rajgopal, University of Pittsburgh, USA
Marlin H. Mickle, University of Pittsburgh, USA

Radio frequency identification (RFID) and Real Time Location Systems (RTLS) provide a wireless means to identify, locate, monitor, and track assets and people. RFID technology can be used for resource and patient location, to reduce costs, improve inventory accuracy, and improve patient safety. A number of pilot deployments of RFID and RTLS technology have yielded promising results, reduced costs, and improved patient care. However, there are three major issues facing RFID and RTLS systems: privacy, security, and location accuracy. As described in this chapter the privacy and security issues can be eas-

ily addressed by employing standard security measures. Location accuracy issues are physics-related and new advances continue to improve this accuracy. However, in hospital applications accuracy to the room level is sufficient.

Both during and after the recent reform efforts, healthcare delivery has been identified as the key to transforming the U.S. healthcare system. In light of this background, we borrow from systems engineering and business management to present the concept of service co-production as a new paradigm for healthcare delivery and, using the foresight afforded by this model, to systematically identify the barriers to healthcare delivery functioning as a service system. The service co-production model requires for patient, provider, insurer, administrator, and all the related healthcare individuals to collaborate at all stages – prevention, triage, diagnosis, treatment, and follow-up – of the healthcare delivery system in order to produce optimal health outcomes. Our analysis reveals that the barriers to co-production – the misalignment of financial and legal incentives, limited incorporation of collaborative point of care systems, and poor access to care – also serve as the source of many of the systemic failings of the U.S. healthcare system. The Patient Protection and Affordable Care Act takes steps to reduce these barriers, but leaves work to be done. Future research and policy reform is needed to enable effective and efficient co-production in the twenty-first century. With this review, we assess the state of service co-production in the U.S. healthcare system, and propose solutions for improvement.

Discrete-event simulation (DES) is an effective tool for analyzing and improving healthcare processes. In this chapter we discuss the use of simulation to improve patient flow at an outpatient procedure center (OPC) at Mayo Clinic. The OPC addressed is the Pain Clinic, which was faced with high patient volumes in a new, untested facility. Simulation was particularly useful due to the uncertain patient procedure and recovery times. We discuss the simulation process and show how it helped reduce patient waiting time while ensuring the clinic could meet its target patient volumes.

Chapter 11
Reducing Consultation Waiting Time and Overtime in Outpatient Clinic:
Challenges and Solutions 229
Zhu Zhecheng, Health Services & Outcomes Research, Singapore
Heng Bee Hoon, Health Services & Outcomes Research, Singapore
Teow Kiok Liang, Health Services & Outcomes Research, Singapore

Outpatient clinics face increasing pressure to handle more appointment requests due to aging and growing population. The increase in workload impacts two critical performance indicators: consultation waiting time and clinic overtime. Consultation waiting time is the physical waiting time a patient spends in the waiting area of the clinic, and clinic overtime is the amount of time the clinic is open beyond its normal opening hours. This chapter analyzes the complexity of an outpatient clinic in a Singapore public hospital, and factors causing long consultation waiting time and clinic overtime. Discrete event simulation and design of experiments are applied to quantify the effects of the factors on consultation waiting time/clinic overtime. Implementation results show significant improvement once those factors are well addressed.

Chapter 12
Reducing Patient Waiting Time at an Ambulatory Surgical Center.. 246
David Ben-Arieh, Kansas State University, USA
Chih-Hang Wu, Kansas State University, USA

This chapter describes a methodology to reduce patient waiting time in a for-profit ambulatory surgical center. Patients in this facility are scheduled in advance for the various operations, and yet operations start late, last longer than expected creating undesired delays.

Although this facility is limited to ambulatory surgery, it provides a large number of different surgeries, which are scheduled using "block" scheduling approach. The methodology presented generates a more accurate schedule by creating better time estimates for the operations and with lower variability. The effect of sequencing the surgeries, such that the ones with lower variability are performed earlier in the day, is also discussed.

Chapter 13
Scheduling Healthcare Systems: Theory and Applications 261
Arben Asllani, The University of Tennessee - Chattanooga, USA

This chapter offers a series of scheduling techniques and their applications in healthcare settings. Healthcare administrators, physicians, and other professionals can use such techniques to achieve their operational goals when resources are limited. The chapter covers a wide spectrum of scheduling models, from single server and deterministic models to the more difficult ones, those which consider several servers and stochastic variables. A strong emphasis is placed on the practical aspects of scheduling techniques in healthcare.

Chapter 14
Appointment Order Outpatient Scheduling System with Consideration of Ancillary
Services and Overbooking Policy to Improve Outpatient Experience 287
Yu-Li Huang, New Mexico State University, USA

Patient wait time and access to care have long been a recognized problem in modern outpatient healthcare delivery systems. In spite of all the efforts to develop appointment rules and policies, the problem of long patient waits persists. Despite the reasons, the fact remains that there are few implemented models for effective scheduling that consider patient wait times, physician idle time, overtime, ancillary service time, as well as individual no-show rate, and are generalized sufficiently to accommodate a variety of outpatient clinic settings. The goal of this chapter is to improve the quality and efficiency of healthcare delivery by developing a physician schedule that meets the clinical policies without overbooking using an innovative 'wait ratio' concept, a patient arrival schedule from the physician schedule accounting for ancillary services, an evidence-based predictive model of no-show probability for individual patient, and a model-supported dynamic overbooking policy to reduce the negative impact of no-shows.

Section 3
Electronic Health Records

Over the last two decades there has been considerable deliberation, experience, and research in the arena of Health Information Technology (HIT), Electronic Medical Records (EMR), Electronic Health Records (EHR) and more recently Electronic Personal Health Records (PHR). This chapter attempts to synthesize the vast amount of information, experience and implementation perspectives related to Electronic Health Records with the intent of assisting healthcare institutions and key stakeholders make informed choices as they embark on designing, developing and implementing an EHR. EHR considerations, challenges, opportunities and future directions are also addressed. The chapter highlights the power of management engineering to facilitate planning, implementation and sustainability of the EHR, a critical asset for a healthcare organization and the overall healthcare industry.

For many years the electronic medical record has been the holy grail of hospital system integration. Hundreds of millions of dollars have been spent in attempts to develop effective electronic medical records (EMR) to provide clinical care for patients. The advantages of an EMR are listed as reducing error, streamlining care, and allowing multiple people to provide simultaneous care. Unfortunately, most current EMR implementations are developed without completely understanding the processes that are being automated. In some implementations, there is an effort to first outline the process, and then try to create software that will facilitate the existing process, but this effort is not typically done systematically and with the discipline of an engineer. We will discuss the areas that management systems engineers can facilitate the design and implementation of the EMR, reducing the errors in the current processes and preparing the healthcare system for further improvements.

Chapter 17
Health Information Exchange for Improving the Efficiency and Quality of Healthcare Delivery 352
Jing Shi, North Dakota State University, USA
Sudhindra Upadhyaya, North Dakota State University, USA
Ergin Erdem, North Dakota State University, USA

In healthcare industry providers, patients and all other stakeholders must have the right information at the right time for achieving efficient and cost effective services. Exchange of information between the heterogeneous system entities plays a critical role. Health information exchange (HIE) is not only a process of transmitting data, but also a platform for streamlining operations to improve healthcare delivery in a secure manner. In this chapter, we present a comprehensive view of electronic health record (EHR) systems and HIE by presenting their architecture, benefits, challenges, and other related issues. While providing information on the current state of EHR/HIE applications, we also discuss advanced issues and secondary uses of HIE implementations, and shed some light on the future research in this area by highlighting the challenges and potential.

Section 4
Patient Flow

Chapter 18
Evaluating Patient Flow Based on Waiting Time and Travel Distance for Outpatient Clinic Visits.......376
S.Reza Sajjadi, North Dakota State University, USA
Jing Shi, North Dakota State University, USA
Kambiz Farahmand, North Dakota State University, USA

Patient flow greatly affects the quality of service delivered to the patients. Among the various performance measures identified for patient flow, the chapter focuses on the analytical modeling of two key measures, namely, patient waiting time and travel distance. Waiting time is analyzed by a promising yet simple analytical tool – queuing theory. Three queuing models including single station, multiple serial stations, and network systems are presented. Meanwhile, patient travel distance is investigated by an analytical model to evaluate the patient flow. For both measures, the applicability of models is illustrated with numerical examples.

Chapter 19
Using Patient Flow to Examine Hospital Operations 402
Renata Konrad, Worcester Polytechnic Institute, USA
Beste Kucukyazici, Zaragoza Logistics Center, Spain
Mark Lawley, Purdue University, USA

Adopting an admission-to-discharge patient flow perspective has the potential to improve hospital operations. Flow paths provide insight regarding patient care needs, support resource allocation and capacity planning decisions, and improve the operational performance of the hospitals. Studying patient flow through systems engineering tools and applications can help decision makers assess and improve care delivery. This chapter presents current research and techniques used to describe, measure, and model

inpatient flow. We formally define patient flow from an operational standpoint and discuss why it is crucial for operational decisions. Systems engineering techniques that describe and analyze inpatient flow are introduced. However, these techniques present certain modeling challenges, which we address. The chapter concludes with a discussion of emerging approaches to capture patient flow.

Section 5
Cost Management

Chapter 20
A New Cost Accounting Model and New Indicators for Hospital Management
Based on Personnel Cost..419
Yoshiaki Nakagawa, Kyoto University, Japan
Hiroyuki Yoshihara, Kyoto University, Japan
Yoshinobu Nakagawa, Kagawa National Children's Hospital, Japan

Specified hospital accounting systems in a hospital are necessary for a manager to determine the proper management strategy. We developed a new cost accounting model based on new allocation rules of personnel cost. The model presented in this chapter offers a manager useful tools to calculate the medical cost not only for an individual patient and for each clinical department, but also each DRG system for a specific period.

New financial indicators were developed based on personnel costs which were calculated using this new cost accounting system. Indicator 1: The ratio of the marginal profit after personnel cost per personnel cost (RMP). Indicator 2: The ratio of investment (=indirect cost) per personnel cost (RIP). Operation profit per one dollar of personnel cost (OPP) was demonstrated to be the difference between the RMP and RIP. The break-even point (BEP) and break-even ratio (BER) could be determined by combining the indicators. RMP demonstrates not only the medical efficiency, but also the medical productivity in the case of DPC/DRG groups. OPP can be utilized to compare the medical efficiency of each department in either one hospital or multiple hospitals. It also makes it possible to evaluate the management efficiency of multiple hospitals.

Compilation of References 435

About the Contributors 468

Index...479

Foreword

To paraphrase a very important speech made by British Prime Minister Harold McMillan in South Africa in February of 1960, "*The wind of change is blowing through Healthcare...*"

Healthcare in the US is in crisis. Report after report has chronicled the poor quality of care provided on average, the exorbitantly high costs of care (which are rapidly leading the US into a fiscal nightmare), poor health outcomes and poor health status as compared with other industrialized countries, and – more recently – a decrease in consumer trust in the healthcare system.

This is happening despite the continued and even accelerating technological and therapeutic advances that have occurred in medical devices, surgical techniques, and imaging technologies, as well as the dramatic biologic advances such as the use of stem cells.

Frankly, this situation is not all that surprising if you consider its root causes, i.e. the use, almost exclusively, of the centuries old "medical model" of thinking to drive change in healthcare, and perpetuating an incentive system among almost all stakeholders that results in precisely the outcomes it is designed to give, but which are not those compatible with a highly functioning, cost-efficient, consumer-friendly system of healthcare.

In our current US healthcare sector we have highly trained, superbly skilled clinicians and healthcare professionals functioning at the top of their skill levels, but who are by and large not supported by an equally high-functioning operational system(s) that effectively prevent errors, insure high reliability of outcomes in the population, appropriately conserve resources, and incentivize all those in the system to "do the right thing." Further, largely because of the perpetuation of the "medical model" approach to change, few healthcare professionals are exposed to concepts outside the medical "comfort zone" such as systems thinking, process engineering, change management, et cetera, either in their formal education or in their practical training.

In addition, in healthcare, we now have many highly paid, well-trained executives and administrators who – in accordance with their training – are focused almost exclusively on the business of developing, acquiring, maintaining, and financing new healthcare products, services, and treatment facilities. Motivated by recent regulatory and legislative changes requiring more efficiency, more accountability, and better results, these executives and administrators are just beginning to realize the potential of developing a total culture of quality (e.g. Virginia Mason) and of the systematic use of process and systems engineering tools and techniques (e.g. Theda Care, Virtua Hospital and others).

Almost five years ago, the Institute of Medicine (IOM) and National Academy of Engineering (NAE) published the third in a series of IOM reports on the sad state of our healthcare system. This report noted that "a real impact on quality, efficiency and sustainability of the health care system can be achieved only by using health care delivery engineering." Sadly, this report was all but ignored.

Dr. Kolker and Mr. Story are to be congratulated for bringing this text to those working in healthcare at this time, when – as never before – the potential for our nation's people to have accessible to them needed healthcare services, depends on the degree to which all those working in the healthcare system can expeditiously and successfully abandon their disciplinary silos and traditional modes of thinking to embrace and actualize a team-based approach to facing and overcoming the ills of our system.

Such a team must include not only those who have always been there (doctors, nurses, hospital administrators, etc.) but now must also include professionals from fields that have a huge potential to contribute effective solutions such as industrial engineering, cultural anthropology, health informatics, etc. whose practitioners use proven, validated tools that have been successfully deployed elsewhere in science, industry, government, and even in the military.

I do not mean to imply that for there to be success in the use of engineering sciences and methodologies in the transformation of our health system that every physician, nurse or healthcare administrator has to possess advanced engineering skills sets, or – conversely – that process engineers, change management professionals, etc. need to be able to practice medicine. Far from it! Rather, what needs to happen, and what I think is the beauty and genius of this text, is that everyone working in healthcare needs to have some familiarity and a working awareness of the power and utility of system thinking when applied correctly and adequately to health care.

This text is easy-to-understand, authoritative, and includes twenty well-referenced chapters, authored by leaders in their respective fields. It helps to those in healthcare faced with the current chaotic situation, at whatever level in whatever venue, to begin to understand how engineering principles can be applied to the situations and settings that everyone knows need to be improved but which have not been – due largely to bias against and/or ignorance of the solutions that the Institute of Medicine and National Academy of Engineering Report indicates can and must be applied.

I believe that this text ushers in a "New Dawn" of understanding and teamwork. I believe that in a short time (because we do not have very much time), if effectively and widely used, this text can contribute toward realizing the dream of the authors of the Institute of Medicine and National Academy of Engineering Report for creating and sustaining a new "partnership between engineering and medicine".

As such, I believe that this book should become *de rigueur* reading for healthcare professionals in training and/or in practice.

Joseph A. Fortuna
Prism, USA & Healthcare Division of the American Society for Quality (ASQ)

Joseph A. Fortuna *is the Co-Founder and CEO of PRISM, a non-profit corporation providing sustainable transformative services to medical practices. He is also the current Chair of the Health Care Division of the American Society for Quality, is a member of the Executive Committee of the Michigan Primary Care Consortium (MPCC), and is a member of the Steering Committee of the Detroit Beacon Communities Program funded by the Office of the National Coordinator of HIT. Dr. Fortuna has also served as a Divisional Medical Director of the DELPHI Corporation where he supervised the medical and occupational health activities in 73+ facilities worldwide, and where - using process improvement tools - he directed the design, development, and implementation of Delphi's Corporate Medical-Safety-Workers Comp Health Information System. He is also a member of the Patient Centered Primary Care Coalition (PCPCC) Executive Committee. He has served as the Speaker of the House of Delegates of the American college of Occupational and Environmental Medicine (ACOEM) and as a member of its Board of Directors.*

Foreword

MEDICAL EDUCATION AND THE NEW MEDICAL PRACTICE

Calls from the IHI, Leapfrog Group, health plans, purchasers, patients, and physician groups for improving quality and safety make it untenable to continue medical education as a status quo. Physicians and health care administrators must have a new skill and knowledge set to effectively manage and direct the change that is well upon the U.S. health care system. Challenges faced by health care professionals include low efficiency of delivery of care, low level of public accountability, unsustainable rate of rising cost of health care, quality and outcomes issues and the rising burden of chronic illness/disability.

Healthcare management engineering is the foundation of the new model for delivery of care. It is based on quantitative, engineering approach to analyzing, changing and improving the systems with complex interdependencies within hospitals and clinics. There is a visible increase in demand for healthcare management engineers, which are sometimes called performance engineers, process engineers, operation improvement or process improvement specialists. Yet, such specialists remain in short supply. They have to possess both the knowledge of engineering and mathematical disciplines and the knowledge of hospital and clinic operations.

While this book is not intended to serve as a college textbook, it provides the current state of affairs in methods and knowledge required today for the efficient healthcare management. This book can serve as the basis for both formal and informal education demonstrating a wide area of topics for the application of healthcare management engineering methodology.

On top of that, this book provides an international exposure to this challenging area. Researchers and healthcare practitioners not only from USA but also from Australia, Singapore, Japan, Italy, and Spain have contributed to this book. Despite different models of care delivery in these countries, the authors appreciate the power of healthcare management engineering and illustrate its use as a means of improving efficiency of care delivery and cost containment. These issues are not unique to USA, and international experience is instructive.

In summary, healthcare education system cannot afford to produce another generation of health care administrators and leaders in the current paradigm of traditional practice of management. This book contributes toward achieving the goal of producing that new generation.

Ernest Lee Yoder
Central Michigan University College of Medicine, USA

Ernie Yoder *is currently Professor and Founding Dean, Central Michigan University College of Medicine. Prior to this, Dr. Yoder was Vice President for Medical Education and Research at St. John Health System and Clinical Professor of Medicine at Wayne State University School of Medicine. Ernie completed medical school at WSU in 1978, residency in internal medicine in 1981, and following a year as Chief Medical Resident, joined the WSU full time faculty. He completed his PhD in Education at WSU in 1997. Dr. Yoder has received many awards including the Association of American Medical colleges – CGEA Laureate, WSU – School of Medicine Academy of Scholars, and multiple times Best Doctors in America. His main clinical and academic efforts focus on improving primary care medical practice, medical education, educational program evaluation, evidence based medicine (EBM), and continuous quality improvement (CQI). He has published in these areas. Dr. Yoder has served on numerous Boards, including Governor for the MI Chapter of the American College of Physicians, a term on the Executive Committee of the ACP Board of Governors, Chair of the AAMC Central Group on Educational Affairs, and Chair for the AAMC-GEA Section on Undergraduate Medical Education. In 2006 Dr. Yoder was inducted as a Fellow of the Detroit Medical Academy, and in April 2010 was honored as a Master of the American College of Physicians. He was active in leading quality improvement studies and teaching CQI and EBM to students, residents, and faculty at St. John Health.*

Preface

Modern medicine has achieved great progress in treating individual patients. This progress is based mainly on life science (molecular genetics, biophysics, biochemistry) and the development of medical devices, surgical techniques and imaging technologies. However, according to a report 'Building a Better Delivery System: A New Engineering & Healthcare Partnership' published jointly by National Academy of Engineering and Institute of Medicine in 2005, relatively little material resources or technical talent have been devoted to the proper functioning of the overall healthcare delivery as an integrated system in which access to efficient care should be delivered to many thousands of patients in an economically sustainable way.

As this report strongly points out in its Executive Summary, a real impact on quality, efficiency, and sustainability of the healthcare system can be achieved only by using methods and principles of healthcare delivery engineering. At the same time, this report states in an unusually blunt way, "In fact, relatively few healthcare professionals or administrators are equipped to think analytically about healthcare delivery as a system or to appreciate the relevance of engineering tools. Even fewer are equipped to work with engineers to apply these tools."

Thus, it is often difficult for many administrators to appreciate the role of management engineering methodology to the healthcare delivery process analysis. On the other hand, engineering professionals do not always have enough knowledge of healthcare delivery processes or the role of the physicians in making management decisions. Healthcare has a culture of rigid division of labor. This functional division does not effectively support the methodology that crosses the functional areas, especially if it assumes significant change in traditional relationships.

A systematic way of developing managerial decisions for efficient allocating of material, human and financial resources needed for delivery of high quality care using quantitative methods is the scope of what is called healthcare management engineering.

It is now imperative for healthcare administrators and executives to become familiar with the quantitative decision-making techniques and tools offered by management engineering. Fixing the healthcare system requires decision-makers who are 'bilingual' both in hospital operations and in management and system engineering principles.

While there is much work to do, especially at the hospital level, some changes addressing the recommendations for the dissemination of management engineering and system thinking are already under way. There are some journal publications in which the role and importance of management engineering in developing efficient decisions is discussed. However, many of them lack concrete, specific examples of practical applications and decision-making methodology. Therefore these publications are somewhat declarative.

The objective of this book is to illustrate the powerful methodology for making predictive efficient managerial decisions in different areas of healthcare, as well as fundamental management engineering principles for healthcare settings.

The distinct feature of this book is that it provides an international exposure to this challenging area. Researchers and healthcare practitioners not only from U.S., but also from Australia, Singapore, Japan, Italy, and Spain have contributed to this book. Despite different models of care delivery in these countries, the international contributors demonstrate the power of healthcare management engineering and its use as a means of improving efficiency of care delivery and cost containment. These issues are not unique to U.S. healthcare, and highlighting international experience and approach is instructive.

Prospective audience for this book includes healthcare and clinic administrators, managers, directors, vice-presidents for improvement and chief operating officers, i.e. those stakeholders who have the power to make managerial decisions. Another perspective segment of readers are graduate students pursuing a Master of Business Administration (MBA) or Master of Public Health (MPH) programs. These students are on the forefront in developing and providing economically viable processes of healthcare delivery.

This book is organized in 5 sections.

Section 1, **Efficient Managerial Decision-Making and Management of Operations**, includes 9 chapters.

Chapter 1, *Efficient Managerial Decision-Making in Healthcare Settings: Examples and Fundamental Principles,* provides an overview of the overall domain of healthcare management engineering. Management engineering domain includes capacity management, staffing, scheduling, patient flow, probabilistic resource allocation, patient volume forecasting, techniques for reduction of the number of variables for large patient data bases, as well as optimization of the geographic location of facilities and facilities layout, engineering (design) of the facility optimized workflow, defining and measuring productivity, supply chain and inventory management, quality control techniques, advanced multivariate statistical data analysis for marketing and budgeting purposes.

Four types of problems are illustrated in particular in this chapter: (i) dynamic supply and demand balance using discrete event simulation, (ii) the probabilistic resource optimization, (iii) variables reduction technique for identifying a few significant contributing variables (factors), and (iv) the recursive forecasting of a time series. Traditional managerial decision-making and management engineering methodology are applied side by side to analyze the same problems in order to illustrate and explain their differences. Some fundamental management engineering principles are summarized in conclusion.

Chapter 2, *Dynamic Capacity Management (DCAMM™) in a Hospital Setting,* illustrates that hospitals are dynamic systems and must be analyzed and managed as such. Therefore, it is needed dynamic analytical tools and thinking to fix hospitals' most pressing issues. Concepts such as "Dynamic Standardization" and "Outlier Management" can augment the existing, static process improvement methods such as Lean and Six Sigma. This chapter provides an overview of the concepts and structures necessary to profoundly change the way our hospitals, and health systems, are managed.

Chapter 3, *Simulation Modeling of Healthcare Delivery*, points out that healthcare has delivered incredible improvements in diagnosis and treatment of diseases but faces challenges to improve the delivery of services. This chapter reviews the current challenges and methods including the use of simulation modeling. Analysis of emergency patient flows through a major hospital shows the capability of simulation modeling to enable improvement of the healthcare delivery system. This chapter enables healthcare managers to understand the power simulation modeling brings to the improvement of healthcare delivery.

Chapter 4, *Simulation Applications in a Healthcare Setting,* will broaden the engineer's perception in regards to the gamut of simulation implements. This ranges from paper-and-pencil and board-game reproductions of situations to complex computer-aided interactive systems. Some of the problem-solving models discussed include labor and delivery room utilization, neonatal intensive care unit expansion, emergency department staffing and process improvement, radiology process improvement, patient transport, operating room elective case surgery optimization, partial pediatric unit conversion to Intermediate Medical Care unit, family practice, and women's health clinics.

Chapter 5, *Modeling Clinical Engineering Activities to Support Healthcare Technology Management,* discusses that in order to assure patient safety medical devices must be correctly managed and used, and that the quality of healthcare delivery is related to the suitability of the available technology. The activities that guarantee a proper management are carried on by the people working on a Clinical Engineering (CE) Department.

The chapter describes a model to estimate the number of clinical engineers and biomedical equipment technicians (BMET) that will constitute the clinical engineering department staff. It was used by managers of Regione Piemonte (Italy) to start a regional network of clinical engineering departments.

Chapter 6, *Intensive Care Unit Operational Modeling and Analysis*, illustrates that the outcome of critical illness depends not only on life threatening disturbances, but also on several complex "system" dimensions. Systems engineering tools offers a novel approach which can enable the emergence of a "systems understanding" of patient-environment interactions facilitating advances in the science of healthcare delivery. Patient variation and uncertainties present an additional challenge to investigators wishing to model and improve healthcare delivery processes. A system engineering approach is presented to modeling critical care delivery using sepsis resuscitation as an example.

Chapter 7, *Human-Centered Systems Engineering: Managing Stakeholder Dissonance in Healthcare Delivery,* discusses that deploying new tools and technologies often results in creating new problems while solving existing problems. A root cause is the interaction between tool design and organizational deployment. One undesirable result is the creation of stakeholder dissonance (SD). SD is a term for the conflict between the needs, wants, and desires (NWDs) of different stakeholders. In healthcare delivery systems, it is evidenced by errors, workarounds, and threats to patient safety and organizational profitability.

Human-Centered Systems Engineering (HCSE) is the foundational paradigm for managing SD. HCSE emphasizes the criticality of the interfaces between humans, their tools, and their organizations, offering methods to recognize, measure, and control SD. It is complimentary to Lean, Six Sigma, Balanced Scorecard, and Quality Function Deployment approaches.

Chapter 8, *Enabling Real-Time Management and Visibility with RFID,* indicates that Radio frequency identification (RFID) and Real Time Location Systems (RTLS) provide a wireless means to identify, locate, monitor, and track assets and people. RFID technology can be used for resource and patient location, to reduce costs, improve inventory accuracy, and improve patient safety. A number of pilot deployments of RFID and RTLS technology have yielded promising results, reduced costs and improved patient care. However, there are three major issues facing RFID and RTLS systems: privacy, security, and location accuracy. As described in this chapter, the privacy and security issues can be easily addressed by employing standard security measures. Location accuracy issues are physics-related and new advances continue to improve this accuracy. However, in hospital applications accuracy to the room level is sufficient.

Chapter 9, *Healthcare Delivery as a Service System: Barriers to Co-Production and Implications of Healthcare Reform,* discusses issues of healthcare delivery as a system. The authors borrow from systems engineering and business management to present the concept of service co-production as a new paradigm for healthcare delivery. Using the foresight afforded by this model the authors systematically identify the barriers to healthcare delivery functioning as a service system. The service co-production model requires for patient, provider, insurer, administrator and all the related healthcare individuals to collaborate at all stages – prevention, triage, diagnosis, treatment, and follow-up – of the healthcare delivery system in order to produce optimal health outcomes. Analysis presented in this chapter reveals that the barriers to co-production – the misalignment of financial and legal incentives, limited incorporation of collaborative point of care systems, and poor access to care – also serve as the source of many of the systemic failings of the U.S. healthcare system. The Patient Protection and Affordable Care Act takes steps to reduce these barriers, but leaves work to be done. The authors assess the state of service co-production in the U.S. healthcare system, and propose solutions for improvement.

Section 2, **Outpatient Clinic Management and Scheduling**, includes 5 chapters.

In Chapter 10, *Using Simulation to Design and Improve an Outpatient Procedure Center,* the authors discuss the use of simulation to improve patient flow at an outpatient procedure center (OPC) at Mayo Clinic. The OPC addressed is the Pain Clinic, which was faced with high patient volumes in a new, untested facility. Simulation was particularly useful due to the uncertain patient procedure and recovery times. The authors discuss the simulation process and show how it helped reduce patient waiting time while ensuring the clinic could meet its target patient volumes.

Chapter 11, *Reducing Consultation Waiting Time and Overtime in Outpatient Clinic: Challenges and Solutions,* analyzes the situation for an outpatient clinics that face increasing pressure to handle more appointment requests due to aging and growing population. The increase in workload impacts two critical performance indicators: consultation waiting time and clinic overtime. Consultation waiting time is the physical waiting time a patient spends in the waiting area of the clinic, and clinic overtime is the amount of time the clinic is open beyond its normal opening hours. This chapter analyzes the complexity of an outpatient clinic in a Singapore public hospital, and factors causing long consultation waiting time and clinic overtime. Discrete event simulation and design of experiments are applied to quantify the effects of the factors on consultation waiting time/clinic overtime. Implementation results show significant improvement once those factors are well addressed.

Chapter 12, *Reducing Patient Waiting Time at an Ambulatory Surgical Center,* describes a methodology to reduce patient waiting time in a for-profit ambulatory surgical center. Patients in this facility are scheduled in advance for the various operations, and yet operations start late and last longer than expected, creating undesired delays. Although this facility is limited to ambulatory surgery, it provides a large number of different surgeries, which are scheduled using "block" scheduling approach. The methodology presented generates a more accurate schedule by creating better time estimates for the operations and with lower variability. The effect of sequencing the surgeries, such that the ones with lower variability are performed earlier in the day, is also discussed.

Chapter 13, *Scheduling Healthcare Systems: Theory and Applications,* offers a series of scheduling techniques and their applications in healthcare settings. Healthcare administrators, physicians, and other professionals can use such techniques to achieve their operational goals when resources are limited. The chapter covers a wide spectrum of scheduling models, from single server and deterministic models to the more difficult ones, those which consider several servers and stochastic variables. A strong emphasis is placed on the practical aspects of scheduling techniques in healthcare.

Chapter 14, *Appointment Order Outpatient Scheduling System with Consideration of Ancillary Services and Overbooking Policy to Improve Outpatient Experience,* points out that patient wait time and access to care have long been a recognized problem in modern outpatient healthcare delivery systems. In spite of all the efforts to develop appointment rules and policies, the problem of long patient waits persists. Despite the reasons, the fact remains that there are few implemented models for effective scheduling that consider patient wait times, physician idle time, overtime, ancillary service time, as well as individual no-show rate, and are generalized sufficiently to accommodate a variety of outpatient clinic settings.

The goal of this chapter is demonstrating how it is possible to improve the quality and efficiency of healthcare delivery by developing a physician schedule that meets the clinical policies without overbooking using an innovative 'wait ratio' concept, a patient arrival schedule from the physician schedule accounting for ancillary services, an evidence-based predictive model of no-show probability for individual patient, and a model-supported dynamic overbooking policy to reduce the negative impact of no-shows.

Section 3, **Electronic Health Records**, includes three chapters.

Chapter 15, *Electronic Health Record: Adoption, Considerations and Future Direction,* points out that over the last two decades there has been considerable deliberation, experience, and research in the arena of Health Information Technology (HIT), Electronic Medical Records (EMR), Electronic Health Records (EHR) and more recently Electronic Personal Health Records (EPHR).

This chapter attempts to synthesize the vast amount of information, experience, and implementation perspectives related to Electronic Health Records with the intent of assisting healthcare institutions and key stakeholders in making informed choices as they embark on designing, developing, and implementing an EHR. EHR considerations, challenges, opportunities, and future directions are also addressed. The chapter highlights the power of management engineering to facilitate planning, implementation, and sustainability of the EHR, a critical asset for a healthcare organization and the overall healthcare industry.

Chapter 16, *Electronic Medical Records (EMR): Issues and Implementation Perspectives*, presents the views and experience of the practicing physician. The author indicates that for many years the electronic medical record has been the holy grail of hospital system integration. Hundreds of millions of dollars have been spent in attempts to develop effective electronic medical records (EMR) to provide clinical care for patients. The advantages of an EMR are listed as reducing error, streamlining care, and allowing multiple people to provide simultaneous care. Unfortunately, most current EMR implementations are developed without completely understanding the processes that are being automated. In some implementations, there is an effort to first outline the process, and then try to create software that will facilitate the existing process, but this effort is not typically done systematically and with the discipline of an engineer. We will discuss the areas of the EMR that management systems engineers can facilitate to design and implement, reducing the errors in the current processes and preparing the healthcare system for further improvements.

In Chapter 17, *Health Information Exchange for Improving the Efficiency and Quality of Healthcare Delivery,* it is pointed out that in healthcare industry providers, patients and all other stakeholders must have the right information at the right time for achieving efficient and cost effective services. Exchange of information between the heterogeneous system entities plays a critical role. Health information exchange (HIE) is not only a process of transmitting data, but also a platform for streamlining operations to improve healthcare delivery in a secure manner. In this chapter, the authors present a comprehensive view of electronic health record (EHR) systems and HIE by presenting their architecture, benefits, challenges, and other related issues. While providing information on the current state of EHR/HIE applications, the authors also discuss advanced issues and secondary uses of HIE implementations, and shed some light on the future research in this area by highlighting the challenges and potential.

Section 4, **Patient Flow**, includes 2 chapters.

Chapter 18, *Evaluating Patient Flow Based on Waiting Time and Travel Distance for Outpatient Clinic Visits,* discusses how and why patient flow greatly affects the quality of service delivered to the patients. Among the various performance measures identified for patient flow, the chapter focuses on the analytical modeling of two key measures, namely, patient waiting time and travel distance. Waiting time is analyzed by a simple analytical tool – queuing theory. Three queuing models, including single station, multiple serial stations, and network systems are presented. Meanwhile, patient travel distance is investigated by an analytical model to evaluate the patient flow. For both measures, the applicability of models is illustrated with numerical examples.

Chapter 19, *Using Patient Flow to Examine Hospital Operations*, points out that adopting an admission-to-discharge patient flow perspective has the potential to improve hospital operations. Flow paths provide insight regarding patient care needs, support resource allocation and capacity planning decisions, and improve the operational performance of the hospitals. Studying patient flow using systems engineering tools and applications can help decision makers assess and improve care delivery. This chapter presents current research and techniques used to describe, measure, and model inpatient flow. The authors formally define patient flow from an operational standpoint and discuss why it is crucial for operational decisions. Systems engineering techniques that describe and analyze inpatient flow are introduced. However, these techniques present certain modeling challenges, which the authors address. The chapter concludes with a discussion of emerging approaches to capture patient flow.

The last section 5, **Cost Management**, includes chapter 20, *A New Cost Accounting Model and New Indicators for Hospital Management Based on Personnel Cost.* This chapter discusses that specified hospital accounting systems are necessary for a manager to determine the proper management strategy. A new cost accounting model based on new allocation rules of personnel cost is presented in this chapter. The model offers a manager useful tool to calculate the medical cost not only for an individual patient and for each clinical department, but also each DRG system for a specific period.

New financial indicators were developed based on personnel costs which were calculated using this new cost accounting system. Indicator 1: The ratio of the marginal profit after personnel cost per personnel cost (RMP). Indicator 2: The ratio of investment (=indirect cost) per personnel cost (RIP). Operation profit per one dollar of personnel cost (OPP) was demonstrated to be the difference between the RMP and RIP. The break-even point (BEP) and break-even ratio (BER) could be determined by combining the indicators. RMP demonstrates not only the medical efficiency, but also the medical productivity in the case of DPC/DRG groups. OPP can be utilized to compare the medical efficiency of each department in either one hospital or multiple hospitals. It also makes it possible to evaluate the management efficiency of multiple hospitals.

In conclusion, this book illustrates the power of management engineering for quantitative managerial decision-making in healthcare settings. Management engineering helps in understanding responses of processes and systems to different inputs with random and non-random variability. This understanding makes it possible, in turn, to predict performance and/or real resource requirements, allowing decision-makers to be truly proactive rather than reactive.

This book illustrates to healthcare administrators the importance of understanding quantitative decision-making techniques offered by management engineering. The editors hope that this book will help to reduce barriers between healthcare practitioners and engineering professionals.

Acknowledgment

The editors would like to acknowledge the support and encouragement of the IGI Global Development Division team, as its help and patience have been indispensible. We would like to especially acknowledge the role and help of Mike Killian, Editorial Assistant, for his continual readiness to answer multiple questions and supply all the materials and templates required for the timely completion of this complex project.

It is well known that reviewers have a critical role for producing high quality books. The editors express their sincere gratitude to the reviewers of these chapters for their time, expertise, and highly valuable suggestions that, as we believe, significantly increased the value of the entire book.

Last but not least, no book can be produced without the support, encouragement and patience of loved ones. The lead editor (AK) would like to express his indebtedness to his wife, Rosa, and to his daughter, Julia, for their moral support and understanding during the long evenings and many weekends spent working on this book.

Alexander Kolker
Children's Hospital and Health System, Wisconsin, USA

Pierce Story
GE Healthcare, USA

Section 1

Efficient Managerial Decision-Making and Management of Operations

Chapter 1
Efficient Managerial Decision-Making in Healthcare Settings:
Examples and Fundamental Principles

Alexander Kolker
Children's Hospital and Health System, Wisconsin, USA

ABSTRACT

This chapter illustrates the predictive and analytical decision-making power of healthcare management engineering compared to traditional management reasoning. An overview of the domain of healthcare management engineering is provided. Four types of problems are illustrated in details: (i) dynamic supply and demand balance using discrete event simulation, (ii) the probabilistic resource optimization for specimen screening testing, (iii) principal component analysis for identifying a few significant independent contributing variables (factors) for a large patient demographic data-base, and (iv) recursive forecasting of a time series using its auto-correlation function to identify the strongly correlated past data-points.

Traditional managerial decision-making and management engineering methodology are discussed and applied side by side to analyze the same problems in order to illustrate and explain their differences. Some fundamental management engineering principles are summarized in conclusion.

DOI: 10.4018/978-1-60960-872-9.ch001

The irony of the Information Age is that it has given new respectability to uninformed opinion.

Michael Crichton, Airframe, New York, 1996

INTRODUCTION

Modern medicine has achieved great progress in treating individual patients. This progress is based mainly on life science (molecular genetics, biophysics, biochemistry) and the development of medical devices and imaging technology.

However, according to a report published jointly by National Academy of Engineering and Institute of Medicine, relatively little material resources and technical talent have been devoted to the proper functioning of the overall health care delivery as an integrated system in which access to efficient care should be delivered to many thousands of patients in an economically sustainable way (Reid et al, 2005).

As this report strongly points out, a real impact on quality, efficiency and sustainability of the health care system can be achieved only by using methods and principles of system engineering or healthcare delivery engineering (Reid et al, 2005).

At the same time, this report states in an unusually blunt way, "In fact, relatively few health care professionals or administrators are equipped to think analytically about health care delivery as a system or to appreciate the relevance of engineering tools. Even fewer are equipped to work with engineers to apply these tools."

Thus, it is often difficult for many administrators to appreciate the role of management engineering methodology to the health care delivery process analysis. On the other hand, engineering professionals do not always have enough knowledge of health care delivery processes or the role of the physicians in making management decisions. Healthcare has a culture of rigid division of labor. This functional division does not effectively support the methodology that crosses the functional areas, especially if it assumes significant change in traditional relationships (Reid et al, 2005).

A systematic way of developing managerial decisions for efficient allocating of material, human and financial resources needed for delivery of high quality care using quantitative methods is the scope of what is called healthcare management engineering. (The term 'management engineering' is sometimes substituted by the terms 'operations research', 'system engineering', 'industrial engineering', or 'management science'. All these terms have practically the same meaning).

Management engineering methodology is indispensable in addressing *typical* pressing hospital issues, such as:

- **Capacity:** How many beds are required for a department or unit? How many procedure rooms, operating rooms or pieces of equipment are needed for different services?
- **Staffing:** How many nurses, physicians and other providers are needed for a particular shift in a unit (department) in order to best achieve operational and service performance objectives?
- **Scheduling:** What are the optimized staff schedules that help not only delivering a safe and efficient care for patients but also take into account staff preferences and convenience?
- **Patient flow:** What patient wait time at the service stations is acceptable (if any at all) in order to achieve the system throughput goals?
- **Resource allocation:** Is it more efficient to use specialized resources or pooled (interchangeable) resources (operating/procedure rooms, beds, equipment, and staff)?
- **Forecasting:** How to forecast the future patient volumes (demand) or transaction volumes for the short- and long-term budget and other planning purposes?

This list can easily be extended. Other issues that belong to the management engineering domain are, for example, optimized geographic location of facilities and facilities layout, engineering (design) of the facility optimized workflow, defining and measuring productivity, supply chain and inventory management, quality control techniques, advanced multivariate statistical data analysis for marketing and budgeting purposes, and so on. The ultimate goal of management engineering methodology is providing an aid and guidance to efficiently managing hospital operations, i.e. reducing the costs of using resources for delivery of care while keeping high quality, safety and outcomes standards for patients.

As Butler (1995) states, it is imperative for healthcare management to become familiar with the quantitative decision-making techniques and tools offered by management engineering.

Carter (2002), in the article with the revealing title "Diagnosis: Mismanagement of Resources", summarizes that "…Ailing health care system desperately needs a dose of operations research…".

Fabri (2008) supports this assessment, saying "…fixing healthcare will require individuals who are 'bilingual' in healthcare and in systems engineering principles".

For the last few years some positive signs have been observed as management engineering makes its way into hospital settings. Story (2009) notices in his strongly articulated article "…while we still have much work to do, especially at the hospital level, some change addressing the recommendations for the dissemination of systems engineering and systems thinking is already under way". A similar conclusion on advancing the role of management engineering in healthcare settings is made by Buttell Crane (2007).

Although the above references on the role and importance of management engineering for healthcare are insightful and to the point, they lack concrete specific quantitative examples. This makes them somewhat declarative.

The objective of this chapter is to illustrate the predictive and analytical decision-making power of management engineering methodology compared to traditional management reasoning. Both management engineering and the traditional management approach are applied side by side to analyzing the same concrete problems. The focus is on explanation of why management engineering results are usually different from the typical traditional "common sense" management approach. The problems are taken from a real hospital and clinical practice. They are somewhat simplified and adapted to focus on the fundamental principles of quantitative decision-making. However, even simplified, most of the problems are not trivial.

It is not possible to illustrate all of the above-mentioned management engineering applications in one chapter. This chapter includes in details four types of problems.

The first type is one of the most practically important and widespread issues of dynamic supply and demand balance, such as an analysis of the required capacity, patient flow, department staffing and scheduling. It is widely acknowledged that the most powerful and versatile methodology for analyzing this kind of problems is discrete event simulation. The following examples of quantitative managerial decision-making based on discrete event simulation modeling are included: (1) outpatient scheduling order for appointments with different duration variability, (2) 'excessive' capacity, 'improved' efficiency and delay for access to care, (3) centralized discharge vs. individual unit discharges, (4) capacity, costs and staffing for an outpatient clinic, (5) staffing of hospital receiving department, (6) relative efficiency of specialized vs. pooled (interchangeable) operating rooms (resources), (7) daily load leveling (smoothing) of scheduled elective procedures, (8) special procedure operating rooms capacity, and (9) entire hospital system patient flow and interdependency of hospital departments/subsystems.

The second type of problems is the probabilistic resource optimization, such as optimized pooled specimen screening testing aimed at reducing an overall number of tests per specimen.

The third type of problems is advanced multivariate data analysis for reducing the number of variables and identifying only a few significant independent contributing variables (factors); for example, identifying a few demographic population variables (factors) that most contribute to the hospital financial contribution margin. Application of the advanced statistical data analysis for decision making is illustrated using principal component decomposition of the large matrix of the original observational data. Because of inevitable inter-correlation of some variables in large observational data sets, regression analysis with dozens of the original variables usually fails. In contrast, regression analysis with totally uncorrelated principal components is one of the most powerful methodologies for identifying only a few significant independent contributing variables (factors).

The fourth type of problems is forecasting of a time series using past data-points. It is discussed that the past data-points used for forecasting the future data-points should be strongly correlated to each other (in contrast to uncorrelated variables in the previous type of problems). It is illustrated that the strongly correlated past data-points can be identified from the autocorrelation function of the time series. It is further illustrated that a powerful forecasting procedure for the time series is a recursive technique. Its application is demonstrated using, as an example, an annual patient volume forecasting. In conclusion, some fundamental management engineering principles for efficient managerial decision-making in healthcare settings are summarized.

A step-by-step description of discrete event simulation performed manually for a simple process is presented in Appendix 1. Some mathematical methods that can be used for the various management engineering applications are summarized in Appendix 2.

Traditional Management and Management Engineering

There are many possible definition of management. For the purpose of this chapter, we define management as controlling and leveraging available resources (material, financial and human) aimed at achieving the system performance objectives.

Traditional healthcare management is based on past experience, feelings, intuition, educated guesses, simple linear projections and calculations based on the average values of input variables.

In contrast, management engineering is the discipline of building mathematical models of real systems and analysis thereof as a basis for developing justified managerial decisions. Management decisions for leveraging resources that best meet system performance objectives are based on outcomes of validated mathematical models.

Although no formal definition can capture all aspects of the concept, it follows that management engineering typically includes the following elements (steps): (i) the goal that is clearly stated and measurable, (ii) identification of available resources that can be leveraged (allocated) in different ways, (iii) mathematical models (analytic or numeric computer algorithms) to quantitatively test outcomes (scenarios) for the different ways of using resources, and consequences of the different use of resources (especially unintended consequences) before finalizing the decisions.

The underlying foundation of the management engineering approach is that an outcome of a valid mathematical model forms a basis for truly justified managerial decisions.

Decisions based on management engineering methodology are often different compared to traditional managerial decisions. Sometimes, they even look counterintuitive. There are several factors that contribute to this difference.

First, most managerial decisions in healthcare settings are being made in highly variable and random environments. It is a general human tendency to avoid the complications of incorporating uncertainty and randomness into the decision making by ignoring it or turning it into artificial certainty. For example, the average procedure time or the average patient length of stay or the average numbers of patients are typically treated as if they are fixed values, ignoring the effect of variability around these averages. This practice usually results in highly inaccurate conclusions made by traditional management decision-making.

Another factor is that healthcare systems usually contain internal hidden interconnections and interdependencies of units, departments, physicians, nursing and other staffing, regulators and so on. These multiple interconnections make healthcare systems truly complex. Traditional management lacks a means of capturing such interconnections and predicting their effect on the response of one unit to the change in other units. After all, a hospital or a large clinic looks more like, say, a chaotic, busy airport than an automated manufacturing assembly line. This is a root cause of the frequently observed unintended and undesired consequences of managerial decisions that look reasonable on the surface.

One more factor that contributes to the difference between traditional management and management engineering decision-making is a non-linear scaling effect (size effect) of most healthcare systems. Larger systems can function at a much higher utilization level and lower patient waiting time than smaller systems even if the patient volume relative to their size is the same (Green, 2006; Kolker, 2010a). Such non-linear relationships are not easy to incorporate into traditional decision-making.

Only analytic mathematical models (if applicable) or computer simulation models offer a means of capturing all these factors into the efficient managerial decision-making.

Problems included in this chapter represent a number of typical examples taken from the hospital and clinic practice for which efficient managerial decisions should have made. It is illustrated how truly efficient managerial decisions can be developed and why traditional management approaches often result in unsatisfactory and short-lived outcomes.

Dynamic Supply and Demand Balance Problems

Problem 1: Scheduling Order for Appointments with Different Duration Variability

An outpatient clinic manager has to schedule two groups of patient appointments for one physician-specialist: one group is new patient appointments and another group is follow-up patient appointments. On average, a new patient appointment takes about 60 min but could be in the range from 45 min to 90 min. The follow-up appointment takes on average 30 min and its duration is usually from 25 min to 35 min.

On a typical day, 5 new and 6 follow-up appointments are scheduled. Using the average appointment time 60 min and 30 min, respectively, it is estimated that the clinic's total work time will be 5*60+6*30= 480 min, or 8 hours.

The following managerial problem arises: does appointment order affect patient wait time and clinic daily total work time? In other words, is it better to schedule new appointments first and then the follow-up appointments, or the way around? Or does the appointment order make a difference at all?

Traditional Management Approach

All other factors being equal, the schedule slots should be filled in the order in which they are received (whoever first called for an appointment gets the first available slot).

For example, if a new patient is scheduled first at 8:00 am and appointment time is 60 min on average, then the next follow-up patient will be scheduled at 9:00am, and next patient will be scheduled at 9:30 am, and so on. If the follow-up

Table 1. Simulation of scheduling rules for one clinic operational day

Scheduling rule	99% CI of the average patient wait time, min	99% CI of the number of patients with NO wait	99% CI of the total clinic time, hours
Smallest variability first	6.0 – 7.3	3.1 - 3.6	9.6 – 9.9
Random order	9.4 – 11.6	2.6 – 3.1	10.2 – 10.8
Largest variability first	17.7 – 21.6	1.6 – 2.0	11.9 – 12.8

patient is scheduled first at 8:00 am and appointment time is 30 min on average, then the next new patient will be scheduled at 8:30 am, and so on. There is no preference for appointment order. Indeed, the total clinic time for the average 60 min appointment followed by 30 min appointment would be the same as that for a 30 min appointment followed by a 60 min appointment.

Management Engineering Approach

The appointment duration times of 60 min and 30 min are only the average values. There is a significant variability around these averages that affect the clinic's operational performance. In order to capture an effect of the variability a model of clinic operations should be developed using simulation methodology. The outcomes of scheduling scenarios can be quantified, and comparative conclusions on their efficiency can be made.

The simulation model layout is very simple and straightforward for this particular case (see Appendix 1). Every patient (entity) has a descriptive attribute "appointment type": new or follow-up. If the attribute is "new" then the appointment variability is captured using a simple triangle statistical distribution from 45 min with the most likely value being 60 min to the maximum 90 min; if the attribute is "follow up" then the appointment variability is captured using a triangle distribution from 25 min with the most likely value being 30 min to the maximum 35 min. A total of 11 appointments are included: 5 new and 6 follow-up. For simplicity, simulation for one typical operational day is performed using 300 replications to capture an effect of the variability accurately enough. The first appointment is scheduled at 8 am and the last one is scheduled at 3:30 pm. Results are presented in Table 1.

Thus, appointment order does make a difference. Scheduling rule with the smallest variability first is much better both in terms of lower patient wait time and a higher number of patients who do not wait at all. This is in contrast to traditional management expectation of no effect of appointment order.

Notice also that the total clinic work time significantly exceeds the 8 hours expected based on the average appointment duration, i.e. overtime is required to serve all scheduled patients (unless there is a non-filled cancellation or no-show). This is a consequence of the appointment duration variability around the average, not the average duration itself.

Another example of the effect of appointment sequence is presented by the Institute for Healthcare Improvement on its website (IHI, 2005). This example includes Monte-Carlo simulation for 25 days of clinic operations. It is assumed that new appointments take 45 min, plus or minus 15 min (30 to 60 min range); follow-up appointments take 30 min, plus or minus 5 min (25 to 35 min range). Results for one random sample of 25 days are represented in Table 2.

These data also demonstrate that appointment sequence with the smallest variability first (follow-up appointments) results in the smallest patient wait time and the largest number of patients who do not wait at all, followed up by appointment

Table 2. Summary of 25 days of clinic operations

Scheduling rule	Average wait time, min	Standard deviation of wait time, min	Average number of patients with NO wait	Standard deviation of number of patients with NO wait
Smallest variability first	6.3	4.4	3.2	2
Random order	12.2	12.1	2.5	1.9
Largest variability first	19.2	17.4	1.4	1.6

sequence with random order and largest variability first (new appointments).

These simple examples illustrate a fundamental management engineering principle (proven in manufacturing): scheduling appointments (jobs) in the order of increased variability (jobs with lower variability come first) results in a lower overall cycle time and patient wait time (Klassen and Rohleder, 1996; Cayirli, et al, 2006; Teow, 2009). The reason for the erroneous traditional management expectation is, already mentioned, lacking a means to take into account the effect of the appointment length variability around the average.

Problem 2: Excessive Capacity, Improved Efficiency and Access to Care

There is a 10-bed unit. The average daily patient arrival rate is 2 patients per day but actual daily arrival rate varies depending on the day of week. Patient length of stay (LOS) is in the range from 1 day to 3 days, with 2.5 days being the most likely. It is observed that the daily average number of patients in the unit (average census) is 5. The manager believes that the average daily utilization of 5 beds out of total available 10 beds, i.e. 50%, is too low. The manager wants to improve the efficiency of the unit.

Traditional Management Approach

Because the available capacity of 10 beds is not fully utilized, the manager decides to trim the 'extra' capacity, i.e. to take out of service at least 4 'extra' beds leaving only 6 active beds (one bed above the daily needed average 5 is left as a precaution, just in case it is suddenly needed). This way, daily utilization will be 5/6=83% instead of 50%. Also, because there is no need to staff four beds any more, the nursing and cleaning services budget will also be trimmed. This looks like a good management decision.

Management Engineering Approach

Due to variations around the average daily number of patients in the unit, this average value will be exceeded on a regular basis, and operational problems will occur regularly.

For example, a random sample with the daily average of 5 patients in the unit (average census) for one week can be: Monday- 7, Tuesday- 6, Wednesday- 4, Thursday- 8, Friday -4, Saturday- 3, Sunday- 3. Thus, there will not be enough capacity for two days of this particular week (Monday and Thursday), i.e. about 28% of time.

What is the probability that more than 6 beds will be needed with the average daily 5 patients, *P(#beds>6)*? Patient admissions are often (but not always) independent random time arrivals. A Poisson type process is widely used to model such random events. Using a Poisson formula, it is easy to find that

$$P(\#\, beds > 6) = 1 - \exp(-5)\sum_{n=0}^{n=6} \frac{5^n}{n!} = 24\%$$

Thus, more than 6 beds will be needed for about a quarter of time. Therefore, the traditional management approach would create a regular bed shortage.

Capacity and staffing decision/planning based only on averages is called the flaw of averages (Costa et al, 2003; Marshall et al, 2005; de Bruin et al, 2007, Savage, 2009).

A more detailed picture of unintended consequences of trimmed capacity for a highly variable process could be performed using a very simple simulation model (without resorting to assumptions needed for the use of analytic mathematical formulas for the Poisson process). The model design was similar to the one used in Problem 1.

The unit capacity was trimmed to 6 beds. Patient daily arrival pattern was: Monday-4; Tuesday- 4; Wednesday- 1; Thursday- 3; Friday- 1; Saturday- 1; Sunday- 0. Thus, the average daily patient arrival rate was (4+4+1+3+1+1+0)/7=2 patients/day.

Patient LOS was from 1 to 3 days with the most likely 2.5 days that was fitted by the triangle distribution.

Simulation was performed for one week (168 hours) with warm-up period 8736 hours to get stable steady-state results and 300 replications to capture accurate enough the process variability.

The following simulation results were obtained. The 99% confidence interval for the average admission wait time was 3.1 - 3.6 hours. About 24% of patients waited more than 3 hours to get in, and 18% - 21% of time more than 6 beds (full capacity) was needed, i.e. patients remained in the queue area. Apparently, such performance of the unit with trimmed bed capacity would not meet operational safety and quality standards.

This example illustrates a fundamental management engineering principle: because of variability of the number of patient arrivals and length of stay, some degree of reserved capacity (sometimes up to 40%) is needed in order to avoid regular operational problems (Green, 2006).

Another possible way of improving the unit's operations is the daily load leveling (smoothing) of the number of elective surgical procedures scheduled for patients with required post-surgical unit admission, as illustrated in Problem 7 and also in (Kolker, 2009).

Problem 3: Centralized Discharge vs. Individual Units Discharges

Inability to discharge patients in a timely fashion is a typical hospital problem.

Let's consider an ICU with four nursing units. Discharges occur daily Monday to Friday, usually in the afternoon between 2 pm and 9 pm. The number of discharges from each unit is a random quantity with the average 4 daily discharges, i.e. the number of discharges on a particular day could be less or more than 4. The most likely time to complete discharge is about 30 min, but the time could range from 20 min to as high as 60 min. So, on average about 2 hours of nursing time is spent on the discharge process for each of 4 units. This nursing time is taken away from direct patient care. The ICU manager wants nurses to spend more time for direct patient care rather than for discharge paperwork.

Traditional Management Approach

After a brainstorming session, the idea of hiring a dedicated discharge nurse was proposed. This was considered a good management solution for all units because (PHLO, 2008):

i. the unit nurse would be free from a paper-intensive discharge process to maximize their time for direct patient care
ii. bed management could rely on one contact person who would notify cleaning services to clean beds after discharge
iii. case management would get a resource to help coordinate and plan their activities
iv. patient flow and throughput would improve because of a more timely discharge process

Figure 1. Simulation model layout of current discharge arrangement. Each nurse RN_A, RN_B, RN_C, and RN_D discharges patients individually from each separate unit

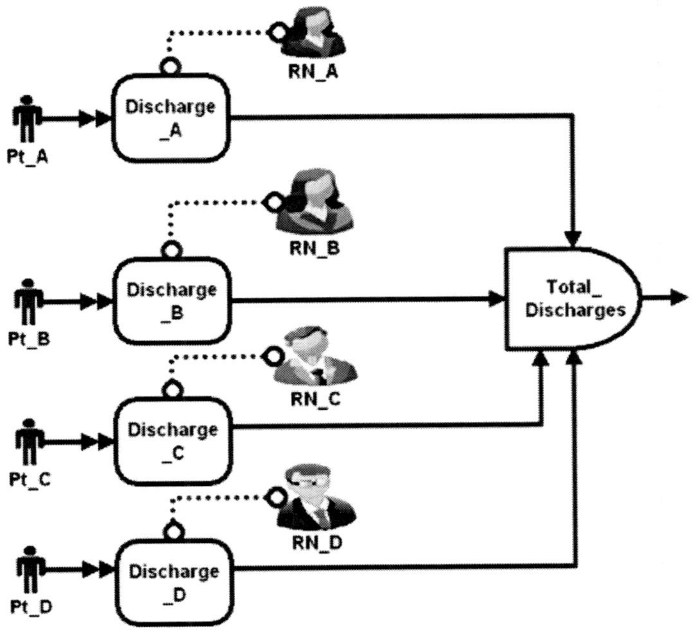

Management Engineering Approach

The centralized discharge should be analyzed quantitatively and then compared to the performance of the current process before creating an additional discharge nurse position. Let us consider two scenarios.

Scenario 1

Current process: there are four independent units. Each unit has its own nurse who handles discharges as they ordered. Four random discharges take place daily in the afternoon from 2 pm to 9 pm. A model layout is depicted on Figure 1.

Simulation of the discharge process indicates that the total number of discharges for one typical week is about 74.

Scenario 2

Proposed discharge process: one dedicated nurse who performs discharges for all units as they ordered. The nurse's shift duration is 8 hours, from 1 pm to 9:30pm with 30 min lunch break, as indicated on the panel layout on Figure 2.

Simulation of this discharge process indicates that the total number of discharges for a similar typical week is only about 60.

This is a rather unexpected result: a newly hired dedicated discharge nurse would make significantly less discharges than nurses in the current process, creating additional discharge backlog and waiting time.

Why does this seemingly good management idea actually create a worse problem?

In the current process, at least four nurses perform discharges independently. Each nurse has her own path to discharge. If there is a delay with a particular patient in a particular unit, none of the other nurses in other units are affected.

With the new centralized discharge process, all discharges from all units form a so-called series of dependent events (Goldratt, 2004; Motwani et al, 1996). In a series of dependent events, a random

Figure 2. Simulation model layout of the proposed discharge arrangement. One centralized nurse (Central discharge) discharges patients from all units. Central discharge nurse shift is from 1 PM to 8:30 PM with 30 minute lunch (light band) as presented on the shift editor panel

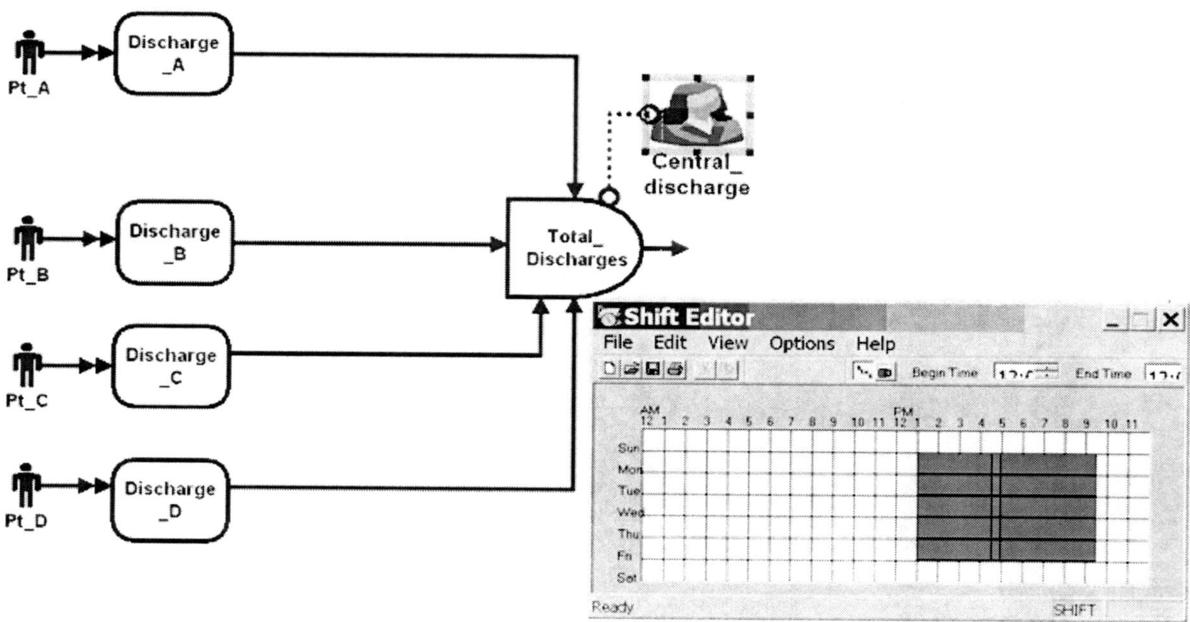

delay with the discharge of a particular patient would inevitably impact the rest of the patients. In other words, hiring a dedicated resource would likely create a system bottleneck. By definition, a system bottleneck is a resource whose capacity is less than or equal to demand placed on it (Goldratt, 2004).

Based only on averages, a dedicated nurse would be able to perform 80 discharges for a week (4 discharges*4 units* 5 days), and, spending on average 30 min for each discharge, this would take 40 work hours for a week. This makes the capacity of the dedicated discharge nurse equal to demand place on her/him, i.e. makes this resource a bottleneck according to the above definition. In reality, the situation is even worse because of the demand variability, and the nurse availability is less than 100% due to additional breaks, meetings, etc.

On the 'good' days, when the demand for discharges is less than nurse capacity to perform them (fewer than 4 discharges per unit that take less than 30 min per discharge), the extra capacity cannot be 'stored' to serve the next day demand. Such an extra capacity on a particular 'good' day is lost. On the other hand, on the 'bad days', when demand for discharges exceeds nurse capacity, the unserved demand is not lost; it has to be fulfilled in the next day, forming a backlog (unless there is overtime). Thus, effect of 'bad' days is accumulated while effect of 'good' days is not.

This illustrates the following fundamental management engineering principles: (i) in a series of dependent events, only the bottleneck defines the throughput of the entire system regardless on the throughput and capacity of non-bottlenecks; (ii) an unfulfilled service request backlog (appointments, discharges, document processing, etc) can exist and remain stable even if the average high variability demand is less than service capacity.

There are possible solutions that can elevate the bottleneck constraint of the centralized discharge nurse, e.g. scheduling easy discharges with lower variability first (see Problem 1) or the use of the shared staff. However, discussion of the techniques for elevating the bottleneck's constraint is beyond the scope of this chapter.

Problem 4: Outpatient Clinic Operations: Costs, Capacity and Staffing Planning

An outpatient flu clinic is open during the flu season to provide the flu vaccine shots on a walk-in basis. The clinic stays open from 8 am to 6 pm. On the average day patient arrival rate in the morning from 8 am to 10 am is about 9 patients per hour. From 10 am to 2 pm the patient traffic picks up to the average of 15 patients per hour. From 2 pm to 4 pm it slows down back to 9 patients per hour. It increases again late in the afternoon from 4 pm to 6 pm to 12 patients per hour. Thus, the average patient arrival rate is highly variable during a typical day.

Giving a shot (including filling out the paper work) takes on average about 8 min but could be in the range from 6 min to 10 min.

The clinic charges the patient $20 for the flu shot; the clinic's cost of one vaccine dose and supplies is $1, and staffing pay rate is $14/hour.

Clinic's management should decide: how many medical providers are needed to staff the clinic on a typical day, and what is the projected net revenue (on a weekly basis)?

Traditional Management Approach

The projected total average number of patients for a typical day is 120 (=9*2+15*4+9*2+12*2). One provider is going to serve on average 60 min/ 8 min = 7.5 patients/hour. Hence 120/7.5 =16 hours of staffing time is needed to daily serve all patients. Therefore, two medical providers should be scheduled to staff the clinic on a daily basis. One can be scheduled to work from 8 am to 5 pm. Another provider can be scheduled to work from 9 am to 6 pm.

Both medical providers have unpaid 30 min lunch time and an additional paid 30 min off for a few short breaks (not overlapped to each other). Practically no (or very short) patient waiting time is expected.

The weekly revenue is going to be 5*120*$20=$12,000. Weekly labor cost for two providers is ($14/hour*8.5 hours*5days)*2=$1,190, and the total weekly vaccine and supplies costs is $120*5=$600. Hence, the average clinic's weekly net revenue is expected to be $12000 - $1190 - $600 = $10,210.

Management Engineering Approach

Because of inevitable variability in the daily number of patients coming for the shots, and the variability of the time it takes to give a shot, the actual staffing needs and the actual estimated net revenue will differ significantly from the average values. On top of that, it is observed that some patients leave without a shot if their waiting time is longer than 20 min.

In order to develop a realistic evaluation of the clinic performance, the process variability and patients leaving without a shot should be taken into account. This is possible only using the clinic process simulation.

The model design and layout is similar to the one described in Problem 1 with an additional routing for 'inpatient' patients leaving after waiting more than 20 min (of course, any other numbers and input data can be used).

Simulation with one provider working from 8 am to 5 pm (1 FTE- full time equivalent) and another one starting later from 9 am until the end of the day 6 pm (1 FTE) results in 99% confidence interval for the weekly number of served patients, which ranges from only 509 to 513. This is much lower than the expected average value 600. On top of that, 105 to 109 patients (about 17%) will leave weekly without a shot because of waiting longer than 20 min.

The 99% confidence interval for the weekly net revenue is going to range from $8,483 to $8,560,

Figure 3. Net revenue vs the number of served patients and corresponding FTE

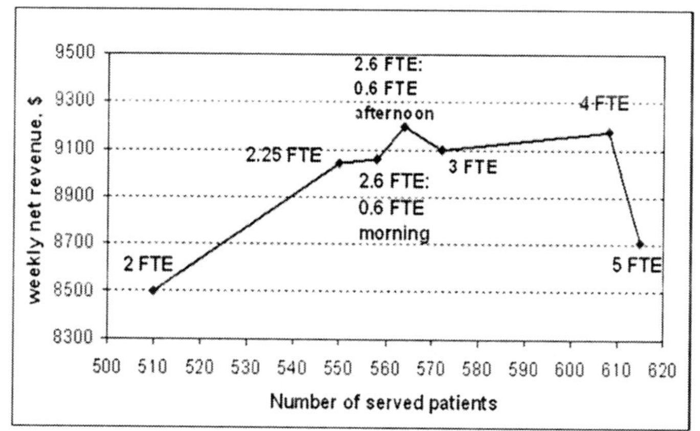

which is much less than the expected average value $10,210. This significant decreasing of revenue results from the inevitable process variability as well as patients leaving without the shot because they have to wait too long.

The next management step might be deciding how much it would help to increase the net revenue and reduce the number of leaving patients if an additional part time provider is available.

From a traditional management view it is not needed because 16 hours of working time on average should be enough to meet the average patient demand for service time. Therefore, an additional provider would result in staff underutilization.

However, simulation with an additional part-time provider (on top of 2 FTEs) working five hours in the morning from 8 am to 1 pm (0.6 FTE) with 30 min paid time off for short breaks indicates that 556 to 559 patients will be served weekly and 58 to 61 patients would leave. Total net revenue is going to range from $9,026 to $9,088, which is much better than the original amount of $8,483 to $8,560.

Certainly, an additional provider (additional 0.6 FTE) results in an additional operational and staffing costs; however, these costs are amply offset by the clinic's higher revenue because more paying patients are served.

What if this additional part-time provider is placed for the same five hours (0.6 FTE) for the second shift, from 1 pm to 6 pm? Simulation with this staffing arrangement results in serving more patients, from 561 to 565, and even fewer patients leaving without a shot, from 52 to 56. The net revenue 99% confidence interval is going to range from $9,158 to $9,238, which is better than that for the morning staffing hours.

Thus, simulation modeling indicates that a third provider (0.6 FTE) placed in the right shift does help to serve even more patients and increase the net revenue despite the higher costs of keeping one more additional provider.

Of course, many other scenarios of staffing shifts and clinic's operation modes are possible to analyze using a simulation model. The clinic's manager might be interested, for example, in knowing what staffing is needed to serve all projected weekly patient volume. Simulation modeling indicates that almost all weekly patient volume (99% CI from 614 to 616) will be served using 5 FTE. However, the net revenue in this case will range only from $8,698 to $8,722.

A graphical summary that illustrates these results is presented on Figure 3.

It follows from Figure 3 that the maximum weekly net revenue is generated from serving about 564 patients using 2.6 FTEs with 0.6 FTE in the afternoon. However, practically the same net revenue can be obtained using 4 FTE that serve many more patients, about 608. The cost of additional 1.4 FTE is practically offset by revenue from serving about 45 more patients. Therefore the latter staffing arrangement with 4 FTE would be preferred. Notice, that although 5 FTE serve even more patients, about 615, the net revenue would be much lower because in this case the cost of one more FTE is not offset by the additional revenue from serving just a few more patients (only about 7 more).

This summary illustrates an important general trade-off between the number of served patients, cost of resources to serve them and the net revenue. (The net revenue is defined here as the difference between the revenue generated by the served patients and the staffing costs and supplies required to provide this service). The net revenue increases if the revenue growth from serving more patients offsets the growth of staffing and supplies costs (resources) to serve them. However, at some point the growth of the costs of resources exceeds the growth of the revenue generated by serving only a few more patients; hence, the net revenue goes down.

Problem 5: Staffing of Hospital Receiving Center

The hospital receiving center is projected to receive annually 127,139 packages. The time to process one package (screen, scan, store, etc) could range from 7 min to 15 min with the average time of 10 min. The department works Monday to Friday from 8 am to 4:30 pm, with a 30 min lunch time and two 15 min breaks for each staff member during a typical day. (Total annual number of work days is 255).

The manager should develop a staffing plan for the receiving department with no overtime.

Traditional Management Approach (Langabeer, 2007)

The daily average number of packages is 127,139/255= 498.6.

Because each staff member has 30 min off for lunch and two 15 min breaks, the total daily time off is 60 min. Hence each staff member is available for 7.5 hours, i.e. the daily availability is 88.2%.

Using the average time of 10 min to handle a package and the available daily work time 7.5 hours*60=450 min, each staff member can handle 450 / 10= 45 packages per day. Hence 498.6/45= 11.1 staff members are needed to handle the projected work volume without delay and overtime.

Management Engineering Approach

A typical traditional approach to calculate the average daily productivity is based on dividing the total available time by the average time per package. Such an approach always results in underestimating of the required resources. This is another illustration of the flaw of averages (Savage, 2009; Costa et al, 2003). Notice that in the above calculation the variability range from 7 min to 15 min per package is not used at all.

However, it is a rigorous mathematical fact (theorem) that the average value of a non-linear function is not equal to the function of the average values of its arguments.

If the low limit of the time range 7 min is used, then only 7.7 staffing FTEs would be needed, while the use of the high limit of 15 min per package results in 16.6 staffing FTEs. The average of these values is not the same as the average staffing 11.1 FTEs based on the average time of 10 min per package.

It is not possible to make a correct staffing calculation without taking into account the frequency of each possible time to handle a package. Only simulation modeling methodology allows one to directly take into account the handling time variability.

The simulation model layout to get the correct staffing in this case is very simple and it is similar to the one discussed in Problem 1. A time range from 7 min to 15 min with the most likely 10 min is the model input in the form of a triangle statistical distribution (in the absence of a more accurate data collection).

Another model input is the daily variable number of packages. While the daily average number of packages is 498.6, the actual number should be of integer type and it varies around this average. It is typically assumed that the daily number of packages is independent of each other, and there are no periods during the year with systematically very high or very low daily package arrivals. Therefore, the daily package arrivals can be represented as a random number from a discrete Poisson distribution with the constant average value parameter 498.6. A number of random samples from this distribution are generated. Each sample consists of 255 random integer numbers (each number represents one work day load of package arrivals). Because samples are random, only the sample that sums up to 127,139 is picked up as the model input- daily package arrival volume. Simulation results indicate that 11 FTEs (calculated with the traditional approach based on the average time without variability around the average) would not be able to process the required annual work load of 127,139 packages: the maximum number of packages that could be processed is only 118,869 with 99% confidence interval from 118,295 to 118,492. Thus, department staffing of 11 FTEs was significantly underestimated.

According to simulation results, staffing of minimum 13 FTEs is needed to process the required annual workload: the 99% confidence interval of the number of packages will range from 127,138 to 127,139, i.e. practically all packages will be processed. The daily staff utilization would be rather healthy, about 85%.

Thus, the traditional management approach would result in chronic department understaffing, and, consequently, underestimated the staffing budget. This, in turn, would result in staff burnout, overstress, and possible increasing in staff turnover.

If budgeting and hiring of the staff is strictly limited, for example, to 11 FTEs, then the department management should provide some additional training or other means that would result in a reduction of the processing time per package and, more importantly, its variability by process standardization.

Simulation modeling easily demonstrates how much reduction of the process time and its variability per package is needed in order to process the required workload with only 11 FTEs.

For example, if the average processing time is reduced to 9 min and the variability is in the range from 7 min to 12 min, then 11 FTEs would be able to process practically all package volume, from 127,136 to 127,139.

Of course, many other operational scenarios are possible to analyze to develop and budget a realistic staffing plan using a simulation model, such as different work shift length for different staff members, part time shifts, unplanned staff absence, seasonal or quarter variability of package volume, different processing times for different package types, different package handling priorities, and so on.

Problem 6: Emergency and Elective Surgeries: Separate Specialized Operating Rooms vs. Pooled Operating Rooms

The issue of specialized vs. pooled (interchangeable) Operating Rooms (OR) caused a controversy in literature on healthcare improvement. Specifically, if surgical cases include both elective (scheduled) and emergency (random arrival) surgeries, is it more efficient to reserve specialized operating rooms (OR) dedicated separately for elective and emergency surgeries, or is it better to perform both types of surgeries in any available OR (make pooled or interchangeable resources)?

Traditional Management Approach

Haraden et al (2003) recommends that hospitals that want to improve patient flow should designate separate ORs for scheduled and unscheduled (emergency) surgeries. The authors state that in this arrangement "...Since the vast majority of surgeries is scheduled, most of the OR space should be so assigned. Utilization of the scheduled rooms becomes predictable, and wait times for unscheduled surgery become manageable". The authors imply that this statement is self-evident, and provide no quantitative analysis or any other justification for this recommendation.

Management Engineering Approach

In contrast to the above traditional approach, Wullink et al (2007) developed a discrete event simulation model (DES) of OR suite for the large Erasmus Medical Center hospital (Rotterdam, The Netherlands) to quantitatively test scenarios of using specialized dedicated ORs for emergency and for elective surgeries vs. pooled (interchangeable) ORs for both types of surgeries. These authors concluded that based on DES model results "... Emergency patients are operated upon more efficiently on elective ORs instead of a dedicated emergency ORs. The results of this study led to closing of the emergency OR in this hospital".

In contrast to the intuitive 'common sense' recommendation of Haraden et al (2003), Wullink et al (2007) presented specific data analysis to support their conclusions: pooled use of all ORs for both types of surgery results in the reduction of the average waiting time for emergency surgery from 74 min to 8 min.

In this section a simple generic simulation model is presented to address the same issue and to verify literature results. For simplicity, we consider an OR suite with two operating rooms, OR1 and OR2. Both emergency (random) and elective scheduled surgeries are included.

Let's first consider the situation when the majority of cases are scheduled elective surgeries. Six elective surgeries are scheduled 5 days a week, Monday to Friday at 7 am, 9 am, 11 am, 1 pm, 3 pm and 5 pm.

Emergency surgeries are assumed to arrive independently randomly 24 hours a day with the average inter-arrival time of 6 hours (a Poisson arrival rate is 0.166 patients/hour).

The most likely scheduled surgery duration is 2.4 hours, and emergency surgery duration is 2.1 hours (Wullink et al, 2007). The assumed variability is from 1.5 hours to 3 hours for scheduled surgeries and from 1.5 hours to 2.5 hours for emergency surgeries.

Using these arrival and service time data, let us consider two scenarios.

Scenario 1: there are two ORs, one is specialized dedicated only for elective surgeries (OR1) and stays open from 7 am to 7 pm; another one is specialized dedicated only for emergency surgeries (OR2) and is open 24 hours a day, as shown on Figure 4. If the dedicated OR is not available, then the new patient waits in the queue area until the corresponding dedicated OR becomes available.

Scenario 2: there are also two ORs. However, they are pooled, i.e. fully interchangeable: both emergency and scheduled patients go to any available OR, as indicated on Figure 5. If both ORs are not available, then patients wait in the queue area until one of the ORs becomes available. Emergency patients have higher priority and move first to the available OR.

Simulation was performed for 5 days (120 hours) Monday to Friday using 300 replications. Results for these two scenarios are given in Table 3.

An examination of the results is instructive. While the number of performed surgeries is practically the same for both scenarios, the wait time for elective surgery for pooled ORs is more than an order of magnitude (!) lower than that for dedicated ORs. The wait time for emergency surgery is also lower for pooled ORs by about a factor of 2. Practically no patients wait in queue for pooled ORs. This means that, contrary to expectation of Haraden et al (2003), specialized

Figure 4. Simulation model layout of dedicated operating room for scheduled elective surgeries OR1 and dedicated operating room for emergency unscheduled surgeries OR2

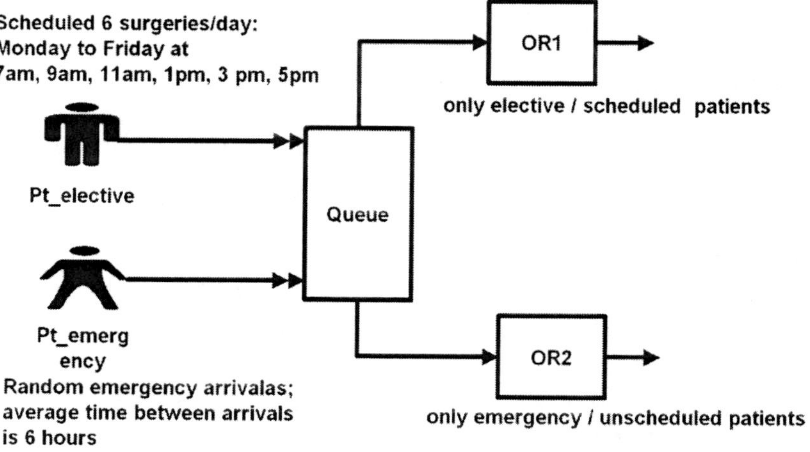

Figure 5. Simulation model layout of interchangeable emergency and scheduled elective operating rooms (ORs)

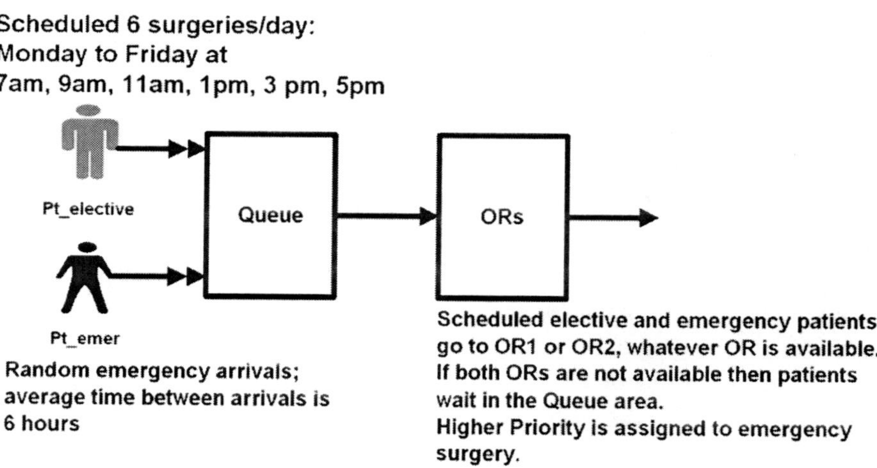

Table 3. Specialized ORs vs. Pooled ORs. Most surgeries are scheduled elective

Characteristics	Dedicated OR		Pooled OR	
	Elective	Emergency	Elective	Emergency
95% CI of the number of performed surgeries	28 – 29	20 - 21	30	20 - 21
95% CI of the average wait time, hours	2.3– 2.9	0.4 – 0.49	0.14 – 0.17	0.16 - 0.2
95% CI of the average number of patients in Queue	0.65 – 0.8	0.08 – 0.1	0.035 – 0.044	0.03 – 0.04
Average weekly OR utilization, %	99%	35%	46%	

dedicated ORs arrangement results in inevitable overtime in order to perform the same number of surgeries as in the pooled (interchangeable) ORs arrangement.

The reason for such an unexpected result for OR specifically dedicated to elective scheduled surgeries is the actual surgery duration variability. Therefore scheduling elective surgeries every 2 hours inevitably results in delays and/or required OR overtime. At the same time scheduled surgeries cannot be moved into another standby OR that is dedicated only for emergency patients, even though this OR is currently available. This situation is also reflected by the highly uneven weekly OR utilization, 99% and 35%, respectively.

Now, let us consider the situation when the majority of cases are unscheduled emergency surgeries. We have the same two scenarios with two ORs (dedicated and pooled) with the same surgeries duration variability.

However, this time only 4 daily elective surgeries are scheduled three days of week, Tuesday, Wednesday and Thursday at 8 am, 10 am, 1 pm, and 3 pm. Dedicated scheduled OR stays open from 8 am to 6 pm. Emergency (random) surgeries are more frequent, with the average inter-arrival time of 2 hours, Monday to Friday, 24 hours a day.

Simulation results for 120 hours (5 days), 300 replications are given in Table 4.

Notice that in this case, the number of performed emergency surgeries is higher for pooled ORs. Although the average waiting time for scheduled elective surgeries increased up to about 1 hour for pooled ORs, the average wait time for emergencies dropped dramatically by more than an order of magnitude, from about 7 hours down to about 0.5 hours (Compare this dramatic drop to Wullink et al (2007) result). A similar picture is observed for the average number of patients in the queue.

Overall, these results support the conclusions of Wullink et al (2007) that performing emergency surgeries in the pooled ORs scenario is more efficient than in the reserved dedicated emergency OR. These authors provided a detailed instructive discussion on why the dedicated OR scenario performs worse, especially for emergency surgeries, while intuitively it seems that it should perform better, as Haraden et al (2003) assumed.

Wullink et al (2007) pointed out that besides reserving OR capacity for emergency surgeries arrivals, ORs need to reserve capacity to cope with the variability of surgery duration. In the pooled ORs scenario, the reservation might be shared to increase the flexibility for dealing with unexpected long case duration and emergency surgery, whereas the dedicated scenario does not offer the opportunity to use the overflow principle.

On top of that, a dedicated OR scenario may cause queuing of emergency surgeries themselves because of their random arrival time. If emergency surgeries were allocated to all available ORs (pooled ORs scenario), then it would be possible to perform them simultaneously, thereby reducing the waiting time.

Table 4. Specialized ORs vs. Pooled ORs. Most surgeries are unscheduled emergencies

Characteristics	Dedicated OR		Pooled OR	
	Elective	Emergency	Elective	Emergency
95% CI of the number of performed surgeries	12	53 - 54	12	59 – 60
95% CI of the average wait time, hours	0.16 – 0.18	6.3 – 7.7	0.96 – 1.3	0.55 – 0.65
95% CI of the average number of patients in Queue	0.017 – 0.02	3.5 – 4.4	0.11 – 0.14	0.3 – 0.35
Average weekly OR utilization, %	55%	92%	62%	

Wullink et al (2007) acknowledge that "... interrupting the execution of the elective surgical case schedule for emergency patients may delay elective cases. However, inpatients are typically admitted to a ward before they are brought to the OR. Although delay due to emergency arrivals may cause inconvenience for patients, it does not disturb processes in the OR".

As simulation modeling indicates, delay in scheduled cases in the pooled ORs (if the majority of surgeries are emergencies) is usually not too dramatic (e.g. up to 1 hour), while reduction of waiting time for emergency surgeries is very substantial (from 74 min to 8 min according to Wullink's model, or from about 7 hours to 1 hour, according to our simplified simulation model with generic input data described in this section).

If the majority of surgeries are scheduled, then there is not much delay in pooled ORs at all, both for scheduled and emergency surgeries.

At the same time, it is still possible a situation when the pooling of resources is not always beneficial with regard to the waiting times for urgent patients. This can happen if there is a relatively large difference in process (surgery) time for different types of patients, or due to significantly different performance targets (waiting time) because of a different level of urgency. A trade-off line can be developed that indicates whether the use of pooled or separate resources is more beneficial (Joustra et al, 2010). For example, Joustra et al (2010) demonstrated that the separation of urgent and regular patients in a radiotherapy outpatient department becomes beneficial if the target wait time for urgent patients is much shorter than that for regular patients.

Problem 7: Daily Load Leveling (Smoothing) of Scheduled Elective Procedures

In most hospitals, random (emergency) surgeries compete for the same operating rooms (OR) resources with scheduled (elective) surgeries. While the variable number of daily emergency surgeries is beyond hospital control (this is a natural variability), there is a significant variation in the number of daily scheduled elective surgical cases that could be actively managed using hospital scheduling system (Litvak and Long, 2000; Kolker, 2009).

It is possible to manage the scheduling of the elective cases in such a way that smoothes the overall patient flow variability. A daily load leveling of elective cases would reduce the chances of excessive peak demand for the system's capacity (operating rooms and ICU) and, consequently, would reduce patient waiting time.

The managerial decision problem is to see whether the daily load leveling of elective surgeries is worth of implementing. In other words, what is a quantitative effect of the daily load leveling of elective surgeries on delay to start the case in the presence of the competing demand from random emergency surgeries for OR resources?.

Traditional Management Approach

It is generally known that elective scheduling smoothing could help reduce delay (Litvak and Long, 2000; McManus et al, 2003; McManus et al, 2004).

For example, McManus et al (2003) concluded "...variability in scheduled surgical caseload represents a potentially reducible source of stress on the ICU in hospitals and throughput in the healthcare delivery system generally". Further, they stated "...the data demonstrated that bed availability was more strongly determined by variation in scheduled demand than by variation in requests for unscheduled admissions". The authors repeat several times that "...artificial variability is best managed by elimination wherever possible", and that "...we propose that hospitals first seek to control artificial variability as much as possible". However, the authors provide no specific information on how to quantitatively evaluate an effect of smoothing on availability and delay of care.

Management Engineering Approach

While the number and timing of emergency cases are truly random by their nature, elective procedure scheduling is usually within the hospital management control. In order to quantitatively analyze the effect of daily load-leveling it is required to make two simulation models: (i) baseline model that uses current elective and emergency admission schedules to calculate the delay for emergency and scheduled patients; (ii) model with load-leveled (smoothed) elective schedule and the same emergency admissions to calculate the delay for emergency and scheduled patients.

A comparison of the difference in the delay (if any) helps to make a conclusion.

An example of the number of elective and emergency admissions, as well as a possible smoothed (load-leveled) elective schedule for four weeks time period is given in Table 5.

A smoothed schedule (last column in the Table 5) has the same number of cases over the four-week period as the original un-smoothed schedule, i.e. not a single case was dropped but they are rather re-arranged over the time period to smooth daily peaks and valleys.

It is assumed that three interchangeable operating rooms (OR) are available in this case. The emergency surgery duration is in the range from 1.5 to 2.5 hours, with this most likely time of 2.1 hours. Elective surgeries duration is in the range from 1.5 to 3 hours, with the most likely time of

Table 5. Elective, emergency and daily load leveled admissions for the 4-week period

Week	Day of week	Number of elective admissions	Number of emergency admissions	Number of daily-leveled (smoothed) elective admissions
1	Monday	9	16	6
1	Tuesday	11	14	7
1	Wednesday	8	14	7
1	Thursday	5	20	7
1	Friday	5	15	7
2	Monday	10	18	7
2	Tuesday	13	20	7
2	Wednesday	11	9	7
2	Thursday	8	11	7
2	Friday	3	20	7
3	Monday	5	17	7
3	Tuesday	9	11	7
3	Wednesday	8	15	7
3	Thursday	6	15	7
3	Friday	6	20	7
4	Monday	7	15	7
4	Tuesday	4	13	7
4	Wednesday	3	12	7
4	Thursday	4	11	7
4	Friday	3	20	6
	Total	138	306	138

2.4 hours. Both are represented by corresponding triangle distributions similar to those used in the previous section (Problem 6).

The simulation model layout is also similar to the one presented in the previous section (Problem 6) on Figure 5.

Simulation for 672 hours (4 weeks) for the original un-smoothed elective schedule along with competing emergency cases results in the average patient waiting time of 0.64 hours for emergency cases (99% CI is 0.62 – 0.66 hours) and 0.99 hours for elective cases (99% CI is 0.96 – 1.0 hours).

Simulation with a smoothed (load-leveled) elective schedule along with the same competing emergency cases results in the average patient waiting time of 0.53 hours for emergency (99% CI is 0.51 – 0.54 hours) and 0.68 hours for elective cases (99% CI is 0.66 – 0.70 hours).

Thus, in this particular example, the elective daily load leveling results in about 17% reduction in waiting time for emergency surgeries and about 31% reduction in waiting time for elective surgeries.

Elective schedule smoothing (daily load-leveling) is indeed a very powerful approach of reducing patient waiting time and improving efficiency.

A simple simulation model also allows testing an effect of the different smoothing schemes. For example, if nearly the same daily number of elective cases is not possible due to some practical limitations, it is possible to test another less perfect smoothing scheme to make sure that the end result is still worth the effort of its implementation (or maybe not). No traditional management methods are capable of providing such insights for decision-making.

Kolker (2009) provided a more detailed analysis of the effect of daily load leveling of elective surgeries on ICU performance.

Ryckman et al (2009) reported the results of practical implementation of load-leveling of elective surgical admissions at Cincinnati Children's Hospital. New elective surgical admissions to the pediatric ICU were restricted to a maximum of five cases per day. As a consequence of the smoothing of elective surgical cases, it was observed that there was a near elimination of ICU diversion and cancellation of elective surgeries due to lack of ICU beds.

Problem 8: Surgical Capacity of Special Procedure Operating Rooms

A specialized procedure operating rooms (SPR) unit is being planned to unload the volume of outpatient day surgeries from the main surgical department's general operating rooms. At the end of the current year, 1844 special surgical procedures of type 1 and type 2 were performed. Projected additional procedure volume for the next year is 179 procedures of type 1 and 13 procedures of type 2.

Patients get prepared for procedures in the preparation bed area; then they move to the available SPR for the procedures and come back into the same bed area (not necessarily into the same bed) for post-procedure recovery. After initial post-anesthesia recovery time (phase 1), inpatients are moved to a regular nursing unit for full recovery. Outpatients stay in the bed area for the full recovery time (phase 1 and phase 2).

The average post-procedure recovery time is 3.3 hours. The average time to perform a procedure is 0.82 hours. SPR turnover time ranges from 10 to 20 min (cleaning the room, re-stocking it with supplies and making it ready for the next patient). Bed turnover time (cleaning, changing linens and making the bed ready for the next patient) is also from 10 to 20 min. The SPR unit is supposed to work annually 255 days from 7 am to 5 pm (10 hours daily, no weekends); the target average annual utilization is 85%.

The following operational SPR performance criteria have been established: (i) patient wait time to get into SPR for a procedure is not more than 1 hour for 95% patients; (ii) post-procedure patient wait time to get back into the recovery bed from SPR is not more than 5 min for 95% patients.

Management should decide on the minimal number of beds and SPRs that are needed in order to meet the established operational performance criteria. This information is required by an architectural firm hired to design a floor plan needed for the unit construction.

Traditional Management Approach

The number of beds and the number of SPR is calculated using a simple formula (See Box 1).

Thus, four preparation and post-procedure recovery beds and 1 procedure room would be enough.

Because the projected annual patient volume will be served for the available annual time, no or very little patient wait time is expected.

Management Engineering Approach

The typical SPR procedure time and patient recovery bed time have wide and skewed distributions with long tails that are much larger than the average values, as indicated on Figure 6 (panels

Box 1.

$$\#beds = \frac{Annual\_Patient\_Volume * Average\_Bed\_Time}{Total\_Annual\_Available\_time * utilization} = \frac{2036*(3.3+0.25)}{2550*0.85} = 3.3 \cong 4$$

$$\#SPR = \frac{Annual\_Patient\_Volume * Average\_(SPR+TurnOver)\_Time}{Total\_Annual\_Available\_time * utilization} =$$

$$\frac{2036*(0.82+0.25)}{2550*0.85} = 0.99 \cong 1$$

Figure 6. Special procedure room (SPR) procedure time (a) and recovery bed time (b)

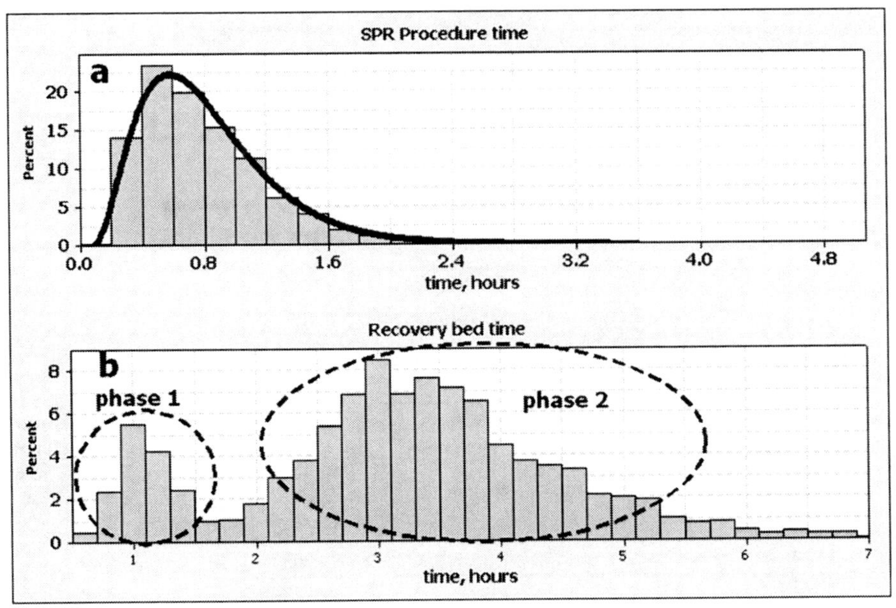

a and b). Therefore, the use of the average time in the above formulas produces a misleading estimation of the required number of beds and SPR (resources).

The only way of capturing this wide time variability is by using a simulation model of SPR operations. The model layout is presented on Figure 7.

The model incorporates patient preparation time variability (best fit statistical distributions) separately for inpatients and outpatients. The post-procedure recovery time is also incorporated separately for inpatients and outpatients, as well as the SPR best fit procedure time variability. Simulation modeling results are presented in Table 6.

It follows from this table that 4 beds and 1 special procedure room calculated using the average preparation and recovery and procedure time are badly underestimated: 23% of patients will wait longer than 1 hour to get to SPR, and 23% of patients will wait longer than 5 min to get back into bed from SPR for recovery (vs. acceptable limit 5%).

The simulation model that takes into account natural variability indicates that the minimal 6 beds and 2 SPR are required to meet operational performance criteria. In this case only about 2% of patients will wait longer than the acceptable limit.

Thus, the correct amount of resources in healthcare settings with highly variable demand can only be predicted by using process simulation methodology. This is another illustration of the flaw of averages, as it was already discussed earlier.

Figure 7. Simulation model layout of patient flow for special procedure operating rooms (SPR) and preparation and post-procedure recovery beds

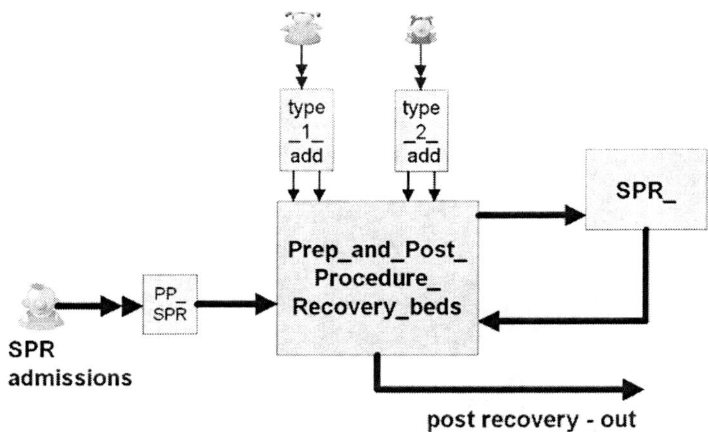

Table 6. Effect of the number of preparation and post-procedure recovery beds and special procedure rooms (SPR) on operational performance characteristics

Number of beds	Number of SPR	Average patient wait time to get to SPR	Percent of patients waiting longer than 1 hour to get to SPR, %	Average post-procedure wait time to get back to bed for recovery	Percent of patients waiting longer than 5 min to get back to bed for recovery, %	Performance criteria met?
4	1	53 min	23%	9.5 min	23%	No
6	2	9.2 min	2.2%	5.5 min	2.2%	Yes

Problem 9: The Entire Hospital System Patient Flow: Effect of Interdependency of ED, ICU, OR and Regular Nursing Units

A typical large community hospital includes main units: an Emergency Department (ED) with 30 beds; an Intensive Care Unit (ICU) with 51 beds; a Surgical Department with 12 Operating Rooms (OR); and Regular Nursing units (NU) with a total capacity of 380 beds.

The overall hospital performance needs significant improvement. A large percent of time ED is on ambulance diversion and there are long ED patient lines and wait time. The ICU frequently does not have beds for ED patient admissions or delays admission of post-surgical patients. The Surgical Department is often at capacity, and elective surgeries are frequently cancelled or re-scheduled.

The hospital management needs to decide: what unit/department to start with for process improvement projects; what type of projects to select; and decide on process improvement performance metrics.

Traditional Management Approach

Because the most patient crowding is visible in ED, it is believed that inadequate ED capacity is an issue. The management wants to increase ED throughput and capacity by reducing patient length of stay (LOS). A process improvement team is formed. After a lot of invested time and efforts, the project improvement team finally reports a 25% reduction of the average length of stay (LOS) and a significant reduction of ED diversion time. The management praises great ED improvement success.

However, both the ORs and ICU start reporting increased patient wait time to get in due to 'no ORs or no ICU beds'. This, in turn, results in increased cancellation rate for scheduled surgeries and keeps more post-surgical patients boarded in ORs waiting for ICU beds. Hence, more surgical cases are now delayed.

The hospital management wants to repeat ED improvement success by initiating ICU or Surgical Department process improvement projects. But the management is not sure anymore that departmental process improvement will be translated into the overall hospital patient flow improvement. They are looking for a better analysis and solution.

Management Engineering Approach

The entire hospital system consists of interdependent departments/units that interact to each other. ED is not a stand-alone unit. Increased patient flow out of ED cannot consistently be supported by available ORs and ICU capacity to handle it. Therefore ED improvement is not necessarily translated into the overall hospital system improvement although this is the actual goal. It turns out that patient flow is a property of the entire system rather than the property of the separate departments/units. A detailed analysis is required of the overall hospital system patient flow and the interdependency of subsystems/units in order to establish right units for process improvement projects. Such an analysis can only be performed using a system simulation methodology (Kolker, 2010a; Kolker, 2010b).

A high-level flow map (layout) of the entire hospital system is shown on Figure 8.

Patients admitted into the ED by ambulance or by walk-in form an ED input flow. Some patients are treated, stabilized and released home. ED patients admitted into the hospital (ED output) form an inpatient input flow into the ICU, OR and/or NU. The length of stay distribution best fit was identified separately for patients released home and patients admitted to the hospital (Kolker, 2008). Patients waiting longer than two hours in the ED waiting room leave the ED without being seen (lost patients). About 60% of admitted patients are taken into operating rooms (OR) for emergency surgery, about 30% of admitted patients move into the ICU, and about 10%

Figure 8. Simulation model layout of patient flow for a typical entire hospital system

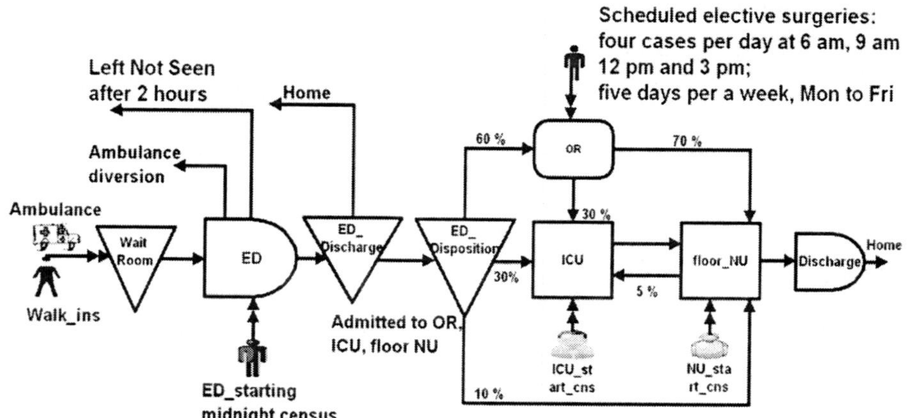

of patients are admitted from ED into the floor nursing units (NU).

OR suite has 12 interchangeable operating rooms used both for ED emergency and scheduled surgeries. There are four daily scheduled OR cases at 6 am, 9 am, 12 pm and 3 pm, Monday to Friday (there are no scheduled surgeries on weekends). Scheduled cases form a separate OR admissions flow, as indicated on the diagram Figure 8.

Elective surgery duration depends on surgical service type, such as general surgery, orthopedics, neuro-surgery, etc. For the simplicity of this particular model, the elective surgery duration was weighted by each service percentage, and the best statistical distribution fit was identified (inverse Gaussian in this case). Emergency surgery duration best fit distribution was Pearson 6.

About 30% of post surgery patients are admitted from OR into the ICU (direct ICU admission), while 70% are admitted into the floor NU. However, some patients (about 5%) are readmitted from the floor NU back to the ICU (indirect ICU admission from OR). ICU length of stay is assumed to range from 1 day to 3 days, with the most likely of 1.5 days, represented by a triangle distribution. Kolker (2009) developed a detailed ICU simulation model and analysis.

Patient length of stay (LOS) in NU is assumed to range from 2 days to 10 days, with the most likely of 5 days, also represented by a triangle distribution.

When ED, OR, ICU or NU are completely full (at full capacity), diversion status is declared. The units stay on diversion until at least one bed in the unit is freed. Total unit diversion is defined here as the percentage of operational time when the unit is at full capacity and can no longer accept new patients.

At the simulation start, the ED, ICU and NU were pre-filled with the midnight census of 15, 46 and 350 patients, respectively. (Pre-filling was used to shorten a simulation warm-up period). Simulation was run for 1 month (31 full days) using 300 replications.

A summary of simulation results for the hospital system is given in Table 7.

Seven performance metrics used to assess the system operational performance indicated in column 1. Baseline (current state) results are presented in column 2. Aggressive improvement efforts in the ED resulted in reducing LOS for patients admitted into the hospital to less than 6 hours compared to the baseline state of 20 to 24 hours (from ED registration to ED discharge). However, because of interdependency of the

Table 7. A summary of simulation results for the hospital system patient flow performance metrics

1	2	3	4	5	6
Performance metrics	Baseline state	Too aggressive ED improvement: patients admitted within 6 hrs	Downstream units: better or worse than baseline?	Less aggressive ED improvement: patients admitted within 10 hrs	Downstream units: better or worse than baseline?
99% CI of the number of patients waiting to get to ED	23 – 23.5	9.6 -10.4	Much Better	21 – 22	Better
99% CI of the number of patients waiting hospital admission	59 - 61	66-68	*Worse*	61 – 63	Not much different
99% CI of number of patients left not seen after waiting 2 hrs	25.5 -28.5	0	Better	11 –13	Better
99%CI for percent ED diversion	23% -23.4%	1.7% - 1.9%	Much Better	17.9% - 18.3%	Better
99% CI for percent ICU diversion	28% -30%	31% - 33%	*Worse*	29% - 30%	Not much different
99%CI for percent OR diversion	14%-14.8%	15.5% - 16.5%	*Worse*	14.6% - 15.7%	Not much different
99%CI for percent NU diversion	11.2% -11.6%	11.1% -11.5%	Not much different	11% - 11.4%	Not much different

downstream units, three out of seven metrics became worse (column 4). The ED bottleneck just moved downstream into the OR and ICU because of their inability to handle the increased patient volume from ED.

Thus, aggressive process improvement in one subsystem (ED) resulted in worsening situation in other interrelated subsystems (OR and ICU). If, instead of too aggressive ED LOS reduction, a less aggressive improvement is implemented, e.g. LOS not more than 10 hours for patients admitted to the hospital, then none of the seven metrics become worse than the baseline state (columns 5 and 6). While in this case ED performance is not as good as it could be, it is still better than it is at the baseline state level. At the same time, this less aggressive local ED improvement does not, at least, make the ICU, OR and floor NU worse. In other words, less aggressive ED improvement is more aligned with the ability of the downstream subsystems to handle increased patient volume.

Thus, from the entire hospital system standpoint, the primary focus of process improvement should be on the ICU because of its highest percent diversion followed by the ED and OR. At the same time, ED patient target LOS reduction program should not be too aggressive, and it should be closely coordinated with that for OR and ICU. Otherwise, even if the ED reports a significant progress in its patient LOS reduction program, this progress will not translate into improvement of the overall hospital system patient flow. In order to improve the entire system do not 'over-improve' locally.

Of course, many other scenarios could be analyzed using the simulation model to find out how to improve the entire hospital system patient flow rather than those for each local hospital subsystem/department.

Patient flow (throughput) is a general dynamic supply and demand balance problem. This is not a one-time snapshot. The system's behavior depends on time. There are three basic components that should be accounted for in these type of problems: (i) the number of patients (or, generally, any items) entering the system at any point of time (admissions); (ii) the number of patients (any items) leaving the system at any point of time after spending some variable time in the system (discharges), and (iii) limited capacity of the system which limits the flow of patients (items) through the system. All three components affect the flow of patients that the system can handle. A lack of the proper balance between these components results in the system over-flow, bottlenecks or, sometimes, underutilization. Simulation methodology provides the only means of quantitative analysis of the proper balance and dynamic variability in complex systems.

This analysis illustrates the following important management engineering principles: (i) improvement of the separate subsystems (local optimization or local improvement) does not necessarily result in the improvement of the entire system, (ii) a system of local improvements (local optimums) could be a very inefficient system (Goldratt et al, 2004), and (iii) analysis of an entire complex system is usually incomplete and can be misleading without taking into account the *subsystems' interdependency.*

The Probabilistic Resource Optimization Problems

Problem 10: Optimized Pooled Screening Testing

The US Center for Disease Control and Prevention (CDC) has revised its recommendations for screening for human immunodeficiency virus (HIV) and now recommends HIV screening for all patients age 13 to 64 years in all health care settings, including hospital emergency departments, urgent care clinics, inpatient services, sexually transmitted disease clinics, tuberculosis clinics, and primary care offices (Armstrong and Taege, 2007; Bozzette, 2005).

A large testing laboratory is staffed and equipped to the testing capacity of 60 HIV specimens per day. Due to new CDC recommendations the specimen daily volume has increased to about 100 per day. This results in a testing backlog and frequent staff overtime.

The management is eager to increase the testing capacity in order to reduce the backlog and staff overtime.

Traditional Management Approach

Because specimen testing is largely automated and must follow a standard operating procedure, testing time per specimen cannot be much reduced. The only option is budgeting additional laboratory staffing and equipment even though the budget is tight, and might not be approved in full.

Management Engineering Approach

The specimen testing capacity cannot be directly increased due to budgeting issues. However, it is possible to reduce the expected overall number of tests per specimen, thereby increasing the overall laboratory capacity.

Indeed, in the current testing arrangement one specimen requires one test (assuming that there is no rework for the same specimen). Thus, the daily workload of 100 specimens requires 100 individual tests that are beyond current laboratory capacity.

However, if prevalence of the disease to test for is low, then most tests come back negative. Therefore, a combined batch of samples pooled together will frequently result in a negative test. A negative test for the batch allows one to declare each individual specimen used to make up this combined batch negative as well, using a single test. If a batch is positive then each individual specimen used to make up this batch should be retested to identify a positive specimen.

There is a trade-off between the overall reduction of the number of tests if the batch is negative and additional retesting if the batch is positive. The problem is identifying an optimal batch size that results in the overall reduction of the number of required tests compared to the original arrangement for testing each individual specimen.

It is assumed that test results of each sample are independent events. The expected total number of tests is the probability of a positive batch times the number of necessary tests *(batch size* +1) plus the probability of a negative batch times 1.

Let n be a batch size and let P be the probability that each individual specimen is tested positive. The expected number of tests per specimen, N, is going to be (Saraniti, 2006)

$$N = \frac{[1-(1-P)^n]*(n+1)+(1-P)^n}{n}$$
$$= 1-(1-P)^n + 1/n$$

Reduction of the number of tests compared to the current arrangement of one test per specimen is possible only if N is less than 1. In order for this to happen, the probability of a positive specimen should satisfy the inequality condition

$$P < 1 - n^{-1/n}$$

The maximum of the right-hand side for this inequality for integer numbers is about 0.306 for n=3. Therefore, a reduction of the number of tests per specimen is theoretically possible only if the probability of a positive specimen (disease prevalence), P, is less than about 30%. For each P in this range N has its minimal value. If 12.4% $< P <$ 30.6% then the optimal batch size which minimizes N is exactly $n = 3$. If $P <$ 11.1% then the optimal batch size which minimizes N can be approximated by the formula (rounded to the nearest integer number)

$$n \cong \frac{1}{\sqrt{P}} + 0.5$$

For example, according to a CDC report (2008), the HIV prevalence in the USA population at the end of 2006 was about P=0.447% with 95% CI from 0.427% to 0.468% (without breaking down by risk groups). Using the above formulas, the optimal batch size for this prevalence is 15 and the expected number of tests per specimen is about N=0.13. This gives 87% reduction of the number of tests per specimen; instead of 100 required daily specimen tests only about 100*(1-0.87)≅ 13 tests (!) would be needed.

If the probability of a positive test (prevalence) is much higher, e.g. P=10% for high risk population group, the optimal batch size is 4, and the number of tests per specimen is about 0.594. Thus, even in this case only about 100*0.594≅59 daily tests are needed. This is within the current laboratory capacity of 60 daily tests.

In a practical implementation of this technique some additional factors should be taken into account. A particular concern is batch dilution due to sample pooling that could result in reduced tests' analytic specificity and/or sensitivity. This issue has been addressed in the literature (Saraniti, 2006).

On the other hand, the basic principle of pooled specimens testing can be further enhanced under certain circumstances by two variations: sorting and multistage testing. Sorting patient specimens into high and low risk groups allows for additional savings when easily identifiable high risk groups have a much greater prevalence than larger low risk groups.

In multistage testing, positive batches are rearranged into new smaller batches, which are then retested (instead of individual sample retesting). This approach is most efficient if prevalence is very low and the analytic sensitivity loss from large pools is minimal (Saraniti, 2006).

Notice that this basic test per specimen reduction methodology can be applied to mass testing of any fluids/specimens.

Thus, management engineering demonstrates how to get more by doing less through smarter and more efficient managing of the available resources.

Reducing the Number of Variables and Identifying a Few Significant Independent Contributing Variables (Factors)

Problem 11: Strategic Market Share Expansion Analysis: Population Demographic Factors that are the Most Significant Contributors to the Hospital Contribution Margin

This problem illustrates another area of application for management engineering: an advanced statistical multivariate data analysis methodology for decision-making. This area can also be viewed as Business Intelligence and Data Mining application.

A hospital plans a major market share expansion to improve its long-term financial viability. The management would like to know what population demographic factors and population disease prevalence specific to the local area zip codes are the most important contributors to the financial contribution margin (CM $). Contribution margin is defined as the difference between all payments collected from patients and the patient variable costs.

A set of population demographic data was collected for ten local area zip codes and corresponding median contribution margins from each zip code (CM $).

The following groups of demographic variables and disease prevalence data were collected for each zip code as the percentage of the total zip code population (actual data are not shown here because of limited space):

- Four Age categories: 18-34, 35-54, 55-64, 65+
- Four Educational categories: BS/BA degree and higher, Associate/Professional degree, high school diploma, no high school diploma
- Four Income categories: less than $50K, $50 - $75K, $75K - $100K, $100K +
- Five occupational categories: Healthcare, Labor, Professional/Administrative, Public Service, Service industry
- Gender: male, female
- Five Race categories: African American, Native American, Asian, White, Other
- Fourteen disease categories: BMT, Medical Oncology, Surgical Oncology, Cardiology, Cardiothoracic surgical, Vascular surgical, Digestive, Medicine/Primary care, Musculoskeletal, Neurology, Transplant, Trauma, Unassigned, Women Health

There are total 38 data variables included in the database.

Traditional Management Approach

Because of the large number of variables, it is difficult to select the most important factors for the zip codes with the largest CM $. For example, it could be expected that older and more affluent patients (e.g. 65+ years old and in annual income category $100K+) contribute more to CM $ than younger and / or lower income patients.

However, data indicate that the zip codes with the largest CM $ have lower percentage of the above categories than the other zip codes with lower CM $.

On top of that, many of these categories are highly correlated. This means that there is a redundant information and uncertainty in the data that makes it difficult to attribute the contribution of one or more variables to CM $.

For example, it is reasonable to expect a high positive correlation of low education and low income, and a negative correlation of high education degrees (say, BS/BA+) and low income. Indeed, using demographic data, it was calculated that a linear correlation coefficient of the categories 'No high school diploma' and 'annual income less than $50K' is 0.93, while the same income and BS/BA+ degree are correlated negatively at

-0.79. This means that it is very likely that those with 'No high school diploma' earn less annually than $50K, while there is a tendency that those with BS/BA+ educational level earn more annually than $50K.

Obviously, performing such a paired correlation analysis for all 38 variables (703 pairs!) is impractical. Besides, knowing the linear correlation coefficient does not help to reduce redundant information and extract meaningful information for separate contributing factors.

Attempt to perform a linear regression analysis using 38 variables as predictors and CM $ as a response function results in a regression equation with low goodness of fit (R-sq(adj) about 10%), and all coefficients that are not statistically significant at the 5% significance level (p-value is in the range from 0.2 to 0.8) with the huge variance inflation factors (VIF) that are in the range from a few dozen to a few millions. This is an obvious indication of a serious multicollinearity problem in the original data set that leads to the failure of the traditional regression analysis to extract meaningful information for contributing factors (variables).

Therefore, an alternative technique should be employed. One of the most powerful methodologies for multivariate data analysis is based on principal component decomposition of the original data base matrix (Jobson, 1992).

Management Engineering Approach

Principal component decomposition methodology allows one to perform a multivariate correlation analysis and identifies redundant variables that carry little or no information while retaining only a few mutually uncorrelated principal variables. This technique is a special case of a matrix approximation procedure called singular value decomposition. The higher the level of correlation between the columns of data of the original matrix, the fewer the number of new (principal) variables is required to describe the original data set.

More formally, given an original data matrix **X** representing *n* observations on each of *p* variables X_1, X_2, …., X_p, the purpose of principal component analysis is to determine *r* new variables PC_r (PC-principal component) that can be used to best approximate variation in the *p* original *X* variables such as linear combinations

$$PC_1 = v_{11}X_1 + v_{21}X_2 + ... + v_{p1}X_p$$

....

$$PC_r = v_{1r}X_1 + v_{2r}X_2 + ... + v_{pr}X_p$$

(Best approximation is calculated as the minimized the sum of squared deviations of the PCs approximations and the variables in original data matrix **X**).

The solutions to the problem are the eigenvalues, λ_j, *j=1,2,..,s*, and the corresponding eigenvectors, v_j, *j=1,2,..,s*. The elements of the *j*-th eigenvector define the *j*-th PC associated with the data. The *j-th* eigenvalue is a measure of how much information is retained by the *j-th* PC. A large value of λ_j (compared to 1) means that there is a substantial amount of information retained by the corresponding *j-th* PC, whereas a small value means that there is little information retained by *j-th* PC.

All eigenvalues must add up to the total number of the original independent variables, *p,* i.e. $\sum_{j=1}^{s}\lambda_j = p$. Thus, if some eigenvalues are large, then the others should be small. This illustrates the principle of information conservation: the total amount of information in the original data set is not changed because of PC decomposition; rather, it is rearranged in the form of a number of linear combinations of the original variables in such a way that main information holders (linear combinations - PCs) are clearly identified, significantly reducing thereby the number of independent variables that retain the same amount of information.

Table 8. Eigen value analysis of the demographic data correlation matrix

Eigen value	16.44	11.19	4.63	2.73	1.15	0.853	0.63	0.307	0.067
Proportion	0.433	0.295	0.122	0.072	0.03	0.022	0.017	0.008	0.002
Cumulative	0.433	0.727	0.849	0.921	0.951	0.974	0.990	0.998	1.000

For this particular problem, the principal component analysis of the demographic matrix has been carried out using the Minitab statistical software package (version 15). Results are presented in Table 8.

Thus, it can be concluded that only nine principal components (nine linear combinations of the original variables) are required to account for all 38 original variables. Only five principal components are enough to approximate 95% of the original data. This indicates that a lot of variables in the original data matrix are indeed highly correlated and contain no new information; most of them form a so-called information noise that hampers extracting meaningful information for contributing factors.

Notice also that the sum of all nine eigenvalues in Table 8 is equal to the number of the original data variables, i.e. 38, as it is required by the PC decomposition technique.

The next step is to perform regression analysis in order to relate CM $ (response function) to mutually uncorrelated PC variables, and then to determine the original variables (factors) that contribute the most to CM $.

Regression analysis with PC has a lot of advantage over regular regression analysis with original data, and it is much more reliable (Jobson, 1992; Glantz and Slinker, 2001).

Because PCs are mutually uncorrelated, the variation of the dependent variable (CM $) is accounted for by each component independently of other components, and their contribution is directly defined by the coefficients of the regression equation. Since PCs are mutually uncorrelated, the presence of any one PC does not affect the regression coefficients of the other PC.

Usually, if the purpose of PC analysis is reduction of the number of independent variables and the search for the underlying data pattern, the PCs with the eigenvalues close to zero (minor PCs) can be omitted because they carry on little or no information. However, in multiple regression with PC it is not a good idea to drop the minor PC because doing so can introduce an uncertain bias in the regression coefficients (Jobson, 1992; Glantz and Slinker, 2001). In this particular case, the number of PC that account for all original data is relatively small (nine). Therefore, all nine PCs have been retained for performing multiple regression.

In order to perform the regression, we first find the best subset using all nine PC as independent variables. Results for PC2 to PC9 are presented in Table 9. (A subset analysis with predictors PC1 to PC8 results in the overall lower R-sq(adj), and it is not presented here).

The best subset regression identifies the best-fitting regression models that can be constructed with as few predictor variables as possible. All possible subsets of the predictors are examined, beginning with all models containing one predictor, and then all models containing two predictors, and so on. The two best models for each number of predictors are displayed.

Each line of the Table 9 represents a different model. An X symbol indicates predictors that are present in the model.

In this case, the best subset includes eight predictors PC2 to PC9 because this subset has the highest R-sq (adjusted), as well as the Mallow coefficient C_p that is close to the number of predictors.

Table 9. Best subsets regression with PCs

Vars	R-sq (adj)	Mallow Cp	PC2	PC3	PC4	PC5	PC6	PC7	PC8	PC9
3	87.0	128	X	X					X	
3	64.9	349		X	X				X	
4	90.1	83.0	X	X	X				X	
4	88.1	99.6	X	X				X	X	
5	92.2	54.4	X	X	X			X	X	
5	91.3	60.3	X	X	X	X			X	
6	94.5	31.7	X	X	X	X		X	X	
6	93.4	37.2	X	X	X			X	X	X
7	97.4	14.5	X	X	X	X		X	X	X
7	94.0	26.2	X	X	X	X	X	X	X	
8	99.4	9.0	X	X	X	X	X	X	X	X

The regression equation with predictors PC2 to PC9 is

CM \$ = 12.8 + 0.0101 PC1 + 0.201 PC2 - 0.387 PC3 + 0.171 PC4 + 0.190 PC5 + 0.122 PC6 + 0.286 PC7 + 1.95 PC8

with R-sq (adj) = 99.4%. Thus, this equation is rather accurate in what it accounts for 99.4% of the response function (CM \$) variability.

At the same time, only three predictors turn out to be statistically significant at the 5% significance level: PC2 (p-value=0.039), PC3 (p-value=0.031) and PC8 (p-value=0.024). Because PC predictors are orthogonal (mutually uncorrelated), all terms that are not statistically significant can be removed from the regression equation without affecting the remaining coefficients, and we arrive to the much simpler regression equation,

CM \$ = 12.8 + 0.201 PC2 - 0.387 PC3 + 1.95 PC8

An examination of this equation indicates that the predictor PC8 has a much higher contribution coefficient than PC2 and PC3 (almost by a factor of 10 for PC2 and by a factor of 5 for PC3). Also, because PC3 regression coefficient is negative, only relatively large negative PC3 eigenvector coefficients contribute positively into CM \$.

The eigenvector coefficients for PC2, PC3 and PC8 are presented in Table 10.

These coefficients represent the weight of each variable into each PC.

An examination of the eigenvector coefficients from Table 10 combined with the regression equation coefficients results in the following primary contributing variables (factors) to CM \$: Age 55-64; Annual income \$50 K - \$75 K; Occupations Public Service and Service Industry; Race- Other. Relative contributions of diseases are: neurology, cardiology and musculoskeletal, followed by cardiothoracic surgery, primary care, transplant and trauma.

There are some possible demographic and societal explanations of these results, but they are beyond the scope of this chapter.

Thus, in order to increase the contribution margin, hospital management should focus the marketing campaign on attracting more patients from the zip codes with a higher level of the above primary contributing factors.

Table 10. Eigen vector coefficients for statistically significant principle components

Variable	PC2	PC3	PC8
Age 18-34	0.26	0.037	-0.034
Age 35-54	-0.084	0.331	0.037
Age 55-64	-0.229	-0.173	0.236
Age 65+	-0.058	-0.185	0.015
BS/BA+ degree	-0.269	-0.137	0.049
Assoc/Prof degree	-0.237	0.081	-0.18
High school	0.097	0.332	0.101
No high school	0.286	-0.084	-0.078
Income < $50K	0.275	-0.105	0.025
Income $50K-$75K	-0.059	-0.013	0.256
Income $75-$100K	-0.27	0.125	-0.183
Income $100K+	-0.259	0.097	-0.012
Occupation: Health	-0.21	-0.176	-0.206
Labor	0.265	0.116	-0.133
Professional/Adm	-0.275	-0.059	-0.104
Public Service	0.029	-0.328	0.463
Service Industry	-0.125	0.264	0.542
% male	0.059	0.210	0.017
% female	-0.059	-0.210	-0.017
Race: African American	0.235	-0.123	0.007
Asian	0.157	0.142	-0.337
Native American	-0.033	-0.339	-0.253
Other	0.263	-0.114	0.158
White	-0.252	0.128	-0.087
Disease: Cancer-BMT	0.012	0.108	0.002
Med Oncology	0.012	0.107	0.01
Surgical Oncology	0.011	0.108	0.012
Cardiology	0.014	0.103	0.012
Cardiothoracic Surgery	0.014	0.103	0.011
Vascular surgery	0.018	0.104	-0.001
Digestive disease	0.014	0.103	0.005
Medicine/Primary Care	0.015	0.103	0.01
Musculoskeletal	0.014	0.105	0.012
Neurology	0.014	0.104	0.013
Transplant	0.016	0.106	0.008
Trauma	0.015	0.104	0.006
Unassigned	0.014	0.103	0.000
Women Health	0.015	0.103	-0.002

Forecasting of a Time Series Using Past Data-Points

Problem 12: Forecasting Patient Volumes Using Time Series Data Analysis

Forecasting the future patient volume (demand) is an important step in managerial decision-making, such as planning facility capacity and properly budgeting and allocating resources needed to meet the demand.

As an example, let us consider a problem of forecasting the future patient volumes for a facility using its annual patient volumes for a number of previous years.

The annual patient volumes for 13 years, from 1997 to 2009, are presented in Table 11.

For planning budgets and staffing, the facility management needs to forecast annual patient volumes for the future years, from 2010 to 2015.

Table 11. Annual Patient Volumes

Year	Patient Volume
1997	9,400
1998	9,100
1999	9,966
2000	8,900
2001	10,052
2002	9,700
2003	11,200
2004	10,090
2005	12,772
2006	13,130
2007	16,867
2008	17,725
2009	18,225

Traditional Management Approach

The simplest method to forecast the annual patient volume trend (or some workload volume tend) is to assume some percent of annual growth from the last year on the record, say 2% or 3%. Using this assumption, the calculations are simple and sometimes presented as plausible 'scenarios' for different growth percents. However, such scenarios are actually a wild guess; they assume unlimited growth and provide no insights into trends or the pattern in the data.

Some simple enough smoothing statistical methods are recommended to use, such as polynomial regression for extrapolation (linear and non-linear), Box-Jenkins, exponential smoothing (single and double), Holt-Winter's, weighted moving averages, autoregressive integrated moving averages (ARIMA), and some others (Ozcan, 2009; Langabeer, 2007).

Smoothing statistical forecasting methods are based on the idea of finding a pattern in the time series data, and then extrapolating this pattern to the future in order to generate forecast.

However, before applying any forecasting method, the number of previous data-points that have to be used to make the future predictions should be identified.

The Number of Past Data-Points that Have to Be Used for Making a Forecast

It seems reasonable to assume that too 'old' data-points do not practically affect the most recent data-points, let alone the future data. For example, it is unlikely that the 13-years-old patient volume data from 1997 would affect the 2009 patient volume, and beyond. On the other hand, it is likely that the 2008 patient volume is more closely related (i.e. correlated to some extent) to the 2009 patient volume. Therefore, it is reasonable to expect that the 2008 data-point will affect to some extent the future data-points (forecasts).

The maximum number of 'steps back to the past', at which the older data-points are still strongly correlated to the newer data-points (the correlation cut-off time lag k), can be estimated using an autocorrelation function (ACF) of a time series. The data-points that are strongly correlated to the newer ones can be included for making the forecast. The data-points that are weakly correlated to the newer ones (or not correlated at all) should not be included for forecasting; otherwise, the forecast will likely be skewed.

An autocorrelation function of a time series is a measure of a linear interdependency between the data-points separated by k time units (time lag). For a discrete time series of length n with the data-points y_i (i= 1, 2, ..., n), the normalized unbiased ACF for each time lag k (k=0, 1, 2, ...,m<n) is calculated as

$$ACF(k) = \frac{1}{(n-k)\sigma_1(k)\sigma_2(k)} \sum_{i=1}^{n-k} (y_i - m_1(k)) * (y_{i+k} - m_2(k)),$$

where $m_1(k)$ and $\sigma_1(k)$ are the population average and the standard deviation of the first n-k data-points, i.e.

$$m_1(k) = \frac{1}{n-k}\sum_{i=1}^{n-k} y_i,$$

$$\sigma_1^2(k) = \frac{1}{n-k}\sum_{i=1}^{n-k} (y_i - m_1(k))^2$$

The $m_2(k)$ and $\sigma_2(k)$ are the population average and the standard deviation of the last n-k data-points

$$m_2(k) = \frac{1}{n-k}\sum_{i=k+1}^{n} y_i,$$

$$\sigma_2^2(k) = \frac{1}{n-k}\sum_{i=k+1}^{n} (y_i - m_2(k))^2$$

ACF(k) as a function of time lag k goes from 1 (at k=0) to close to 0 for larger k-values, usually (but not always) with some oscillations around the time-lag axis k with the decreasing amplitude.

A possible measure of a correlation cut-off value k is the first zero-crossing of the time-lag axis (if the crossing occurs). Sometimes, the correlation cut-off lag is defined as the smallest value k that makes ACF(k) < K, where K = 0.5 or K=e^{-1}=0.37 (Schuster, 1988).

However, it is more justified to compare the computed ACF(k) with the critical level required to reject the null hypothesis that ACF(k) at the specific lag k was generated by a completely random time series, i.e. it is statistically indistiguishable from zero at some level of significance.

It turns out that the statistic

$$t = ACF(k) * [\frac{n-k-2}{1-ACF(k)^2}]^{1/2}$$

is distributed as t-distribution with n-k-2 degrees of freedom (Press et all, 1988). Thus, the correlation cut-off lag is the maximum value of k at which the above t-statistic becomes less than the critical t-distribution value at, say, 95% confidence level (at the α level of significance 0.05).

The autocorrelation function ACF(k) of the patient volume time series from Table 11 is presented on Figure 9.

The ACF(k) values are statistically different from zero according to the above statistic for the values k=1 to k=4. Hence, the data-points that are strongly correlated in this case go back to the past for about 5 years (ACF(0)=1 at 2009 corresponds to k=0, i.e. no time lag; each consecutive year corresponds to one time lag unit, i.e. k=1,2,...,10). Thus, only the most recent five patient volume data-points from 2005 to 2009 with strong interdependency (linear correlation larger than about 0.8) should be used to generate the forecast for the future years.

Validation of Some Typical Forecasting Models

In order to check how good some forecast generating models are, the patient volume data-points for the years 2005 to 2008 from Table 11 were used

Figure 9. Autocorrelation function of the patient volume time series. Panel (a) – ACK(k) statistically different from zero. Panel (b) – ACF(k) are not statistically different from zero at 0.05 significance level

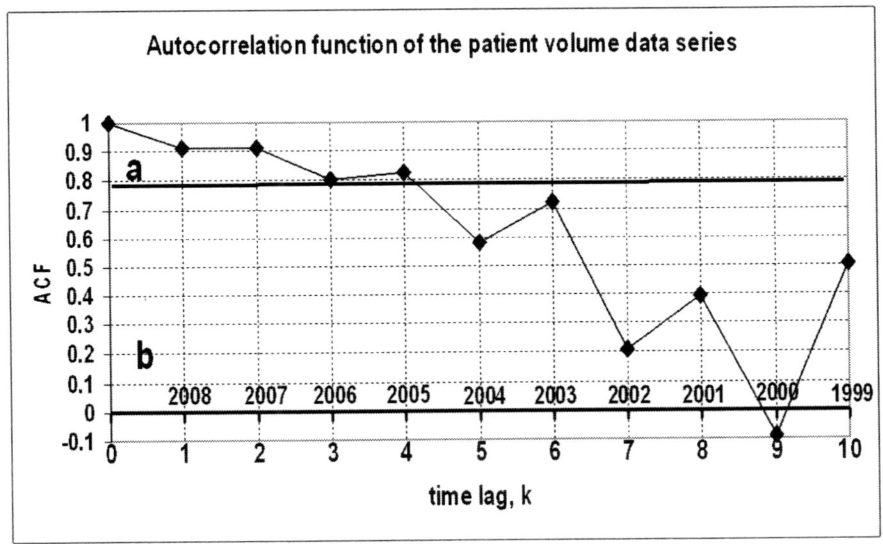

Table 12. Prediction capability of some traditional smoothing forecasting models

Forecasting Model	Forecasted value for 2009 using the data-points for 2005-2008	Forecasting error
Growth curve	20,369	11.8%
Single Exponential	15,427	15.3%
S-Curve Trend	17,880	1.9%
Winter's	20,449	12.2%
Polynomial Quadratic	20,397	11.9%
Moving Average	17,296	5%
ARIMA	16,903	7.2%

to predict the data-point for the 2009 year. This data-point was compared with its known actual value, 18,225. The forecasts, presented in Table 12, were generated using the statistical software package, Minitab 15 (with the default software parameters, where applicable).

As can be seen from Table 12, none of these traditional models are particularly good at predicting even one year ahead. Therefore, it is unlikely that they will provide a reasonably reliable forecast for a longer period of time.

Examples of application of four forecasting models for six consecutive years from 2010 to 2015 using the last five data-points from Table 11 are presented on Figure 10.

Regression polynomials (2-nd and 3-rd order) resulted in an apparent strong downward trend after the year 2011. These models are not shown on Figure 10 due to limited space, as well as Moving Average and ARIMA models.

None of the longer term forecasts generated by these models seem reliable. Indeed, the growth curve and Winters' models forecast that by the end

Figure 10. Smoothing forecasting models for patient volume

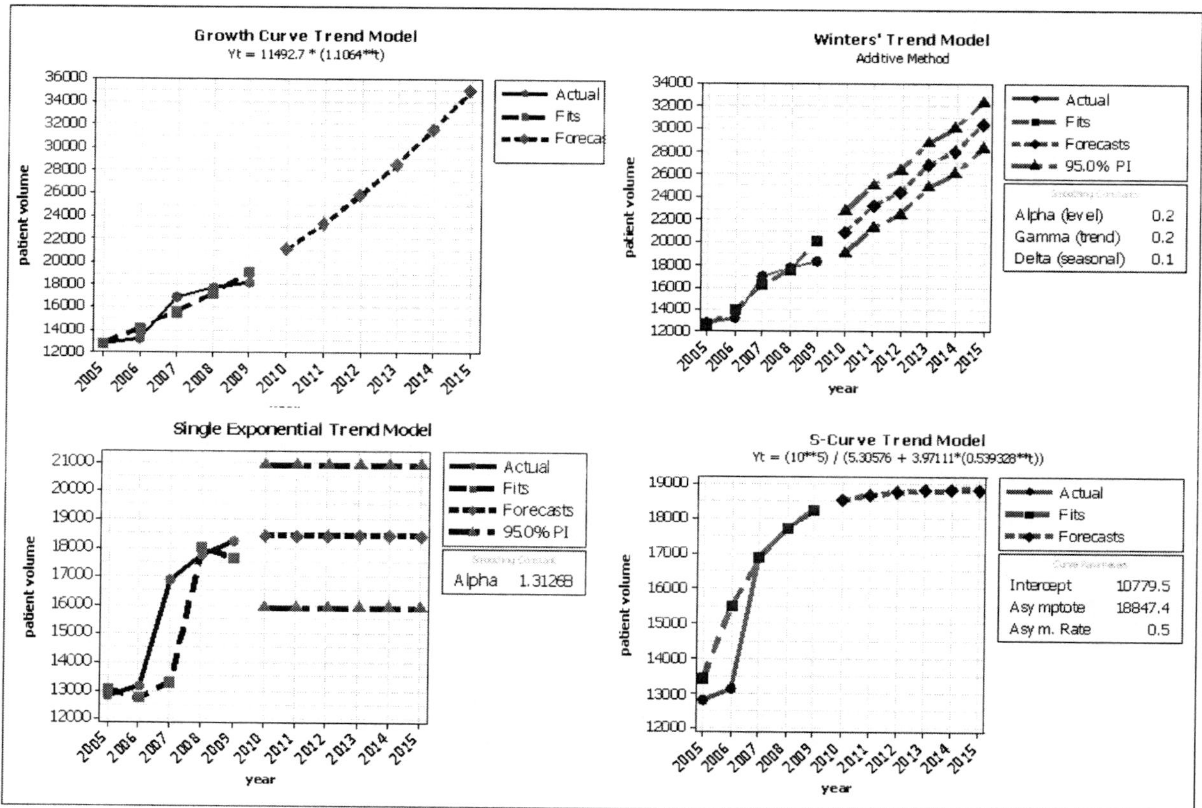

of 2015 the patient volume will be about 35,000 or 30,500, accordingly. These forecasts seem way too large and unlikely.

On the other hand, the single exponential model predicts the constant patient volume at the 18,500 level for all years from 2010 to 2015, while S-curve model predicts a very slow growth with asymptotic constant value at the 18,847 level. These longer term forecasts are also seem unreliable because they indicate practically no change in patient volume at all for the years ahead.

Management Engineering Approach

Since traditional forecasting methods are apparently not adequate enough in this particular situation, another technique can be used. This technique is based on the theory of digital recursive linear filters that are widely used in digital signal processing applications (Press et al, 1988).

Let y_i (i= 1, 2, ..., n) are the data-points that are equally spaced along a time line, and one wants to use n consecutive values of y_i to predict $n+1$ data-point. The equation for predicting the next data-point of a time series from the previous values is

$$y_n = \sum_{j=1}^{m} d_j y_{n-j} + x_n,$$

where d_j is a set of prediction coefficients, m is the number of coefficients, and x_n is the discrepancy of the prediction at time-step n and the true value, y_n.

Prediction coefficients, d_j,are calculated in a way that minimizes the discrepancy, i.e. makes |

$x_n| << |y_n|$, or $\sum_n |x_n|^2 << \sum_n |y_n|^2$. Thus, using a right set of coefficients d_j, one can predict the future data-points of a time series from a record of its past.

Because the predicted future data-points, y_n, are generated using previously calculated data-points, y_{n-j}, such a procedure is called the *recursive* procedure; its predicting behavior quickly becomes much more complex than a straight line, or a polynomial. It is especially successful at predicting time series that are rather smooth and oscillatory, though not necessarily periodic (Press et al, 1988).

However, in order to achieve its full usefulness, recursive procedure must be stable. Recursive procedures feed on their own output; therefore they are not always stable, i.e. some particular 'bad' sets of coefficients, d_j can generate an exponentially growing output.

The condition that the recursive prediction procedure is stable is that all n complex roots of the characteristic polynomial equation

$$z^n - \sum_{j=1}^{n} d_j z^{n-j} = 0$$

are inside the unit circle, i.e. satisfy the condition $|z| \leq 1$. Press et al (1988) provide a detailed description of the computational procedure for using recursive prediction of the future data-points of a time-series using the above equations.

Similarly to the traditional smoothing forecasting models illustrated above, the recursive procedure was tested using the previous four patient volume data-points for the years 2005 to 2008 in order to predict the fifth data-point for the year 2009, which was compared with the known actual value. Forecasted 2009 patient volume was 18,275, while the actual value for 2009 was, 18,114. The prediction error in this case was very small, about 0.6%. Thus, this forecast is much better than that provided by smoothing forecasting methods.

Of course, one should not always expect such a good predicting accuracy. However, Press et al (1988) pointed out that in many situations the recursive forecasting turns out to be vastly more powerful than any kind of a smoothing or polynomial extrapolation used in a traditional forecasting.

Forecasted values for six consecutive years from 2010 to 2015 using the most recent five data-points from Table 11 are presented on Figure 11.

It is seen that the recursive linear forecasting is more reasonable than some traditional smoothing forecasting models presented on Figure 10. Indeed, recursive forecasting predicts neither an unlimited growth in patient volume over the years, nor its constant value. Instead, the forecast indicates some growth in patient volume up to the year 2013, flattening it and then a slight decline from 2014 to 2015.

Of course, no forecast can be very accurate; forecasting errors are inevitable. In general, it is impossible to accurately predict the future based on the past.

Nonetheless, if the underlying factors are stable enough for the forecasting time horizon, and the most recent data-points from the past are used that are strongly correlated to each other, then a recursive forecasting is capable of providing a reliable enough forecast that can be valuable for efficient managerial decision-making.

CONCLUSION

This chapter illustrates the power of management engineering for quantitative managerial decision-making in healthcare setting. Using a number of problems adapted from hospital and clinic practice, traditional management reasoning and management engineering methodology are applied side by side in order to illustrate and explain the differences between them. It is emphasized that traditional managerial decision-making does not have a proper means to take into account the inevitable process variability, unit interdependency

Figure 11. Patient volume forecasting based on recursive linear prediction model

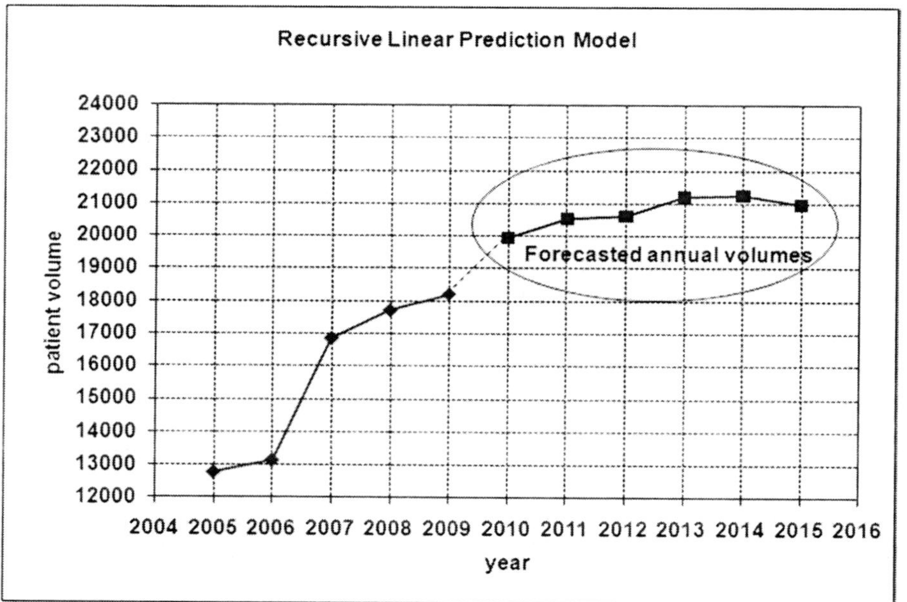

and scaling. Traditional approach is based on past experience, simple linear projections or calculations with the average input values.

In contrast, management engineering methodology reveals the deep hidden interconnections between the elements of a complex system. Management engineering is indispensible in understanding responses of the processes and systems to different inputs with random and non-random variability. This understanding makes it possible, in turn, to predict performance and/or real resource requirements, allowing decision-makers to be proactive rather than reactive.

There is a general human tendency to avoid the complications of incorporating uncertainty in decision-making by ignoring it or turning it into artificial certainty. It is illustrated in this chapter how such a practice often results in misleading conclusions made by traditional management decision-making.

As it is highlighted in a number of publications and illustrated in this chapter, it is imperative for the healthcare management to become familiar with the quantitative decision-making techniques offered by management engineering.

Some fundamental management engineering principles in healthcare settings are summarized below. These principles have been illustrated both by examples presented in this chapter and in examples published elsewhere (Kolker, 2010a). Knowledge and understanding of these fundamental principles alone would help the decision-makers to steer in the right direction even without building detailed complex simulation operational models, or conducting a sophisticating multivariate data analysis.

Summary of Some Fundamental Management Engineering Principles

- Scheduling appointments (jobs) in the order of their increased duration variability (from lower to higher variability) results in a lower overall cycle time and patient waiting time (illustrated in Problem 1)
- Size matters. Larger systems can function at a much higher utilization level and lower

patient wait time than smaller systems with the same patient volume relative to their size-scaling effect (illustrated in Problem 2).

- Because of variability of patient arrivals and service time, a reserved capacity (sometimes up to 30% or more) is usually needed to avoid regular operational problems due to excessive waiting time and long lines (illustrated in Problem 2).
- In a series of dependent activities, only a bottleneck defines the throughput of the entire system. A bottleneck is a resource (or activity) whose capacity is less than or equal to demand placed on it (illustrated in Problem 3).
- An unfulfilled service request backlog (appointments, discharges, document processing, etc) can exist and remain stable even if the high variability average demand is less than service capacity (illustrated in Problem 3).
- For low disease prevalence (less than 30%), pooled screening specimen testing is more efficient than individual specimen testing (illustrated in Problem 10).
- Capacity, staffing and financial estimations based on average input values without taking into account the variability around the averages result in significant underestimation or, sometimes, overestimation of required resources (except for strictly linear relationship between the input and output). This is called the flaw (deception) of averages (illustrated in Problems 1, 2, 5, 6, 9).
- Generally, the higher utilization level of the resource (good for the organization), the longer the waiting time to get this resource (bad for patients). Utilization levels higher than 80% -85% usually result in a significant increase in waiting time for random patient arrivals and random service time (illustrated in Problem 2).
- For systems with a similar type of service, mutually interchangeable (pooled) resources are more efficient in terms of waiting time performance and / or required capacity than specialized (dedicated) resources with the same total capacity/workload (illustrated in Problem 6).
- If specialized (dedicated) resources are needed due to patient privacy, infection control, non-movable equipment or other special factors, then some additional capacity should be planned and budgeted to cover the loss of resources' efficiency. Specialized resources (staff, operating or procedure rooms, beds, etc) typically cost more than mutually interchangeable (pooled) resources (illustrated in Problem 6).
- Workload leveling (smoothing) of elective scheduled procedures is an effective strategy for reducing waiting time and improving patient flow (illustrated in Problem 7).
- Improvement of the separate subsystems (local optimization or local improvement) does not necessarily result in the improvement of the entire system; a system of local improvements (local optimums) could be a very inefficient system (illustrated in Problem 10).
- Analysis of an entire complex system is usually incomplete and can be misleading without taking into account the *subsystems' interdependency* (illustrated in Problem 10).
- Reduction of process variability is the key to patient flow improvement, increasing throughput and reducing delays (illustrated in all dynamic supply and demand balance Problems in this chapter).
- Identifying separate significant independent contributing factors (variables) from a large observational data set that contains the mutually correlated data is not possible. In order to determine the significant

contributing factors, the original data set should be decomposed into the mutually uncorrelated components using principal components methodology or another appropriate advanced multivariate data analysis technique (illustrated in Problem 11).

- In order to generate the forecast of a time series, only the most recent strongly correlated past data-points should be used. The data-points that are weakly correlated to the newer data-points (or not correlated at all) should not be used for making the forecast (illustrated in Problem 12).

Note: Material and views presented in this chapter are developed solely by the author. They do not represent in any way the views of the current author's affiliation, Children's Hospital and Health System, WI, as well as management engineering work performed in this organization.

REFERENCES

Armstrong, W., & Taege, A. (2007). HIV screening for all: The new standard of care. *Cleveland Clinic Journal of Medicine*, *74*(4), 297–301. doi:10.3949/ccjm.74.4.297

Bozzette, S. (2005). Routine screening for HIV infection-timely and cost effective. *The New England Journal of Medicine*, *352*, 620–621. doi:10.1056/NEJMe048347

Butler, T. (1995). Management science/Operations research projects in healthcare: Administrator's perspective. *Health Care Management Review*, *20*(1), 19–25.

Buttell Crane, A. (2007). Management engineers. *Hospitals & Health Networks (H&HN), April*, 50. Retrieved from http://www.hhnmag.com/hhnmag_app/jsp/

Carter, M. (2002). Healthcare management-Diagnosis: Mismanagement of resources. *Operation Research/Management Science (OR/MS). Today*, *29*(2), 26–32.

Cayirli, T., Veral, E., & Rosen, H. (2006). Designing appointment scheduling systems for ambulatory care services. *Health Care Management Science*, *9*, 47–58. doi:10.1007/s10729-006-6279-5

CDC. (2008). HIV prevalence estimates-USA, 2006. *MMWR Weekly*, *57*(39), 1073–1076.

Costa, A., Ridley, S., Shahani, A., Harper, P., De Senna, V., & Nielsen, M. (2003). Mathematical modeling and simulation for planning critical care capacity. *Anesthesia*, *58*, 320–327. doi:10.1046/j.1365-2044.2003.03042.x

De Bruin, A., van Rossum, A., Visser, M., & Koole, G. (2007). Modeling the emergency cardiac inpatient flow: An application of queuing theory. *Health Care Management Science*, *10*, 125–137. doi:10.1007/s10729-007-9009-8

Fabri, P. (2008). Can healthcare engineering fix healthcare? *American Medical Association Journal of Ethics*, *10*(5), 317–319.

Glantz, S., & Slinker, B. (2001). *Applied regression & analysis of variance* (2nd ed.). McGraw-Hill, Inc.

Goldratt, E., & Cox, J. (2004). *The goal* (3rd ed., p. 384). Great Barrington, MA: North River Press.

Green, L. (2006). Queuing analysis in healthcare. In Hall, R. (Ed.), *Patient flow: Reducing delay in healthcare delivery* (pp. 281–307). New York, NY: Springer.

Haraden, C., Nolan, T., & Litvak, E. (2003). *Optimizing patient flow: Moving patients smoothly through acute care setting*. Cambridge, MA: Institute for Healthcare Improvement Innovation.

Institute for Healthcare Improvement (IHI). (2005). *Office practices*. Retrieved from http://www.ihi.org/IHI/Topics/OfficePractices/SpecialtyCareAccess/EmergingContent/Appointment+Sequence+Simulation.htm

Jobson, J. D. (1992). *Applied multivariate data analysis, vol. 2: Categorical and multivariate methods*. New-York, NY: Springer-Verlag, LLC.

Joustra, P., van der Sluis, E., & van Dijk, N. (2010). To pool or not to pool in hospitals: A theoretical and practical comparison for a radiotherapy outpatient department. *Annals of Operations Research, 178*, 77–89. doi:10.1007/s10479-009-0559-7

Klassen, K. J., & Rohleder, T. R. (1996). Scheduling outpatient appointment in a dynamic environment. *Journal of Operations Management, 14*, 83–101. doi:10.1016/0272-6963(95)00044-5

Kolker, A. (2008). Process modeling of emergency department patient flow: Effect of patient length of stay on ED diversion. *Journal of Medical Systems, 32*(5), 389–401. doi:10.1007/s10916-008-9144-x

Kolker, A. (2009). Process modeling of ICU patient flow: Effect of daily load leveling of elective surgeries on ICU diversion. *Journal of Medical Systems, 33*(1), 27–40. Retrieved from http://dx.doi.org/10.1007/s10916-008-9161-9. doi:10.1007/s10916-008-9161-9

Kolker, A. (2010a). Queuing theory and discrete events simulation for healthcare: From basic processes to complex systems with interdependencies. In Abu-Taieh, E., & El Sheik, A. (Eds.), *Handbook of research on discrete event simulation technologies and applications* (pp. 443–483). Hershey, PA: IGI Global.

Kolker, A. (2010b). System engineering and management science for healthcare: Examples and fundamental principles. *Proceedings of the SHS/ASQ Conference and Expo*. Atlanta, GA, February 26, 2010.

Langabeer, J. R. (2007). *Health care operations management* (p. 438). Sudbury, MA: Jones and Bartlett Publishers.

Litvak, E., & Long, M. (2000). Cost and quality under managed care: Irreconcilable difference? *The American Journal of Managed Care, 6*(3), 305–312.

Marshall, A., Vasilakis, C., & El-Darzi, E. (2005). Length of stay-based patient flow models: Recent developments and future directions. *Health Care Management Science, 8*, 213–220. doi:10.1007/s10729-005-2012-z

McManus, M., Long, M., Cooper, A., & Litvak, E. (2004). Queuing theory accurately models the need for critical care resources. *Anesthesiology, 100*(5), 1271–1276. doi:10.1097/00000542-200405000-00032

McManus, M., Long, M., Cooper, A., Mandell, J., Berwick, D., Pagano, M., & Litvak, E. (2003). Variability in surgical caseload and access to intensive care services. *Anesthesiology, 98*(6), 1491–1496. doi:10.1097/00000542-200306000-00029

Motwani, J., Klein, D., & Harowitz, R. (1996). The theory of constraints in services: Part 2-Examples from healthcare. *Managing Service Quality, 6*(2), 30–34. doi:10.1108/09604529610109738

Ozcan, Y. (2009). *Quantitative methods in health care management*, (2nd ed., p. 438). San Francisco, CA: Jossey-Bass, a Wiley imprint.

PHLO. (2008). *Creating and running proactive hospital operations website*. Retrieved from http://phlo.typepad.com/phlo/2008/01/the-worst-thing.html

Press, W., Flannery, B., Teukolsky, S., & Vetterling, W. (1988). *Numerical recipes in C: The art of scientific computing* (p. 735). New York, NY: Cambridge University Press.

Reid, P., Compton, W., Grossman, J., & Fanjiang, G. (Eds.). (2005). *Building a better delivery system: A new engineering / healthcare partnership. National Academy of Engineering and Institute of Medicine*. Washington, DC: The National Academy Press.

Ryckman, F., Yelton, P., Anneken, A., Kissling, P., Schoettker, P., & Kotagal, U. (2009). Redesigning intensive care unit flow using variability management to improve access and safety. *Joint Commission Journal on Quality and Patient Safety, 35*(11), 535–543.

Saraniti, B. (2006). Optimal pooled testing. *Health Care Management Science, 9*, 143–149. doi:10.1007/s10729-006-7662-y

Savage, S. (2009). *The flaw of averages* (p. 392). Hoboken, NJ: John Wiley & Sons, Inc.

Schuster, H. G. (1998). *Deterministic chaos: Introduction*. Weinheim, Germany: Physik Verlag.

Story, P. (2009). *Are we thinking systems yet?* American Society for Quality (ASQ), January, 2009. Retrieved from http://www.asq.org/pdf/healthcare/are-we-thinking-systems-yet.pdf

Teow, K. L. (2009). Practical operations research applications for healthcare managers. *Annals of the Academy of Medicine, Singapore, 38*(6), 564–566.

Wullink, G., Van Houdenhoven, M., Hans, E., van Oostrum, J., van der Lans, M., & Kazemier, G. (2007). Closing emergency operating rooms improves efficiency. *Journal of Medical Systems, 31*, 543–546. doi:10.1007/s10916-007-9096-6

KEY TERMS AND DEFINITIONS

Complex System: A system that exhibits a mutual interdependency of components and for which a change in the input parameter(s) can result in a non-proportional large or small change of the system output.

Discrete Event Simulation: One of the most powerful methodologies of using computer models of the real systems to analyze their performance by tracking system changes (events) at discrete moments of time.

Flow Bottleneck / Constraint: A resource (material or human) whose capacity is less than or equal to demand for its use.

Management Science: A quantitative methodology for assigning (managing) available material assets and human resources to achieve the operational goals of the system. Based on Operations research.

Operations Research: The discipline of applying mathematical models of complex systems with random variability aimed at developing justified operational business decisions.

Principal Component Methodology: A methodology that allows one to perform a multivariate correlation analysis and identifies redundant original variables that carry little or no information while retaining only a few mutually uncorrelated new variables. These new variables called principal components; they are linear combinations of the original variables.

Queuing Theory: Mathematical methods for analyzing the properties of waiting lines (queues) in simple systems without interdependency. Typically uses analytic formulas that must meet some rather stringent assumptions to be valid.

Simulation Package: Also known as a simulation environment. A software with user interface used for building and processing discrete event simulation models.

APPENDIX A

What is a simulation model and how does a simple discrete event simulation model work?

A discrete event simulation model (DES) model is a computer model that mimics the dynamic behavior of a real process as it evolves with time in order to visualize and quantitatively analyze its performance. The validated and verified model is then used to study behavior of the original process and its response to input variables in order to identify ways for its improvement (scenarios) based on some improvement criteria. This strategy is significantly different from the hypothesis-based testing widely used in medical research (Kopach-Konrad et al, 2007).

DES models track entities moving through the system at distinct points of time (events). The detailed track is recorded for all processing times and waiting times. Then the system's statistics for entities and activities are gathered.

To illustrate how a DES model works step by step, let's consider a very simple system that consists of a single patient arrival line and a single server. Suppose that patient inter-arrival time is uniformly (equally likely) distributed between 1 min and 3 min. Service time is exponentially distributed with the average 2.5 min. (Of course, any statistical distributions or non-random patterns can be used instead). A few random numbers sampled from these two distributions are, for example see Table 13.

Let's start our example simulation at time zero, t=0, with no patients in the system. We will be tracking any change or event that happened in the system.

A summary of what is happening in the system looks like Table 14.

These simple but tedious logical and numerical event-tracking operations (algorithm) are suitable, of course, only for a computer. However, they illustrate the basic principles of a typical discrete events simulation model, in which discrete events (changes) in the system are tracked when they occur over the time. In this particular example, we were tracking events at discrete points in time t=2.6, 4.0, 4.8, 6.2, 8.6, 13.6, 22.7.

Once the simulation is completed for any length of time, another set of random numbers from the same distributions is generated, and the procedure (called replication) is repeated. Usually multiple replications are needed to properly capture the system's variability. In the end, the system's output statistics is

Table 13.

Inter-arrival time, min	Service time, min
2.6	1.4
2.2	8.8
1.4	9.1
2.4	1.8

Table 14.

Event #	Time	Event that happened in the system
1	2.6	First customer arrives. Service starts that should end at time = 4.
2	4	Service ends. Server waits for patient.
3	4.8	Second patient arrives. Service starts that should end at time = 13.6. Server idles 0.8 minutes.
4	6.2	Third patient arrives. Joins the queue waiting for service.
5	8.6	Fourth patient arrives. Joins the queue waiting for service.
6	13.6	Second patient (from event 3) service ends. Third patient at the head of the queue (first in, first out) starts service that should end at time 22.7.
7	22.7	Patient #4 starts service…and so on.

calculated, e.g. the average patient and server waiting time, its standard deviation, the average number of patients in the queue, the confidence intervals and so on.

In this example, only two patients out of four waited in the queue. Patient 3 waited 13.6-6.2=7.4 min and patient 4 waited 22.7-8.6=14.1 min, so the simple average waiting time for all four patients is (0+0+7.4+14.1)/4=5.4 min. Notice, however, that the first two patients did not wait at all while patient 4 waited 2.6 times longer than the average. This illustrates that the simple average could be rather misleading as a performance metric for highly variable processes without some additional information about the spread of data around the average.

Similarly, the simple arithmetic average of the number of waiting patients (average queue length) is 0.5. However, a more informative metric of the queue length is the time-weighted average that takes into account the length of time each patient was in the queue. In this case it is (1*7.4+1*14.1)/22.7=0.95. The time-weighted average is often a better system performance metric than the simple average.

DES models are capable of tracking hundreds of individual entities, each with its own unique attributes, enabling one to simulate the most complex systems with interacting events and component interdependencies.

Typical DES applications include: staff and production scheduling, capacity planning, cycle time and cost reduction, throughput capability, resources and activities utilization, bottleneck finding and analysis. DES is the most effective tool to perform quantitative 'what-if' analysis and play different scenarios of the process behavior as its parameters change with time. This simulation capability allows one to make experiments on the computer, and to test different options before going to the hospital floor for actual implementation.

The basic elements (building blocks) of a simulation model are:

- Flow chart of the process, i.e. a diagram that depicts logical flow of a process from its inception to its completion
- Entities, i.e. items to be processed, e.g. patients, documents, customers, etc.

- Activities, i.e. tasks performed on entities, e.g. medical procedures, exams, document approval, customer check-in, etc
- Resources, i.e. agents used to perform activities and move entities, e.g. service personnel, equipment, nurses, physicians
- Entity routings that define directions and logical conditions flow for entities

Typical information usually required to populate the model includes:

- Quantity of entities and their arrival time, e.g. periodic, random, scheduled, daily pattern, etc. There is no restriction on the arrival distribution type.
- The time that the entities spend in the activities, i.e. service time. This is usually not a fixed time but a statistical distribution. There is no restriction on the distribution type.
- Capacity of each activity, i.e. the max number of entities that can be processed concurrently in the activity
- The maximum size of input and output queues for the activities
- Resource assignments: their quantity and scheduled shifts

APPENDIX B

Summary of some mathematical methods used for the various management engineering applications

- Data Envelopment Analysis-to compare relative efficiency of units/organizations
- Graph theory-for facilities layout, location, ambulance routings
- Linear programming-optimization of linear systems subject to a linear set of constraints
- Non-linear optimization problem (optimization function and/or constraints are non-linear)
- Mixed/Integer programming- some or all decision variables are only integer numbers
- Stochastic programming (linear, integer, mixed/integer, nonlinear with random input variables)
- Just-in time (dynamic pull system- based on actual usage)
- Materials requirement planning and inventory control–optimal Order Quantity
- Network analysis (critical path -for total duration of interrelated activities)
- Theory of Constraints: the concept of a bottleneck in a series of interdependent events (activities) – illustrated in this chapter (Problem 8)
- Decision trees (probabilistic analysis of different options)
- Forecasting a time series (linear and/or non-linear), as well as recursive forecasting technique-illustrated in this chapter (Problem 12)
- Markov processes (chains)
- Sampling Quality control
- Monte-Carlo Simulation (static probabilistic analysis)
- Queuing analytic theory
- Discrete Event Simulation modeling - illustrated in multiple examples in this chapter (Problems 1 - 9)
- Regression analysis with principal components for multiple mutually correlated factors- illustrated in this chapter (Problem 11)

Chapter 2
Dynamic Capacity Management (DCAMM™) in a Hospital Setting

Pierce Story
GE Healthcare, USA

ABSTRACT

"Hospitals are dynamic systems and must be analyzed and managed as such. Therefore, we need dynamic analytical tools and thinking to fix hospitals' most pressing issues" (Story, 2010).

This is the premise of the chapter on Dynamic Capacity Management (DCAMM). In the near future, healthcare providers will be expected to achieve even better results with reduced compensation, fewer resources, lower capital expenditures, even stricter regulations and restrictions, and more litigation. This means that there must be a radical operational transformation away from the traditional, static management and improvement methodologies towards a dynamic, high-capacity approach. DCAMM is an analytical methodology and (non-proprietary) toolset that is meant to profoundly change the way hospitals are managed.

DCAMM starts with an analysis of dynamic demand, matched against dynamic capacity. This brings forth simple yet important operational concepts that take a dynamic, "systems" level view of the entire care structure (e.g. a hospital or a community). Using specially designed simulation models and the power of predictive analytics, we can achieve a very different perspective on the variability and interdependencies that were once considered chaos. By "managing to" the variation, and understanding and predicting the dynamism of the system, concepts such as "Dynamic Standardization" and "Outlier Management" can augment the existing, static process improvement systems such as Lean and Six Sigma. This chapter will provide an overview of the concepts and structures necessary to profoundly change the way our hospitals, and health systems, are managed.

DOI: 10.4018/978-1-60960-872-9.ch002

INTRODUCTION

As I outline in my recently published book, Dynamic Capacity Management for Healthcare: Advanced Methods and Tools for Optimization, (Story, 2010) healthcare is a dynamic environment in which to work, changing every hour of every day in a seemingly constant state of flux. Short of a battlefield, few environments are as dynamic and complex as healthcare. The processes required to take thousands of these unique patients from sick and diseased to cured or improved are perhaps as complex as any, with care provision specialized for each patient with the individuality of a snowflake. Thus our systems are known more for their complexity and chaos than their standardization and regimen. Our nurses, doctors, and administrators are therefore correct to claim that healthcare is indeed different from other industries.

But because we are caring for fellow human beings, with lives and loves and livelihoods at stake, our systems are expected to yield results that are nothing short of perfection. Though they may not be designed to achieve the desired results, patients, insurers, and regulators expect our systems to function flawlessly and inexpensively. Cost controls therefore cannot dictate lowered quality standards or become excuses for errors. Product recalls don't apply here, and well-heeled, greed-inspired lawyers await every mistake.

Furthermore, in the future, healthcare providers will be expected to achieve even better results with reduced compensation, fewer resources, lower capital expenditures, stricter regulations and restrictions, and more litigation. As U.S. "healthcare reform" (a.k.a. "Obamacare") is slowly implemented, the financial struggles ahead for healthcare provision have never looked more troubling. This means that efficiency and performance optimization will be of even greater importance as we try to perfect the processes of the care we provide within the constraints of reduced or existing capacity, higher per-patient costs, and reduced compensation. The provision of services must yield high quality and optimal clinical outcomes yet be provided at the lowest possible cost. Therefore, improving the efficiency of the complex and dynamic operations of care delivery may be one of the best ways to ensure the survival of our facilities.

It's Up to Us

Read the following three quotes, and see if they sound familiar:

"We need legislation which reorganizes the system to guarantee a sufficient volume of high quality medical care, distributed equitably across the country and available at reasonable cost to every American. It is going to take a drastic overhaul of our entire way of doing business in the health-care field in order to solve the financing and organizational aspects of our health crisis. One aspect of that solution is the creation of comprehensive systems of health-care delivery".

"I think that this new system will be successful and give us exciting and constructive alternatives to our existing programs of delivering better health services to Americans."[1]

"I have strongly advocated passage of legislation to assist the development of [these concepts] as a viable and competitive alternative to fee-for-service practice.... This bill represents the first initiative by the Federal Government which attempts to come to grips directly with the problems of fragmentation and disorganization in the health care industry.... I believe that [this approach] is the best idea put forth so far for containing costs and improving the organization and the delivery of health-care services."[2]

The year was 1973. The speakers were [the late] Sen. Ted Kennedy, (D-MA), and Rep. Harley Staggers (D-WV). The subject...HMOs! The similarities between this sort of language and that of the recent "healthcare reform" discussion are eerie, at best. Clearly, over the years, government has done little to improve the delivery of healthcare through its mandates and "clever" solutions. Indeed, one could argue that the Federal Government created the HMO, instigated and promoted the fee-for-service business model, and the gives ongoing support to the employer-based private insurance industry, all of which have done tremendous disservice to the provision of care.

Therefore, with Healthcare Reform on the books with no chance of repeal, it will be up to the healthcare industry, and specifically healthcare providers, to "save the system" and prevent it from burdening the U.S. economy with costs to great to bear.

A Child of Our Own

Given the dynamic world of the provision of healthcare and the inherent uniqueness of our operations and processes, it is ironic that we haven't developed our own performance and process improvement (PPI) methodologies. We tend to try to improve healthcare systems with tools and methodologies adopted from other, very different and less dynamic industries. Throughout the last twenty years, we have seen various and sundry manufacturing performance and process improvement methodologies become the "play of the day" or the "flavor of the month". We commonly adopt the latest improvement concepts without enough customization to the unique environs of care delivery, resulting in frustration and reduced impact. We might tweak them, or "blend" several concepts together, so as to force relatively "static" methodologies to fit into our dynamic systems.

Some of these methodologies can and have worked well, bringing with them new thinking and perspectives which have allowed healthcare systems to experience dramatic improvements. Often, however, they fail in the face of healthcare's ever-dynamic complexities. Too much simply doesn't apply well to healthcare to allow for the achievement of the desired, dramatic, and sustainable results. As when learning to speak an alien language, much can be lost in the translation between one environment or industry and another, leaving us constantly groping for the "next big thing". This is a testament to the need for better applicability.

The history of healthcare PPI is thus replete with great leaps forward, frustrating setbacks and wasted effort, and far too much stasis. While we can and should learn from the improvement efforts, tools, and methodologies of other, less dynamic industries, we should expect that our unique environment requires us to create our own PPI systems. In fact, since our world is so much different…

We Need Tools and Methodologies Which Won't Apply at all to the World of Manufacturing!

That, essentially, is the premise and the reason behind this chapter. Herein, I would like to shed some light on the nuances and uniqueness of healthcare operations, challenge the current thinking about healthcare performance improvement, and offer some new ways to think about the management of hospitals and healthcare systems. With these new concepts added to other methodologies, philosophies, and tools, I hope we can profoundly change with way hospitals are managed!

DCAMM: Dynamic Capacity Analysis, Matching, and Management: Concept Overview

The purpose of this chapter is to bring forward some new thinking and analysis to persistent and consistent issues in healthcare PPI, specifically within hospitals[3]. The essentials are summed up in the following paragraphs:

Our systems are dynamic. Variable demand comes to us from our communities through various entry points, and changes every hour of every day. This demand is met with our variable service capacity, which also changes through the day, week, and season. Because these elements are ever-changing, our environments are inherently difficult to manage since "dynamically matching dynamic demand with dynamic capacity" can be quite problematic. Thus, while we may improve individual departments, we may not have improved the system as a whole. We need to develop something more like a Swiss watch, with dynamically interconnected components, rather than a box of individually optimized gears.

Our most common analytical tools and our use of "averages" to represent the performance of our systems fail us, often terribly. In fact, averages can deceive us because they fail to capture the real variability and dynamics of the systems. Instead, averages can yield incorrect conclusions and misguided solutions. The "dynamism" (defined herein as the combination of the inherent variability and interdependencies in our complex systems) in the "demand-capacity continuum" is simply too complicated to be effectively represented by averages. Thus, it begs for better analytics by which we can better understand our complex systems, proactively manage them, and better care for our patients. Fortunately, at least some of the system's variability has patterns by which we can discern current and future behavior. Indeed, in many instances, some 80%-90% of the variability (and its related dynamism) occurs within relatively tight ranges around our commonly-used-yet-misleading averages. It can therefore be more accurately patterned and thus more thoroughly understood if we use the right analytical tools.

These patterns offer us the realization that our systems are not as random and chaotic as we might think. More importantly, the patterns are the key to "predictive analytics" by which we can predict our system's behavior by hour-of-day, day-of-week, week-of-month, and season-of-year. These patterns, when and where they exist, offer us the means by which to study our systems within the context of their inherent dynamism. This in turn lets us *manage to* the ever-changing environment, rather than being managed by it.

This leads us to new ways to understand and better manage the capacity we make available for our communities…herein known as Dynamic Capacity Management. As we see the demand-capacity continuum and its impact on performance, we begin to see how we can influence the up- and downstream demand patterns in the system so as to have a truly systemic impact. Through new analytical concepts, we can now understand that some of our processes need to become "dynamically standard", flexing as needed to the dynamism of the system performance. This "dynamic standardization" helps us to cope better and even control some of the processes and systems that we heretofore considered unmanageable. We also come to the realization that the patternable dynamism…that 80%-90% of the dynamism that commonly occurs…can and should be dealt with as commonplace, standard, and "in-range". This in-range variability, represented by the 80%-90% of the conditions in the patterns, does and will occur in a high number of instances and thus must be managed well in order to manage the system optimally. The remaining, relatively small percentage are the truly random and unpredictable events which drive the systems over the edge and cause breakdowns. These are our nearly inevitable "outliers". They are the reason that averages so deceive us and are so unreliable as metrics.

At certain points, the system may tip into an "outlier status"…circumstances and conditions which are among the more rare and unusual, but which are relatively unpredictable and cause great impacts on the system's overall performance. The points at which the system leaves its standard range and moves into outlier status are the system's "break points". Break points must therefore be recognized and their causality predicted, so as to help us discern and predict when the in-range performance can no longer be expected, and when perhaps some change to the standardized processes needs to occur.

Using a combination of tools, new ways of thinking, and existing process improvement methodologies, outliers must and can be dealt with as the unique events that they are… as outliers. Our thinking must change from managing every day *as if* it's an outlier to managing "outliers as outliers". Since it is the outliers which cause us the most pain and suffering, and since the "in-range" metrics can be predicted relatively well, we should focus on the former and not the latter. This becomes a new way of thinking about the management of dynamic systems, known as "outlier management", and should be the locus of our tactical and strategic analytical and managerial efforts. Thus we move from reacting to static averages towards dynamically and proactively managing the dynamic demand-capacity continuum based on a better and more realistic understanding of the system's actual dynamic performance. Therefore, we can indeed create the "Swiss-watch" of interdependent components, rather than relying on a more randomized proper alignment of demand and capacity.

This is the heart of DCAMM: Dynamic Capacity Analysis, Matching, and Management.

In order to proceed through this chapter, we will need to define some specific terms (some of which will be elaborated on later). Here are some definitions of a few of the concepts above which we'll be discussing in the coming pages:

- **DCAMM:** Dynamic Capacity Analysis, Matching, and Management. The proactive, predictive management of dynamic capacity to meet, with the precision possible, the dynamic demand of the communities we serve.
- **Service Capacity.** The sum of the ability to meet some level of demand for a given service. In this text, "capacity" will be synonymous with service capacity.
- **Variability.** The range of performance measurements, values, or outcomes around the average which represents all the possible results of a given process, function, or operation.
- **Interdependencies.** The causal impact of one process or operation on another within a given process flow or system.
- **Interdependency.** Those links between one system component and another which result in some sort of impact(s) on either, both, or other components of the system. Or, stated another way, the causal impact of one process or operation on another within a given process flow or system.
- **Dynamism:** The product and state of a system's performance capabilities resulting from the combination of process variability and system interdependencies.
- **In-range.** A range of performance measurements, values, or outcomes of a given process, function, or operation which falls within a specified degree of commonality or rate of occurrence. The range may vary, depending on the degree of variability of the system in question. Commonly, it is the 80%-90% of all occurrences.
- **Outlier.** A performance measurement, value, or outcome of a given process, function, or operation which falls outside a specified degree of commonality or rate of occurrence.
- **Break-Point.** A condition or set of conditions which result in the performance measurements, values, or outcomes varying outside a given range of expectations, (a.k.a. "in-range" performance). Break-points occur as performance gives way to outlier status. The consistent presence of a break-point and an outlier can indicate the evolution of the system.
- **Evolution.** In this text, evolution will refer to the changes within and/or to the system which take a performance measurement, value, or outcome of a given process, function, or operation from an outlier to some new standard and expected level of occur-

rence, or vice versa. Systems evolve as the outliers become in-range metrics, or in-range metrics become outliers.

- **Dynamic Standardization.** The use of a variety of standardized processes or operations for the same given function to achieve a specific performance standard for that function.
- **Predictive Analytics.** The use of data, modeling, and an understanding of a system's dynamic behavior to predict future performance based on current performance or a hypothetical combination of input variables.
- **"What-If?" Scenario.** The construction of a hypothetical situation created from the combination of system input variables so as to generate an understanding of the expected performance measurements, values, or outcomes of a given process, function, or operation in that situation. Used with a variety of simulation and other analytical tools.

Lean, Static Analytical Tools and DCAMM

It is worthwhile to stop here to discuss the differences between dynamic analytical tools as we will purport herein and the common, static performance improvement systems such as Lean. This chapter is not meant to deride or criticize the more commonly used methodologies and philosophies, including Lean, Six Sigma, LSS, TOC, TQM, etc. Indeed, we strongly support the use of waste reduction, variability reduction, workflow standardization, throughput mapping, and other tenets of these systems. However, because the nature of many of the analyses and tools of common performance improvement methodologies are "static", they are of inherently limited value in analyzing and improving complex, dynamic systems such as healthcare. This is due to the inherent need to use averages or similar analytical benchmarks, which is in turn due to the inability to effectively account for the variability and its inherently impact on interdependencies within complex systems. Unable to account for these dynamically, Lean and the others commonly use at worse an average, and at best some static visual or statistical representation of variance. This leads to the inability to effectively replicate dynamic systems and account for the impacts of outliers in and on outcomes, and the resulting failure to precisely quantify the impacts of future change, system evolution, and general ongoing dynamism. Indeed, dynamic analytical tools such as simulation were developed specifically to analyze and predict the future performance of altered dynamic and complex systems.

This does not, however, mean that the common though static analytical methodologies such as Lean are either worthless or incompatible with more dynamic analytical tools and methodologies. As mentioned previously, these could and perhaps should be blended together for a more holistic approach to solutions development. Lean, having been in use for many years across many industries, requires less technical training and software programming techniques than do tools such as simulation. However, the tenets and concepts that make Lean a valuable though static analytical methodology and philosophy offer benefits when those same tenets and concepts are applied using dynamic analytics. Furthermore, performance improvement is not all about "the numbers". "Soft" changes, as are brought about through visual cues, tidier workplaces, work involvement in change decisions, and statistical representation of variances are all highly valuable in the journey towards optimization of system performance. Yet, these latter changes are not readily analyzed using dynamic analytics, begging the need for a truly holistic approach that involved "hands on" changes to culture, workspace, and worker perspectives as well as a more precise and accurate analysis of the systems' dynamic performance capabilities. The blending of the "static" and the "dynamic" is required if complex systems are to be truly optimized, which will demand the blending of multiple tools, approaches, philosophies, and methodologies.

For instance, such tools as Value Stream Maps (VSMs) are greatly enhanced when "made dynamic " and brought to life by simulation technologies. According to Aiken, "Basic lean tools, including Value Stream mapping are fine for analyzing simple, linear processes with relatively consistent demand patterns. [However], static approaches are less appropriate for analyzing processes which incorporate [elements such as] volatile demand dynamics, product mix complexity or the shared use of specialist resources (machines or labor). Where such [complexities are present], a Process Simulation model can more accurately describe and visually explain the dynamics of the process, its performance and resource requirements and show what the main drivers for end-to-end process performance are." (Aiken, 2008).

Furthermore, writes Woehrle, et. al., "The fusion of simulation with VSM has countered the limitations of traditional VSM. McDonald et al (2002), and separately, Lian and Van Landeghem (2002), showed in their case studies that discrete event simulation can provide important information for implementing [solutions] in complex production systems (Braglia et al.,2006). This way, the limitation of using traditional VSM for complex systems is eliminated by integrating simulation with VSM." (Woerhle, Abu-Shady, 2010). Additionally, "simulation also supports the reduction of uncertainty and the creation of shared consensus about the process since it helps visualize the process dynamic views of given future states before implementation." (Woerhle, Abu-Shady, 2010). Narasimhan et al. (2007) also support the use of Lean in analysis and consensus-building, demonstrating that the dynamic analytics of simulation helps to increase confidence in solutions sought, specifically in the application of lean solutions. Detty and Yingling (2000) point out that simulation can help in the adaptation of adopt lean by quantifying the expected outcomes, a common use of dynamic simulation tools. Furthermore, Detty and Yingling state that discrete event simulation, combined with Value Stream Maps, can help quantify the expected benefits of changes created by lean manufacturing systems before changes are actually made. (Detty and Yingling, 2000). As is common in dynamic analytics such as discrete-event simulation, this can allow for the precise analysis of cost versus benefits, long- and short-term issues and concerns, unforeseen problems, and future constraints to system performance. Importantly, "the information generated from the [discrete event simulation] can be used as a benchmark to measure the effectiveness of implementing the lean changes" (Detty and Yingling, 2000).

Thus, the blending of methodologies to include dynamic analytics of the complex interdependencies, variability, evolution, and outliers is required if we are to truly solve for the difficulties facing healthcare delivery.

DCAMM, Variability, and Patterning

Variability can have a tremendous impact on human process. It is also a key culprit in driving down productivity, throughput, and efficiency. Consider how long it takes you to do a reasonably lengthy task, such as going to the store, getting a cup of coffee from your office pantry, or walking your dog. Then consider how much variability there is between each iteration of these tasks. Consider even simple tasks, such as writing an email or folding a load of laundry. These, too, can take differing amounts of time. The variance in the time it takes you to do a task can have a significant impact on the other tasks you have to do during your day. For instance, encountering traffic while going to the store could cause you to miss a favorite television show. Nearly all human process has some degree of variability. That variability can have a significant impact on the many other tasks we perform in a given day or

Figure 1. Variability in a process time or arrival pattern

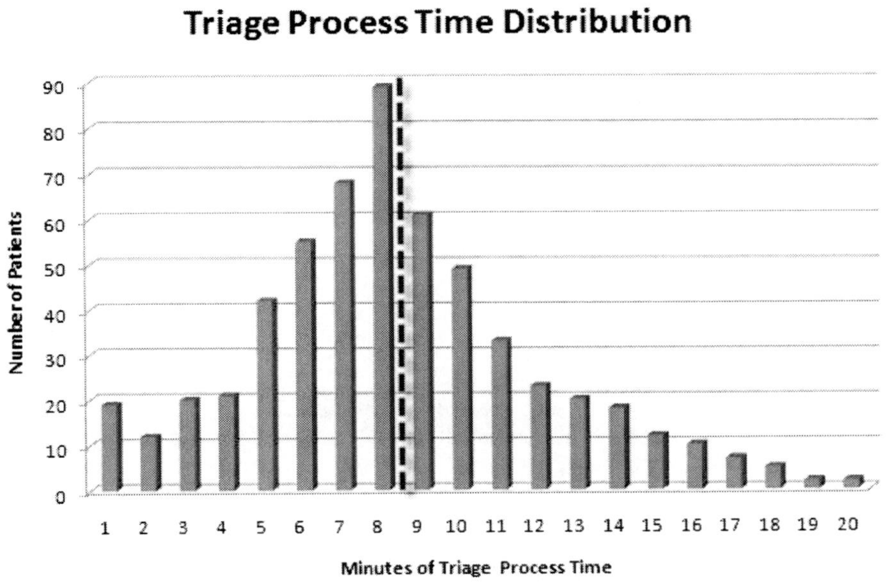

Triage Process Time Distribution

Number of Patients

0 10 20 30 40 50 60 70 80 90

1 2 3 4 5 6 7 8 9 10 11 12 13 14 15 16 17 18 19 20

Minutes of Triage Process Time

week, as well as tasks performed by those with whom we interact.

Variability has this inevitable deleterious impact on system performance, throughput, and capacity because the system often doesn't "catch up" when a given process takes longer than its average. The system is thereby inevitably slowed. This builds up over time, and ultimately reduces system performance. This is why the average is a dangerous metric. The average only gives a single "snapshot" of the system's performance, but doesn't tell us anything about the performance variance, or how often and to what degree the system may perform differently.

Fortunately, variability does not equate to randomness. Variability commonly comes within definable "ranges" around the commonly used average. It is this range around the average which is so critical to understanding system performance, since the ranges form distinct patterns. These patterns can be detected, and more importantly predicted, such that we can predict the variability in our systems rather than merely predicting a relatively useless average. The range is therefore a far more telling piece of information, though it is also more difficult to obtain and relate (See Figure 1).

Imagine trying to predict the volume in your ED tomorrow. Let' assume the average is 127 patients. Would you be able to accurately predict the exact number of arrivals? Unlikely. However, if you knew that 85% of the time, the range of arrivals was between 105 and 148, would you feel comfortable making a prediction about the range? Of course! Indeed, we don't need to know the exact numbers, unless we could consistently expect it. Since we cannot rely on a consistent single number, it is better to know the range and the degree of "in range" variance, since this will tell us more about what we should expect to see from day to day, how to plan everything from staffing to workload and workflow, and when we have a truly unusual day. Ranges are made predictable based on historical data, and become more relevant as we slice our data by day of week (DOW) and hour of day (HOD). While growth

Figure 2. Averages and the patterns of ranges of demand

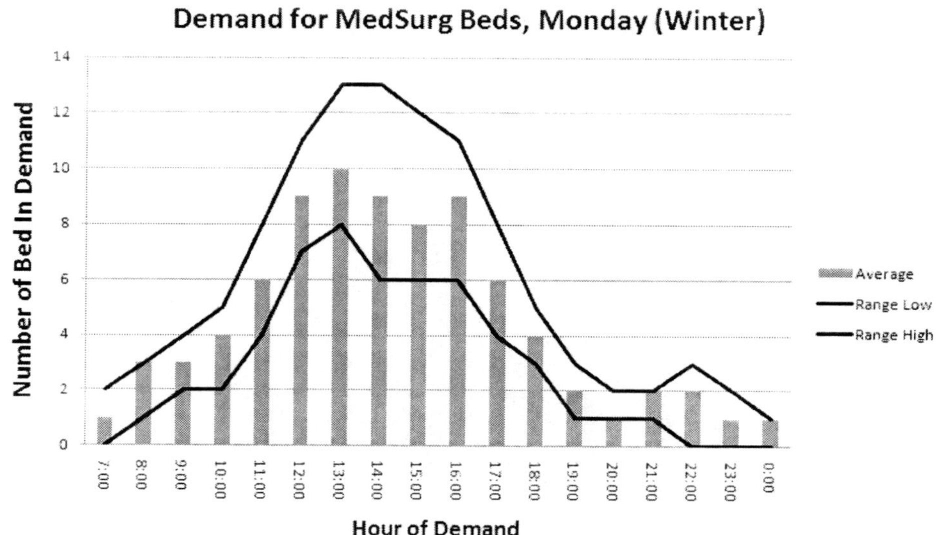

and demographics change the numbers as years go by, there are nonetheless surprisingly accurate patterns trends which we can glean from historical data (See Figure 2).

Ironically, most department managers know little if anything about the common range of demand for their departments. They are often too concerned about far less-important average metrics, which they can usually quote from memory.

These ranges give us the opportunity to understand how our systems perform most of the time. Without needing precise numbers, we can plan for the variability if it confidently known. If we can detect the patterns, we can more accurately predict them and therefore plan for their occurrence. This allows us to use tools such as discrete-event simulation (DES) to predict the precise outcomes of specific points within the range, and therefore predict how we need to react to each one. To the extent necessary, we can alter processes, staffing, task allocations, etc., to better be able to manage specific points within the range, knowing the likelihood of their occurrence.

Of course, there may be "outliers" which go beyond the typical range of performance. In healthcare, these are almost inevitable, though largely unpredictable. Because our systems are so highly variable, the common ranges rarely hold forever, if for no other reason than market growth and demographic trends.

In a hospital setting, this might be a "bus crash day" in the ED, when volumes spike to unusually levels, or, on the other end of the spectrum, unexpectedly drop to a very low level. This might also occur when the acuity on the inpatient units spikes and causes extended LOS. Outliers, by their definition and nature, cannot be accurately predicted, though their impacts on the rest of the system can. Indeed, these outliers commonly cause the system to feel "out of control". But, they should always be understood within the context of their relationship to the more common and predictable ranges. Outliers must be dealt with for what they are…unique events that create occasional havoc. Since they can do such damage to our performance, we need to develop specific remedies to help us define outliers, understand their impact, and manage them for what they are. Indeed, if the rest of the system can be relatively easily predicted, based on the typical [historic] range of performance, and if the outliers are what actually makes they system less manageable, our focus should be on managing the outliers if and when they occur. This will allow us to better manage the overall system performance by focusing on those scenarios and situations in which the system would normally be more chaotic and cause the system to perform poorly. If we can use "outlier management" to detect and manage unique outlier scenarios, the rest of the system will be allowed to perform more smoothly within its more typical performance ranges. Controlling the outliers can help us control the entire system, since they are what cause the system to become more chaotic.

Examples of the Use of Patterns and Outlier Management

A simple example of the use of these concepts occurred at a mid-sized community hospital near St. Louis, MO. The hospital suffered from poor ED throughput, high ED service wait-times, and off-benchmark LWOT (left without treatment) metrics. Before the ED Manager set about the task of improving operations, she decided to first analyze the demand patterns coming from her community. At first glance, the variance in arrivals was stunning, from the mid 70's per day to over 130. However, as she broke down the patterns into DOW and hours of day, she began to see week-to-week patterns in the daily volumes. The ranges tighten substantially, and offered her the ability to analyze her system within the context of daily variance rather than total variance.

She set about to plan resource and task allocations according the ranges she saw by DOW. She employed the used of DES to accurately predict the outcomes of the specific volumes within her ranges, and determined if, where, when, and by how much she needed to change processes, staffing, and task allocations. On specific days of week, she saw that the high end of the common ranges of demand overloaded her system and caused significant back-ups in throughput, higher LOS, and higher wait-times. She realized, through statistical analysis provided by a consultant, that the top 20% of the common range caused issues. Therefore, she developed remediation strategies which called for special process changes as the arrival patterns on certain days (Tuesdays through Fridays) exceeded a specific point (95).

After that "break point", she deployed specific resources to the front-end of the ED to process low-acuity patients, even though this strategy was financially unfeasible if consistently applied. She was willing to accept the higher cost to improve the throughput and maintain performance standards, since the likelihood of a 95+ arrivals day was relatively low (since it was at the high end of the common range). Remedies included a moving a Physician to the triage area when arrivals hit certain specific quantities on certain days (she called them "alarms").

Interdependencies of Hospital-Wide Systems and Flow

Examine Figure 3.

This image is a relatively simple but effective visual aid to describe the complex interdependencies of hospital-wide flow, resource allocations, and capacity requirements. It is important to remember that each component, (e.g., the ED, Surgical Services), all contain variability in their arrival patterns, performance, and capacity. The demand from the community is, of course, variable, depending on seasons, days of week, and other external variables. This combination of variable demand and variable capacity is, of course, what makes the healthcare systems more difficult to improve and maintain.

A good example of the use of DCAMM analysis is in redesigning an OR schedule. Let's use an example of a hospital with eight (8) current surgical suites, which will add three additional suites, and furthermore increase the utilization of the existing capacity. Commonly, this would be done in relative isolation, with the Surgical

Figure 3. The complex interdependencies of the hospital-wide demand-capacity continuum

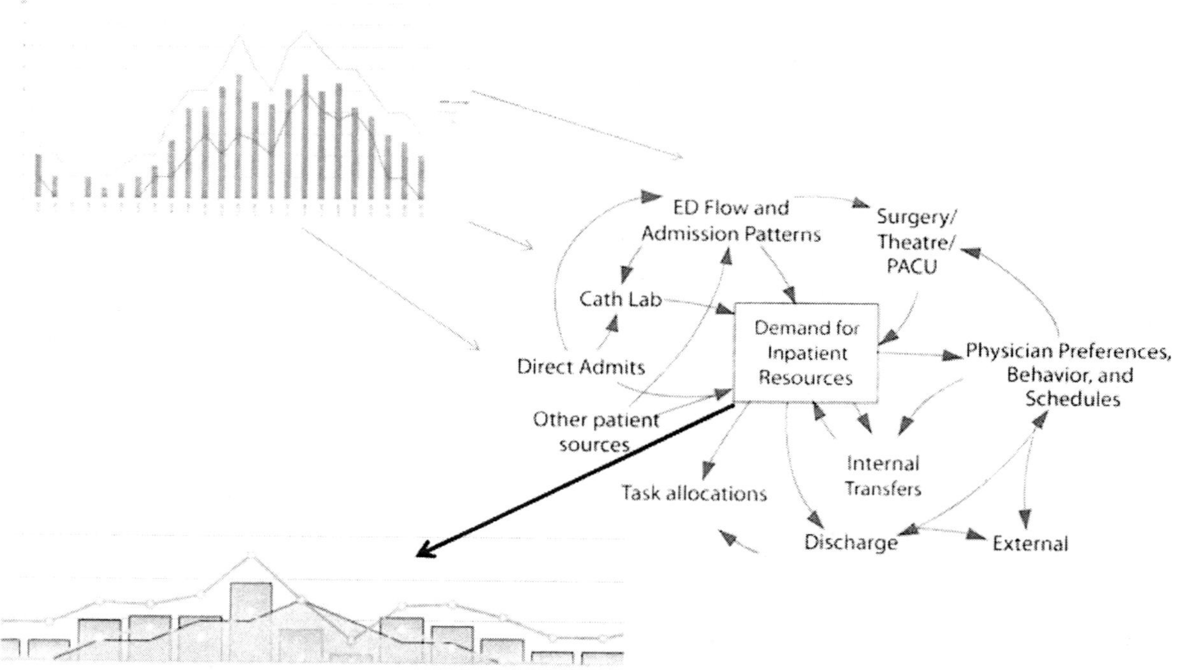

Services management team creating the new block schedule in conjunction with Physicians and their preferences for case times. New cases would be added, with the current block schedule redesigned to allow for accommodation of the additional capacity and increased utilization of allocated block time.[4] However, rarely are the complexities of the "downstream" demand patterns or the other areas of inpatient and/or resource demand accounted for. Therefore, bottlenecks and constraints can be created from what was supposed to be a means by which to increase system capacity.

A simple examination of the Figure 3 offers us some insights into what is required for these sorts of changes to be optimally effective. First, we must discern the new demand patterns for inpatient resources based on the new surgical schedule. We should do this recognizing the variability in case time for each Physician, case type, and PACU LOS. (Even without accounting for the variability in case time and PACU LOS, we can at least have a reasonable understanding of the new capacity which will be required to accommodate the new demand patterns). We should do this by hour of day (HOD) and day of week (DOW), so as to capture the changes that take place from day to day.

In the case of this sample hospital, the goal was to add a new group of Orthopedists to create an Orthopedic Center of Excellence. The new ORs would allow for the new Physician group to maximize their potential case load, while also allowing the expansion of other case types through an optimization of utilization of the entire facility. So, we would need to analyze the case types, how they fit into the schedule, and the downstream resource requirements for each case, by HOD and DOW. (In this instance, the pre-operative resource and sterile processing availability and utilization is assumed to be adequate, though certainly this is not always the case. Efficiencies here can mean impacting on-time starts, proper materials and supply management, and intra-case delays). This analysis would take the typical variability (with or without any outliers, depending on their frequency and severity) of the length of each case type, by Physician, to determine the appropriate placement in a block schedule. Even if the schedule is normally managed by blocks rather than individual cases, we will still need to initially assess the downstream demands so as to properly set up the schedule for the future. Using simulation models, or other tools if these are not available, cases can be analyzed within various configurations of blocks, so as to study how to optimize the capacity of the available suites. This work will be iterative, since optimizing for Surgical Services must be done within the context of the rest of the hospital's demand and capacity, so as to optimize total system capacity. Thus, before settling on a new case/block schedule, we should first look downstream. The block schedule should never be created in isolation, but rather through its inclusion in the grander scheme of total system capacity.

Next, we combine these new surgically-based hourly and daily demand patterns with those from the other "feeder" departments, such as ED, Cath Lab, Direct Admissions, etc. We will want to look within the total demand pattern for potential conflicts wherein the inpatient resources might become overloaded by concurrent admissions, discharges, and workloads. This will also help us gauge where, when, and to what extent variability in the less-predictable feeder departments might impact the system's performance.

Then we want to analyze any and all potential conflicts for variability. By determining the extent of the variability of the demand patterns, by HOD, DOW, and demand source, we can better understand the conditions under which conflicts and constraints in capacity arise. This may only happen under certain circumstances or certain days of the week, and be caused by certain excesses in demand from specific feeder departments such as the ED. Or, it might occur only under specific conditions of variance, such as a combination of high but in-range ED demand and slower than average case lengths. Furthermore, we will also want to examine where and when *reduced* demand might cause us to shutter excess capacity, even for short periods.

Importantly, the use of averages will *rarely if ever* show us this kind of information, and therefore will leave us guessing as to possible issues and remediation. Since the average never shows us the range of demand possibilities, we are left to deal with the variation, and combinations of variance, as they arise throughout our operations. Depending on the variance in demand, this can be significant, especially when combining demand patterns from multiple feeder components (e.g. ED, OR, and Cath Lab).

Once we understand the potential conflicts in demand, and before moving to make any corrections or adjustments, we want to examine the available downstream capacity. Look to the bottom right of Figure 3, beyond the "inpatient bed" block. You will see the many downstream capacities which need to be accounted for in order to optimize flow and eliminate capacity constraints. Starting at the point of admission and moving to inpatient, observation, and short-stay units, we can look for possible constraints in a variety of critical resources, inclusive of beds, nurses and other staff, pumps and equipment, etc., under a variety of circumstances. This should happen by HOD and DOW, such that we can balance the necessary capacity with the incoming demand.

Since we can control capacity more readily that we can demand (we purchase and allocate our own resources), we can "manage to" the variable demand patterns coming at us by varying capacity as needed. If studied within the context of the demand-capacity continuum, and given the relative predictability of demand patterns, we should be better able to allocate capacity such that it effectively matches variable demand.

We should keep in mind that it is not just the *numbers* of resources that matters, particularly as it relates to staff. It is the way in which they are deployed and what they do that offers us potential capacity flexibility. This is essentially "Who does what, where, when, and how frequently", hereinafter simply "4WF". Demand creates requirements for service tasks. In a restaurant, service demand created by arriving customers obviously includes cooking, but also includes cleaning, serving, advertising, purchasing, garbage pick-up, and accounting. If a single resource type, say cooks, did everything necessary to run the restaurant, their capacity would be limited and/or they would work a lot of hours doing non-cooking tasks. Similarly, if nurses do a great deal of non-nursing tasks, they reduce their capacity to do the work for which they were hired.

Before going further, let's differentiate between workload and workflow. *Workload*, as used here, refers to the totality of tasks for a given process or set of processes. *Workflow* is the order in which we do those tasks. Before determining the flow, we need to understand the load. Now that we understand at least some of the latter, we can construct the former around the significant tasks. We can construct the workflow around the workload (known tasks and task times), whether that is an admission, expected discharge, med distribution, or shift change. Work with patients already on the unit, including those just admitted, is obviously part of the day's activities. The care for these patients must be considered in the overall scheme of the workload analysis and placed into the day's workflow. To manage our capacity properly, prioritization should be made for the processes that are most important to patient care and those that are mission-critical to the hospital: admissions and discharges. Processes such as med req's, rounding, and shift change can be filled in around other, mission-critical tasks, so that we can actually begin to organize the day around our mission-critical processes. This will allow nursing staffs to split up responsibilities among themselves and other staff members, and prioritize their work according to the predicted workload and necessary tasks to be done. The key point here is as we move away from feeling that our environments are randomized and out of control, we can move towards a more scheduled and prioritized flow of tasks and work.

For instance, if a nurse comes out of a patient room after having just spent some time changing dressings and so forth, the next task she chooses should not be randomly selected. There should be some science to the choices, because her workload has already been anticipated by HOD. The nurse may need to pull from a list of (scheduled) choices, perhaps on a cheat sheet she keeps in her pocket, with prioritization given to specific tasks and times such that care is optimized and patient flow is steadied.

Furthermore, we can use analysis and task modeling to determine the appropriate staff for certain tasks. Just because the nurse does a task doesn't make it a nursing task. In an inevitable future of more expensive resources, the growth of unions, and the reduction in the numbers of qualified resources, task allocation will be critical to the effective function and financial viability of our facilities. This methodology will aid us in maximizing the patient care with the resources available through the predictive analysis of the important and time-consuming tasks.

Task Allocation

The optimal configuration of care patterns while minimizing the cost of care is in part dependent on the task assignments of our resources. If all our care resources were nurses, we'd have much more expensive operations. There are a number of other resources we can tap, which might be more readily available in the marketplace, and who can support operations effectively.

In an assembly line environment, a given worker does a specific tasks or set of tasks, and repeats. The worker, with a standardized set of specific tasks, produces products faster and more efficiently and allows for better workflow and reduced stress. The best example is an automobile assembly line, wherein a pile of parts moves slowly from one end of the plant to another, slowly becoming a shiny new vehicle along the way. This concept can teach us a little about *work breakdown structure*, or the breaking up of a large collection of tasks into individually assigned subtasks that yield the completed project. Work breakdown structure can apply, to a limited degree, to the work of patient care. The overall care of a patient during his or her stay on a unit, as the aggregate work to be done, is split into tasks and assigned, as needed, to the various resources on the unit. The appropriate allocation of these tasks among care providers is the key to optimizing care while reducing the total cost of care provision.

Even nursing tasks can be split up so as to offer greater efficiency, reduce travel time and stress, and improve care provision. A good example of this is the revitalization of the med nurse (MRN). The MRN was popular many years ago, but went away as nurses became more ubiquitous in the overall work of patient care. The MRN is assigned the task of ensuring that all patients receive the right meds at the right time throughout the day. Proper distribution of medications can be an issue for nurses who get caught up in the work of the day, resulting in delayed medications, displeasing both physicians and patients. Furthermore, the MRN can individualize the med distribution to accommodate more options, such as two, four, five, or more meds per patient day. By being the sole resource in charge of med distribution, the MRN reduces errors, improves timeliness, and reduces workload and stress on other nursing staff.

Other tasks can be allocated to support staff, who can work in teams with the nursing staff to achieve more efficient care with reduced stress and cost. Yet many team environments fail due to lack of proper planning, failure to communicate effectively, and distrust among team members, which leads to confusion about roles and responsibilities. Thus, teams become no more efficient than a group of "lone rangers" all doing the tasks that pop up. Instead, proper process mapping of care requirements, study of scheduled events and tasks, proper allocation of tasks based on skill, and effective communications and documentation are critical. One recommendation for this kind of analysis is the common "swimlane" process map. This map allows users to see the task assignments and even the timing of the tasks within a given process flow, so as to determine the best sequence of events to alleviate delays and optimize efficiencies or other key metrics. Simulation is an excellent follow up to a static swimlane diagram. By incorporating the appropriate dynamism, simulations offer a much more realistic vision of how a task allocation will actually work for a given team. Simulation can locate and quantify the bottlenecks in such an allocation and allow for "what-if?" testing of scenarios for possible improvement opportunities. Simulation also allows for the dynamic analysis of the processes and resource allocations, so as to develop any necessary dynamic reactions to the changes in the environment. Importantly, we can test resource and task allocations for quality, appropriateness, and cost-benefit. By altering the allocation of tasks within a resource pool and using a variety of resource types, we can allocate tasks and understand the outcomes for a variety of performance metrics, whether they be productivity- or cost-related. Then, we select those that offer the best outcomes for our particular goals and situation, while accounting for constraints such as 1) tact times and skill-set trade-offs, and 2) quality and task requirement legalities.

Thus, the best way to analyze 4WF is with a computer simulation, since it can account for the variability in each task time (including resource-specific variance and skill requirements), the variability in the tasks requirements for each patient type, and the variance in the demand for these tasks. Using a properly constructed simulation model, one can effectively "play" with the 4WF and determine the best mix of resources to optimize patient care time, minimize tasks done which are unrelated to resource qualification, improve quality and reduce staff stress. This allows the building of a "care team" concept which allows the tactical cooperation of resources on a given unit, based on specific demand patterns, to optimize the work done while minimizing the stress on a given resource type.

Naturally, we do not expect to be able to schedule every minute of each day. Nursing work can be quite chaotic, given the immediate and seemingly random requests of patients, arrivals of patients' Physicians, and other distractions from critical flow-related tasks. The way to achieve any amount of control over this is to analyze the important tasks expected within a given period of time, determine what can be scheduled (including patient admissions and discharges), then align the tasks with the resources.

Thus, several inputs to decision making are coming together for this new management style. These include predictable boluses of care activity in the form of:

- HODDOW admissions and discharges
- Known tasks that must be achieved throughout the staff's day
- Patient types, acuity patterns, and other workload-related data on the specific patients in the system

With this, we can begin to both proactively manage the expected workload and the flow of tasks throughout the day, based on the predictive analysis of demand and the knowledge of resource capacity. We can also begin to allocate tasks more effectively, examining resource allocations and staffing patterns along the way.

This may require drastic cultural change. Nurses, to their credit, often do not want to give up much, if any, of their patient care tasks to others. Nurses must sometimes to retrained to think in teams and resource/task allocations if these concepts are to take hold and be effectively maintained.

As final step in this process, we will want to re-evaluate the demand-capacity continuum, and see where, when, and if better management of both the demand and capacity might be possible. Two concepts need to be introduced here: Entitlement and Dynamic Standardization.

Dynamic Standardization

The concept of *standard work* comes from decades of process improvement expertise, though it was codified as a concept in the Lean methodology. Intuitively, it makes sense. Essentially, standard work refers to the elimination of process variation and intra-process waste, and the creation of repeatable, standard processes that all workers follow. The goal is the achievement of standard and expected output and results. Structured and followed properly, standard work reduces or eliminates output variation, and thus rework and waste. This concept applies well to many processes where workers might take liberties in performing a task in their own way or in which there might be multiple ways in which to accomplish a task. When this happens, variances in productivity can erupt as one worker's methods are more or less efficient than another's. Furthermore, any errors that occur are more difficult to trace back to a root cause, since it may be difficult to tell which process produced an error and which did not. Lack of standardization can also yield too much flexibility in the way tasks are performed, which can yield takt or process time variation, resulting in up- and downstream bottlenecks. The outputs can therefore see more defects, waste, and errors. Standard work says that there should be a single way to complete a process, such that the expected result is ensured.

In healthcare, standard work can be important to process flow and the reduction in process time variation, reduction in errors, management of quality in caregiving, and training of new staff. However, we must remember that we are working in very dynamic environments. This dynamism has been shown to lead to changing parameters and circumstances, both internal and external to our systems.

If processes remain rigid in the new environments, the processes themselves may contribute to a breakdown in system performance. In other words, a process flow that performs admirably under a given set of conditions may not perform as well under another. Therefore, while standardization of the actual performance of a process is still needed to ensure quality and proper outcomes, certain process flows may need to dynamically flex to meet the variations in demand, capacity, and other inputs.

Therefore, in certain circumstances, what may be needed is *dynamic standardization*. That is, the use of multiple versions of standard work, the use of which depends on the circumstances under which the work is performed. Dynamic standardization could and should be employed when some system variation might cause a single version of standard work to fail to offer its expected outcome.

Take, for instance, ED triage. Let's assume that under normal circumstances, standard work dictates that a triage nurse manages all incoming patients, with a specific set of tasks. However, in outlier volume scenarios, this triage nurse may become overwhelmed, reducing her ability to effectively manage the incoming stream, possibly putting the emergent patient at risk. Under this outlier scenario, several options might be offered. First, the number of triage nurses performing the standard work of triage could be increased. Or, alternatively, an entirely new process might be developed in which an ED physician comes to the triage area to manage the patient streams. While both processes might be standardized, their dynamic use can be based on specific criteria, such as number of patients awaiting triage, door-to-triage time, or door-to-physician time.

Standard work, used dynamically, allows for quality to remain high under varying circumstances of parameters and variables. To set up a dynamically standardized workflow, one can use simulation models, value stream maps, or flowcharts.

Knowing the breaking points in the system, the outcomes of various processes, and the required quality and performance metrics are all critical to the implementation of this concept. It is important to remember that if dynamic standardization leads to lower quality, lesser care, or inefficiencies; it is not achieving its goals. The goal is the same as that of standard work: to reduce variation and increase the likelihood of an expected or desired outcome. One of the important reasons for dynamic standardization is to establish clear and structured processes and operations that will apply in a number of different circumstances. This eliminates the "this happened, so I had to do it this way" excuse, which is the same as violating the standard work principle. The reason isn't variation in the process itself, rather in variables related to the process. In fact, the use of dynamic standardization might serve to improve quality, as it gives staff a way to deal with the dynamic environments in which they work in ways that still allow for the maintenance of quality.

As an example of the need for this concept, according to Dr. Jeffrey Liker, Lean advocate, author, and guru, "many manufacturers lose their … gains after a few years because managers fail to monitor their variability as sales volumes or other conditions change." In other words, gains are lost because manufacturing systems vary and fail to evolve. Because of the volatility of healthcare environments, and the dynamism within healthcare systems, the loss of gains Liker describes could happen in hours rather than years. External variables, such as arrival patterns or downstream flow constraints, can cause our current standard work to break down leading to confusion and frustration. Since the healthcare environment is more susceptible to the vagaries of dynamism, it makes sense to allow for a dynamic reaction. So, we need to meet the dynamism with dynamic standardization, producing the quality and outcomes we expect through a variety of standard work configurations.

Managing Demand

The natural inclination at this stage would be to create capacity to effectively meet demand. However, before we go through this step, we will want to evaluate whether or not we can manage the demand coming into the units. Look again at Figure 3, this time to the upper left side where the demand is generated from the feeder components, (e.g. the ED, Direct Admissions, etc.). We will want to examine whether or not capacity can be made to match demand. Or, perhaps demand can be managed to better allow it to be matched by available capacity.

Capacity Entitlement is simply that amount of capacity that should be expected to be made available, based on the historical patterns of demand, regardless of the current demand. Simply put, if the optimized, dynamic capacity patterns show available capacity of, say, between 4 and 6 beds on Unit 4-West on Tuesdays between 2p and 5p, we should expect that this can and will be made available each week. The Entitlement for capacity then becomes at least 4 beds. The onus is then on Unit 4-West to make the Entitlement available, such that the upstream components can anticipate available capacity.

Similarly, patterns of capacity can also be anticipated, even in the most over-crowded facilities. Even if, again, the demand far exceeds capacity, there is *some degree* of capacity made available though it may not fully satisfy the demand. The patterns by which this capacity is made available should be as consistent as possible, so as to allow for smooth and predictable flow within the system. Acceptance Patterns are simply the patterns by which downstream components accept the demand from upstream components, based on a well-matched DCAMM system. As the components are dynamically meshed together, the dynamically optimized capacity matches as much dynamic demand as possible, thus eliminating the typical scrambling we are used to in crowded hospitals.

However, in order to achieve these two concepts, the demand side of the system must be better managed. If we are to ask for a capacity entitlement, we must be expected to manage the flow of demand to match that entitlement. So, if the ED's entitlement allows for, say, one admitted patient every hour to Med Surg on Tuesday afternoons, we must manage the patients flowing into the ED such that we plan for our entitlement "slot". When our slot opens, we should have a patient ready to go. Of course, outliers on the "low end" of demand will occur, and there will be days when our entitlement goes unneeded. But the establishment of this concept will allow for better planning and patient flow if used effectively.

Outlier Management and DCAMM

This alters the analysis we would do and the way we think about improving the system. Thus we come to realize that healthcare systems are dynamic yet still manageable. We can begin to discern how one component's dynamism impacts others upstream and downstream, and how the initial demand patterns drive all other system demand and the requirements for capacity. As we understand this dynamic demand–capacity continuum and its impact on performance, we begin to see how we can influence the up- and downstream demand patterns in the system so as to have a truly systemic impact. And furthermore we can more effectively and proactively allocate resources (remember to include staff, equipment, supplies, etc.) to dynamically match dynamic demand.

Since the standard range does and will occur in a high number of instances, it must be managed well in order to manage the system optimally. The remaining, relatively small percentage is the truly random and unpredictable events that drive the systems over the edge and cause breakdowns. These are the outliers, and they are caused by the dynamism of the system that occasionally goes beyond the norm. Outliers can have a tremendous impact on system performance, and are often the root cause of process bottlenecks and breakdowns. Furthermore, because they are relatively unpredictable, they are inherently more impactful. However, they should be recognized for what they are: relatively unique events.

The points at which the system leaves its standard range and moves into these more unusual circumstances are the *"break points"*. Break points must be recognized and quantified, so as to help discern when the in-range performance can no longer be expected and when perhaps some change to the standardized processes needs to occur. Beyond a break point, the system may tip into an outlier status—circumstances and conditions that are among the more rare and unusual, but that are relatively unpredictable and cause great impacts on the system's overall performance. The system's flow and balance begin to fall apart, and bottlenecks seem to appear everywhere as the demand-capacity continuum ceases to mesh. The interdependencies cause the outliers to ripple throughout the system wherever causal impacts lead. Planning for the normal range of circumstances fails us, as the unexpected circumstances cause in unanticipated results, leading to a feeling of chaos.

Look at Figure 4. A demand outlier appears outside the normal expected range, occurring less than 20% of the time. As you probably know, outliers can appear on the "low" and "high" side of the range, but are most commonly associated with the end of the range that causes us the most angst. An outlier in demand can overwhelm the capacity before it has time to react, while an outlier on the capacity side can constrain incoming demand like a pinched hose. While outliers are relatively uncommon, they are often the situations we remember most. We can all rattle off stories of a few favorites.

Outliers are so impactful in part because of the interdependencies of the system. If a bolus of arrivals of patients to the ED only impacted triage, we might not complain. If slower-than-normal discharges only impacts families awaiting the release of their loved ones, it wouldn't be so bad. However, because surgical services demand impacts demand for hospital discharge (a portion of

Figure 4. Outliers and their appearance

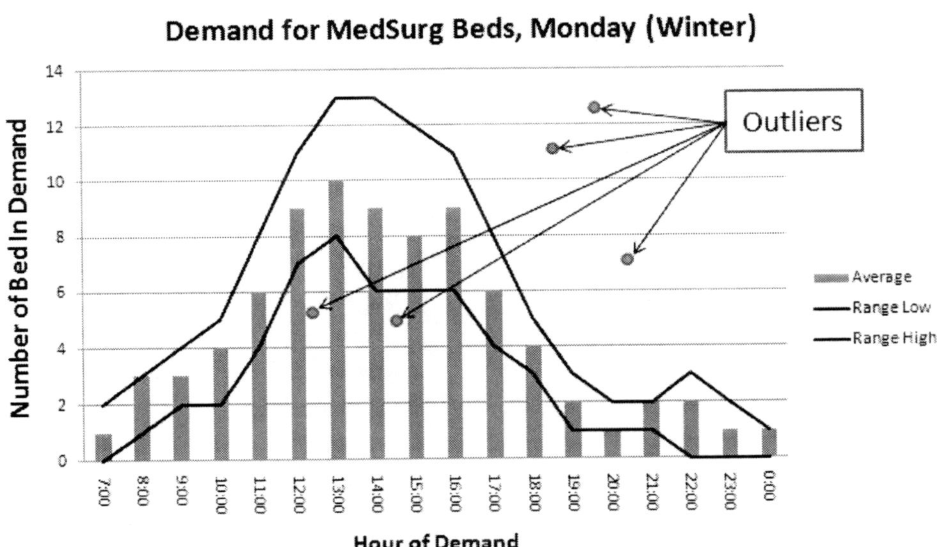

our capacity), we must be concerned about the systemic nature of outliers as they erupt.

Outliers can erupt wherever there is variability. The degree to which outliers impact us depends on several factors, including:

- The relative variability of the process or system. For processes with "tight" distributions (meaning, little variability around the average), outliers may not be very impactful except in high-volume, high-speed processes. For instance, if the registration time distribution is between three and four minutes 90% of the time, a five minute outlier will likely have little impact.

A process or system with a wider range of variability is likely to see most distant outliers. Recall some of the Figures we've used in this chapter, and recall the long "tails" on the distributions. Of course this concept can apply to arrival patterns, process times, system performance metrics, etc. The importance of outliers and the degree of their impact can depend on many factors, including:

- Their relative degree and probability of occurrence. A 1-in-20 occurrence is closer to the "typical" than a 1-in-1000 occurrence. The further an outlier is from its norm, the more likely its impact will be more widely felt.
- The degree of up- and downstream dependencies. If an outlier occurs at, say, registration throughput time due to a staff member calling in sick, it is unlikely that hospital discharge processes will be affected three days later. However, other upstream outliers could have impacts from end to end. Thus is it critical to fully grasp the nature and quantifiable impact of the system's interdependencies.
- The complexity of the interdependencies. The ED touches so many areas of the hospital that its outliers are widely noticed. A high volume outlier in the ED can impact demand on ancillary services, transport, inpatient and observation units, Physician rounding, Hospitalist and/or admitting Physician demand, case management, and discharge. The same degree of an outlier in direct admits or cath lab might not have similar systemic impacts.

Examples of outlier scenarios include:

- "Bus crash day" in the ED, in which a higher than normal volume and/or acuity of patients arrive.
- A high number of add-on or emergent cases in the OR. Though we might accommodate them, they can still throw off the normal patterns of workflow as demand overwhelms capacity throughout surgical services as well as downstream components and resources.
- Longer than expected LOS for a high number of patients on a unit causes upstream bottlenecks and shuts down the normal flow from the feeder components.

As we have discovered, the interdependencies of the system cause the impact of outliers to be felt throughout. Bottlenecks from the above scenarios can last for hours or even days. For instance, the above "bus crash day" in the ED may result in a higher-than-normal number of admissions, which clog inpatient or observation units for several days. Same with a high number of add-on's from the OR. The inpatient unit LOS example may result in worse-case impacts such as cancelled cases in the OR, or ED diversion and high wait-times.

Ironically, extreme outliers, such as disaster scenarios, are often studied. While their occurrence is perhaps the rarest, we tend to spend a relatively large amount of time and energy planning for them, while we ignore planning for the more common "really really bad day". Indeed, it is not uncommon to see cities and towns run a "live scenario" meant to mimic a terrorist attack, earthquake, or other natural disaster. I recall vividly the city of Chicago spending some $16 million of Federal and State dollars to run a half-day disaster scenario, complete with fire trucks, ambulances, and hundreds of "volunteer dead and wounded". For the minimal lessons and information gathered, I would suggest it was not money well-spent. What a simulation could have built with those same dollars! Remember, however they are studied and understood, disasters are just outliers in the extreme.

Outlier Management

Outliers must be dealt with as the unique events that they are—as outliers—such that we do not manage each and every day as if it's an outlier. Since the in-range metrics can be predicted relatively well, and since it is the outliers that cause us the most pain and suffering, we should focus on the latter and not the former. This becomes *outlier management*.

Of course, everyone remembers "bus-crash day" in the ED, or flu season on the med units. Too many bad days are remembered as normal when they are not. We need to discern specifically what makes up an outlier, as indicated by the performance and outcomes of the circumstances, and the statistical analysis of the data. What is important about this concept is that we can quantify what constitutes an outlier, rather than assuming that a tough day is always an outlier day.

Outlier management is simply the focus on impacting outliers in order to significantly improve performance. Since much of a process' or system's performance can be managed through the predictive analytics derived from the analysis of the patterns of dynamism, in-range performance is inherently more manageable than the random outlier. Furthermore, altering the in-range parameters presumably has a finite and inherently limited impact on the results, since there is only a limited amount of change available—the parameters are already within a given range. However, any outlier is a risk to not only performance metrics, but also breakdowns in quality, patient satisfaction, costs, and revenues. Since a small number and degree of outliers can have such a significant impact on system performance and metrics, outliers should become the locus of analytical, tactical, and strategic analysis and efforts. Eliminating an outlier can have a tremendous impact on the system's overall performance as well as quality and cost.

Outlier management does not mean that we ignore the in-range performance or the parameters that lead to dynamism. In-range performance will still be of concern, so long as there is room for improvement. Outlier management should be the first goal of the management team so as to minimize outliers and their impacts to the extent possible. (This section, up to this point, seems out of place ... like you're explaining it long after you first introduced the concept.)

There are a number of ways of proceeding into outlier management. The first step is to understand what outliers are and what their impact(s) might be. This requires the kind of analysis already recommended in this chapter. Assuming you have already begun your DCAMM analysis, then you'll have already likely found some of the instances of outliers and their outcomes. Since any variable component or process can have an outlier, we also need to ascertain which outliers do or might cause significant impact(s) on performance standards and metrics.

Once this step is achieved, you should begin to ascertain the root cause(s) of their occurrence. There may be several interdependent causes, so each should be isolated for analysis (this, as we have seen, is readily achieved using a simulation model). Assess what can be changed, and by how much, and to what degree any associated variability can be reduced or eliminated. Running the "new outliers" through a DCAMM model will tell us the [predicted] systemic impact of the changes made by the outlier. Furthermore, it will aid us in determining the source(s) and extent of the root cause(s) of outlier appearance. Knowing the root cause(s) will then aid in the development of meaningful and effective remediation steps. Of course, some will cause greater impact than others, and should be prioritized for removal or prevention. And as we determine those outliers that impact us most, we can then proceed to develop the necessary PI improvement solutions. We can also use our simulation scenarios to test possible dynamic solutions, including dynamic standardization, dynamic staffing, and other measures. These scenarios aid us in determining several key elements of proactive management:

1. What are the break points? In other words, what triggers the tip over into outlier status?
2. How can these break points be detected? How quickly can they be detected? And what mechanism gives the indicators of performance change?
3. How granular do we need to be in the definition of the outlier? Is a single number enough or do we need to go deeper into the characteristics of the numbers?
4. What dynamic changes need to take place to accommodate them?

For instance, in an ED, a break point for admission volume to med-surg on a given Tuesday winter afternoon between 1 p.m. and 5 p.m. is seventeen. After this break point, (as we should have already determined through root cause and simulation analysis using "what-if?" simulation scenarios), the current OR schedule and the resulting total demand for inpatient beds begins to create conflicts and constraints on certain inpatient units. The key questions become: (1) How early can we detect this condition in the ED? (2) What can we do to proactively alleviate it, so as to mitigate the impact of the outlier?

Perhaps the answer might be to look all the way back to triage arrival patterns (by volume, acuity, etc.) to discern what a seventeen-admission afternoon looks like at the front end of the system. Is there any discernable difference between a seventeen admission afternoon or, say, an in-range fourteen-admission afternoon in triage? What makes the front end of the system different? Perhaps the difference lies in morning flow bottlenecks, which lead to a bolus of afternoon admissions not seen on in-range days. Before we charge forward with solutions, we need a solid understanding of the impacts of perhaps a variety of causes.

Using a DCAMM simulation model, we could test various combinations of the actual timing of demand so as to discern how the capacity is made available for patients being admitted. As another example, capacity analysis might reveal incongruities in discharge patterns between days, which can be traced back to physician rounding caused by a busy Tuesday surgical schedule. Importantly, *testing scenarios can reveal how much capacity needs to be made available during specific hours, so we can use the entitlement concept to appropriate a specific additional amount of capacity such that the outlier is eliminated and becomes "in range".*

There are myriad ways to go about this analysis. However, as described earlier, you will be inherently limited in your analysis without simulation and a systems approach. The sort of root cause analysis described herein is very simple, for demonstration purposes. But management engineers are schooled in the art and science of many methodologies of complex and sophisticated root cause analytics, and can guide your facility to these sorts of revelations. Once the revelations are made, then the task of discovering how to better proactively manage them, as or preferably before they occur, will be a tremendous help in improving the overall performance of the system.

Focusing on the outliers, and bringing out-of-range performance into range will enhance the overall performance of the system.

CONCLUSION

Dynamic Capacity Analysis, Matching, and Management (DCAMM) is a relatively new concept for healthcare managers and providers, though many "feel" it or know it intuitively. Since our systems are so clearly dynamic, it is not surprising that these concepts would seem quite reasonable, even if new. However, it is this dynamism that requires us to leap beyond what other industries have brought us, and develop our own mechanisms, tools, analytical methodologies, and concepts for performance optimization. Since the systems in which we work as so dynamic, so too must be the way we approach, analyze, and improve them.

DCAMM offers a simple, methodical, and systemic approach to the improvement of the dynamic systems of healthcare. Through the adoption of its concepts, tools, and methodologies, we should be able to profoundly change the way hospitals are managed.

REFERENCES

Aiken, A. (2008). *Lean: Concepts and realities*. Lanner Corporation Publication.

Braglia, M., Carmignani, G., & Zammori, F. (2006, September 15). A new value stream mapping approach for complex production systems. *International Journal of Production Research*, *44*(18/19), 3929–3952. doi:10.1080/00207540600690545

Detty, R., & Yingling, J. (2000, January 20). Quantifying benefits of conversion to lean manufacturing with discrete event simulation: A case study. *International Journal of Production Research*, *38*(2), 429–445. doi:10.1080/002075400189509

Lian, Y., & Van Landeghem, H. (2007, July). Analyzing the effects of Lean manufacturing using a value stream mapping-based simulation generator. *International Journal of Production Research*, *45*(13), 3037–3058. doi:10.1080/00207540600791590

McDonald, T., Van Aken, E., & Rentes, A. (2002, July). Utilizing simulation to enhance value stream mapping: A manufacturing case application. *International Journal of Logistics: Research & Applications*, *5*(2), 213–232. doi:10.1080/13675560210148696

Narasimhan, J., Parthasarathy, L., & Narayan, P. S. (2007). Increasing the effectiveness of value stream mapping using simulation tools in engine test operations. *Proceedings of 18th IASTED International Conference '07: Modeling and Simulation*. Montreal, Quebec, Canada

Story, P. (2010). *Dynamic capacity management for healthcare: Advanced methods and tools for optimization*. Productivity Press/Taylor and Francis Publishing. doi:10.1201/b10393

Woehrle, S., & Abu-Shady, L. (2010). Using dynamic value stream mapping and lean accounting box scores to support lean implementation. *2010 EABR & ETLC Conference Proceedings,* (pp. 839-840).

ENDNOTES

1. Representative Harley O. Staggers, Sr., speech on floor of the U.S. House of Representatives Congressional Record, December 18, 1973, p. 42229.
2. Senator Edward M. Kennedy, speech on the floor of the U.S. Senate, Congressional Record, December 19, 1973, p. 42505
3. Though these concepts could apply to Physician offices, clinics, nursing homes, and other care areas, the foci of these tools will be the hospital and its many departments.
4. This can be done using sophisticated simulation tools, such as those offered by GE Healthcare's Performance Solutions group. These tools take into account the variability of each case length, allowing for a much more realistic and functional case/block schedule

to be developed which reduces wait times and staff overtime, and increases Physician satisfaction. Most hospitals, unfortunately, use traditional static methodologies available from their schedule management software provider. Or, they may simply use a spreadsheet or manual analysis.

Chapter 3
Simulation Modeling of Healthcare Delivery

Ian W. Gibson
Health Delivery Modeling, Australia

ABSTRACT

Healthcare has delivered incredible improvements in diagnosis and treatment of diseases but faces challenges to improve the delivery of services. Healthcare is a complex system using expensive and scarce resources. Benchmarking, experience, and lean management techniques currently provide the basis for developing service delivery models and facility planning. Simulation modeling can supplement these methods to enable a better understanding of the complex systems involved. This provides the basis for developing and evaluating options to provide improved healthcare delivery. Simulation modeling enables a better understanding of the processes and the resources used in delivering healthcare services and improving healthcare delivery systems. Options to improve the cost effectiveness can be evaluated without experimenting with patients. This chapter reviews the current challenges and methods including the use of simulation modeling. Analysis of emergency patient flows through a major hospital shows the capability of simulation modeling to enable improvement of the healthcare delivery system. This chapter enables healthcare managers to understand the power simulation modeling brings to the improvement of healthcare delivery.

DOI: 10.4018/978-1-60960-872-9.ch003

INTRODUCTION

This chapter takes the perspective of a manager responsible for improving healthcare delivery. This may be management of a large health system; integrated healthcare service; hospital; health service or hospital department. Managers in such positions face the daily challenge of delivering services with highly variable and increasing demand; limited staff, equipment and facilities; increased expectations; changes in regulations and cost pressures. Managers need an analytical method, which improves understanding of the system, facilitates input from the disciplines involved and rigorous analysis to test options to improve delivery of health care. Current methods use experience, benchmarking, and process mapping to develop improvements. However, these methods lack a rigorous analytical method than enables analysis of the current systems and testing of options. Simulation modeling can supplement these methods to enable a better understanding of the complex systems involved. This provides the basis for developing and evaluating options to provide improved healthcare delivery.

The chapter commences with a review of the challenges facing health services, current methods and the emerging direction for delivery of health care. A brief description of simulation modeling provides the basis for an improved approach to the challenges. The approach focuses on the delivery of healthcare services rather than the health science or technology involved in providing health care. For example, the focus is on the staffing, equipment and facility requirements to deliver high quality healthcare and not the life science or medical technology involved in the diagnosis and treatment of disease.

The objective of the chapter is to enable readers too understand simulation modeling and its capability to improve delivery of healthcare services. The chapter also provides approaches, which can be used in improving healthcare delivery.

BACKGROUND

The background section provides the context for the example of using simulation modeling on the emergency patient flows through a major hospital.

Crossing the Quality Chasm: Identifying the Needs

There are a many reports that consider the challenges in providing health care. The Institute of Medicine (2001) report "*Crossing the Quality Chasm*" focused on the healthcare delivery system to provide preventative, acute, chronic and end of life healthcare for individuals.

The report summarized the US healthcare system as follows:

- "*The American healthcare delivery system is in need of fundamental change. Many patients, doctors, nurses, and healthcare leaders are concerned that the care delivered is not, essentially, the care we should receive. The frustration levels of both patients and clinicians have probably never been higher. Yet the problems remain. Healthcare today harms too frequently and routinely fails to deliver its potential benefits.*" (p 1)
- While healthcare knowledge and technology have advanced in the last 50 years, healthcare delivery has been unable to provide consistent high quality care. The system is frequently unable to translate knowledge into practice and apply new technology safely and appropriately. The healthcare delivery system does not make best use of the available resources.
- The delivery of safe healthcare is a major issue. It is estimated that in the US, between 44,000 to 98,000 patients die each year from errors in delivery of healthcare services. The total cost of preventable adverse events was estimated to be $17 to

$29 billion. (Kohn 2000) Adverse events are associated with 10% of hospital separations in Australia and other developing nations. Adverse events are incidents involving harm to persons receiving healthcare including infections, injuries, reactions or complications due to surgery, medication, or medical devices. About 2% of separations associated with serious adverse event, resulting in major disability in 1.7% of separations and 0.3% with death. Some of these are preventable. (AIHW 2008)

- Fragmentation of the delivery system and lack of clinical information results in poorly designed care processes with duplication of services, long waiting times, and delays. Little progress was being made in restructuring healthcare systems or using information technology to improve administration or clinical processes. The needs for healthcare are changing from acute episodic care to care for chronic diseases. Coordinated care is essential as over 40% of these have more than one condition, however frequently healthcare operates in silos of disciplines, departments, or organizations.

"*Crossing the Quality Chasm,*" (Institute of Medicine 2001) concluded, "*The current care systems cannot do the job. Trying harder will not work. Changing systems of care will.*" (p 4)

Institute of Medicine 2001 (p 5-6) proposed six aims for improving healthcare systems:

- ***"Safe***—*avoiding injuries to patients from the care that is intended to help them.*
- ***Effective***—*providing services based on scientific knowledge to all who could benefit and refraining from providing services to those not likely to benefit (avoiding under use and overuse, respectively).*
- ***Patient-centered***—*providing care that is respectful of and responsive to individual patient preferences, needs, and values and ensuring that patient values guide all clinical decisions.*
- ***Timely***—*reducing waits and sometimes-harmful delays for both those who receive and those who give care.*
- ***Efficient***—*avoiding waste, including waste of equipment, supplies, ideas, and energy.*
- ***Equitable***—*providing care that does not vary in quality because of personal characteristics such as gender, ethnicity, geographic location, and socioeconomic status".*

Improved performance to achieve these aims depends on new system designs. "*Such systems must facilitate the application of scientific knowledge to practice and provide clinicians with the tools and support necessary to deliver evidence-based care consistently and safety*". (p 8)

The major challenges facing organizations implementing this approach are:

1. Redesign of care processes to serve effectively the needs of the chronically ill thorough coordinated, seamless care across setting, service providers, and time.
2. Making effective use of information technology to automate clinical information and improve its accessibility.
3. Knowledge management to maintain the workforce's skills.
4. Coordination of care for patient conditions, care services, and care settings.
5. Continually advancing the effectiveness of teams.
6. Incorporating care process and outcome measures into the daily work of clinicians.

Consequences of Inadequacies in Health Systems

A number of papers outline the consequences of inadequacies in the health systems.

Bernstein (2008) studied Emergency Department crowding and patient outcomes through a systematic review of English language articles published between 1989 and 2007. The study concluded that overcrowding of Emergency Departments at least compromised the quality and timeliness of care. Overcrowding is also associated with increased risk of in hospital mortality, longer treatment times for patients with pneumonia and acute pain.

Ehsani (2006) sought to identify the main hospital acquired conditions and estimate the cost of these complications on the Australian health system. The study considered 979,834 admitted episodes of care that resulted in 67,435 adverse events. The total additional cost of the adverse events was estimate to cost 15.7% of the direct hospital costs.

Sprivulis (2006) examined whether high hospital occupancy and emergency access blockage is associated with increased mortality in hospitals in Perth, Western Australia. The study considered 62,495 first emergency admissions over a three-year period from 1 July 2000 to 30 June 2003. The mortality rate at 30 days after admission increased by 0.6% for patients arriving at the emergency department when it is operating at more than 90% of capacity. The increase appears to be independent of patient age, season, diagnosis or urgency. Sprivulis (2006, p 211) states "*The estimate of 120 deaths per annum associated with overcrowding in metropolitan Perth hospitals suggests that overcrowding should be regarded as a patient safety issue rather than simply an issue of hospital workflow.*" This compares with an average of 70 road accident fatalities per year for the same area for a comparable period in Perth. (Office of Road Safety, (2006, p 15) A target of 85% occupancy at a midnight census is suggested as an appropriate target.

Cost of Avoidable Deaths in Healthcare

Avoidable deaths such as associated with overcrowding in hospitals impose a large human and financial cost on society. These costs are similar to the cost of road fatalities considered by the Bureau of Infrastructure, Transport, and Regional Economics (2009) and the Department of Finance and Deregulation, Australian Government Best Practice Regulation, *Value of a statistical life* (2010). The cost of fatalities, injury, and the cost of a fatal crash are noted as key inputs in the policy development and cost benefit analysis of safety programs and infrastructure projects.

This approach is worthy of consideration in considering healthcare delivery.

The value of a statistical life is estimated to be $2.4 to $3.5 Million per fatality in 2006$AUD (approximately $2.7 - $3.6 million USD). This cost is estimated using a hybrid human capital model. The estimate considers the possible future earnings and the other consequential costs of the loss of life. The cost of property and vehicle damage is not included in this cost..

Design Healthcare Facilities to Improve Patient Safety

Barch et al (2009) considers the physical environment a key part of a systemic approach to improving patient safety in healthcare facilities. Although there is significant evidence that the building design has a significant effect on health and safety, these aspects are not generally integrated into the design process. Studies show impressive reduction in patient falls, hospital-acquired disease, and medical errors being attributed to improved building design in individual hospitals. Patient focused care and evidence-based building design are now being considered, but the approach has not touched many aspects of facility planning that effect safety and quality of care. Some examples are the stress of visiting a hospital, poor environmental design increasing hospital acquired infections, and lighting levels affecting patient depression.

Barch et al (2009) argues that the range of factors being considered requires complex system theory to provide the basis for a *"new principled approach to optimizing hospital design, performance and outcomes, managing risk and guiding health policy."* Traditional hospital design methods start with the hospital managers providing the architect with the function and health services to requirements. The architect then develops a space programme (or schedule of accommodation) and the adjacencies between the departments. This provides the basis for laying out the rooms within the department, which in turn provides the basis for contract documentation to enable building pricing and construction. Equipment and technology planning occur late in the design process. Patient safety is rarely considered. This creates latent conditions from existing hospitals into new hospitals as described by Reason (2000). *"Human factors, the interface, and impact of equipment, technology, and facilities is also not typically discussed or explored early in the process."*

To address these issues a systems approach is proposed. It is expected that this approach will improve patient safety and support the development of a safety-oriented organizational culture. The new approach considers the *"physical environment for healing is an integral sub component of the care delivery process."* The system needs to be designed to support delivery of health care. This requires changes to the process to include briefing by clinicians on critical design factors such as infection control, patient identification, surgical techniques, staff accommodation, patient transfer, utility systems, and systems coordination.

Developing Safe Systems

Reason (2000) reviews the personal and systems approaches to human error in the context of health care.

The personal approach is the common approach to safety generally and in healthcare in particular. When applied to health, the personal approach focuses on the people delivering the health care, the doctors, nurses, pharmacists and others. This approach considers that failure is the result of the person being careless, poorly motivated, negligent, or reckless. Blaming individuals absolves the organization of responsibility for the mishap. The solutions focus wholly at the people responsible through posters, disciplinary measures, litigation, and procedures. The personal approach inhibits the development of trusting reporting and a just culture that learns from safety incidents and builds a system to avert future, and possibly more serious, incidents. The personal approach also isolates the unsafe acts from their systems context and impedes the process of seeking and removing the error-provoking properties from the system.

The systems approach focuses on the working conditions of the individuals and develops defenses to avoid errors and mitigate their effects. This approach recognizes that people are fallible and errors are to be expected. Errors are seen as the result of human nature and system factors. The solution is to build systems defenses that provide barriers against errors occurring and, when errors occur, to focus on why and how the system failed rather than the people involved in the situation. Barriers and safeguards are key parts of developing a systems approach to safety. These include physical barriers, people, procedures, and administrative controls. However, there are always points of weakness that can lead to adverse events. These can occur through active failures where people make slips, mistakes, or violate procedures. They can also occur through latent conditions, which cause time pressure, understaffing, inadequate equipment, fatigue, and inexperience. Latent conditions may be dormant in the system until an active failure triggers an adverse event. Latent conditions need to be identified and remedies developed before mishaps occur.

Error management seeks to limit the incidence of errors, improving error tolerance and containing the damage of errors. Study of highly reliable organizations, which deal with major safety issues shows they are concerned with the possibility of failure of the safety system. This includes anticipating the worst possible scenario and equipping the organization to deal with the possibility of errors.

Medical Research and Healthcare Design

Eriksson, (2009) considers the changes affecting healthcare building design largely from medical research, information, and communications technology. This includes diagnostics using imaging and genetics to improve detection and treatment of cancer, heart and vascular disease and psychiatric disorders. Other changes include rising costs, ageing population, patient's expectations, lifestyle, and political factors.

Healthcare is expected to become a process-oriented system where continuum of care replaces fragmented services; managing health rather than treating illness; prevention and primary care replace acute inpatient care and integrated IT systems replace individual IT systems. This is expected to result in larger institutions with integrated networks using information and communications technology. This will have a fundamental impact on the way in which healthcare professionals work together and with the patient. These changes will have a profound effect on the healthcare design and the buildings requirements. Utilization of these advanced technologies will lead to concentration in larger hospitals with expensive technology and specialized clinicians. These hospitals will services as nodes and integrated networks of healthcare providers with information and communications technology connecting to smaller centers.

Kolker (2009) considered the relative merits of queuing theory and simulation modeling as methods for qualitative analysis of patient flow. Queuing theory uses formula to describe the processes assuming limited statistical distributions of arrival times. The paper concludes that queuing theory cannot deal effectively with the interactive nature of complex healthcare systems. For instance, arrival times at emergency departments vary with the season, day of the week and hour of the day. Another shortcoming of using queuing theory is that elective or scheduled services that are non-random cannot be considered. Simulation modeling provides a flexible approach that can deal with a wide variety of arrival times and variation in the times for particular activities. Simulation modeling can better consider the complexity of patient flow by considering the variability of demand, complexity and variability of service delivery, and complex resource requirements.

Fomundam (2007) surveyed the application of queuing theory to healthcare organizations considering waiting times, utilization and appointment systems. Queuing theory methods have the advantage of requiring less information than simulation modeling. However, simulation modeling has an advantage in considering complex patient flow. Use of both techniques has advantages with queuing theory providing an initial analysis and a basis for more detailed analysis using simulation modeling. The paper concludes that variability in demand and services times meant that simplistic rules, such as mandating nurse to patient ratios, will only lead to congestion and poor quality services and are unlikely to contain or reduce costs. Analysis also needs to consider how queues interact within the organization. For example the interaction between the operating theatre and the post-operative recovery unit. Developing models of the links between the queuing systems is identified as an important direction for research.

Nason (2009) reports on the Canadian conference, *Taming the Queue VI-Improving Patient Flow*. The conference concluded demand needed to be understood to provide a basis for making more efficient and effective use of resources. Supply management includes improved collaboration and use of technology. Increasing capacity can lead to increased demand such as when emergency department services improve and attract more demand. Improvement to process covers the activities in providing health services. Reduction of current queues requires re-engineering of the health system. However, this is restrained by lack of people with experience in health and process engineering. Re-engineering guidelines need to be developed and applied across the health system. They need to understand where waiting times, inefficiencies, and ineffectiveness occurs in the health system. Addressing waiting times must be based on mapping the process that focuses on improving the quality of the health care. Reducing waiting times is essential to providing timely access to appropriate, safe, competent, effective, and efficient care.

Simulation Modeling

Dittus (2001) considers the use of discrete event simulation in the redesign of the healthcare delivered, the process of delivery, and how healthcare systems are organized. This method complements biomedical and clinical research in achieving the improvements sought by the Institute of Medicine for the US health system.

Biomedical and clinical research provide the majority of advances in health care. Traditional research methods consider the specificity and sensitivity of diagnostic tests and the efficacy and effectiveness of treatment. However many clinical management questions cannot be easily addressed by traditional health research methods such as clinical trials. The paper describes a study of healthcare delivery using discrete event simulation to develop a decision model and examine the cost-effectiveness of one-time screening for colorectal cancer. The wide range of possible solutions and size of clinical study made use of traditional research approaches impractical. The model considered the biology, risk factors, and healthcare system for screening and treating the disease. The model included cost effectiveness of alternative screening strategies and description of the outcome of the disease. Clinical trails and literature searches assisted in developing the model. Analysis of the data provided insights into the effectiveness and efficiency of care options and informed the biomedical science. The discrete event simulation model enabled the cost effectiveness and efficiency of screening for colorectal cancer to be determined. Efficient use of the resources for screening is critical, as there is insufficient capacity to meet the demand of testing everyone.

The process of care or how care is delivered is not amenable to biomedical research. Continuous quality improvement has provided some improvements in the quality of care. The "plan, do, study and act' approach is often not appropriate when new methods are required quickly in response to new regulations. A discrete event simulation study to consider redesign of workforce and related schedules for resident medical officers is described. Change in work rosters were required by new regulations aimed at improving patient safety by reducing doctor fatigue. The objective of the study was to make predictions of the hours of sleep resident medical officers would experience while on call with the new roster proposals. The model included prioritized tasks and considered interruption of tasks and changes in priority with time. Discrete event simulation is able to consider these factors and flexibility in the input data. This is not possible with other methods of analysis. The model was used to compare the quality metrics of the new roster, designed to reduce fatigue and the old roster. The study showed that rather than reducing the fatigue, the new roster would increase fatigue. The model allowed changes to the process of delivering care to be considered. Analysis of the interruptions to sleep showed that starting intravenous lines and drawing blood were frequent tasks. Allocating these tasks to a specialist team improved the sleeping time for the doctors significantly.

Use of Simulation in Healthcare: The Future

Oden et al (2006, p xiii) considered the challenges and potential benefits of simulation modeling in a number of sectors including medicine. Simulation modeling is the representation of a real life system using a computer. Simulation in health can also mean the the use of physical models and mock rooms to consider clinical practice situations.

"Simulation (modeling) also provides a powerful alternative to the techniques of experimental science and observation when phenomena are not observable or when measurements are impractical or too expensive." Simulation has advantages in dealing with real world situations, cost, or restrictions from health and environmental concerns. Advances in hardware and software have made simulation an effective tool. Computer simulation is beginning a new period with advances in software, computer speed, and storage.

Simulation-based Engineering Science (SBES) promises significant improvement in fields including health. Challenges to achieving this outcome include changing the way simulation is used including simplifying and enabling complex simulations; advances in computation, education and research.

SBES can study diseases and improve treatments. Medical practice and engineering are both problem-solving disciplines that require understanding of complex systems. Medicine may be able to use simulation to design optimal treatments with predicable outcomes.

Simulation aims to predict the behavior of the system to support decisions. Verification and validation (V&V) methods are use to consider the reliability of the model. Validation considers the accuracy of the depiction of the real events in the model. Verification checks the equations used in the model. Further development of V&V is critical to the further development of simulation modeling. Uncertainty about the data that provides the basis for the model is critical part of V&V. Use of stochastic models to address uncertainty increases data management and complexity. Developing methods to address these challenges is critical to the development of SBES.

Linking measuring devices directly to simulations to provide predictions is a very promising, but difficult application of SBES. Research on "*dynamic data-driven application systems*" describes application simulations using online data to provide the basis for decisions with major benefits to medicine. "*This synergistic and symbiotic feedback control loop among applications, simulations, and measurements hasthe potential to transform the way science and engineering are done*". (page 37) Implementation of such systems is a challenging multi-disciplinary task with immense potential benefits.

Development of SBES needs new approaches to simulation software. Computing has created an exponential growth in information. New methods are required to make better use of the data. Improved visualization is the key to people comprehending complex data more rapidly than considering the raw numbers. New methods are needed to enable the visualization of time-dependent data. The massive amounts of data from simulation require visualization to enable comprehension.

Oden et al (2006, p49) "*Visualization and data management are key technologies for enabling future contributions in SBES. In addition, they hold great promise for scientific discovery, security, economic competitiveness, and other areas of national concern. Computer visualization will be integral to our ability to interpret and utilize the large data sets generated in SBES applications*".

USING SIMULATION MODELING TO IMPROVE DESIGN OF HEALTH SERVICES AND FACILITIES

Overview

The preceding pages have outlined the challenges in healthcare and the shortcomings of current methods for analysis and design in healthcare services and facilities.

This section illustrates the capability of simulation modeling in the improvement of health services by considering the emergency patient flow through a major medical / surgical hospital and the facility requirements to enable service delivery. The objective of the study is to demonstrate the capability of the simulation modeling to improve decisions on the resources required for delivering patient service safely, efficiently and effectively. This approach is relevant to improvement of existing health services, development of new models of care and planning of new health facilities. The model also provides a template for studying emergency patient flows in major hospital including default values from various studies and assumptions.

The model considers the variability of the demand for emergency department services, the major activities in delivering these services and the patient flow through the system. The model is patient–focused,using the patient as the basis of the model. Establishing the major resources is fundamental to delivering a high quality and safe health service.

Although this model deals with the patient flows from the emergency department, the principles used may be applied to any patient flow. It aims to prove the value of using simulation modeling to study patient flows and the resource requirements.

Major Patient Flows in an Acute Hospital

The major patient flows in a modern acute care hospital are illustrated in Figure 1. The public may access the health system directly as emergency patients or as elective patients referred by their General Practitioner or Specialist for a scheduled admission for outpatient consultation or diagnostic investigation. The patients diagnosis and treatment may flow between a number of departments shown be the arrows. Patients move through the hospital using the specialist resources of the department to receive their treatment including personnel, facilities, and other services.

The emergency function used to illustrate the approach considers the patient flow from entering the hospital to discharge. In addition to being a major part of healthcare delivery, emergency health services are variable and challenging to resource.

The emergency patient flow through the system is a major component of the health service. It has variable demands within days, weeks, and the seasons. Often patients have health conditions and trauma, which are immediately life threatening. Quick delivery of appropriate diagnosis and treatment is often essential. There are also specialist staff that move between the departments providing health services.

Simulation Model of Emergency Patient Flows

The patient flows from the emergency department have been developed into the simulation model shown in Figure 2. The patient demand considers the five categories of emergency patients (resuscitation, emergency, urgent, semi-urgent and non-urgent). The variability of the patient flow with time and the attributes of age are included

Figure 1. Major patient flows within a major acute hospital

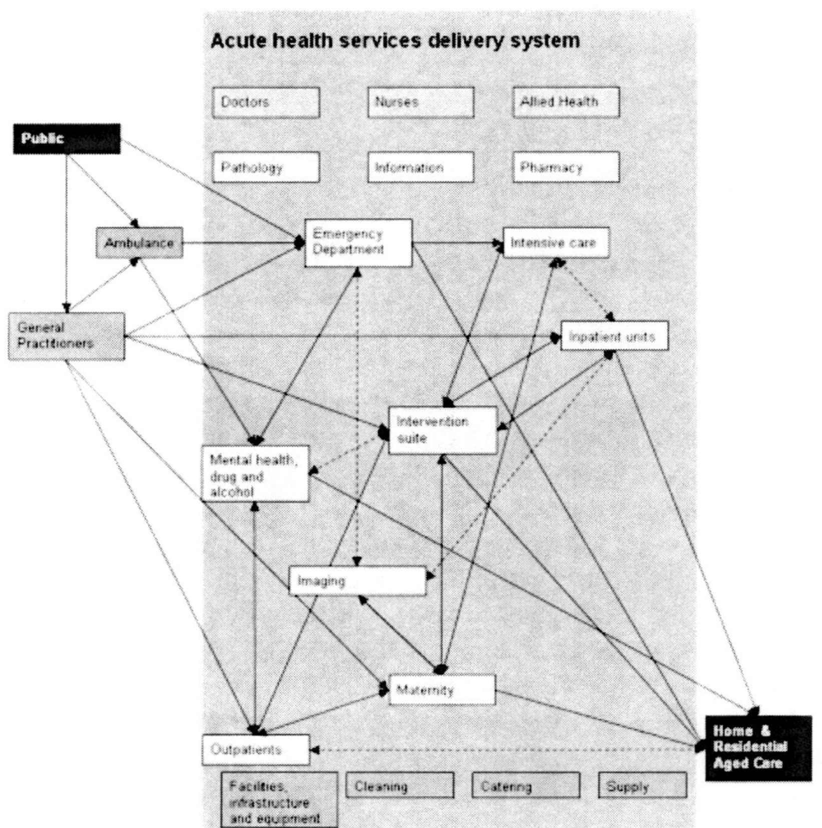

in the model. Each of the patient groups creates a patient flow through the waiting for admission; diagnosis and treatment; theatre and recovery; inpatient wards and discharge.

This model provides the basis for understanding emergency patient flows through the hospital and experimentation to develop and test options to improve the health service delivery. The simulation model uses ExtendSim 7. It includes 16 activities, seven queues and four resource pools.

A patient entering the ED waits until an ED cubicle is available before commencing diagnosis and treatment. Progress of patients through the model relies on resources being available for diagnosis, treatment. The resources are emergency cubicles, operating rooms, and recovery and inpatient beds for children, adults, and aged patients. A resource is a proxy for the range of facilities and resources required for patient diagnosis and treatment. For instance, ED cubicles include consult examination cubicles, treatment rooms, and other spaces in the ED. It also implies that staffing and logistics are adequate to provide services for the ED cubicles. Ensuring that these resources are adequate could be subject of further detailed studies.

Progressing to the next activity relies on the required resource being available. If the resource is not available, the patient waits and continues to use their current resource until the required resources is available. For instance, if an inpatient bed is not available then an ED patient requiring

Figure 2. Model of emergency patient flows

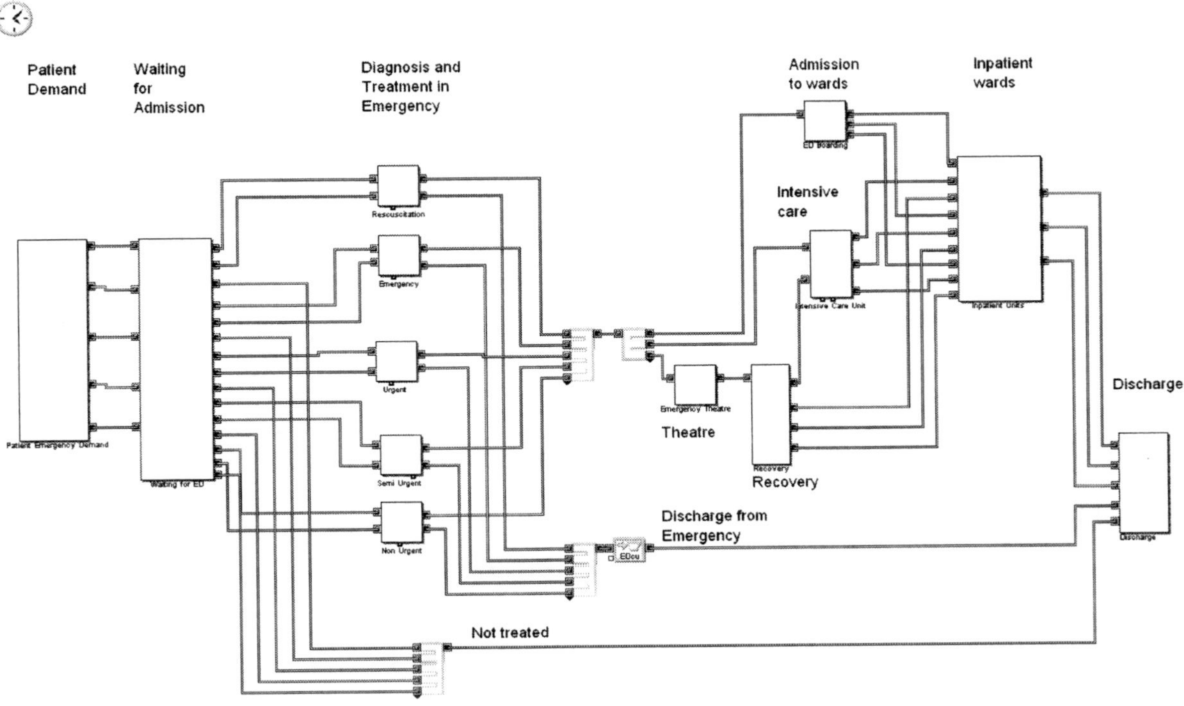

admission will continue to use the ED Cubicle, until a bed is available, If there are insufficient ED cubicles to provide for arriving patients, they continue to wait for ED cubicles.

Once the occasion of service in the Emergency Department is complete, the patient maybe discharged or admitted to inpatient accommodation, intensive care, or surgery.

Estimate of Patient Demand

The estimate of the patient demand uses large data sets to provide the basis for simulation modeling. The data sets provide default values to provide a preliminary data for preliminary analysis and proof of the concept. In studying a major hospital, the data would be derived from current patient flows and forecast growth and changes..

Table 1. Summary of typical emergency department use for a US population of 100,000 people in 2010

	Percentage of population	**Population by age category**	**Visits to ED**	**Emergency Category**				
				Resuscitation	Emergency	Urgent	Semi Urgent	**Non Urgent**
Child	20%	20,000	7,200	259	652	2,927	2,141	**1,221**
Adult	67%	67,000	27,027	1,393	3,226	11,191	7,097	**4,120**
Senior	13%	13,000	6,272	656	1,093	2,934	1,111	**477**
Total		100,000	40,499	2,309	4,972	17,052	10,348	5,818

Table 2. Variation in emergency demand by day of the week

	Percentage of weekly demand
Friday	13%
Saturday	11%
Sunday	15%
Monday	15%
Tuesday	16%
Wednesday	15%
Thursday	15%

The patient demand is modeled on an average US community with a population of 100,000 people. Table 1 shows the emergency patient demand for each of the Triage Categories. The National Health Statistics Reports Number 7 August 2008 provides statistics for the current and future use of Emergency Health services. (http://www.census.gov/popest/national/asrh/NC-EST2009/NC-EST2009-01.xls) On average, 40.5% of the US population uses the emergency department in a year.

The variation of the demand with time is a critical factor in the planning of health services. The simulation model considers the hourly, daily, and monthly variation on the following basis:

- The hourly variation is based on data from Australia Health 2005-06 (Figure 3). The data is based on 4.75 million patient visits. In addition, it is assumed that on 2% of patient arrivals involve two patients and 0.1% involve three patients.
- Bagusta (1999) estimates of the variation of patient flows within a week shown Table 2 in have been used.
- Seasonal variation uses data from Emergency Departments in the United States in 2006 reported in the CDC/NCHS< National Hospital Ambulatory Medical Care Survey.

Simulated Patient Flow

These variations are combined in the simulation model to provide a patient flow illustrated in Figures 3 and 4. Figures are produced by the simulation model to represent the reality incorporated in the data.

Figure 3 shows the average variation in flow per month. Figure 4 shows the comparison of the modeled average daily patient flow and the data used to develop it. The maximum difference between the data and the model is 5.7%. Table 3 compares the total patient flow by category entering the model with the data. The model was run for 100 years and showed a maximum variation within a category of 1.1% and overall 0.1%.

Patient Diagnosis and Treatment

The patient demand flows through the emergency department to either be discharged or receive further treatment in the theatre, intensive care, or inpatient facilities. Table 4 summarizes the basis for the model and sources of the data.

Table 5 details the median service times of patient subsequently admitted or not admitted referenced in Table 4. The duration of the service event is the length of time between when a healthcare professional first takes responsibility for the patient's care and the end of the emergency department patient episode. The table also gives the percentage of patients admitted and not admitted. People not treated were either referred to another hospital, left without medical care, left at own risk, died in the ED, or were not reported.

Figure 5 shows the distribution of the lengths of stay arising from the emergency admissions referenced in Table 4. Most patients have a length of stay of less than eight days. The outliers stay approximately 19 days. These patients are in three groups, either requiring rehabilitation, the result of adverse events or mental health patients. The patient flow includes selecting inpatient accommodation for children, adults, or seniors.

Figure 3. Estimated variation in emergency demand by months

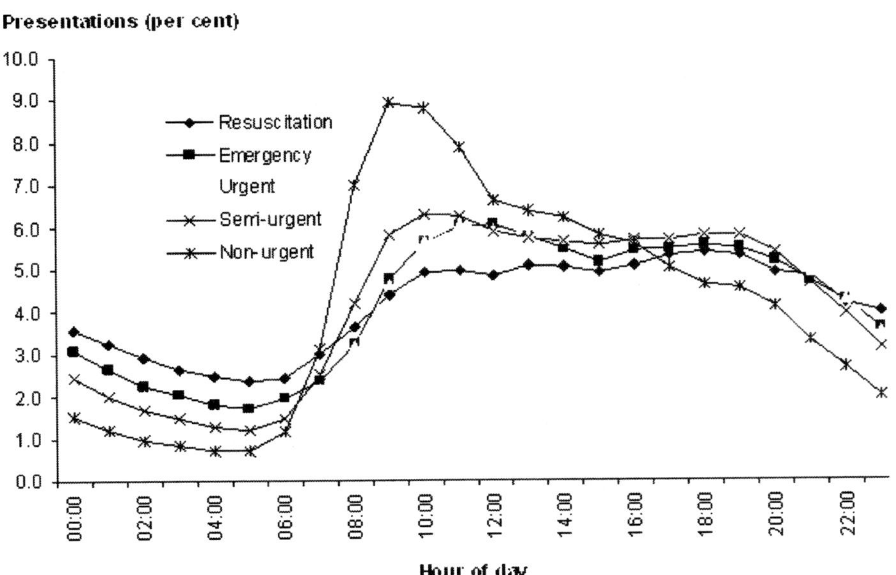

Figure 4. Average daily variability in demand by emergency patients

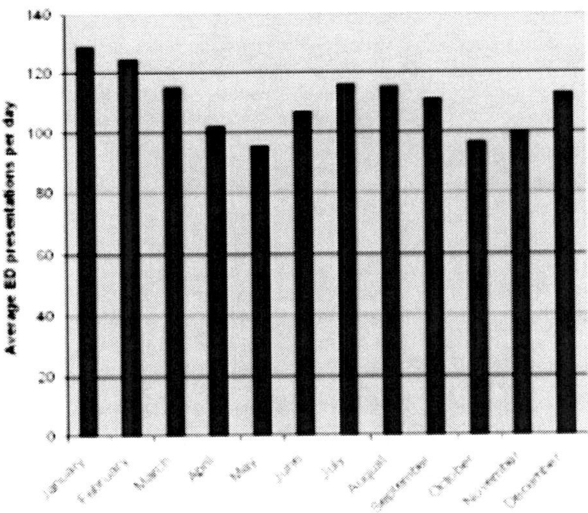

Analysis of Patient Flow

The model has been used to consider the number of Emergency Cubicles to provide safe, efficient, and economical health services. The initial run of the model assumed infinite resources. The model considered 5 years to establish the parameters. Table 6 summarizes the results with a peak demand for 42 ED cubicles.

This initial run then provided the basis for analyzing various numbers of ED cubicles considering various service delivery criteria. The

Table 3. Comparison of the overall patient flow by categories with the data patients

Emergency category	100 year run	Data	Variation
1	23,0576	2309	-0.1%
2	49,6963	4972	0.0%
3	1,687,963	17052	-1.0%
4	1,046,062	10348	1.1%
5	584,295	5818	0.4%
Total	4,045,859	40,499	-0.1%

model provides information on the time on a range of parameters including patients waiting before examination in the ED, waiting time in for admission to the Intensive Care, Operating Theatre or Inpatient accommodation and the use of resources. The model measures the waiting time for each Triage Category. This enables the adequacy of the resources to achieve the required standards. The results of the model runs for between 30 and 40 ED cubicles are summarized in Table 7.

Table 4. Summary of model data and assumptions

Component		Distribution	Reference	Reference
Emergency Department	Percentage of patients admitted or discharged. See Table 5	Constant	Australia's Health 2007 Table 5.8: Non-admitted patient emergency department presentations(a), by triage category and episode end status, public hospitals, states and territories, 2006–07	http://www.aihw.gov.au/publications/hse/ahs06-07/ahs06-07-c05.xls
	Median treatment times for categories See Table 5.	Constant	Australia's Health 2007 Table 5.9: Non-admitted patient emergency department presentation(a)(b) duration (in hours and minutes) for patients subsequently admitted to hospital(c), by triage category, public hospitals, states and territories, 2006-07 Australia's Health 2007 Table 5.10: Non-admitted patient emergency department presentation(a)(b) duration (in hours and minutes) for patients not subsequently admitted to hospital(c), by triage category, public hospitals, states and territories, 2006–07	
Portion of surgical patients admitted to Intensive Care	Percentage of patients	Constant	Assumed	
Theatre	Portion of patients requiring surgery	Constant	Australian Hospital Statistics 2008-09 7 Admitted patient care overview Table S7.8: Separations, by urgency of admission and Medical/ Surgical/ Other care(a), public and private hospitals, 2008–09	http://www.aihw.gov.au/publications/hse/84/11173_c07.pdf
	Operating time	Triangular	Assumed as Triangular distribution of 30/80/150 minutes	
Portion of patients requiring Intensive Care	Portion of patients admitted and from surgery		Assumed as 5% of admitted patients and 50% of surgical patients	
Intensive care	Treatment time	Triangular	Assumed median of 1.8 days, minimum of 0.9 and maximum of 4 days.	
Inpatient	Length of Stay	Distribution in Figure 7	Australia's Health 2010 supplementary tables S16: Separation statistics (a), by principal diagnosis, grouped into ICD-10-AM chapters, public hospitals, 2007–08	http://www.aihw.gov.au/publications/aus/ah10/supplementary/s16.cfm

Table 5. Emergency patient median services times and percentage admitted

	Resuscitation	Emergency	Urgent	Semi Urgent	Non Urgent
	Percentage of patients				
Admitted to Hospital	79%	62%	42%	16%	5%
Discharged from ED	10%	33%	53	75%	84%
Not treated -	11%	5%	5%	9%	11%
	Median Service event time in minutes				
Patient subsequently admitted to hospital	182	245	254	240	156
Patient subsequently not admitted to hospital	188	171	126	60	30

Figure 5. Distribution of the length of stay in inpatient wards

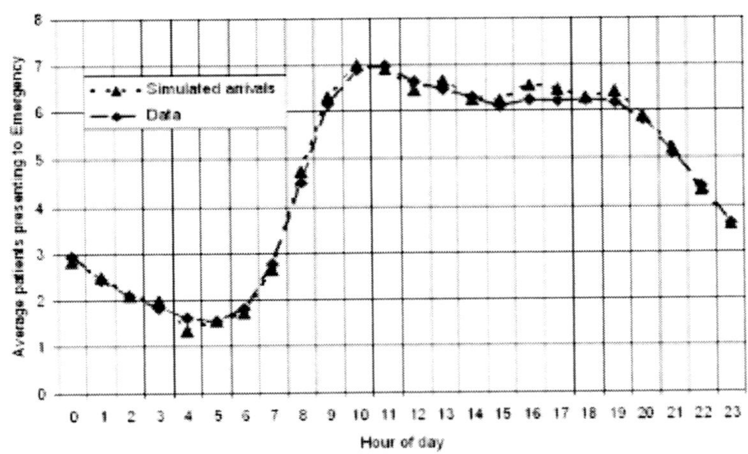

Table 6. Unrestrained resource demand

	Number of unit
ED cubicles	39
Theatre	5
Recovery	4
Intensive Care	23
Inpatient Children	68
Inpatient Adult	209
Inpatient Aged	84
Total Beds	361

This range was chosen as the Capital Development Guidelines estimate the need for 31 to 36 ED cubicles for a demand of 40,500 patients per annum. The upper limit is suggested by the unrestrained initial run.

Sufficient inpatient beds are included in the model, so that bed blocking does not occur. Analysis of the number of inpatient beds required is discussed later in the chapter. The results for each run are summarized and compared to the criteria for each Triage Category in Table 6. The criteria are expressed as a percentage of patients that are treated within specified times. For example, Resuscitation patients are all to be treated immediately. The model showed that this could be achieved with 39 ED cubicles. All the other time related criteria could be satisfied by 30 cubicles.

Table 7. Summary of analysis of emergency department cubicles. Analysis based on the desirable treatment times

					Number of Emergency Department Treatment spaces							
Triage Category	**Number of people in triage category**	**Criteria**	**Desirable treatment times**	**Target percent-ages for desirable times**	30	31	32	33	35	37	39	40
Resuscitation	2,305	People not seen immediately.			44	30	6	5	2	3	0	0
		Percentage of patients delayed more than specified time			1.9%	1.3%	0.3%	0.2%	0.1%	0.1%	0%	0%
		Maximum delay			48	37	44	16	13	16	0	0
Emergency	4,972	People delayed more that	10	80%	76	54	11	11	3	3	0	0
		Percentage of patients delayed more than specified time			1.5%	1.1%	0.2%	0.2%	0.1%	0.1%	0.0%	0.0%
		Maximum delay			48	50	56	34	31	18	0	0
Urgent	16,877	People delayed more that	30	75%	18	21	6	3	0	1		0
		Percentage of patients delayed more than specified time			0%	0%	0%	0%	0%	0%	0%	0%
		Maximum delay			52	54	47	39	29	34	8	0
Semi Urgent	10,272	People delayed more that	60		1	0	0	0	0	0	0	0
		Percentage of patients delayed more than specified time			0%	0%	0%	0%	0%	0%	0%	0%
		Maximum delay			63	56	42	33	32	21	2	0
Non Urgent	5,865	People delayed more that	120		0	0	0	0	0	0	0	0
		Percentage of patients delayed more than specified time			0%	0%	0%	0%	0%	0%	0%	0%
		Maximum delay			58	54	50	36	34	16	10	0

Table 8 summarizes the results considering the number of patients entering the ED when it is operating at more than 90% of capacity.

The 90% capacity criteria can also be considered as a metric describing when the Emergency Department should operate in the bypass mode. This criteria is based on Sprivulis, (2006) which showed that a 0.6% increase in the 30 day mortality of emergency patients when the ED was operating at more the 90%. The analysis shows that with 40 cubicles only 5 people per annum enter the ED when it is operating at more then 90%.

Table 8. Summary of analysis of emergency department cubicles. Analysis based on bypass and overcrowding criteria

Criteria	Number of Emergency Department Treatment spaces								
	30	31	32	33	35	37	39	40	Resource matched
Number of patients entering Emergency Operating at more than 90% capacity - Over 5years	8,533	5,429	3,001	1,699	639	147	29	27	5
Number of patients entering Emergency Operating at more than 90% capacity - average per year	1,707	1,086	600	340	128	29	6	5	1
Percentage of patient affected by Operating at over 90% capacity	4.2%	2.7%	1.5%	0.8%	0.3%	0.1%	0%	0%	0%
Estimated increased in 30 day mortality rate per year due to overcrowding	10.2	6.5	3.6	2.0	0.8	0.2	0	0	0

Figure 6. Emergency Department Cubicle use

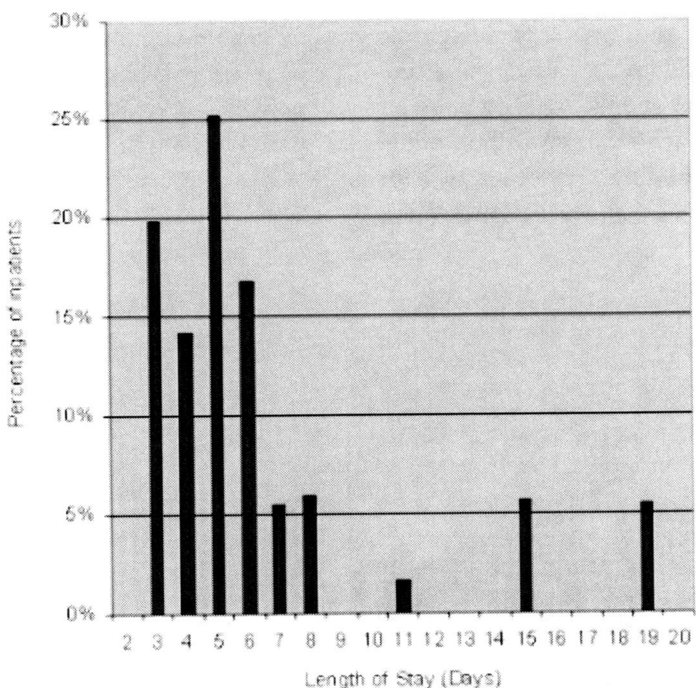

The analysis showed that with 30 ED cubicles 4.2% of patients would enter the ED at over 90% capacity. This reduced to 2.7% with 31 ED cubicles.

Based on this analysis, a resource-matched option that varies the ED capacity available to ensure that the operation was always less than 90% of the available capacity. Figure 6 summarizes the results of this investigation. The left had side of the Figure shows the patient flow for the model over five years. (The modeling is one year by five times, not a five-year period. This provides a better estimate of the distribution of the use of the resource). Note the seasonal and weekly variation with peaks in winter and summer. Peaks occur at 38 cubicles. The upper line is the available capacity developed based on analysis of the resources – the number of ED cubicles is 42/38/40/38/42. Give the limitations of the model, this level of resourcing is considered appropriate. A recent project with similar demands was proposing to provide 59 ED cubicles.

The right hand side of Figure 6 shows that histogram for the use of the ED Cubicles for the resource-matched options. The demand rises to a plateau where the majority of the use is in the range between 7 and 24 ED cubicles in operation. Over 24 cubicles the demand drops dramatically. This provides useful information to design the layout of the ED to provide 24 cubicles in a central efficient work area, and the other 18 cubicles able to be operated when required with minimal inefficiencies. The building services zones for air-condition and lighting could be design on these zones.

Figure 7shows the number of inpatient beds in use by Emergency Patients for five years by age category – children, adult and aged. The simulation shows that the peak demand could be as high as 330 beds. The histogram shows that, for 93% of the time the hospital operates, between 180 and 270 inpatient beds would be devoted to ED patients to maintain free flow condition. Further study will consider the affects of reducing the available beds on the ED patient flow.

FUTURE RESEARCH DIRECTIONS

The simulation model example presented is a work in progress to develop techniques and data to enable economical and powerful models to enable improvements to the design of healthcare delivery services and facilities. Future directions based on the simulation model presented include:

Figure 7. Inpatient bed use over a five year period

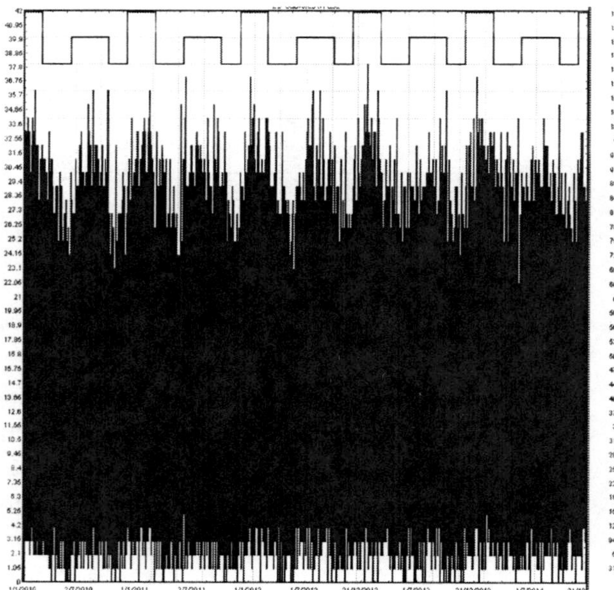

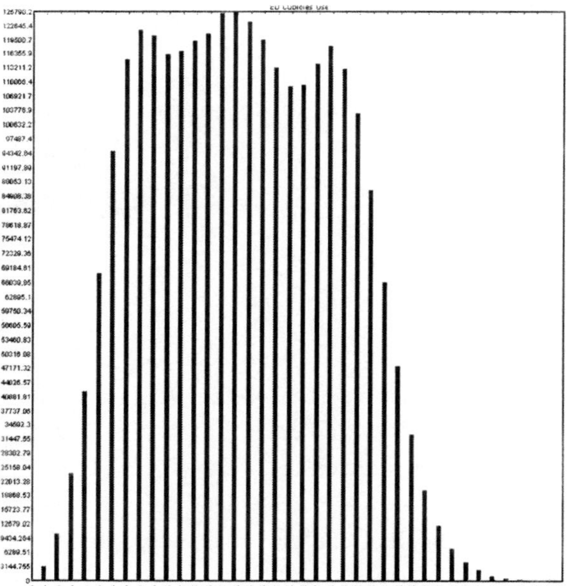

- Distribution of hourly demand and times for emergency department service delivery with further consideration of age category.
- Inpatient bed requirements required to service ED patient flow safely.
- The economics of providing facilities, considering the patient flows and value of saved life.
- Configurations for the ED including 24-hour and holding wards.
- Option for a primary care clinic to service Triage Category 4 and 5 patients.
- Making Category 4 and 5 patients by appointment.
- The affect of ageing of the population on ED demand.
- Disaster scenarios and consideration of the policy options.
- Addition of the elective services and ambulatory care.
- Developing detailed models of the services within the ED on the resource availability approach used in this paper.
- Developing detailed models based on modified clinical pathways to consider resource requirements.
- Development based on a major regional hospital.
- Logistics analysis to support patient flow
- Information and communications technologies based on the patient flow.
- Development of methods of consulting with clinicians to gain their valuable input into the simulation model.
- Develop animated models to represent the patient, staff and goods movement.

In the wider context, simulation modeling seems to be coming of age as a technique. The increased interest in the last five years is phenomenal.

Use of simulation modeling as part of a real-time healthcare operational management tool is futuristic. Oden et al (2006) describe the basis for "dynamic data-driven applications systems". This could be based on Radio Frequency Identification (RFID) technology to identify and track patients, staff, equipment, and supplies. Installation of RFID in a hospital linked to patient medical records and simulation models could provide real time information for the management of delivery of optimal patient care and use of resources. The simulation model could be based on clinical pathways that integrate the best knowledge to the clinicians and operational protocols established with the clinicians. For example, a patient entering the emergency department is assessed by the doctor to require a series of diagnostic tests urgently. The management system automatically schedules them in the optimal order and reschedules other patient tests given their clinical needs and the best use of the hospital resources. When a diagnosis is complete, the treatment plan includes the scheduling of the treatment including the resources and supplies required. Implementation would require major cultural change by clinicians to accept the technology. The pay-offs of improving their working lives and improved delivery of healthcare could provide motivation for such an organizational change.

CONCLUSION

This chapter aims to show how simulation modeling can be used to improve the delivery of health care. It focuses on the coordination and management of the resources to respond to the patient flow and requirements for appropriate care. The challenges to provide improved healthcare are reviewed to provide the context for a demonstration model to consider the concept of resources required to deliver emergency patient care. The model shows the capability of simulation modeling to represent the real life demands and delivery of emergency care. This provides an improved understanding and the basis of considering options for improved delivery of services. The model provides estimates of the physical space requirements to deliver health services and to consider "what if" analysis if interest to management and clinicians. The avenues for further development of the approach list a challenging future for simulation modeling of healthcare delivery. The potential benefits to patients, caregivers, clinicians, and healthcare managers are immense. This chapter describes how healthcare delivery managers may use simulation modeling more effectively for practical day-to-day problem-solving.

REFERENCES

Australia's Health. (2010). *Australian Institute of Health and Welfare*. Retrieved from http://www.aihw.gov.au/publications/aus/ah10/11374-c07.pdf

Bagust, A., Place, M., & Posnett, J. W. (1999). Dynamics of bed use in accommodating emergency admissions: Stochastic simulation model. *British Medical Journal, 319*(7203), 158.

Barach, P., & Dickerman, K. N. (2009). Patient safety: We shape our buildings, then they kill us. *World Health Design*. Retrieved from http://www.worldhealthdesign.com/science.aspx

Bernstein, S. L., Aronsky, D., Duseja, R., Epstein, S., Handel, D., Hwang, U., & Asplin, B. A. (2009). The effect of emergency department crowding on clinically oriented outcomes. *Academic Emergency Medicine, 16*(1), 1–10. doi:10.1111/j.1553-2712.2008.00295.x

Bureau of Infrastructure. Transport and Regional Economics. (2009). *Cost of road crashes in Australia 2006*. Report 118 Australian Government. Retrieved from http://www.bitre.gov.au/publications/48/Files/Cost_of_road_crashes_in_Australia.pdf

Commonwealth of Australia. (2009). *A healthier future for all Australians*. Final report of the National Health and Hospitals Reform Commission. Department of Finance and Deregulation. Australian Government. (2010). *Best practice regulation: Value of a statistical life*. Retrieved from http://www.finance.gov.au/obpr/docs/ValuingStatisticalLife.rtf

Dittus, R. S. (2001). Discrete-event simulation modeling of the content, processes and structures of healthcare. In Institute of Medicine Committee on Quality of Healthcare in America (Eds.), *Crossing the quality chasm: A new health system for the 21st century*.

Ehsani, J. P., Jackson, T., & Duckett, S. J. (2006). The incidence and cost of adverse events in Victorian hospitals 2003–04. *The Medical Journal of Australia, 184*(11), 551–555.

Eriksson, H. (2000). *Medical research and its impact on healthcare design*. International Academy for Design and Health. Retrieved from http://www.designandhealth.com/uploaded/documents/Publications/Papers/Hakan-Eriksson-WCDH2000.pdf

Fomundam, S., & Herrmann, J. (2007). *A survey of queuing theory applications in healthcare. The Institute of Systems Research, A. James Clarke School of Engineering*. University of Maryland.

Forster, A. J., Stiell, I., & Wells, G. (2003). The effect of hospital occupancy on emergency department length of stay and patient disposition. *Academic Emergency Medicine, 10*, 127–133. doi:10.1111/j.1553-2712.2003.tb00029.x

Healthcare at the Crossroads. (2008). *Guiding principles for the development of the hospital of the future*. The Joint Commission. Retrieved from http://www.jointcommission.org/NR/rdonlyres/1C9A7079-7A29-4658-B80D-A7DF8771309B/0/Hosptal_Future.pdf

Hill, D. L., Marchant, R. J., & Gant, P. D. (2007). *Reported road crashes in Western Australia 2005*. Perth, Western Australia: Road Safety Council of Western Australia.

Institute of Medicine. (2001). *Crossing the quality chasm: A new health system for the 21st century*. Committee on Quality of Healthcare in America.

Kohn, L. T., Corrigan, J. M., & Donaldson, M. S. (Eds.). (2000). *To err is human: Building a safer health system. Committee on Quality of Healthcare in America*. Institute of Medicine.

Kolker, A. (2009). Process modeling of ICU patient flow: Effect of daily load leveling on elective surgeries on ICU diversions. *Journal of Medical Systems*, *33*(1). doi:10.1007/s10916-008-9161-9

Nason, E., & Roberts, G. (2009). *Taming the queue VI-Improving patient flow*. Canadian Policy Research Networks.

Oden, J. T., Belytschko, T., Fish, J., Hughes, T. J. R., Johnson, C., Keyes, D., … Yip, S. (2006). *Revolutionizing engineering science through simulation*. Report of the National Science Foundation Blue Ribbon Panel on Simulation-Based Engineering Science.

Office of Road Safety. (2006). *Metropolitan area, road crash and injury summaries including vehicle factors*. Perth, Western Australia: Office of Road Safety. Retrieved from http://www.ors.wa.gov.au/ResearchFactsStats/YearCrashStats/Pages/MetropolitanArea.aspx

Pentecost, R. (2009). *Standpoint: Shaping the future*. Retrieved from http://www.worldhealthdesign.com/Standpoint-Shaping-the-future.aspx

Pitts, S. R., Niska, R. W., Xu, J., & Burt, C. W. (2008). *National hospital ambulatory medical care survey: 2006 emergency department summary. National health statistics reports no. 7*. Hyattsville, MD: National Center for Health Statistics.

Reason, J. (2000). Human errors: Models and management. *British Medical Journal*, *320*, 768. doi:10.1136/bmj.320.7237.768

Reid, P. P., Compton, W. D., Grossman, J. H., & Fanjiang, G. (Eds.). (2005). *Building a better delivery system: A new engineering/healthcare partnership. National Academy of Engineering, Institute of Medicine*. Washington, D.C.: National Academy of Sciences.

Sprivulis, P. C., Da Silva, J.-A., Jacobs, I. G., Frazer, A. R. L., & Jelinek, G. A. (2006). The association between hospital overcrowding and mortality among patients admitted via Western Australian emergency departments. *The Medical Journal of Australia*, *184*(5), 208–212.

State Government of Victoria. (2010). *Capital development guidelines, functional benchmarks*. Retrieved from http://www.capital.dhs.vic.gov.au/Assets/Files/Functional_Benchmarks[1].doc

Chapter 4
Simulation Applications in a Healthcare Setting

Roque Perez-Velez
Management Engineering Consulting Services, USA

ABSTRACT

What is simulation? Most management engineers define simulation as the attempt to predict aspects of the behavior of some system by creating an approximate (mathematical) model of it. Most of the time the engineer writes a special-purpose computer program or uses a more general simulation package, probably still aimed at a particular kind of simulation.

Developing a simulation is often a highly complex mathematical process. Initially the engineer specifies a set of rules, relationships, and operating procedures, along with other variables. The interaction of these phenomena creates new situations, even new rules, which further evolve as the simulation proceeds.

The chapter will broaden the engineer's perception in regards to the gamut of simulation implements. These range from paper-and-pencil and board-game reproductions of situations to complex computer-aided interactive systems.

This proposed chapter will answer the following questions: Why is simulation modeling beneficial as a decision-making tool? When should engineers use simulation modeling as a decision-making tool? Which situations are a good fit for simulation modeling? When is not good to use simulation modeling? Which simulation modeling methods should engineers use? What are other alternatives to simulation modeling? What steps should engineers take in order to develop a sound simulation? Who should be part of the simulation modeling development team? Where are the common pitfalls of simulation modeling? How the engineer can overcome these modeling pitfalls? What should the engineer do when confronted with lack of reliable data?

DOI: 10.4018/978-1-60960-872-9.ch004

The author will attempt to answer the questions above by means of examples, anecdotes, real-case simulation models, and experiences while developing problem-solving models for a healthcare system. Some of the problem-solving models discussed include labor and delivery room utilization, neonatal intensive care unit expansion, emergency department staffing and process improvement, radiology process improvement, patient transport, operating room elective case surgery optimization, partial pediatric unit conversion to Intermediate Medical Care unit, family practice, and women's health clinics.

INTRODUCTION

The purpose of this chapter is to broaden the reader's knowledge in regards to the gamut of *simulation* implements. This chapter is guided towards engineers, neophyte simulation practitioners, analysts and technical staff who, in their daily undertakings, encounter uncertain situations. During their quest for answers to these events or undertakings, the analyst ends with incomplete or inconclusive results. These inconclusive results may be related to the extent of the initial hypothesis. The following real case demonstrates a situation where an inconclusive result showed the need for a simulation:

On a major southeast teaching hospital, an analyst was tasked with determining the optimal space needed to store specialty beds, such as burn, bariatric, orthopedic or other specialty beds, at a storage area of the hospital. These specialty beds are delivered from a rental company when a nursing floor requests it. The standard beds needs to be removed and stored until the specialty bed is no longer needed. A straight forward method, using *static simulation* or analyzing this problem at a finite time, is to account and verify the total number of specialty beds requested at the end of each day. With the total number of beds requested on a daily basis, the analyst can determine the space needed for storage. But, did the analyst perform the most suitable analysis for this situation? In a short answer, no, the analyst failed to take into consideration the dynamic aspect of this specific situation, such as a *dynamic simulation* or analyzing the problem and how it behaves over a known period of time. The analyst may under or overestimated the space needed.

Based on the initial assumption in which beds are requested on a daily basis and are accounted for does not provide the real picture. Specialty beds rental, seen as an independent entity, fails to illustrate the rental process complexity and the relationship to other entities, namely patients. Each specialty bed is allocated to a patient and to the patient's length of stay in the hospital. Using a Gantt chart and plotting each specialty bed's length of stay, gathered from patient's information, will show that some days there are more stored beds on the hospital than beds ordered on the same day.

Following the dynamic simulation analysis performed by the analyst, Figure 1 shows a Gantt chart where two beds were ordered on day 1, an additional two beds were ordered on day 2, one bed on day 3 and one bed on day 4. So, the maximum number of beds ordered on any day is two beds. If the analyst utilizes this process, he will be underestimating the real need. Analyzing this problem from a different perspective by taking into consideration patient's length of stay, the analyst will realize that the number of beds is higher. For instance, there are two beds on day 1, four beds in day 2 (an additional 2 beds compared to the prior method), and three beds on days 3 and 4 (an additional 2 beds each day). Now, the maximum number of beds ordered on any day is four beds instead of two.

The real case analysis, in which the above figure is based on, showed that there was a need for 19 beds at any time instead of the expected 30 beds needed. Savings related to the reduction

Figure 1.

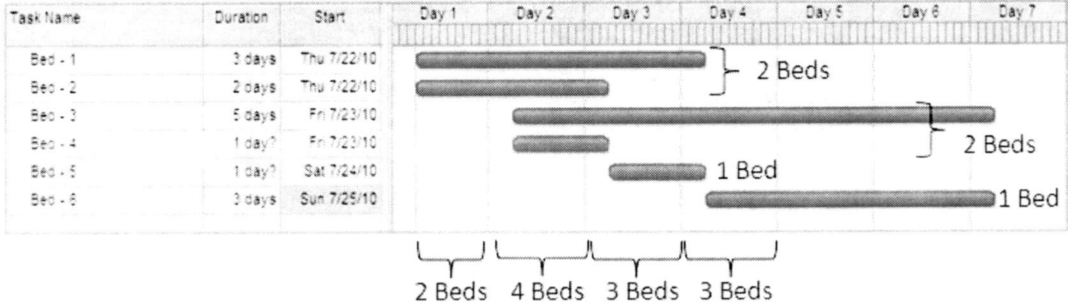

of space utilization of 11 beds, 32 square feet each, at a cost of $300 per square feet of construction, resulted in a reduction of $105,600 in initial costs. This initial cost does not take into consideration the expected long-term maintenance expenses related to this additional space.

As we have seen, there are other methods to solve uncertainty besides typical mathematical methods. An alternative method is simulation applications and these ranges from paper-and-pencil and board-game reproductions of situations, static simulations to complex computer-aided interactive systems.

This chapter will discuss dynamic simulation methods and techniques. Also, this chapter will answer the following questions:

- Why simulation modeling is beneficial as a decision-making tool?
- When should engineers use simulation modeling as a decision-making tool?
- Which situations are a good fit for simulation modeling?
- When is it not good to use simulation modeling?
- Which simulation modeling methods should engineers use?
- What are other alternatives to simulation modeling?
- What steps should engineers take in order to develop a sound simulation?
- Who should be part of the simulation modeling development team?
- Where are the common pitfalls of simulation modeling?
- How the engineer can overcome these modeling pitfalls?
- What should the engineer do when confronted with a lack of reliable data?

The chapter will attempt to answer the questions above by means of examples, anecdotes, real-case simulation models, and experiences while developing problem-solving models for a healthcare system. Some of the problem-solving models discussed include labor and delivery room utilization, neonatal intensive care unit expansion, emergency department staffing and process improvement, radiology process improvement, patient transport, OR elective case surgery optimization, partial pediatric unit conversion to IMC unit, family practice and women's health clinics.

Finally, this chapter is intended for engineers, analysts and technical staff who are not full-time simulation practitioners. The overall intention is to provide a basic understanding of *simulation modeling* and how it can be applied to daily situations or problems.

DEFINITIONS

Before we answer the questions above, first we need to define concepts which will be used throughout this chapter. Let's start with defining the concept of simulation.

What is simulation? Most engineers, simulation practitioners, analysts or technical staff defines simulation as the attempt to predict aspects of the behavior of some system by creating an approximate (mathematical) model of it. Generally, the modeler writes a special-purpose computer program or uses a more general simulation package, probably still aimed at a particular kind of simulation.

Wainer (2009, p. 25) defines simulation "as the reproduction of the dynamic behavior of a system of interest with the goal of obtaining conclusions that can be applied to the system."

Banks and Carson (1984, p.2) said "simulation is the imitation of the operation of a real-world process or system over time. Whenever done by hand or by computer, simulation involves the generation of an artificial history to draw inferences concerning the operating characteristics of the real system."

Maynard's Industrial Engineering Handbook (2001, p. G18) defines simulation as "the technique of using representative data to reproduce in a model various conditions that are likely to occur in the actual performance of a system. Frequently used to test the behavior of a system under varying operating policies."

Developing a simulation is often a highly complex mathematical process. Initially the modeler specifies a set of rules, relationships, and operating procedures, along with other variables. The interaction of these phenomena creates new situations, even new rules, which further evolve as the simulation proceeds.

The process of developing a simulation is called simulation modeling development. This process is similar to a study and, by its very nature, a project. If the analyst hastily jumps into simulation, without taking time to consider complex cause-and-effect relationships that determine the system as well as all steps necessary for a simulation modeling development, the rate of failure increases dramatically.

Many cycles has been proposed on simulation publications and below is a summary of eight simple steps or phases that comprise the simulation development process cycle. These steps are the foundation for a good and sound simulation:

1. Problem formulation
2. Conceptual model
3. Data collection and analysis
4. Modeling phase
5. Model building
6. Verification and validation
7. Experimental phase
8. Output analysis

During the problem formulation phase the modeler determines the need for simulation, defines the scope of the project, identifies the problem and ascertains possible input or output variables which, in turn, can be classified as decisions or parameters. At this point, the modeler decides which of the output variables will become performance metrics.

The conceptual model is a bird's eye view or high level representation of the system that the modeler wants to simulate. This is where we determine which variables are important for the study.

Knowing which input variables are necessary, the modeler proceeds to the data collection and analysis phase. By means of observation, the modeler is able to collect data and analyze it in order to determine statistical features from this data. This data must be tied to time, volume, occurrence or other significant valid values.

At the modeling phase the modeler matches analyzed data with the conceptual model in order to build a detailed representation of the system's behavior and structure. This representation is called the system model.

In the model building phase, the modeler chooses the method to execute the model developed during prior phases. This executable program is called the simulation model. This is the phase where the modeler has the flexibility to choose a simulation method. Examples of several simulation methods will be discussed later in this chapter. Also, this step is time consuming and one of the steps where the analysts will spend a considerable amount of time.

Verification is the process of aligning the conceptual model, system model and simulation model. Validation refers to correlation between models and real systems: how consistent is the model to reality? Analysts must perform formal documentation of results in order to compare the model to reality. This is another step where the analysts will spend a considerable amount of time.

After the model has been verified and validated, the analyst executes the simulation model and evaluates results. These results can be analyzed by means of sensitivity analysis, variance reduction, optimization, and alternatives comparisons (rank and selection).

The goal of output analysis is to provide the analyst with an understanding of system behavior. Since simulation experiments supply a large set of numerical data, visualization techniques are recommended to better understand the results.

These are the steps for a sound simulation. The reader should note that this is not a "step-by-step" process but rather a guide since some of these steps may be performed concurrently. The next section will help the reader determine if simulation modeling is the best approach to solve a problem.

THE SIMULATION SIX W'S: WHY, WHEN, WHO, WHAT, WHICH, AND WHERE?

This section will expand the discussion in regards to the questions presented during the introduction of this chapter. These questions will be answered and tied to the respective step of the simulation development process.

Why Simulation Modeling?

So, why is simulation modeling beneficial as a decision-making tool? Ulgen and Williams (2001, P. 11.101) contend that "simulation modeling and analysis, long the specialized province of mathematicians and computer science specialists, has entered the mainstream of methods available to help organizations increase their efficiency and effectiveness."

Simulation modeling is beneficial for decision-making because this process encompasses all aspects of the system such as decision *variables* (controllable), *parameters* (non-controllable), and changes in the state of a model (also called *events*). Simulation modeling replicates dynamic processes so as to give the analyst a view of all factors affecting the analyzed system. Finally, simulation modeling provides the analyst with an outlook of stochastic and deterministic attributes. Other types of analysis, such as spreadsheets, Monte Carlo simulations, design of experiments and other operation research methods does not encompass all aspects of simulation into one model.

Jacobson, Hall and Swisher (2006) assert that "the application of discrete-event simulation in the analysis of health care systems has become increasingly more accepted by health care decision-makers as a viable tool for improving operations and reducing costs". The contend that this is related to better simulation software applications tied to many successful case studies in the literature.

When to Use Simulation Modeling and Which Situations Are Good Candidates?

If simulation modeling is beneficial for the analyst then, when should analysts use simulation modeling as a decision-making tool? One of the most fundamental drivers of healthcare is cost so there are several targets of opportunity to use simulation modeling as a tool to reduce costs or avoid incurring additional costs. These costs can be related to operational, infrastructure, professional services and equipment as well as costs associated with patient access to services and hospital staff responsiveness to patient needs.

Also, which situations are a good fit for simulation modeling? The analyst must look for opportunities in situations such as capacity analysis, staffing analysis, implementation of new equipment, new construction or facility expansions, transportation matrices, and operational changes.

Finally, when the analyst is assessing a problem and the requirements addresses the possible "what-ifs" games resulting from the problem, Jacobson, Hall and Swisher (2006) assert that changing the rules and policies of patient flow are "an important advantage of discrete-event (dynamic) simulation, over other modeling techniques like linear programming or Markov Chain Analysis, when modeling a health care clinic is the capacity to model complex patient flows through healthcare clinics".

An example of using simulation modeling for the purpose of evaluating a system's capacity is when a healthcare facility expects an increase in volume over time for a known department or service. A Florida-based hospital decided to analyze the capacity of a neo-natal intensive care unit with 58 available and licensed beds running at an average of 90% capacity. The planning department projected a 10% increase for the next year. The analyst used simulation modeling to determine when and if the neo-natal unit will be able to handle the volume increase. The analyst used historical data to replicate arrival times and patient's length of stay. Another viable alternative could have been to randomize the arrival times and / or length of stay duration. Figure 2 illustrates a simple neo-natal intensive care unit simulation model used during this capacity analysis.

Figure 2.

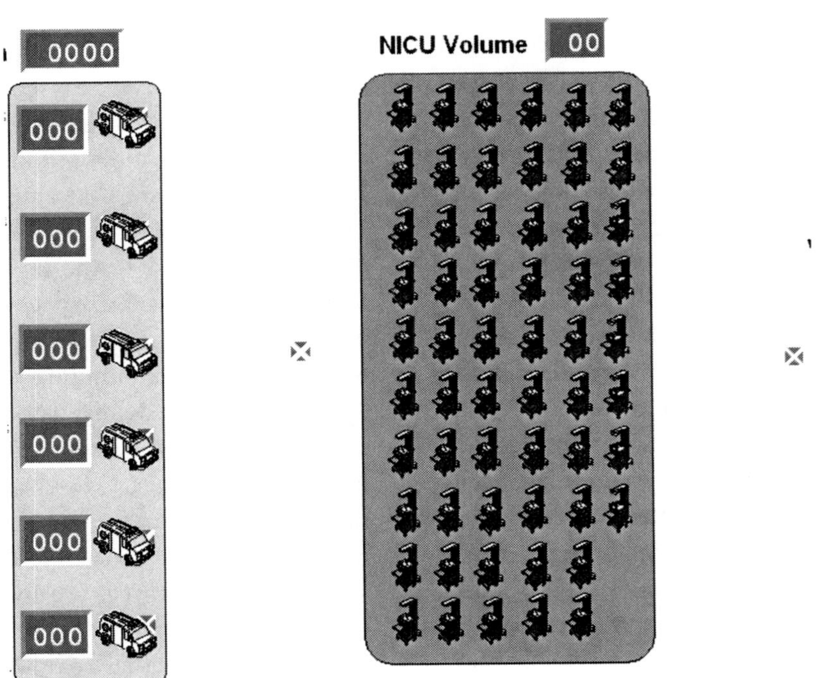

This model shows the arrival of patients, depicted by ambulances, from six sources of which 3 are internal to the hospital. The other arrival sources are external to the system, such as transfers. The overall design of this simulation was to verify the number of patients which may be diverted to other facilities due to capacity issues. The two main variables were patient's arrival time and length of stay.

Staff, such as clerical, technical, nursing, medical, and professional, is one of the major costs drivers in a healthcare facility. It is the author's experience that using simulation modeling for staffing analysis is one of the leading tools generating exceptional outcomes which, in turn, help reduce long-term costs associated to hiring staff.

An example of using simulation modeling for the purpose of evaluating staffing plans is when a southeastern healthcare facility needed to evaluate the need to add or reduce staff due to volume changes. This teaching hospital planned to open a new emergency medicine department. This department consists of 48 exam rooms, 8 specialty rooms such as orthopedics, eye, isolation and ObGyn, and 6 trauma rooms. The emergency medicine medical director wanted to ensure proper coverage and mix of medical staff (attending, residents and practitioners) as well as nursing ratios and technical staff. Simulation modeling helped determine these staffing levels under several conditions and what-if scenarios.

Some of these scenarios included, but not limited to, a varying the number of attending depending on the number of residents and practitioners available. Other tried combinations were varying the number of registered nurses depending on the number of licensed practical nurses (LPN) and ARNP. These scenarios provided the emergency medicine medical director the right mix of staff he felt was needed for patient care coverage.

Major equipment purchases provide many opportunities for simulation modeling. Simulation modeling offers the analyst, if equipment capabilities are available, the prospect of analyzing the cause and effect of replacing, upgrading or automating a current procedure.

The manufacturing industry has been using simulation for decades. Management engineers have used simulation modeling in areas such as radiology services. For example, a hospital is thinking of upgrading a CT-Scan machine and how doing so may shift or create bottlenecks. Simulation modeling can not only expose bottlenecks but can also help determine options to reduce or eliminate them. Using a what-if approach, the analyst can create scenarios, such as adding, re-assigning staff or process changes, which will help mitigate expected and unexpected situation before spending large amounts of money on new equipment.

It is imperative for the analyst or engineer to be closely involved during the early stages of planning and development phases for a new facility construction or expansion of current buildings. Simulation modeling is an immense enhancement during the planning phase. Simulation modeling helps scrutinize alternative layouts for form and functionality. It also can evaluate process, activity and information flows.

As an example, picture a group of medical doctors planning to form a family group practice clinic. Their planning analyst determined that the expected volume will be somewhere in the vicinity of 2,800 visits per month. Preliminary drawings have been provided by the architecture firm who will be in charge of development. The analyst can use simulation modeling to determine if the initial layout will support the expected volume as well as establishing or validating proposed process, activity and information flows.

Simulation modeling has been studied and used successfully extensively in the logistics and transportation industry. Logisticians use simulation modeling in areas such as loading, unloading, route selection and method of transportation. Transportation matrices are quite important on a healthcare facility for two main reasons: horizontal and vertical transportation. In healthcare, horizontal transportation is similar to classical transportation modeling due to the nature of transporting an item or a patient from point A to point B. Also, it is similar when a delivery of clean or medical supplies needs delivery and the analyst's goal is to reduce travel time. The healthcare route replicates the transportation industry on a smaller scale.

As for the vertical transportation, the healthcare industry adds the factor of vertical displacement. This movement is normally conducted by means of elevators. This method of transportation contains other parameters which the analyst needs to take into consideration: elevator wait time and elevator displacement times. The analyst should be cognizant of these parameters when developing a simulation.

Two examples of when it is a good idea to use simulation modeling in regards to transportation are as follow:

A southern state healthcare consortium of one main hospital with several satellite sites desired to reduce the turnaround time for laboratory sample testing. The analysts used simulation modeling to determine the optimal route between sites in order to reduce travel time between locations. This change resulted in an increase of 25% of transported items each day.

The supply chain management would like to determine how to optimize clean supplies deliveries to all hospital locations where these are needed. By studying elevator wait and displacement times, the analyst can perform simulation modeling and determine optimal delivery routes as well as if the hospital needs to allocate a dedicated elevator for these functions. A dedicated elevator may be a permanent allocation as well as on a temporary basis such as during specific blocks of time.

Furthermore, another situation where simulation modeling is a good fit is when there are operational changes on the healthcare facility such as adding or expanding existing services. These services can be of a health, administrative or support nature.

As a case in point, a gastrointestinal and endoscopy service, within a major hospital in north-central Florida, that serves an inpatient population but desired to expand and serve an outpatient population. The analyst used simulation modeling to determine if the service was able to handle the volume increase by analyzing exam room utilization, recovery room utilization as well as how the outpatient flow affected the current facility functionality. Also, the analyst modeled the effect on nursing and medical staff due to delays caused by complications or medical supply availability. The results showed that room utilization increased weekly by 10%.

Finally, Kolb, Schoening, Lee and Peck (2008) used dynamic simulation to characterize the relationship between Inpatient Unit (UI) utilization and Emergency Department (ED) crowding. They found that the sensitivity of ED overcrowding with respect to IU utilization depends on the degree of coupling (pairing) between the two units. They suggest that these findings have potential implications in guiding a hospital's effort to optimize their systems.

Who Should be Part of Simulation Modeling?

It is not expected that the analyst understand and is an expert on all areas or services provided by a healthcare facility. This is not a task to be accomplished only by analysts. Buy-in from the requestor, the process owner as well as a representative from healthcare administration is essential. Then, who else should be part of the simulation modeling development team?

The first candidate to be part of the simulation modeling team should be the system's owner. Also, if is not the same person, the project requestor is a main player. Managers, supervisors or lead personnel should be part of the development team. Another important player on the development team is a person who is knowledgeable on all aspects of the system which needs to be replicated. The analyst must recognize or ask that, if there is a person who knows, possess and can translate organic data for the analyst, such a person must be part of this simulation development team. This is the least possible number of team members involved in simulation modeling development. The analyst may add additional members as the development process evolves.

Also, there are many *subject matter experts* throughout the institution who can provide direct or ad-hoc support. Some of these experts may be representatives from information services, financial analysts, planning department representatives, decision support services technicians and others as needed.

Finally, the analyst must have a subject matter expert on the process being developed and simulated in order to provide guidance and understanding of all related intricacies. This expert will advance the validation process.

Where are the Pitfalls and How Can These be Avoided?

Simulation modeling is a complex procedure. When working with intricate processes to which simulation is applied, it can become a difficult task. By combining an intricate process with a complex procedure the journey will have many pitfalls. So, where are the common pitfalls of simulation modeling? If the analyst can identify these common pitfalls then, how can the analyst overcome them?

There are many pitfalls in simulation modeling but this chapter will illustrate only of the most common pitfalls. For instance, some of the common pitfalls are:

- Wrongly identifies a problem as a possible simulation modeling candidate
- Unclearly defines the project scope
- Poor identification of decision variables
- Incorrectly choosing the simulation modeling method
- Not having the right subject matter experts participation
- Not having buy-in from the process owner or requestor
- Spending excessive amount of time replicating processes which do not affect the overall model's goal or scope
- Being unable to correctly analyze the data collected during the data collection and analysis step
- Not being able to validate the simulation model

The major pitfall is wrongly identifying a problem as a possible simulation modeling candidate. Seasoned analysts rarely commit this error. During the problem definition step, novice analysts tend to mistakenly assess a situation and decide that the problem can be solve by means of simulation modeling. This situation may happen when the analyst or the working group does not clearly define the problem. This can be avoided by carefully analyzing the problem and clearly defining what is the real or perceived problem.

For instance, a southeastern hospital decided to perform a staffing analysis on one of its laboratories. The working group contemplated simulation as a method to solve their problem. After 3 weeks of formulating the problem and developing the conceptual model, the group realized that it was easier to use a workload analysis, using spreadsheets, than a simulation model. The problem definition asked for daily workload to determine staffing level.

When the working group unclearly defines the project scope it causes a similar problem as not clearly defining the problem. Is the project scope to maximize or minimize? If the working group has been able to clearly define the problem, then defining the project scope should be easier.

The identification of decision variables is a subset of problem definition and project scope. These variables must match the project scope. If the project scope is to maximize room utilization, the working group should use decision variables which clearly reflect and are tied to rooms and should be able to collect the necessary information. The overall effect of poor identification of decision variables is to give the analyst wrong or incorrect simulation results.

Another pitfall is incorrectly choosing the simulation modeling method. These methods range from a simple model to a more complex model. A simple model is like a classical queue model: limited numbers of entities and resources, one arrival node, one queue, one activity node followed by an exit node. A complex model may be a model where there are hundreds of activities, nodes and queues with dozens of entities and resources. Also, complex models may include schedules, downtimes and a series of other factors.

The simulation modeling working group should determine what level of complexity is enough and how much detail is needed during development. In other words, does the working group want to see the forest, the trees or scale all the way down to the weeds? Of course, this is dependent on the time available, the problem at hand as well as the objectives for the simulation project. When the group finally agree to the level of complexity and start the modeling phase, the group must avoid scope creep. This creep will turn a simple simulation into a complex simulation in no time.

As part of a designing team, an engineer from a teaching hospital was asked to develop a simulation of the radiology department in order to improve room capacity. After the engineer started the design and development of the simulation model, the working group started to add other features like absenteeism, phone calls, financial counseling, waiting area and machine upgrade. As we can see, a project which started as a simple model turned into a complex project due to scope creep, identification of decision variables and changes related to level of complexity.

Finally, the amount of complexity is directly related to the precision of the results: the more details, the more precise is the simulation results.

If the working group does not have participation from the right subject matter experts, the simulation may be incomplete, may be missing important processes or may not be able to perform verification and validation. Also, the working group may be estimating times, cost or other parameter or variable which readily available data is present but the subject matter expert was not part of the group. Finally, these experts can provide inside information on processes or procedures that are not relevant or necessary to model, thus saving time and money.

Simulation modeling will be an extremely difficult task if the working group cannot attain buy-in from the process owner or project requestor. This buy-in is a must in order to successfully accomplish the task at hand. The owner or requestor plays an important role as the process gatekeeper as well as the contact for internal subject matter experts.

As mentioned above in regards to subject matter experts, the analyst may be spending excessive amount of time replicating processes which do not affect the overall model's goal or scope. If the analyst does not have a process subject matter expert or is not knowledgeable of the system, he may be trying to replicate processes in details which could have been replicated in a simplistic approach. For instance, if the analyst is only concerned with the room utilization of a pediatric nursing unit, does he needs to replicate in detail the nurse's and doctor's activities or a simple delay to account for that time suffice? In some cases a simple delay is enough thus saving time during model building and as well during verification and validation phases.

An engineer was tasked with developing a simulation project, in a southern city hospital, in which a GI Endoscopy suite was analyzed for room utilization. The working group consisted of the department manager, lead nurse, financial analyst and the engineer. When the project was presented to management, the medical staff complaint that they were not involved and that their input was not estimated correctly. This project failed to gain traction and was scratched. This is an example why is important to have subject matter experts involved from the conception and having buy-in from all stakeholders.

Another pitfall to avoid during simulation modeling is incorrectly analyzing the data collected during the data collection and analysis step. This circumstance happens when the collected data is either incorrect or is corrupted.

Corruption happens when data is erroneously transcribed or entered in a database system. These conditions convey inaccurate values for analysis. Careful and detailed analysis of raw data looking for *outliers* shall help the analyst on future statistical analysis. For instance, running the initial data by a commercial statistical analysis package and using distribution fitting capabilities. The analyst will see a graphical representation of the analyzed data and can visually infer the goodness of fit. If the graphical representation or the goodness of fit is not intuitively right, the analyst should proceed to analyze individual data points.

When analyzing individual data points, the analyst should understand where this data does fits on the overall process. For example, consider raw data from a database system where emergency department's nursing triage time has been captured. There are over ten thousand (10,000) data points. The analyst runs the initial data by a commercial statistical analysis package and uses its distribution fitting capabilities. The resulting graph shows a skewed beta distribution with a high peak around the lower bound and then smoothly progresses towards a bell shape. The goodness of fit is in the low seventy percent (70%).

The analyst thinks that there may be some outliers. He confers with the working group's subject matter expert and comes to conclusion that triage time's lower bound is in the vicinity of 4 minutes. When carefully reviewing the raw data, the analyst finds that there are three hundred-fifty eight (358) points that ranges between zero and just under four minutes. The analyst can adjust the data and eliminate those outliers without compromising data integrity. After doing so, the analyst runs again the data by a commercial statistical analysis package and notices that the distribution's goodness of fit increased to ninety-two percent (92%). Now the data will closely resemble actual conditions.

The most worrying of all pitfalls delineated in this chapter is not being able to validate the simulation model. Without validation, the simulation model is useless. During this step the close involvement of subject matter experts will be beneficial for a successful validation. They are the key for validation because these experts will confirm all assumptions and will help with the replication of actual conditions. Also, as mentioned above, data analysis with high goodness of fit characteristics will result in a higher probability of validation.

Which Simulation Modeling Methods to Use?

Which simulation modeling methods should the analyst use? There is no magic test to determine which method to use. The analyst, in conjunction with the working group, should determine how much details are needed when developing the simulation model. As stated above, the modeling methods vary from simple to complex. Choosing the right method is a balance between details, time allotted and cost, definition of problem and project scope.

A case in point of a simple model is when developing a labor and delivery unit. Pregnant women enter and leave hospitals 24 hours a day throughout the year. So, the analyst for this model have to consider the day, the time and the method of arrival, the degrees of emergency, the alternative placement, and the staff availability. If the project scope is to determine if there is a need to expand the unit (number of labor rooms) then simplifying the model by not replicating fully

Figure 3.

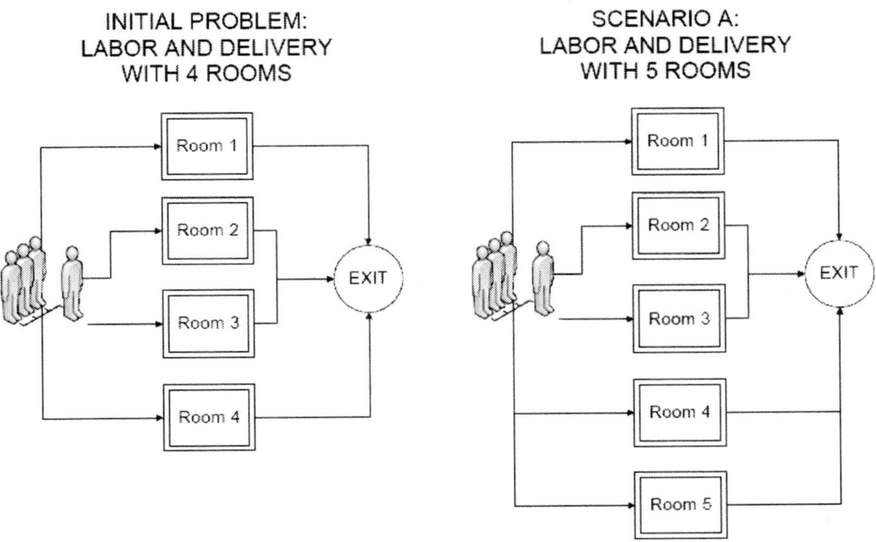

detailed staff activity but by merely using delays will save the analyst substantial development time. Figure 3 shows a simple labor and delivery unit model where minimum details have been used to simulate a clear-cut project scope. This simple model shows an entry point for patients, four delivery rooms and an exit point. There are two main variables: number of patients and time spent on system. Under scenario A the model has been increased to five rooms to determine if this addition will help decongestion in the system. A similar model was used by a southern hospital to determine if they could absorb the workload of a competitor's hospital when it decided to close its doors.

For instance, if the simulation modeling group has been tasked with determining the optimal number of beds for a pediatric nursing unit and the possibility of reconfiguring some of the beds as an intermediate intensive care unit, the group may be able to lessen the simulation development time by reducing the details modeled. One way of doing this is to avoid simulating nursing and medical tasks performed on each room as well as day-to-day ancillary operations. This same process can be modeled by using a grouping delay process in lieu of modeling these resources independently.

There are some cases where additional details must be modeled. In a reception area for a hospital's radiological services department there is a need to model incoming and outgoing phone calls as well as visitors who may be lost and need guidance to locate stairways or elevators. Also, this model includes the CT-scan process and how the reception is influenced by these external factors. This model's development level is moderate to complex. Figure 4 illustrates how upgrading equipment will influence interdependencies among areas.

This simulation model shows that outpatients arrive at the radiology department by means or the elevator or stairways (upper center area identified by the numeral "1"). These patients proceed to the registration desk (upper left quadrant identified as "2") and then proceed to be seated at the waiting area. They wait until called and proceed to an evaluation room (identified as "3"). After the evaluation is performed, the patient moves to the preparation room (center-left quadrant, iden-

Figure 4.

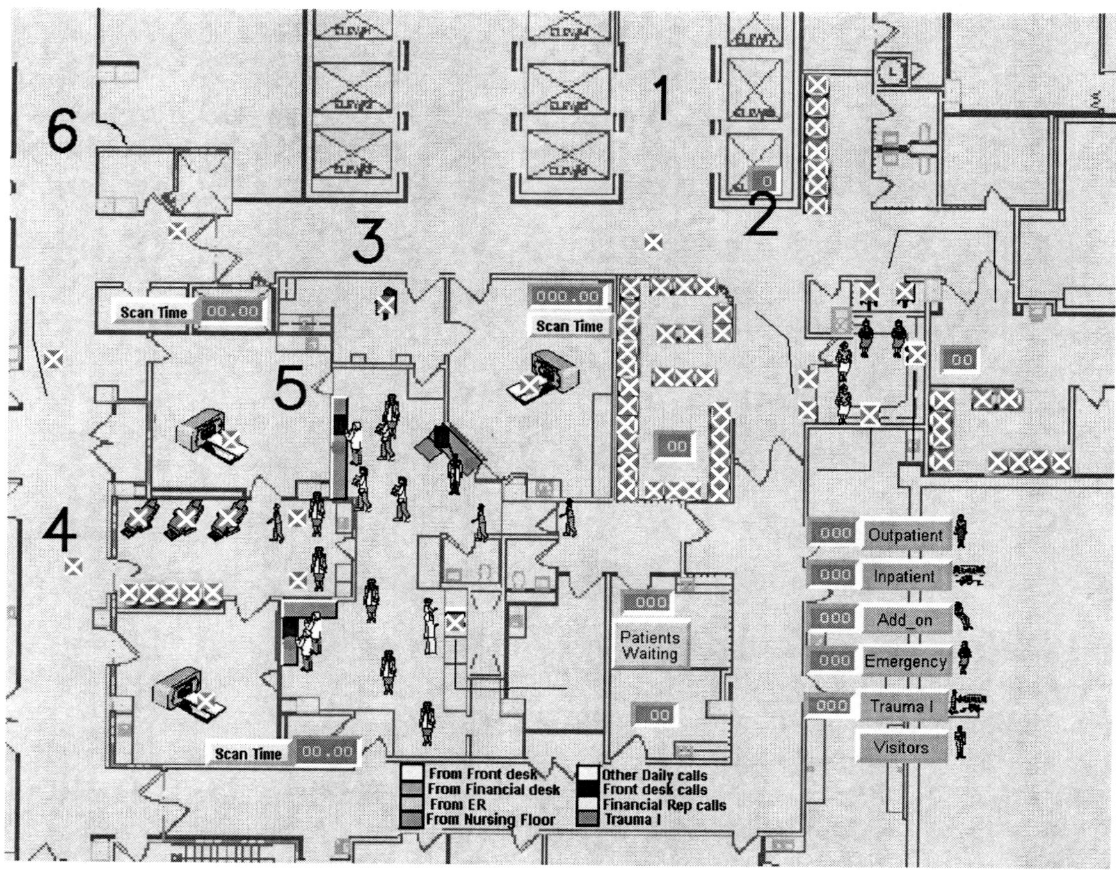

tified as "4") where the patient may receive a contrast solution (for radiological purposes). Finally, the outpatient will proceed to one of the 3 CT-Scan machines (center quadrant, identified as "5".

Some of the factors influencing this process are emergency or trauma patients, with higher priority for service, arriving to the department, straight to a CT scanner, from the hall identified as "6" (upper left quadrant), and inpatients arriving from the elevators (upper center quadrant, identified by "1").

Also, visitors arrive to the front desk (numeral "2") asking for directions and outpatients discussing financial decisions with hospital representatives create a complex system due to increased capacity generated by an upgrade in one of the CT scanners. CT scanning times, due to upgrade on one machine, were reduced by 50% causing an increase in room utilization.

Other complex simulation modeling cases involve details such as absenteeism, multipart work schedules, phone calls, and ancillary services, for instance laboratory test, radiology tests or physical therapy.

An illustration of a complex simulation model is when the analyst is required to model an emergency department staffing and process improvement study. This project requires the modeling of nurses, doctors, transportation staff, rehabilitation therapists, laboratory, x-rays, and many other activities such as triage, minor care,

Figure 5.

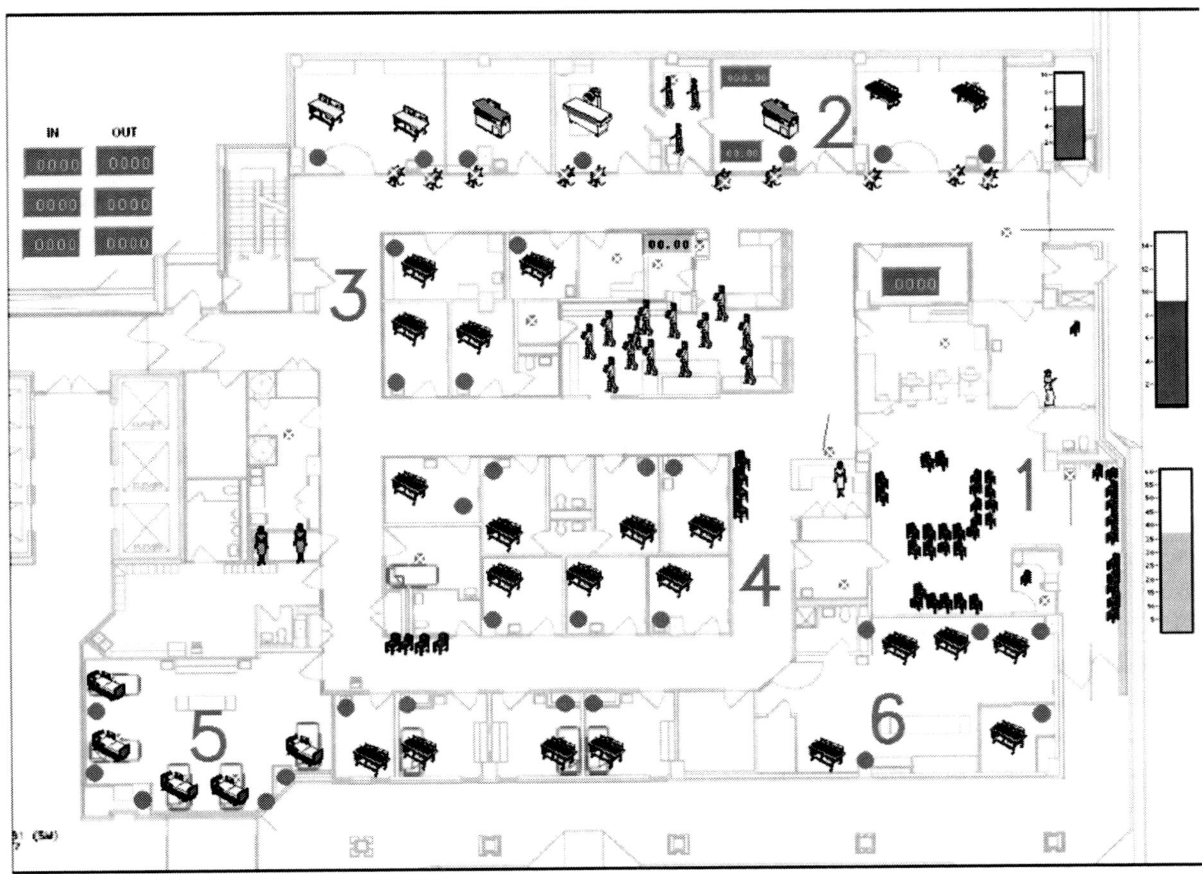

medicine and surgical cases, trauma and even labor and delivery situations. Additional details of this complex system are discussed under the section "When to use simulation modeling?" Figure 5 shows a snapshot of a complex model – a hospital's emergency department.

This model depicts the flow of a patient when arrives at the emergency department. Minor care, pediatric and walk-ins arrive to the main waiting area (right-center quadrant, identified by "1"). They proceed to check-in. If the triage nurse is not busy, patients proceed to triage area (north of waiting area). If triage is not available, the patient waits. Depending on patient acuity and bed availability, the triage nurse takes the patient to trauma/surgery rooms (upper quadrants, identified by "2"), medicine (areas "3" and "4"), minor care (area "5") or pediatrics (area "6").

Ambulance patients arrive through the upper right doors and helo-trauma patients arrive through the center-left quadrant's double doors. Ambulance patients may go to any of the five areas described above. Trauma patients are treated solely in area number 2. Having three methods of arrival (walk-in, ambulance and helo-trauma) and 5 patient classifications (trauma, surgical, medicine, pediatric, and minor care), which in simulation are called patient attributes, compounds the modeling.

Also, this model was developed to replicate the following processes (attributes): portable radiology or transport to radiology department, laboratory samples sent for testing by pneumatic tube or by courier, transport to CT scan area, consults by specialists, nursing assessments, medical doctor assessments, physician assistant and/or resident assessments and bedside patient registration.

As the reader can see, simulating an emergency department, with all possible patients attribute combinations, is a complex and time consuming process. A model of this magnitude will consume extensive hours during model building and validation phases.

When Not to Use Simulation Modeling?

After reading so far, the analyst may be formulating the following question: when is it not good to use dynamic simulation modeling? An answer to the question of when is not good to use simulation modeling is as follow:

If the simulation working group defines a problem and the project scope determines that the need is not related with observing behavior over a period of time, do not use discrete-event simulation modeling. Simulation modeling is a magnificent analysis method if the analyst requires analyzing a system's behavior over time.

If the working group defines a problem and the project scope shows that a possible path towards a solution may be for a single time period or situation, do not use dynamic simulation modeling. For instance, if the hospital's laundry facility receives soiled linen every morning at 8:00 AM, it will be easier to use an alternate method to determine the load size distribution. This is a good example for using Monte Carlo Simulation discussed in the following section.

The most significant factor for not using dynamic simulation modeling is if the working team has cost or time constraints. For instance, if management is requiring a solution in a period of time from 24 hours to one week, it is better to find alternative methods other than dynamic simulation modeling except if the problem is simple and a quick verifiable and validated model can be developed with such short notice.

What Alternatives are Available?

In some instances simulation modeling is not the best method to solve a problem. This section will cover other methods that can be used in lieu of dynamic simulation modeling. If time is of essence and the formulated problem is simple, the analyst can use Monte Carlo simulation, which is a static simulation modeling method. Lee and Matzo (1998) elaborate the use of Monte Carlo simulation on an evaluation of process capability. If the analyst does not have available a commercial simulation software, he may be able to pursue analyzing the formulated problem by means of spreadsheets. Hillier and Lieberman (2000, p.1115) formulate a process in which simple models can be solve by means of spreadsheets. A step-by-step approach is presented with several examples demonstrating this alternative.

Another approach is to use commercial project management software. This method is useful when simulating transportation matrices. Using the Gantt chart view, the analyst models activities on each line, links to preceding activities and then generates activity times with Monte Carlo simulation data or other random generation applications.

Finally, there are other alternatives available in the operation research arena such as linear programming, non-linear programming, game theory, Markov chains and queuing theory. Matthews (2005) employed Linear Programming (LP) in order to determine the effective combination of nurses that would allow for a weekly clinic tasks to be covered while providing the lowest possible cost to the department. By using LP, Matthews demonstrated a reduction of annual staffing costs by 16%. This was accomplished by forcing each level of nurse to be optimally productive by focusing on tasks specific to their expertise. Matthews suggests that LP can be used to solve capacity problems for just about any staffing situation as long as the model is linear.

Anand (2003) contends that non-linear programming can be used to operationalize the integration of claims framework rules to healthcare rationing, though the justifications may not be universally acceptable, concluding that the integration of claims provides a viable framework for modeling healthcare rationing.

Tarrant, Stokes and Colman (2004) have used Game Theory to model the medical consultation process. They agree that the consultation process is an interactive decision process between the doctor and patient. With this in mind, they argue that doctors and patients have identifiable goals and aspirations, and this makes game theoretic models potentially relevant. They concluded that game theory can provide the basis for empirically testable models of the patient-doctor interactions.

Liu, Wang and Guh (1991) used a Markov Chain model to describe the dynamic behavior of the age of medical records associated with patient's visits and provided a method for the long-term planning of record storage facilities based on an optimal disposal and classification policy.

What Data?

Early in the simulation development process, the analyst needs to collect data and analyze it. Sometimes data are not reliable or not readily available. Then, what should the engineer do when confronted with lack of *reliable data*? There are a number of alternatives to overcome this situation.

First, the analyst needs data in order to start the development process. These data may be tied to volume or time factors. If the analyst needs volume data the source can be the subject matter expert involved with forecasting or planning data. This expert can provide expected or forecasted volume.

If the missing or unreliable data are in regards to time, the analyst may be able to interview the process owner or process subject matter expert and estimate these times. The estimated times are valid during the development phase and the analyst should have a data collection method in place to validate these assumptions.

These estimated times should be collected including a minimum, most likely and maximum values. When encountered with similar values, most analysts tend to use a triangular distribution. The author suggests that in lieu of triangular distribution, the analyst should use a commercially available statistical distribution modeler and reproduce these parameters using a bell-shaped distribution such as a beta distribution. When using a triangular distribution to replicate times, it leaves out data points due to its linear shape. Bell shape distributions are better suited for time series. Figure 6 depicts a triangular distribution with minimum value of four (4), most likely at eight (8) and maximum value at fifteen (15). Figure 7 depicts same values using a beta distribution. Note that both distributions' statistical characteristics are within expectations.

Another method to estimate initial parameters close to their true values is called Structured Estimating Technique. Medved (1994) developed a structured estimating technique so as to provide results which are extremely close to real observed times. Cook and Perez (2003) used a variation of this approach to determine discharge planning activity times for case managers and resource managers. Also, Ryan (2007, p. 133) formulates that the analyst can estimate parameters without data. If the analyst knows the minimum and maximum values, he can estimate the variance. Now, with three (3) parameters, the analyst can use a commercially available statistical distribution modeler and estimate a bell-shaped distribution.

Finally, in the case that the analyst is not developing a dynamic simulation model with the aid of a program, and the estimated parameters' lower bound is or approximates zero (0) a random number generator will be of great assistance. Dean and Voss (1999, p. 4) propose a computer program to generate random numbers since "without the

Figure 6.

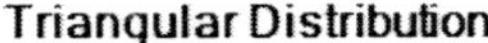

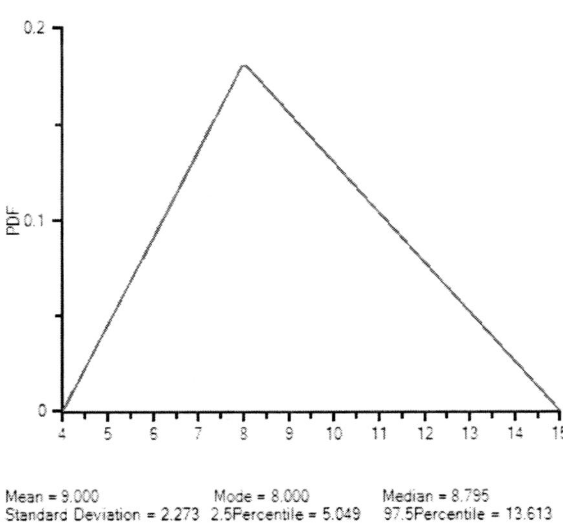

Figure 7.

Beta Distribution

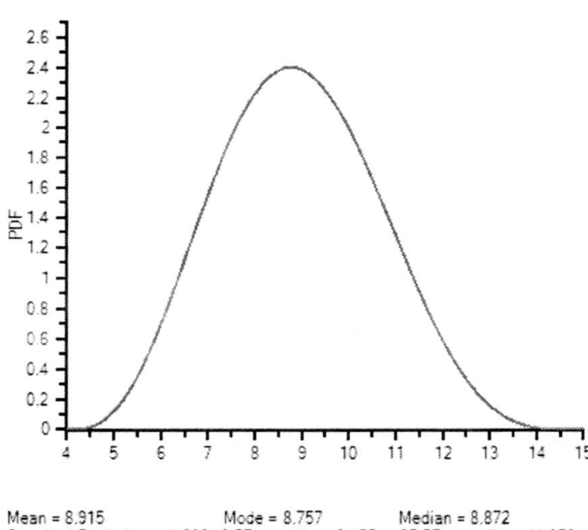

aid of an objective randomizing device, it is not possible for an experimenter to make a random assignment." One of the most desired effects during the development of a dynamic or static simulation is to have random and non-skewed input values in order to get realistic results.

MODEL AND RESULTS PRESENTATION

One of the most important steps of simulation modeling development is presenting the model and results obtained. The author's has observed affirmative response when using a commercial simulation program which uses animation to replicate the system. Process owners, subject matter experts, managers and corporate executives have a tendency to support simulation analysis when able to visually understand cause-and-effect of are recommended alternative processes.

The author presented a complex simulation model of the Emergency Department (ED) to the hospital board members showing various "what-if" scenarios regarding staffing levels. He presented the execution of the model, where several visual indicators were embedded showing location status, to show how various staffing levels affected ED crowding and staff / room utilization. By the time the result tables were presented, the management group was able to understand and buy-in into the final recommendations.

Model and results presentation is extremely important for applied settings and particularly for healthcare. Not only in healthcare but on other sectors as well, an appropriate presentation of the model as well as results can make or break a simulation study.

When presenting results, the analyst wants to present information in a fair and unbiased manner. Information integrity requires that a graphical representation must not show data out of context, and should make important comparisons both visually prominent, and on an equitable basis, all other things should be kept equal.

Tufte (1983) presents a case, Figures 8 and 9, where data is shown out of context presenting a before-and-after comparison of traffic speeding enforcement. The first graph, Figure 8, shows a sharp decline in traffic fatalities from 1955 to 1956. But when a longer period of tabulated data, from 1951 to 1959 (Figure 9), is graphed it shows that there is no sharp decline in fatalities. Instead, it shows a gradual increase in the number of fatalities followed by a gradual decline. This example shows the importance of presenting correct results and in context that can translate to healthcare simulation modeling.

Finally, Wainer, Ryan, and Dean and Voss encourage the analyst to present simulation results using a variety of visually appealing graphical tools for easier comprehension. Straight, to the point, clear and concise presentation of the model and simulation results will surely help the analyst "selling" his recommendations when the time comes. Also, Zelman, Glick and Blackmore agree that "animated-simulation tools offer two major advantages over spreadsheets: they allow clinicians to interact more easily with the costing model so that it more closely represents the process being modeled, and they represent cost output as a cost range rather than as a single cost estimate thereby providing more useful information or decision making". Being able to present interactively the model and results will definitely help the analyst with convincing his superiors of the value of a simulation model.

FUTURE DIRECTION

We see the future of simulation modeling as one with great opportunities in drag-and-drop software applications using random paths, better graphics, and three-dimensional models capable of replicating the real world similar to what can be seen in console games.

Right now the majority of simulation software applications use the tried-and-true method of linear paths for entity or resource movement. Future applications will use an array of paths or move within delineated areas instead of linear paths. This method will replicate human behavior closer to reality.

With the advances in computer processing capabilities and increased memory capacity, we

Figure 8.

Graphics must not quote data out of context.

Nearly all the important questions are left unanswered by this display:

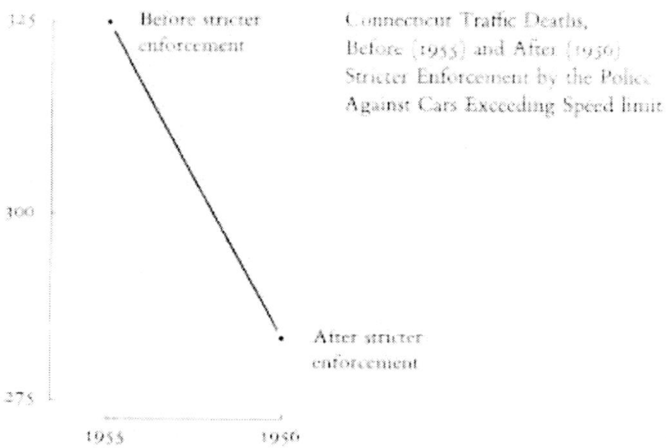

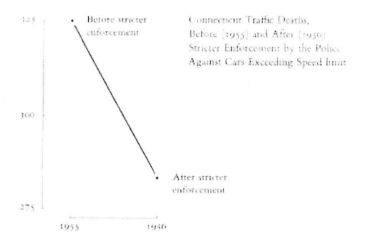

Figure 9.

A few more data points add immensely to the account:

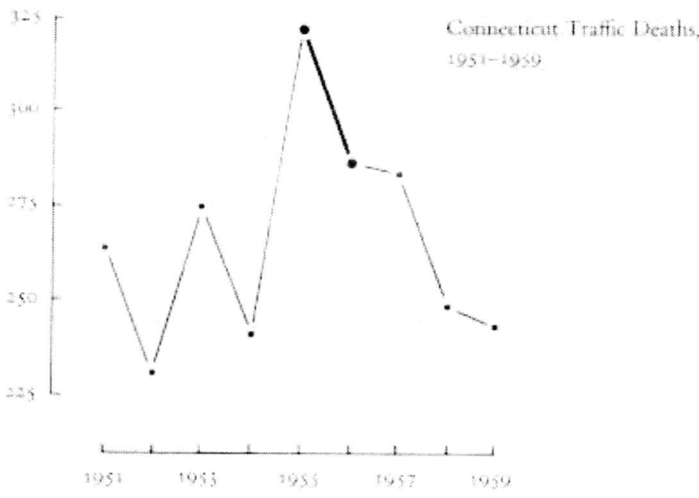

see a leap in computer graphics on simulation software where other applications, such as AutoCad®, Adobe Photoshop®, SketchUp®, will easily merge with simulation software to provide crystal clear graphics. Also, three-dimensional representations will closely resemble current video game consoles. The video gaming industry is the top developer of graphic interface.

Finally, as for software future developments, we see drag-and-drop software applications where the analyst drops icons, paths and other attributes, and add minimal data and the model replicates the system. These characteristics will help novice developers better understand simulation modeling, be more user-friendly, will dramatically shorten development time, and will have an easier and straight-forward method when designing models.

As for other areas, such as data collection, computer interface and hardware, Coles mentions the "recent improvements in the utility of video, time recording of use distribution data, and the ability to download data remotely". Advances in Radio Frequency Identification (RFID) data collection will help the analyst collect real-time data that can interface with the model to provide highly accurate data values. This type of data collection and interface allows the developer to devote more time to simulation concept development as well as model development instead of spending valuable time collecting data. Further development of these technologies will increase the cost effectiveness of model development.

Simulation modeling literature illustrates many models in the most common areas such as emergency department, radiology, material management, nursing units and other patient areas. We see a future direction of simulation modeling in support areas such as finance, human resources as well as at the macro corporate level.

Along these lines, Pitt argues that "future work aims to explore a number of areas within strategic healthcare management which may be accessible to this approach. Of particular interest are changes in the delivery and organization of rehabilitation and intensive care, increased flexibility of resource use, management of waiting lists, emergency contingency planning, and the growing trend towards community care away from institutionalized services".

Healthcare is ripe with many situations where simulation is a great tool to approach optimal solutions to its problems. In order to arrive at Pitt's conclusion, we see a big push by simulation developers educating healthcare practitioner and administrators on how powerful simulation modeling is for the decision-making process. This process must start by researching simulation literature and finding case studies that may apply to their own healthcare system. Formal or informal presentation, to administrator and practitioners alike, of these cases should follow to "sell" the need of simulation modeling in a healthcare environment.

CONCLUSION

This chapter presented an introduction to simulation and its definition, defined the steps necessary for a good and sound simulation and answered common questions asked by many novice simulation practitioners.

The author, using his experience while modeling many healthcare systems, provided insight to questions such as why an analyst should use simulation modeling, when it is appropriate and who should be part of the simulation modeling team.

The chapter also covers common mistakes or pitfalls when using simulation modeling as well as what other alternatives are available when the analyst cannot use simulation modeling. Another area discussed on this chapter is what to do when there is lack of reliable data. Furthermore, the author conferred the importance of presenting simulation execution and analyzed data by means of visually appealing aids.

Finally, the author presents his opinion in regards to the future direction of simulation modeling and the belief that this area of study will advance by leaps and bounds into the upper boundaries of the graphic interface seen in the video gaming industry. Also, the author references to advances in technology that will impact the future of simulation modeling in healthcare.

REFERENCES

Anand, P. (2003). The integration of claims to healthcare: A programming approach. *Journal of Health Economics*, *22*(5), 731–745. doi:10.1016/S0167-6296(03)00024-9

Banks, J., & Carson, J. S. II. (1984). *Discrete events smulation*. Englewoods Cliffs, NJ: Prentice Hall, Inc.

Cole, D. N. (comp). (2005). *Computer simulation modeling of recreation use: Current status, case studies, and future directions*. (Gen. Tech. Rep. RMRS-GTR-143). Fort Collins, CO: US Department of Agriculture, Forest Service, Rocky Mountain Research Station.

Cook, C., & Perez, R. (2003). A management engineering approach to improving throughput and shortening overall LOS: A unique model for efficiency and time studies. *Collaborative Case Management – The Official Publication of the American Case Management Association. 1*(4).

Dean, A., & Voss, D. (1999). *Design and analysis of experiments*. New York, NY: Springer-Verlag, Inc.doi:10.1007/b97673

Hall, R. W. (Ed.). (2006). *Patient flow: Reducing delay in healthcare delivery*. Los Angeles, CA: Springer.

Hillier, F. S., & Lieberman, G. J. (Eds.). (2000). *Introduction to operation research*. New York, NY: McGraw-Hill Companies, Inc.

Kolb, E. M. W., Schoening, S., Peck, J., & Lee, T. (2008). Reducing emergency department overcrowding: Five patient buffer concepts in comparison. *Proceedings of the 40th Conference on Winter Simulation*, December 07-10, 2008, Miami, Florida.

Lee, C., & Matzo, G. A. D. (1998). An evaluation of process capability for a fuel injector process using Monte Carlo simulation. In R. Peck, L. D. Haugh, & A. Goodman (Eds.), *Statistical case studies: A collaboration between academe and industry*. Philadelphia, PA: Society for Industrial and Applied Mathematics/ Virginia: American Statistical Association.

Liu, C.-M., Wang, K.-M., & Guh, Y.-Y. (1991). A Markov chain model for medical record analysis. *The Journal of the Operational Research Society*, *42*(5), 357–364.

Matthews, C. H. (2005). Using Linear programming to minimize the cost of nurse personnel. *Journal of Health Care Finance*, *32*(1), 37–49.

Medved, C. K. (1994, February). *Staffing and labor cost analysis using structured estimating techniques*. Paper presented at the Health Information Management Systems Society, Phoenix, Arizona.

Pitt, M. (1997). A generalised simulation system to support strategic resource planning in healthcare. In S. Andradóttir, K. J. Healy, D. H. Withers, & B. L. Nelson (Eds.), *Proceedings of the 1997 Winter Simulation Conference*.

Ryan, T. P. (2007). *Modern engineering statistics*. Hoboken, NJ: John Wiley and Sons, Inc. doi:10.1002/9780470128442

Tarrant, C., Stokes, T., & Colman, A. M. (2004). Models of the medical consultation: Opportunities and limitations of a game theory perspective. *Quality Safety in Health Care Journal*, *13*, 461–466. doi:10.1136/qshc.2003.008417

Tufte, E. (1983). *The visual display of quantitative information*. Cheshire, CT: Graphics Press.

Ulgen, O. M., & Williams, E. J. (2001). Simulation modeling and analysis. In Zandin, K. B. (Ed.), *Maynard's industrial engineering handbook*. New York, NY: McGraw-Hill Companies, Inc.

Wainer, G. A. (Ed.). (2009). *Discrete-event modeling and simulation: A practitioner approach*. Boca Raton, FL: CRC Press, Taylor and Francis Group.

Zandin, K. B. (Ed.). (2001). *Maynard's industrial engineering handbook*. New York, NY: McGraw-Hill Companies, Inc.

Zelman, W.N., Glick, N. D., & Blackmore, C. C. (2001). Animated-simulation modeling facilitates clinical-process costing - Healthcare organizations finance department use new software. *Healthcare Financial Management, September*.

ADDITIONAL READING

Banks, J. (Ed.). (1998). *Handbook of Simulation: Principles, Methodology, Advances, Applications, and Practice. New Jersey: John Wiley and Sons, Inc. and Norcross*. Georgia: Industrial Engineering, & Management Press.

De Chiara, J., Panero, J., & Zelnik, M. (1991). *Time – saver Standards for Interior Design and Space Planning*. New York, New York: McGraw-Hill Companies, Inc.

Good, P. I., & Hardin, J. W. (2003). *Common errors in Statistics (And How to Avoid Them)*. Hoboken, New Jersey: John Wiley and Sons, Inc. doi:10.1002/0471463760

Grunden, N. (2008). *The Pittsburgh Way to Efficient Healthcare: Improving Patient Care Using Toyota Based Methods*. New York: Productivity Press.

Guerrero, H. (2010). Excel Data Analysis – modeling and Simulation. Berlin, Heilderberg: Springer-Verlag.

Jun, J., Jacobson, S., & Swisher, J. (1999). Application of discrete-event simulation in health care clinics: a survey. *The Journal of the Operational Research Society*, *50*, 109–123.

Law, A. M., & Kelton, W. D. (2000). *Simulation Modeling and Analysis*. Boston, Massachusetts: McGraw-Hill Companies, Inc.

Leemis, L. M., & Park, S. K. (2005). *Discrete-events Simulation: A First Course*. Upper Saddle River, New Jersey: Prentice Hall, Inc.

Montgomery, D. C., Runger, G. C., & Nairn, A. G. (2002). *Applied Statistics and Probability for Engineers*. New York, New York: John Wiley and Sons, Inc.

O'Donnell, J. M., & Goode, J. S. Jr. (2008). Simulation in Nursing Education and practice. In Riley, R. (Ed.), *Manual of Simulation in Healthcare*. Oxford: Oxford University Press.

Perez-Velez. Roque (2005, February) *Improving CT Scan Throughput Using Process Improvement, Analysis and Simulation Methodologies.* Paper presented at the Society for Health Systems Management Engineering Forum. Dallas, Texas.

Tufte, E. R. (2001). *The Visual Display of Quantitative Information* (2nd ed.). Cheshire, Connecticut: Graphics Press.

Tukey, J. W. (1977). *Exploratory Data Analysis*. Reading, Massachusetts: Addison-Wesley, Inc.

Zeigler B.P., Praehofer, H. & kim, T.G. (2000) *Theory of Modeling and Simulation*. New York, New York: Academic Press.

KEY TERMS AND DEFINITIONS

Dynamic Simulation: The recreation of a period of time of the real world: For example: recreating what happened during the last year at the radiology department.

Events: System changes related to cause-and-effect when variables change status or value.

Outliers: Data point outside the +/- 3 δ (sigma) limits of a bell-shape statistical distribution.

Parameters: Simulation factors that are non-controllable which define important elements needed for replicating the system.

Reliable Data: Readily available data which does not have outliers or has been corrupted by any means.

Simulation: The recreation of the real world, in terms of variables and parameters, in order to replicate its behavior and study its performance.

Simulation Modeling: The organized process, in which the analyst plans, develops, executes and analyzes the simulation.

Static Simulation: The recreation of a specific moment of the real world. For example: recreating what happened at 6:00 PM on a Wednesday at the laboratory.

Subject Matter Experts: Is a person who is extremely knowledgeable on a specific topic or work area. The level of expertise is related to educational level, work experience and degree of involvement on the area of study.

Variables: Simulation factors which are controllable and the analyst can modify in order to observe cause-and-effect situations in the system.

Chapter 5
Modeling Clinical Engineering Activities to Support Healthcare Technology Management

Laura Gaetano
Politecnico di Torino, Italy

Daniele Puppato
AReSS Piemonte, Italy

Gabriella Balestra
Politecnico di Torino, Italy

ABSTRACT

Biomedical technology is a valuable asset of healthcare facilities. It is now universally accepted that, to assure patient safety, medical devices must be correctly managed and used, and that the quality of healthcare delivery is related to the suitability of the available technology. The activities that guarantee a proper management are carried out by the people working in a Clinical Engineering (CE) department.

In the chapter we describe a model to estimate the number of clinical engineers and biomedical equipment technicians (BMET) that will constitute the Clinical Engineering department staff. The model is based on the activities to be simulated, the characteristics of the healthcare facility, and the experience of human resources. Our model is an important tool to be used to start a Clinical Engineering department or to evaluate the performances of an existing one. It was used by managers of Regione Piemonte to start a regional network of Clinical Engineering departments.

DOI: 10.4018/978-1-60960-872-9.ch005

INTRODUCTION

Biomedical technology is strategically important to the operational effectiveness of healthcare facilities. During the middle of the 60s technology started to spread inside the hospitals. The instruments were definitively simpler than today but their ability to auto-detect failures was small and the problem of their management was mostly concerned with electrical safety or fixing. In the last fifty years the performances and the potentialities of technology increased dramatically and this change significantly affected biomedical instrumentation. Medical devices became more sophisticated and safer, but the number of devices increased significantly. Testing electrical safety turned into one of the activities, and the principal problems became to correctly manage the devices maintenance, to purchase the most suitable instrument, to plan device substitutions, to ensure the correct functioning of the instruments, and to guarantee the availability of critical devices every time they are needed. It is now universally accepted that to assure patient safety medical devices must be correctly managed and used, and that the quality of healthcare delivery is related to the suitability of the available technology.

The activities related to both technology management and to support physicians and nurses to properly use the devices are carried on by clinical engineers and biomedical technicians, usually employed in Clinical Engineering Department. When a new Clinical engineering department must be established, the healthcare managers must decide the staff composition. In the past, they used to decide the personnel taking into account only the number of beds. With the growing differences among medical devices that are associated to the complexity of the clinical activities this rule is not appropriate. Several more indicators must be taken into account to ensure that the Clinical engineering department has the proper staff.

In our chapter we will describe a model to be used to estimate the number of clinical engineers and biomedical equipment technicians (BMET) that will constitute the Clinical engineering department staff. A simulation model was chosen because we wanted to guarantee not only that the number of working hours needed to perform all the activities was available, but also to guarantee customer satisfaction, meaning that customers will have a quick and right answer to their demands.

BACKGROUND

The Italian National Health Service (NHS) follows a model similar to one developed by the British National Health Service since it provides universal health care coverage throughout the Italian State as a single payer. However, the Italian NHS is more decentralized, because it gives political, administrative, and financial responsibility regarding the provision of health care to the twenty regions (Maio and Manzoli, 2002). Each region must organize its services in order to meet the needs of its population, define ways to allocate financial resources to all the Local Health Agencies (LHAs) within its territory, monitor LHAs' health care services and activities, and assess their performance. In addition, the regions are responsible for selecting and accrediting public and private health services providers and issuing regional guidelines to assure a set of essential healthcare services in accordance with national laws.

The LHAs form the basic elements of the Italian NHS. In addition, in 2000, there were ninety eight public hospitals qualified as "hospital trusts." Hospital trusts work as independent providers of health services and have the same level of administrative responsibility as LHA. Based on criteria of efficiency and cost–quality, the LHAs might provide care either directly, through their own facilities (directly managed hospitals and territorial services), or by paying for the services delivered by providers accredited by the regions, such as independent public structures (hospital agencies and university-managed hospitals) and private structures (hospitals, nursing homes, and laboratories under contract to the NHS).

Each LHA has three main facilities: one department for preventive health care, one or more directly managed hospitals, and one or more districts. Through the districts, the LHAs provide primary care, ambulatory care, home care, occupational health services, health education, disease prevention, pharmacies, family planning, child health and information services.

Both LHA and hospitals build most of their activities on technology, and require a Clinical engineering department to take care of healthcare technology management.

Today clinical engineering may be viewed as a complex system where different elements interact to allow correct healthcare technology management. The papers related to clinical engineering that can be found in literature may be divided into two groups.

The first group includes articles describing the role and the organization of a typical Clinical engineering department. At the beginning, clinical engineering was mainly concerned with the electrical safety of the instruments and the possibility of on-site repair of a damaged device. In the last twenty five years, people started referring to the clinical engineering activities as Healthcare Technology Management (HTM). This change of terminology is due to the fact that attention is now focused on the processes associated with technology management like acquisition, maintenance and so on, and it is greatly justified by the dramatic change of technology characteristics that affected the biomedical instrumentation and, in the last few years, the medical software. According to (David and Janhke, 2004) there are three forces that lead the change: costs, technology, and society expectation. The transition consists of three phases: goal identification, priority definition, and human resources allocation. The correct implementation of the three phases requires procedures able to reduce risks and costs. According to this framework the role of clinical engineering is to support and improve patients care by means of the application of engineering methods to the health technology management.

According to this point of view, we can define a clinical engineer as a professional who supports and advances patient care by applying engineering and management skills to healthcare technology (Grimes, 2003). Clinical engineering is generally considered a specialty of the biomedical engineering profession. Most of clinical engineers work in a hospital or other healthcare provider environment. They may be employed by the healthcare provider or may be an employee of an organization that supplies services to multiple healthcare facilities, and. they must have both technical knowledge and expertise on management procedures. The new vision of clinical engineering also modified the activities carried on by Clinical Engineering (CE) departments. More managerial responsibilities were asked to clinical engineers (Grimes, 2003).

In a Clinical engineering department, all the activities must be supported by a computerized maintenance management system. This system provides several functionalities like "technology inventory" management, preventive maintenance scheduling, work orders creations both automatically according to a schedule or manually, and a lot of data about maintenance history, downtime of a device, purchase orders, and much more.

Moreover, the organization of a Clinical engineering department must take into account the space distribution of the technology. A distributed management is the most appropriate in the current healthcare business environment (Christoffel, 2008). Another important aspect is that health organizations have different sizes and acuity levels, ranging from health clinics to community hospitals to major teaching hospitals. All these aspects impact the staff composition of the department.

The second group of papers is much more numerous and deals with specific activities like healthcare technology assessment (HTA), risk management, medical device software management.

The term HTA is used to designate a multidisciplinary field of policy analysis that studies the medical, social, ethical, and economic implications of development, diffusion, and use of health technology. In the HTA field the word technology has a broad meaning and it is used to indicate all methods applied by health professionals to promote health, prevent and treat disease and improve rehabilitation and long term care. It is a category of policy studies, intended to provide decision makers with information about the possible impacts and consequences of a new technology or a significant change in an old technology. It is concerned with both direct and indirect or secondary consequences, both benefits and disadvantages, and with mapping the uncertainties involved in any government or private use or transfer of a technology. HTA may help decision makers at different levels: from a macroeconomic point of view, by studying the implications that adopting a new technology may have on existing populations, economies, diseases, drugs, procedures, and devices; from a microeconomic point of view when a particular problem is handled, like the acquisition of an equipment.

Risk management (RS) in the healthcare context is a broad subject covering both clinical and non-clinical services. It can be described as the systematic identification, assessment, prioritization and reduction of risk to patients, staff and members of the healthcare facilities (Steele, 2002). The two major causes of clinical RS are drugs and medical instrumentations. Clinical engineers may help reduce the risks by carrying on educational activities, support medical staff in correctly using the equipments, and participating in the development of studies performed by interdisciplinary team to understand how to reduce risks and deploying their results.

Medical software is now frequently used directly for patient care. In this case the software is a medical device and must follow the regulation for medical devices. In this case clinical engineers must cooperate with IT professionals to have it working correctly.

These are activities that usually need people from different departments working together for a specific goal, usually require a specialization of the clinical engineer in that particular field, and are not standardized as the basic activities.

Modeling has been applied in the domain of healthcare both to assist clinical decision making for diagnosis, therapy and monitoring, and to support healthcare managers in facility location and planning, resource allocation, and organizational redesign. Especially the second group of problems benefits also of simulation to understand the consequences of a certain solution. There are three main reasons to choose simulation to analyze healthcare problems: healthcare systems are characterized by uncertainty and variability, healthcare organizations can be hugely complex, and the key role is played by human beings (Brailsford, 2007). Different methodologies are used according to the model objectives. Operational research methods have been successfully used to assist decision makers in analyzing and simulating healthcare organizations. Among the possible methodologies, most of the models are based either on Discrete Event Simulation (DES) or System dynamics (SD). DES represents the operations of a system as a sequence of events. Each event occurs at an instant in time and marks a change of state in the system. Usually the time is simulated by means of probability distributions. DES is widely adopted when the system consists mainly of queues. SD is a methodology for modeling and simulating complex systems, developed by Forrester (Forrester, 1961), based on the idea that the system behavior may be understood by means of the feedback concept, and that it is a function of the activities and interaction of its components. As a consequence, in SD models the system behavior is the result of the interaction of its feedback subsystems that represent its dynamic complexity. A key theme of SD is that policy interventions are diluted, and often fail because decision makers are not fully aware of the feedback structures (Duggan,2008). SD models are deterministic and can be used at a speculative and strategic level. A few mixed models based on both DES and SD may be found in literature (Brailsford, 2007). A new promising tool for modeling in the healthcare domain is Multi Agent System (MAS). Agent technology has become a leading area of research in Artificial Intelligence (AI) and computer science and the focus of a number of major initiatives (Moreno and Nealon, 2003) The features of intelligent agents are aimed at distributing the task of solving problems by allowing different software components to cooperate, each one with its own expertise (Annichiarico et al., 2008). The multiagent systems paradigm is an emerging and effective approach to tackling distributed problems, especially when data sources and knowledge are geographically located in different places and coordination and collaboration are necessary for decision making (Ji et al., 2007).

A multi-agent system offers a natural way of tackling distributed problems, where each agent is a "smart" software program that acts on behalf of human users to find and filter information, negotiate for services, automate complex tasks, and collaborate with other agents to solve complex problems. An important property of intelligent agents is their autonomy. Intelligent agents have a degree of control on their own actions, and under some circumstances, they are also able to make their own decisions, based on their knowledge and the information perceived from the outside environment (Padgham & Winikoff, 2004). Multi-agent systems are a good paradigm for those modeling applications in which each component wants to keep its independence and autonomy from the rest the system.

Another important issue when dealing with organizational problems is process modeling. Various diagrams have been developed and applied to assist the understanding of how people and resources interact to achieve outcomes during a process: different characteristics are modeled with different methods (diagram types) and several diagrams exist for the same characteristic. Methods are frequently supported by software tools. Methodologies were developed to support the user in deciding when to use which modeling method (Jun et al., 2009).

Among the methods used to modeling processes one that is widely used is workflow diagrams. The primary objective of a workflow system is to deal with situations. Similar situations belong to the same category, and usually are dealt with the same way. Moreover, each situation has a unique identity, a limited lifetime, and between its start and end, it always has a particular state. This state may be described by the values of the situation relevant attributes, the conditions that have been fulfilled, and its outcome. To see how far a situation has progressed we use conditions that are also used to determine which tasks have been carried out, and which still remain to be performed. In addition, a condition can be regarded as a requirement that must be met before a particular task may be carried out. Only once all the conditions for a task within a particular situation have been met, that task can be performed.

In general, the workflow system does not contain details about the specific content of the situation, only those of its attributes and conditions. By identifying the process activities and the tasks they consist of, it is possible to structure the workflow representing that process as a series of tasks. A task is a logical unit of work, it is indivisible and thus is always carried out in full. Under particular conditions a task may be skipped or more tasks may be carried out in parallel. A detailed description of workflow diagrams may be found in (van der Aalst and van Hee. 2004).

Among the possible way to represents workflow the most suitable are Petri nets (van der Aalst 1996; Jensen, 1996) that allow the definition of concurrent, asynchronous, distributed, parallel, non deterministic, and/or stochastic processes. Briefly, a Petri net is a directed, weighted, bipartite graph consisting of essentially two kinds of nodes, called places and transitions, and arcs that are either from a place to a transition or from a transition to a place. In the graphical representation, places are drawn as circles, while transitions as bars or boxes. In modelling, using the concept of conditions and events, places represent conditions and transitions represent events. A transition (an event) has a certain number of input and output places representing the preconditions and post-conditions of the event respectively. A marking (called state) assigns to each place a nonnegative integer. If a marking assigns to place p a nonnegative integer k, then p is marked with k tokens. The presence of a token in a place is interpreted as holding the truth of the condition associated with the place. In other words, k tokens are put in a place to indicate that k data items or resources are available. Moreover, some transitions are allowed only if specific conditions are met. These conditions can be represented as triggers of essentially three types: resource, external event or time signal.

THE CED MODEL

Description of the Clinical Engineering Department Activities Model

A model of the basic activities carried on in a typical Clinical engineering department was developed, validated, and applied to start a regional network of Clinical engineering departments. In the following we will refer to it as CED (Clinical Engineering Department) model. As reported in (Balestra et al., 2008) the CED model was essentially based on three elements: the characteristics of the healthcare facility, the activities to be simulated, and the staff expertise and roles. The basic idea was that number and type of required staff people was a function of both the number of the devices to be managed and the complexity of the clinical department of the healthcare facility.

Several parameters that contribute to the definition of the healthcare facility complexity were taken into account: number of hospital with Emergency Department (ED), number of clinical specialist units, number of university departments, number of high-risk devices or complex technologies, and the number of territorial units (hospital and districts). High risk devices are life supports, critical monitoring, energy emitting and other devices whose failure or misuse is reasonably likely to seriously injure patient or staff, while with complex technologies we denotes all the devices that require special set-up (such as for example Positron Emission Tomography) or specialized management procedures.

The number of the devices was described in details taking into account the total number of technologies owned by the facility, the number of technologies not covered by a full-risk maintenance contract,, the number of technologies in hospital with ED, the number of technologies in hospital without ED, and the number of devices used by territorial units.

To define the staff of a clinical engineering department we only considered clinical engineers (CE) and biomedical equipment technicians (BMET). At this stage, any specialization of CE or BMET was not considered. One of the aims was to dimension the staff composition, only in terms of numerousness of CE and BMET. The different specializations could be considered in the next step.

Concerning the activities that were simulated, only activities that were considered fundamental for a Clinical Engineering service were modelled. The basic or core activities were: department management, acquisition procedures, safety and preventive maintenance testing, critical technologies management, inventory management, investments planning, maintenance procedures and end-users training. A brief description of the activities modelled is provided in the following paragraphs.

The CE Department management includes all the organizing tasks necessary for supervising the clinical engineering department, such as the coordination of the staff, and it is performed essentially by the CE director.

The acquisition process consists of several steps starting from the definition of the specifications and ending when the device is installed in the clinical department. In answer to a public call, different companies send their offer. The offers are then evaluated, and the best is chosen. After the arrival of the new device, the BMET installs, tests the new device, and inserts it into the inventory. The end-users training is also scheduled if required.

The aim of preventive maintenance is to keep the safety and quality features of technologies during the entire period of their exercise. In so doing, the planning of safety and functional tests, done periodically according to the laws and technical standards, is mandatory. Also the end-users education is important in this context to avoid the malfunction of a device due to an incorrect use. The people responsible for this activity are both CE, for planning, and BMET, for the execution.

The Clinical engineering department must guarantee the continuous availability of devices defined as critical through the predisposition, update and application of a plan for finding a substitute of the device that is out of order as fast as possible and, in any case, to assure both patient safety and the healthcare essential activities. The clinical engineer has the responsibility of performing this activity.

The inventory management allows the staff to record all the data concerning a device from its insertion into the database to the dismissal: in particular, the technical characteristics, its location, and both preventive and corrective maintenance data. The BMET is responsible of these procedures.

The activity of investments planning, done by CE, deals essentially with a triennial, an annual and three-monthly planning to define the needs of the healthcare facility. Moreover, a monthly review is necessary to check the effective execution of the planning done so far. The investments could be necessary for substituting a technology, for improving the functionalities of an existing one, buying new components, or for acquiring new devices, never owned by the facility so far.

Finally, the corrective maintenance procedures are all the processes that regard the restoration of damaged technologies. This activity is usually performed by BMETs.

The main outputs of the CED simulation are the minimum number of people that must be involved in the staff to guarantee a certain level of service effectiveness, the workload of each kind of staff member in terms of hours, the overtime required for completing tasks, and the answering time to a specific request, i.e. the delays between the arrival of maintenance queries and their solution. Figure 1 shows a schematic representation of the model.

Description of the Management Processes

The first step performed to build the model was to characterize the processes going on in a typical Clinical engineering department with the aim of both describing the tasks that are part of a single process and underlining the connections between tasks and human resources. Among the possible methods that can be used to describe a process we selected workflow diagrams, and in particular the diagram proposed by (van der Aalst and van Hee. 2004) that is based on Petri nets.

It allows the description of different types of jobs or processes, where each process is constituted by a set of tasks that have to be completed following defined rules. One person or a group of people is identified as responsible for each specific task that constitutes the workflow. The diagram consists of transitions, shown as rectangles, and places, represented using a circle. Transitions represent the tasks performed during the process, while places represent the input and output of a

Figure 1. General description of the model. In the center there is the interface. The rectangles describe the input parameters and output variables. A description of them is reported in the text.

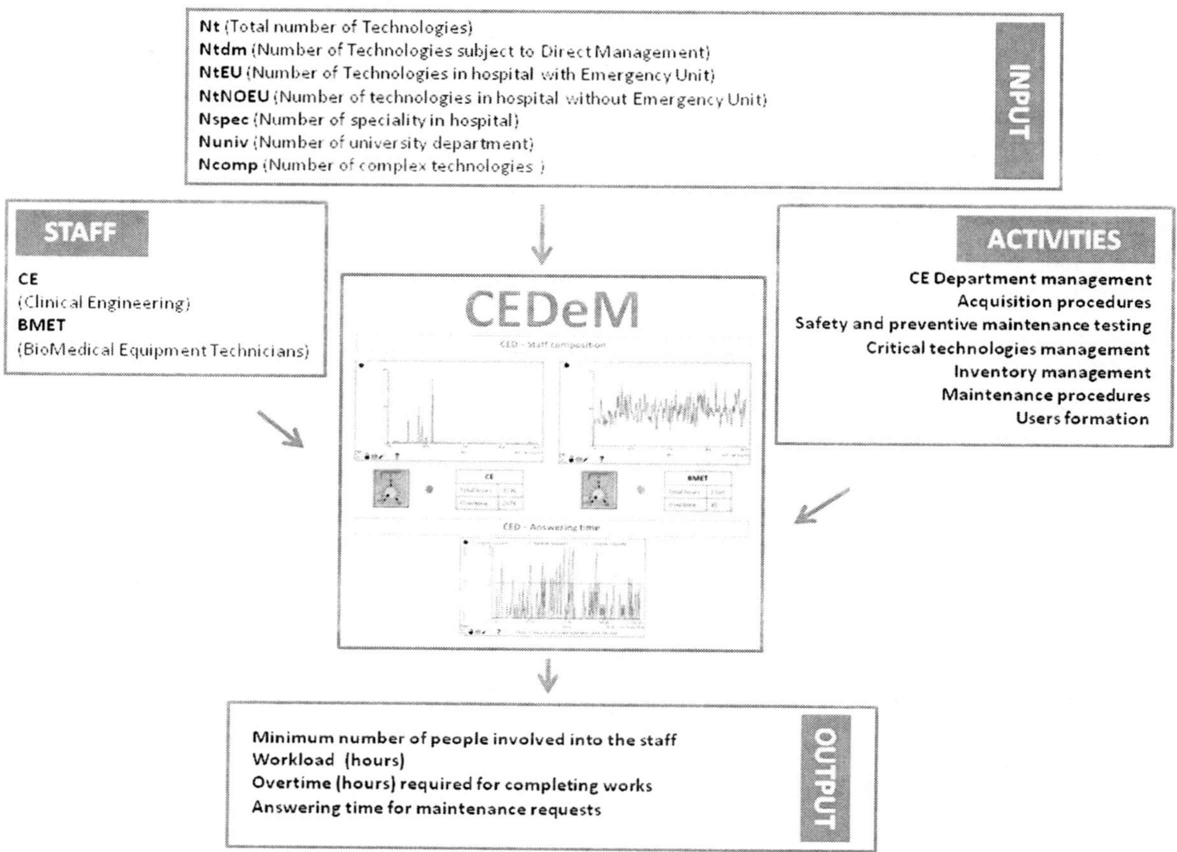

task. Places and transitions are linked by means of a directed arc. Arcs from a place to a place or a transition to a transition are not possible, because they will have no meaning.

As an example Figure 2 presents the workflow of the corrective maintenance process. This is not a scheduled process, but it starts when the Clinical engineering department receives a request to restore any failure of technologies.

The process starts when the call center receives a request of intervention. The BMET that answers the call may be able to solve the problem either because it is only an incorrect use of the device easy to detect or it is a usual problem that may be solved by the user just with a few instructions. If he is not able to solve the problem there are two possibilities. If the technology is covered by a particular maintenance contract by the supplier (called full-risk contract) that guarantees assistance in case of malfunctioning, a call for assistance starts. If the technology do not benefit from a full-risk contract, he asks a BMET assigned to maintenance to go and diagnose the problem. The results of this exploratory assessment may be different. There is no failure, that means that the problem is not caused by device; in this case the intervention is closed. If there is a malfunction, then the BMET decides if he can fix the problem or if the supplier must be called. In the second case, there are two alternatives: either the technol-

Figure 2. Workflow representing the maintenance process. Rectangles represent the tasks while circles stand for the input conditions and output state. Human resources are associated with the tasks by means of dedicated circles. A detailed description of the tasks is reported in the text.

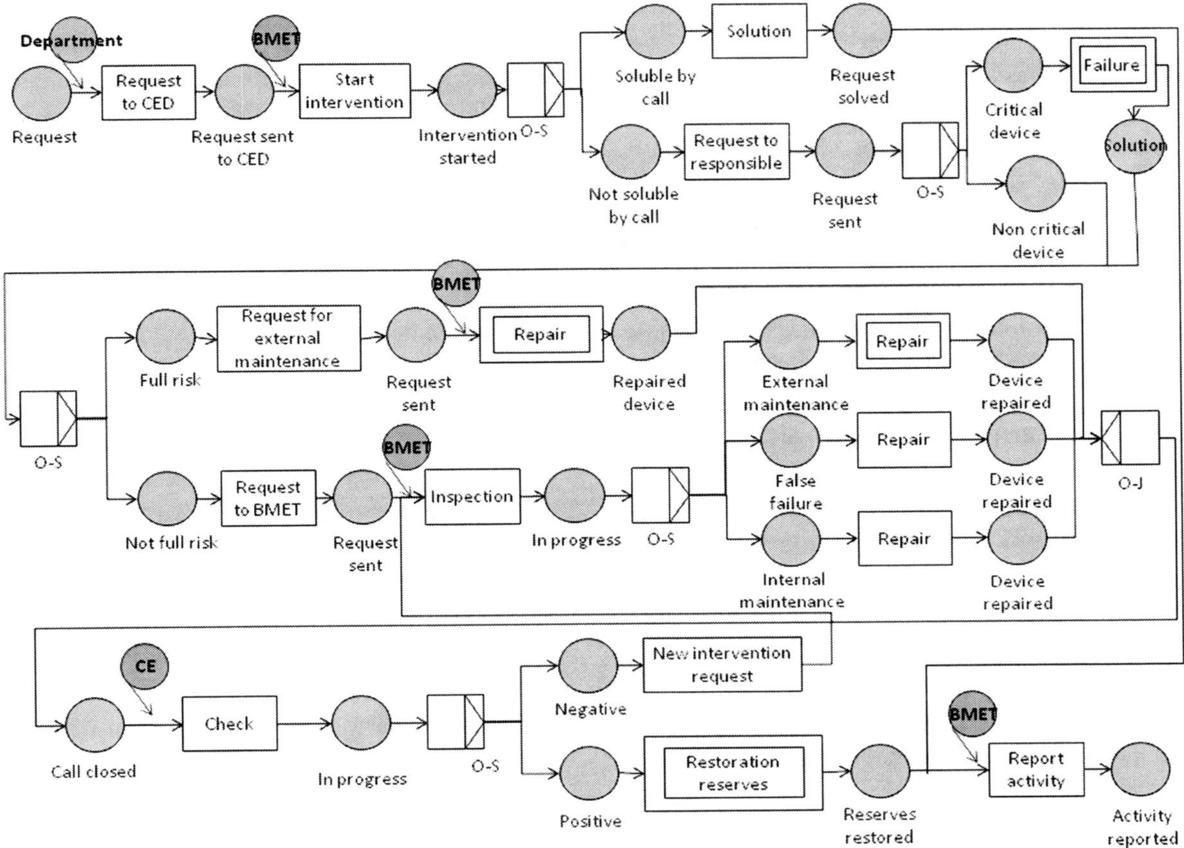

ogy could be repaired in the healthcare facility (in loco) or it must be sent to the supplier. Sometimes, when the external intervention is necessary, the administrative department has to approve that decision and the relative cost. After the repair, BMET verifies the correct functioning of the device: if everything works, the request can be closed, otherwise a new intervention is required. In the end, a report of the intervention with the associated documents is recorded in the inventory database.

Another important task of corrective maintenance is to guarantee the continuity of functioning of devices defined as critical. In this case, when the failure is diagnoses, the BMET uses the plan continuous availability of devices to provide a functioning technology to temporary substitute the damaged one.

The Simulation Model Implementation

The processes previously modelled with workflows diagrams were then simulated using the *iThink* software by ISEE Systems, inc. (http://www.iseesystems.com/), a well known tool for business intelligence that is based on system dynamics. iThink employs the System Thinking approach proposed by Checkland (Checkland, 1981). It allows the design and the simulation of models through four levels that are distinct but also strictly connected: the Interface, the Map, the Model and the Equation layer. Starting with the idea of the system that has to be implemented, the first step is to lay out that idea in a map form through the Map layer. This map can be transformed into a model in the Model layer. Five building blocks are provided in these two layers to define the model: stocks, flows, converters, connectors and modules. Briefly, stocks are measurable accumulations of physical (and non-physical) resources, for example patients, customers and work backlogs. Essentially they are delays which separate and buffer their inputs from their outputs, and are built up and depleted over time as input and output rates into them change. Flows fill and drain accumulations. The directed pipes represent activities. The results of activities flow into and out of accumulations, changing their magnitudes. Converters hold value for constants, define external inputs to the model, calculate algebraic relationship, and serve as the repository for graphical functions. Connectors connect model elements. Modules are self-contained models that you can connect to other models. Each module within a model is cohesive model on its own, which you can run separately or within the larger model. With these building blocks, a map and a model of the system can be created. During model building, a list of equations that makes up the model is automatically generated into the Equation layer. Finally, the Interface layer provides the tools for connecting the end-users interface to the model and to make clear the input/output interactions with the model.

In this environment, the workflow previously described that refers to the corrective maintenance process is translated as reported in Figure 3. Depending on the total number of technologies, a stochastic number of requests of maintenance were generated each day. In this way, we simulated the arrival of various types of demands, concerning essentially failure or malfunctioning of technologies, to the Clinical engineering department call center. Requests were classified according to their urgency, complexity, and the means used (e-mail, phone, letter, or direct call). This meant that demands labelled as urgent must be answered as quickly as possible, while complex demands usually could required an additional time for their solution. For this reason, three accumulations were set with the aim to simulate the waiting time required for the analysis of requests. This time was proportional to the kind of requests. After the analysis, the staff could decide to directly solve some demands or to delegate the corrective intervention to the maintenance technicians of suppliers. In the former case, the hours necessary to the problem solution had to take into account and they had to be referred to the BMET. Concerning the intervention of suppliers, a waiting time was considered simulating the time necessary for the sending of the technology, the repair, and the subsequent arrival at facility, or for the 'in loco' intervention, in which a specialised technicians was sent to repair the device directly at the facility. In both cases, a certain amount of time had to be referred to BMET for the planning activity of these processes. After that, the technology was repaired and the request satisfied.

The model equations are based on time variables, number of devices, and indicators that take into account the different complexity characterizing each facility. All the times involved in the process were composed by the joining of two parts: a fixed part, that indicated the minimum time required for each task, and a stochastic one for considering the differences among the requests or for any possible inconvenient related to that task that could delay the activity. In this way, the time associated to each task was included between a minimum and a maximum that depended on the activity considered. These minima and maxima derived from the experiences of three different experts that guide well-established clinical engineering departments in Piemonte Region. The times generated were then referred to the people

Figure 3. iThink model of the maintenance process as it is defined at the model level. Rectangles represent stocks, red lines are the connectors and the circles the converters. A detailed description of the model is reported in the text.

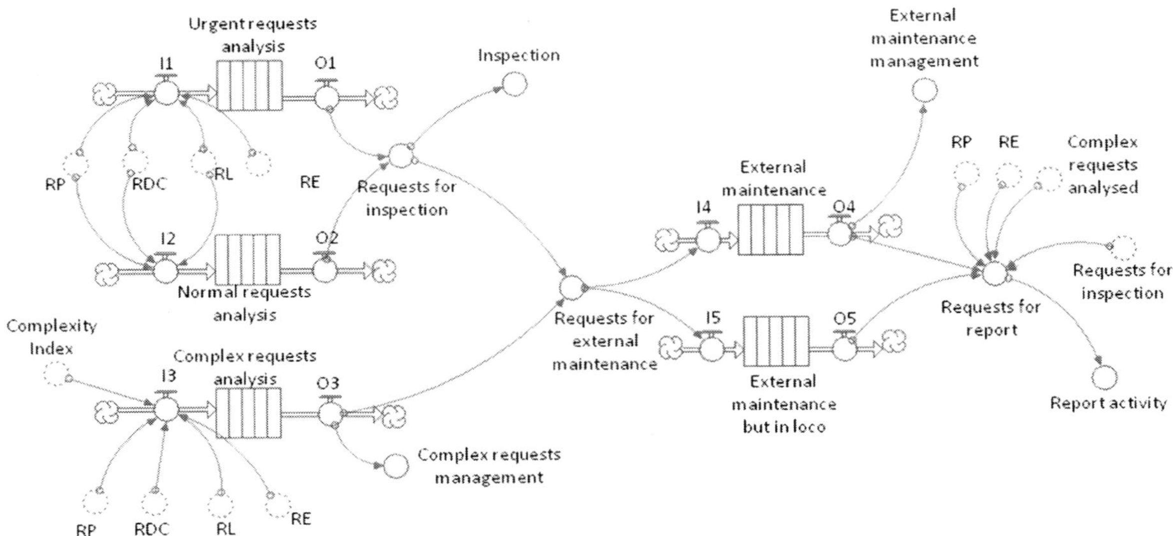

of the staff that were responsible of that task. In particular, those hours were assigned to the person that effectively does the work, completing his daily working time of 7 hours and 21 minutes (as the employment contract regulates). If, after filling the regular working hours, the daily tasks are not finished, overtime started to be counted.

The outputs were showed through an appropriate interface. For every staff member, there were two numeric displays representing the amount of daily workload and the overtime, both in terms of hours. Moreover, a graph showing the daily distribution of the workload was reported. A status indicator was related to each kind of staff people (clinical engineers, BMET working inside a single unit, BMET working across different units) and it was used to point immediately out critical situations. In fact, it acted like a traffic lights depending on the amount of working hours: it changed from green to yellow, before, and then to red if the total amount of work, respectively, not exceeded, slightly exceeded or exceeded in a significant way the daily working hours permitted. In detail, we assumed that, for each person, a year's workload of [0 - 1584] hours was completely sustainable, [1584 - 1900] was moderately sustainable, and finally a workload that exceeded the year's 1900 hours was unsustainable. In addition, the interface showed also the year's distribution of delay in answering customer demands, i.e. the time occurred between the arrival of a maintenance request and its solution. The simulation was performed over a time period of a year, leaving out the number of days off provided for contract. So, the total number of days simulated was two hundred and twenty.

Validation of the CED Simulation System

The validation was aimed to demonstrate that the results of the simulation are reliable, and to understand how general is the model, in order to apply it to every regional healthcare facility. The validation process required data, both input and output, from well working clinical engineering department. For this reason, we chose the data of three different facilities located in Piemonte Region, one for each group previously described (ASOu, ASO, ASL). In order to evaluate the CED ability to model different situation, the three facilities differed from each other in their sizes (such as the number of total technologies owned, the number of university department, and so on) as it can be easily seen in Figure 4: the facility A (a university teaching hospital) was the biggest, the facility C (a LHA) was of middle size and the facility B (a hospital trust) was the smallest.

The starting time of every activity was obtained in a stochastic way. Each day, a certain random number of events related to the different activities occurred. For instance, for the facility A described in Figure 4, approximately 13000 requests (or events) for corrective maintenance were generated in a year. The problem complexity, the waiting time for spare parts, and/or any other possible factor that influenced the considered process were incorporated into the corresponding number of hours that was computed for each event. Regarding the previous example, the 13068 requests generated a total of 26291 hours of work. Those hours were assigned to the person that effectively does the work, completing his daily working time. If extra works remained, overtime started to be counted. Since the BMETs do most of maintenance activities, following the example previously described, they should cover 17928 hours. If we assume that BMETs were 16, each BMET performed a mean of 1120 hours for maintenance issues. Obviously, if the number of BMET increased, the hours associated to each person decreased.

To calibrate the CED model, a first tuning phase was necessary to identify values associated to the parameters and the consensus among three experts was sought. The results obtained were analysed by experts that work directly into these structures and that are able to understand if the results were consistent with their situation. For all three facilities results were correct demonstrating that the simulation provided accurate results and that the model was appropriate to represents different healthcare organizations.

Figure 4. Input data corresponding to the facilities used for the validation process

	A	B	C
Type	ASOu	ASO	ASL
Nt	16995	5619	7642
Ntdm	15495	4103	6979
NtEU	15873	5619	4583
NtNOEU	1122	0	1826
Nspec	49	0	3
Nuniv	17	8	6
Ncomp	14923	4708	6786

After demonstrating that the model was working correctly, a second validation phase could be performed. The same three different kinds of facility were chosen to investigate the model ability to find the minimum number of staff members. Trying different combination of staff composition, in terms of numerousness of each professional figure, the results obtained were reported in Figure 5. As expected, increasing the number of clinical engineers and biomedical equipment technicians led to a decrease of the number of hours associated to each person for completing all occurred events. Both the total number of hours and the overtime obviously followed this trend. Increasing the number of people employed, however, a little bit of overtime generally remained because of the simulation nature: some periods or even only some days, there was a higher concentration of work (such as corrective maintenance, acquisition planning, safety tests to be performed in the same moment) leading to a higher workload that translated into overtime. Depending on the total number of hours necessary to complete all activities and on the overtime, region of sustainable or not sustainable situation could be depicted. The definition of sustainable or not sustainable situation is not settled, because it depends on the employment contract and on the people's needs. According to our definition of sustainable/moderately sustainable/not sustainable, different scenarios could be analysed: for example, if a total coverage of works occurred in facility A was sought, the number of CEs had to be more than 5, and, for BMETs, more than 15. In this case, it was a completely sustainable situation because the hours assigned to each person employed filled the normal working time provided in the contract and the overtime was acceptable. To validate these results with the real situation, the real staff composition was compared with that one come out from CED model. In Figure 5, the dotted lines represented the real number of people employed in clinical engineering department for each facility considered. They were all positioned in the region referred to a sustainable situation. Since the chosen facilities have a well-established clinical engineering department, if the staff composition provided by CED model in sustainable scenario corresponded to the actual staff composition, then the model was able to describe the real situation, even for very different size of facilities. It was possible to compare also the answering time in situations that were unsustainable for the model (Figure 5), and the real situation that sometimes occurred when one or more people were off for illness or vacation. This is a very important parameter, because a clinical engineering department provides an excellent service if it is able to answer every question without any delay. The experts found consistent the CED model results and their real experiences.

Application of the CED Model to Support Piemonte Region Starting the Clinical Engineering Department Network

Piemonte Region has a population of 4,4 million people and its healthcare system is principally based on public structures. The Region is divided in twenty one local health care agencies, managing a total of sixty five hospitals and more than thirteen thousand beds, with an amount of more than 115000 medical equipment items.

The first experiences of Clinical engineering departments, both in Piemonte and in Italy, began during the 80s, when in some hospitals "medical equipment maintenance services" were created, supported by electronic technicians and engineers. In the following decades the diffusion of these services in other hospitals grew rather slowly and in a dissimilar way, even inside the same region.

Until a few years ago, more than a half of health agencies in Piemonte have no structured and acknowledged Clinical engineering department. Medical equipment management was usually in charge of technicians belonging to general maintenance department of the hospital or totally given in outsourcing without any control on quality and costs. Only a few hospitals had specialized BMET and CE being able to face with the complex processes of managing hospital technologies. Even in these case the staff number was not sufficient to deal with all the requests at a reasonably quality level.

In 2005, the growing awareness by regional institutions of the impact of medical technologies in the strategic healthcare choices and costs led the Regional Agency for Healthcare Services (AReSS Piemonte - Agenzia Regionale per i Servizi Sanitari) to start a "Health Technology Management" (HTM) working group, in order to support central planning strategies and to coordinate Clinical engineering departments activities and procedures.

It was soon clear that to ensure a good effectiveness of regional coordinating actions the first

Figure 5. Evolution of total workload and overtime assigned to each person varying the number of CE and BMET of CE Department staff. Depending on the hours amount, it is possible to identify regions of situation that can be unsustainable (US), moderately sustainable (MSS) or completely sustainable (CSS). The definition of sustainability is given evaluating the workload and the answering time to maintenance requests. The dotted line represents the real number of CE and BMET employed in the facilities considered.

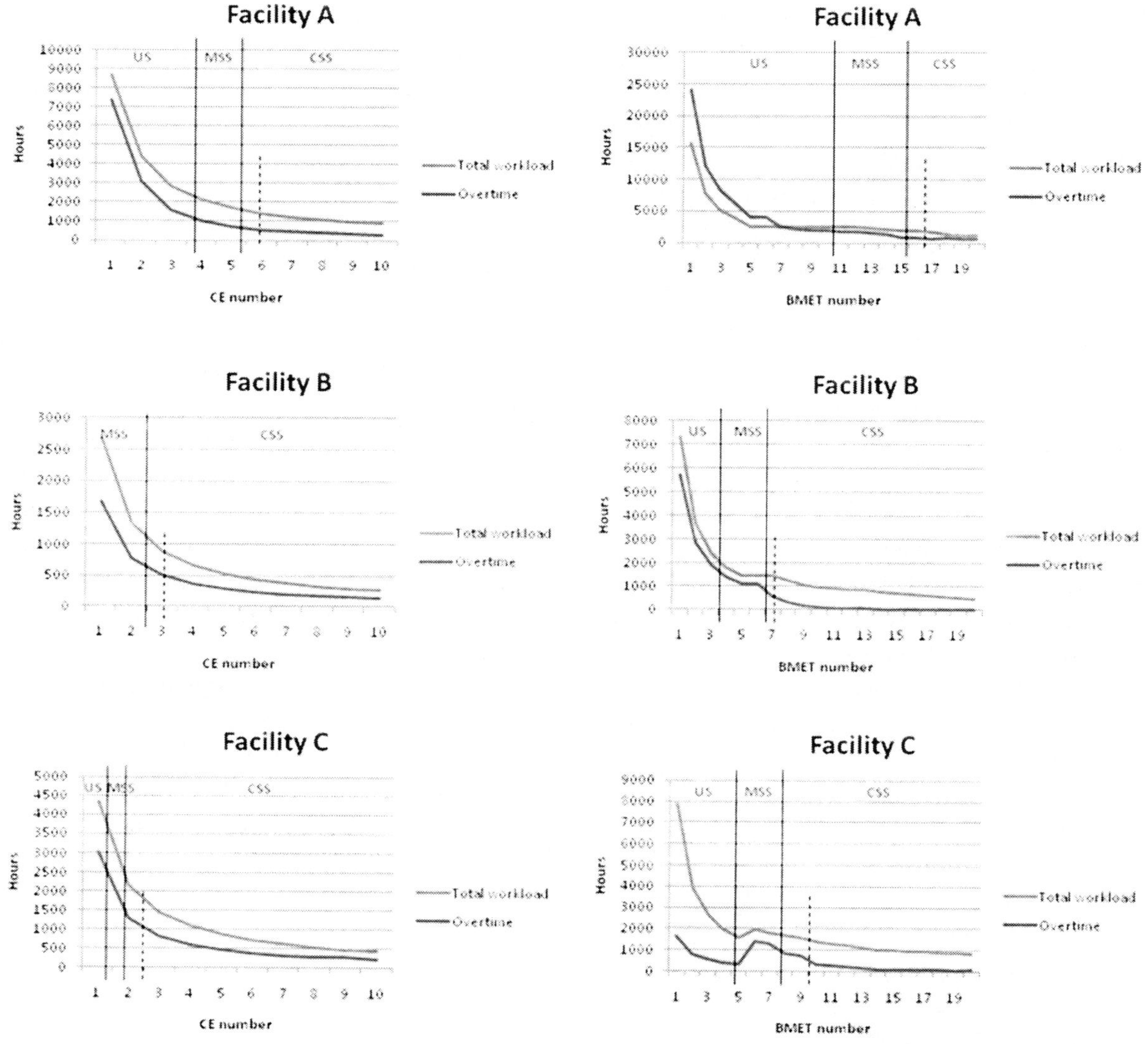

goal was to reach an adequate level of healthcare technology management in every local health care agency of the Region. For this reason in 2006 the AReSS HTM group decided to build a model of a regional network of Clinical engineering departments to be implemented in Piemonte Region (Balestra et al., 2009).

CED model was then constructed, validated, and applied to all the twenty one local health care agencies located in Piemonte Region in order to design the staff composition of the Clinical en-

Figure 6. Number of CE and BMET required to perform the basic activities in each clinical engineering departments of all the healthcare agencies of Piemonte region.

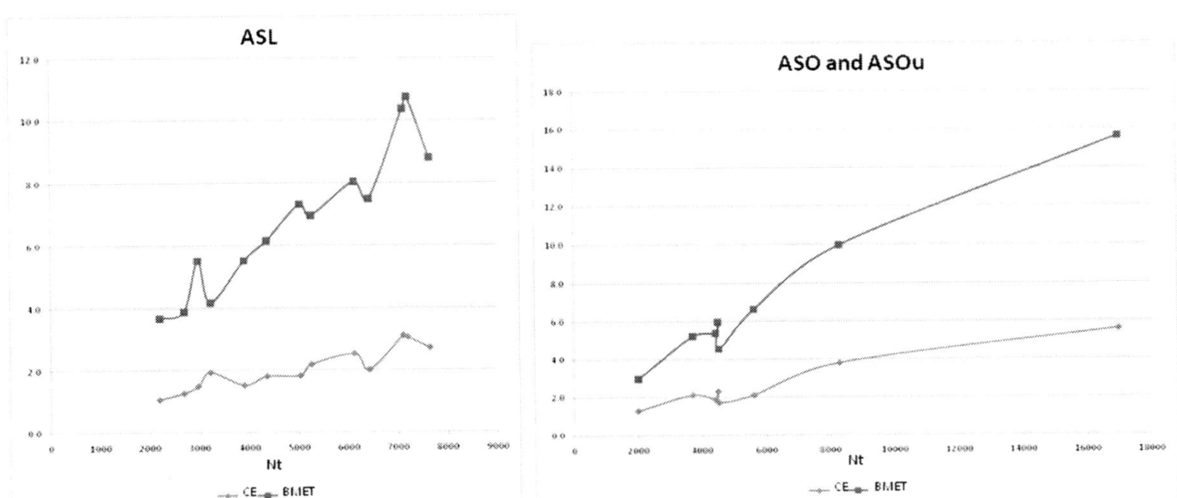

gineering departments that will take part in the network. Moreover, it was possible to simulate different scenarios, characterized by various staff composition, to evaluate drawbacks and benefits of each organizational situation. In so doing, with the model results, every facility could search a good compromise between its Clinical engineering department quality service and the staff composition, in other words between quality service and the costs for setting and maintaining it.

To define the minimum number of staff members necessary for a minimum quality level for each facility, the basic activities occurred in one year were simulated. Some kinds of activities, especially the ones related to planning (such as investment planning), were programmed at the beginning of the year, while others (like corrective maintenance) were modelled during all the simulated time. The results are reported in Figure 6 where, for each facility, the number of CE and BMET are plotted against the number of devices to be managed. The figure shows that there is not a linear trend, and this is consistent with the differences in terms of the organization clinical departments. To understand the impact on the staff composition on the quality level different combinations of number of CEs and BMETs were also tested. These results were published in a AReSS report (Lombardo et al., 2007; Lombardo et al., 2009)

In 2008, Piemonte Region approved an important regional health system reform. This was also the opportunity for many authorities to use these results, and to start establishing the Clinical engineering department or improve the existing one.

In January 2010, the results were used by the region managers to promote a regional guideline for developing the Clinical engineering department network (Determina Dir. Sanità Regione Piemonte n. 41 del 27.01.). The guideline contains the functions and responsibility to assign to Clinical engineering department, classes of equipments to be managed by it, professionals work profiles in terms of activities and educational background, and the global organization of department.

At this time, about 70% of regional healthcare agencies have a properly structured Clinical engineering department. The most usual organisational model used is a "combination model", in which human resources employed by the healthcare agency and other human resources provided by private companies work side by side in the facility. The guide-line encourages this integrated model because of its suitability and sustainability.

The model was developed specifically for the healthcare managers of Regione Piemonte, but with some minor changes can be used by managers interested in evaluating the quality of CE Department performances to compare the actual staff composition with a reasonable one. The managers only have to collect the necessary input data and run the model.

CONCLUSION AND FUTURE RESEARCH DIRECTION

The CED model proved to be adequate to support the healthcare managers in defining the staff of all the Clinical engineering departments that form the network. The applied methodologies not only were able to give accepted results, but they also were sufficiently easily to understand to be used to show these results to the decision makers. The healthcare managers appreciated the possibility to understand and to discuss the results instead of have to take them for true. The authors think that this was one of the characteristics that made the model easily accepted, and that it must be always keep in mind to develop decision aid systems.

The clinical engineering departments networks is growing following the guideline based on our model. A monitoring procedure started a few months ago to trace the changes and to support each facility. The results of the monitoring procedure will be available at the beginning of next year.

While, the application of CED model to start the Clinical engineering departments network demonstrated its usability in terms of estimating human resources, it does not support an advanced tuning of them and it does not constitute a good reference to evaluate the effectiveness of the services provided by each single department. To obtain a more flexible tool we are now developing a new system based on multi agent system (MAS) methodology. This new model will be able to accommodate the combined public-private organization, different expertise of each worker, different kind of organization, and so on.

ACKNOWLEDGMENT

The work herein presented was performed within the project PAS 5.1 founded by AReSS (Agenzia Regionale per i Servizi Sanitari) under the contract # 568/07. The Authors gratefully acknowledge the contribution of the other members of the working group.

REFERENCES

Annichiarico, R., Cortés, U., & Urdiales, C. (Eds.). (2008). *Agent technology and e-health*. Basel, Switzerland: Birkhuser Verlag. doi:10.1007/978-3-7643-8547-7

Balestra, G., Gaetano, L., & Puppato, D. (2008). *A model for simulation of clinical engineering department activities* (pp. 5109–5112). Vancouver, Canada: In EMBC.

Balestra, G., Gaetano, L., Puppato, D., Prato, G., Freda, P., Morena, F., et al. Lombardo, M. (2009). Modeling a regional network of clinical engineering departments. In *Proceeding ORAHS 2009*, Leuven, Belgium July 12-17, 2009.

Brailsford, S. C. (2007). Tutorial: Advances and challenges in healthcare simulation modelling. *Proceeding of the 2007 Winter Simulation Conference* (pp. 1436-1448).

Checkland, P. (1981). *Systems thinking, systems practice*. Chichester, UK: Wiley.

Christoffel, T. (2008). Thinking outside the box. *Biomedical Instrumentation & Technology*, *3*(42), 173.

David, Y., & Jahnke, E. G. (2004). Planning hospital medical technology management. *IEEE Engineering in Medicine and Biology Magazine*, *23*(3), 73–79. doi:10.1109/MEMB.2004.1317985

Duggan, J. (2008). Using system dynamics and multiple objective optimization to support policy analysis for complex systems. In Qudrat-Ullah, H., Spector, J. M., & Davidsen, P. I. (Eds.), *Complex decision making: Theory and practice* (pp. 59–81). Cambridge, MA: Springer.

Forrester, J. W. (1961). *Industrial dynamics*. Productivity Press.

Goodman, C. S. (2004). *HTA 101: Introduction to health technology assessment*. Retrieved August 2010, from http://www.nlm.nih.gov/ nichsr/outreach.html

Grimes, S. L. (2003). The future of clinical engineering: The challenge of change. *IEEE Engineering in Medicine and Biology Magazine*, *22*(2), 91–99. doi:10.1109/MEMB.2003.1195702

Jensen, K. (1996). *Coloured Petri nets. Basic concepts, analysis methods and practical use*. Berlin, Germany: Springer-Verlag EATCS Monographs on Theoretical Computer Science.

Ji, Y., Ying, H., Yen, J., Zhu, S., Barth-Jones, D. C., Miller, R. E., & Massanari, R. M. (2007). A distributed adverse drug reaction detection system using intelligent agents with a fuzzy recognition-primed decision model. *International Journal of Intelligent Systems*, *22*, 827–845. doi:10.1002/int.20230

Jun, G. T., Ward, J., Morris, Z., & Clarkson, J. (2009). Health care process modelling: Which method when? *International Journal for Quality in Health Care*, *21*(3), 214–224. doi:10.1093/intqhc/mzp016

Lombardo, M., Vajo, F., Balestra, G., Freda, P., Gaetano, L., Knaflitz, F. M., et al. Puppato, D. (2009). *Studio di un Modello Sostenibile di Rete Regionale di Servizi di Ingegneria Clinica: Ipotesi di dimensionamento e considerazioni di sostenibilità economica*. AReSS report. Retrieved August 2010, from http://www.aress.piemonte.it/Documenti.aspx

Lombardo, M., Vajo, F., Balestra, G., Freda, P., Knaflitz, M., Prato, G., & Puppato, D. (2007). *Studio di un Modello Sostenibile di Rete Regionale di Servizi di Ingegneria Clinica: I presupposti metodologici*. AReSS report. Retrieved August 2010, from http://www.aress.piemonte.it/ Documenti.aspx

Maio, V., & Manzoli, L. (2002). The Italian health care system: W.H.O. ranking versus public perception. *Pharmacy & Therapeutics*, *6*(27), 301–308.

Moreno, A., & Nealon, J. (Eds.). (2003). *Applications of software agents technology in the health care domain*. Basel, Switzerland: Birkhuser Verlag Whitestein series in software agent technology

Padgham, L., & Winikoff, M. (2004). *Developing intelligent agent systems*. Wiley & Sons Ltd. doi:10.1002/0470861223

Regione Piemonte. (2010). Determina Dir. Sanità Regione Piemonte n. 41 del 27.01.2010. *Linea guida per l'applicazione di un modello organizzativo regionale di servizi di ingegneria clinica.*

Steele, C. (2002). *An introduction to clinical risk management* (pp. 24-27). Retrieved August 2010, from http://www www.optometry. co.uk

van der Aalst, W., & van Hee, K. (2004). *Workflow management: Models, methods, and systems*. The MIT Press, paperback edition.

van der Aalst, W. M. P. (1996). Three good reasons for using a Petri-net-based workflow management system. In S. Navathe & T. Wakayama, (Eds.), *Proceedings of the International Working Conference on Information and Process Integration in Enterprises (IPIC '96)*, (pp. 179–201) Cambridge, Massachusetts, Nov 1996.

ADDITIONAL READING

AA (1989) Completing the transition from clinical engineering to technology management *Health Technology.* Spring;3(1):20-26

Abelson, J., Giacomini, M., Lehoux, P., & Gauvin, F. P. (2007). Bringing 'the public' into health technology assessment and coverage policy decisions: From principles to practice. *Health Policy (Amsterdam)*, *82*, 37–50. doi:10.1016/j.healthpol.2006.07.009

Banta, H. D., & Luce, B. R. (1993). *Health Care Technology and Its Assessment: An International Perspective*. New York, NY: Oxford University Press.

Brown, I., Smale, A., & Wong, M. (2005) Management of Medical Technology – Implementation Issues. *Proceedings of the 27th Annual Conference in Engineering in Medicine and Biology.* 5672- 5675Cohen T (2003) The future of clinical engineering: technology that enables improved patient care *Biomedical Instrumentation and Technoogyl*. 37(2):113-117

De Vivo, L., Derrico, P., Tomaiuolo, D., Capussotto, C., & Reali, A. (2004) Evaluating alternative service contracts for medical equipment *Proceedings of the 26th Annual International Conference of the IEEE EMBS* San Francisco, CA, USA • September 1-5

Gaev, J. A. (2007). Measure for Measure. *Biomedical Instrumentation & Technology*, *4*(41), 267–277. doi:10.2345/0899-8205(2007)41[267:DBFCEA]2.0.CO;2

Gharajedaghi, J. (2006) *System thinking: managing chaos and complexity,* Butterworth-Heinemann, Goldberg, J.R. (2003) The healthcare technologies management program, *IEEE Engineering in Medicine and Biology Magazine*, Jan/Feb 2003, pp.49-52

Grimes, S. L. (2004). Clinical Engineers: Stewards of Healthcare Technologies. *IEEE Engineering in Medicine and Biology Magazine*, (May/June): 56–58. doi:10.1109/MEMB.2004.1317982

Kobielus, J. G. (1997). *Workflow Strategies*. IDG Books Worldwide, Inc.

Kullolli, I. (2008). Selecting a Computerized Maintenance Management System. *Biomedical Instrumentation & Technology*, *4*(42), 276–278. doi:10.2345/0899-8205(2008)42[276:SACMMS]2.0.CO;2

Lo Scalzo, A., Donatini, A., Orzella, L., & Cicchetti, A. Profi li S, Maresso A. (2009) Italy: Health system review. Health Systems in Transition, 11(6)1-216 - Retrieved August 2010, from http://www.euro.who.int/__data/ assets/ pdf_file/ 0006/ 87225 /E93666.pdf

Murata, T. (1989, April). Petri Nets: Properties, Analysis and Applications. *Proceedings of the IEEE*, *77*(4), 541–580. doi:10.1109/5.24143

Rodriguez, E., Miguel, A., Sanchez, M. C., Tolkmitt, F., & Pozo, E. (2003) A new proposal of quality indicators for clinical engineering *Proceedings of the 25 ' Annual International Conference of the IEEE EMBS* Cancun, Mexico September 17-21

Rosow E., Grimes SL (2003) Technology's implications for health care quality. A clinical engineering perspective *Nurs Adm Q.* Oct-Dec;27(4):307-317

Tobey, J., Clark. (2004). Challenges Facing Independent Multihospital Healthcare Technology Management Systems. *IEEE Engineering in Medicine and Biology Magazine*, (May/June): 2004.

Wang, B. (2009) Strategic health technology incorporation. *Synthesis Lectures on Biomedical Engineering*. (32), 1-71

Wang, B., Furst, E., Cohen, T., Keil, O. R., Ridgway, M., & Stiefel, R. (2006). Medical equipment management strategies. *Biomedical Instrumentation and Technology May-Jun, 40*(3), 233–237. doi:10.2345/i0899-8205-40-3-233.1

Zambuto, R. P. (2004). Clinical engineers in the 21st century *IEEE Engineering in Mededical and Bioogyl Magazine. May-Jun, 23*(3), 37–41.

Chapter 6
Intensive Care Unit Operational Modeling and Analysis

Yue Dong
Mayo Clinic, USA

Huitian Lu
South Dakota State University, USA

Ognjen Gajic
Mayo Clinic, USA

Brian Pickering
Mayo Clinic, USA

ABSTRACT

The outcome of critical illness depends not only on life threatening pathophysiologic disturbances, but also on several complex "system" dimensions: health care providers' performance, organizational factors, environmental factors, family preferences and the interactions between each component. Systems engineering tools offer a novel approach which can facilitate a "systems understanding" of patient-environment interactions enabling advances in the science of healthcare delivery. Due to the complexity of operations in critical care medicine, certain assumptions are needed in order to understand system behavior. Patient variation and uncertainties underlying these assumptions present a challenge to investigators wishing to model and improve health care delivery processes. In this chapter we present a systems engineering approach to modeling critical care delivery using sepsis resuscitation as an example condition.

DOI: 10.4018/978-1-60960-872-9.ch006

MEDICAL ERROR IS A GROWING PUBLIC HEALTH PROBLEM IN ACUTE CARE ENVIRONMENT

In 2005, intensive care unit (ICU) costs represented 13.4% of hospital costs, 4.1% of national healthcare expenditures and 0.66% of the gross domestic product in the US (Halpern & Pastores, 2010). With ever-increasing demands and decreasing available resources, the provision of cost-effective healthcare and the elimination of waste is a major focus of policy makers, healthcare providers, and the general public. Indeed, we know today that between \$.30 and \$.40 of every healthcare dollar spent in the US does not contribute to high quality care. Resources are wasted through over-use, misuse, duplication, system failures, poor communication and inefficiency (Lawrence, 2005) and are estimated to cost between \$600 billion and \$850 billion annually (Kelley, 2009). On the other hand, less than one cent (\$.01) of every healthcare dollar is spent on health services research which might eliminate these wasteful activities (Coalition for Health Services Research, 2009). Such spending discrepancies highlight the importance of implementation research proposed as "Blue Highways" on the NIH roadmap (Westfall et al., 2007). There is a dichotomy between science discovery and failure of everyday patient care delivery (Blendon et al., 2002; Grol & Grimshaw, 2003).

Sir Cyril Chantler stated, "Medicine used to be simple, ineffective and relatively safe. Now it is complex, effective and potentially dangerous."(Chantler, 1999). The ICU is a complex environment with multiple team members, interacting with several critically ill patients, many of whom are receiving life supports such as mechanical ventilation and dialysis. With increasing complexity of patient disease, treatment options and technology, the healthcare delivery comes at increased risk of error and poor patient outcome. One of the few studies to systematically examine processes of care delivery and errors in the ICU was carried out in a relatively small (6 bedded) ICU by Israeli investigators. They reported an average of 178 processes of care per day per patient and the absolute number of error was determined to be 1.7 errors/patient per day (Donchin et al., 2003). Given the system complexity, 1.7 errors may not seem to be a large number, however, the consequences of error in this patient population is profound. In addition, more common and complex diagnostic errors have not been considered in this study. Several studies have described increased patient morbidity, increased resource utilization and reduced survival in association with error in the ICU (Bracco et al., 2001; Garrouste-Orgeas et al., 2010).

RATIONALE FOR A SYSTEMS APPROACH TO REDUCING ERROR IN THE ICU

ICU systems are complex. The components of the system include patients, family members, physicians, nurses, allied health staff, support staff, physical and electronic infrastructure, equipment, supplies, processes and culture (Schmidt & Taylor, 1970). Ideally these components work together to optimize patient-centered outcomes. In order to ensure that ICU systems deliver high quality care to patients we need to understand how each system component (patient, provider, equipment, etc.) interacts and works together. This understanding is not easily derived from conventional analytic approaches and optimization of the system can not rely solely on single interventions such as those aimed at improving an individual provider's skills. , Systems-based approaches to error prevention have proven markedly effective in reducing medical errors and iatrogenic complications. For example, Dr. Pronovost's use and distribution of a simple checklist during central line insertion has already "saved more lives than that of any laboratory science discoveries in the past decade" (Gawande, 2007). Similarly, a simple systems intervention, the WHO Surgical Safety Checklist, has been shown to reduce morbidity and mortality in a diverse group of hospitals around the world (Haynes et al., 2009). These examples demonstrate that the systems of care delivery are an important determinant of critical illness outcomes.

Because the metrics of system performance go beyond patient outcome alone, healthcare providers need to adopt methodologies from other disciplines, which handle equally complex systems such as engineering, commercial aviation, aerospace and the nuclear industry. In 2005, the Institute of Medicine and National Academy of Engineering proposed a partnership to advance healthcare delivery research and patient outcomes (Reid et al., 2005). Systems engineering focuses on coordination, synchronization and the integration of complex process components including personnel, data, materials, and financial resources. It provides the appropriate tools to facilitate these tasks as well as provide insights which would normally be beyond the scope of any individual system component to deliver. Modeling and simulation (M&S) are some of the most commonly used tools for system analysis and have been usefully deployed to optimized system's logistics (van Sambeek et al., 2010; Young et al., 2004). These system analysis tools can reveal the mechanisms that influence complex system operation; how well the system meets overall goals and objectives; and model or suggest how system performance can be optimized. NASA, the aviation industry and many high other risk endeavors have employed simulation modeling to dramatically improve quality and safety in manufacturing processes and associated decision making (Allenbach & Huffman, 1998; Barth & Algee, 1996; Bertsimas & De Boer, 2005; Cates & Mollaghasemi, 2005; Schrage, 1999).

ICU OPERATION FROM SYSTEMS ENGINEERING PERSPECTIVE

Characteristics of the ICU as Unique Service Model

A model of the system is used to gain understanding of how the corresponding system behaves (Law & Kelton, 1999). Simulation is the process of building a model for a real system and using the model to conduct experiments to study either the behavior of the system or to evaluate various strategies for system operation. A model may be used to highlight areas of system deficiency and predict the impact of proposed interventions without interrupting normal operations. Simulation has been used in healthcare to support clinical decision-making, facility planning (predict bed occupancy), resource allocation (staffing), evaluation of treatments, and organizational redesign in ED and ICU (Baker et al., 2009; S. Brailsford, 2005; Dittus et al., 1996; Griffiths et al., 2010; A. Kolker, 2009; Kumar et al., 2009).

In a typical ICU patient care is delivered by a group of physicians, fellows/residents, respiratory therapists, pharmacists, working together within the constraints of the physical, electronic and culture environment. Each system component must work effectively and efficiently to delivery high quality care. The system receives multiple inputs (patient data, resource constraints) and generates multiple responses (medical decisions, investigations treatment plan) (Haut et al., 2009) with consequent multi-dimensional outputs: safety, effectiveness, timeliness, patient-centeredness, efficiency, and equality (*Crossing the Quality Chasm: A New Health System for the 21st Century*, 2001).

ICU system operations are centered on the patients admitted to the ICU with critical illness. These operations are very different from those of a manufacturing plant and are characterized by unpredictability. The patient disease state, workload, rate of progress from one health state

Figure 1. The concept of an event driven system

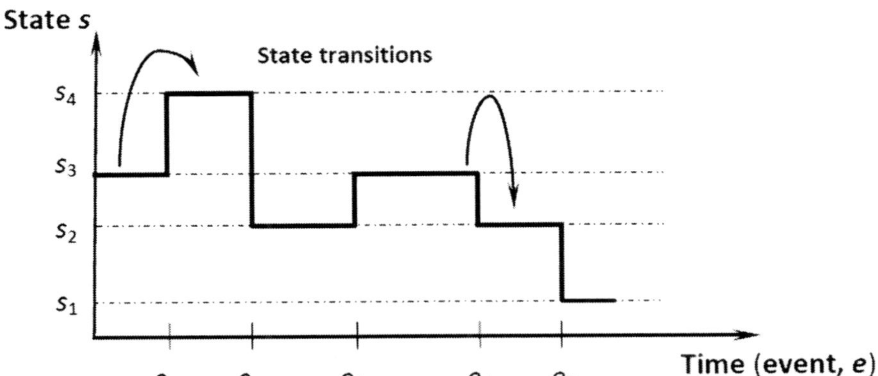

to another, the necessity to deliver simultaneous disparate processes of care, and skills availability are largely outside of ICU operational control. In an attempt to impose some structure on workflow, ICU systems process patients through health states using a number of key operations including admission, rounding, plan of care, hand-off, communication, discharge/ re-admission. These, relatively predictable operations can be significantly disrupted by unpredictable events such as resuscitation or multiple simultaneous admissions. In these circumstances, the system relies heavily on healthcare providers to handle the workload surge and redistribute resources appropriately. The ICU occupies a central position in the health care system with the sickest patients being admitted from and/or discharged to any other part of the health care system. In addition, it interacts with all or most of the ancillary services required to run a modern hospital including laboratory, information technology, transfusion, interventional and diagnostic radiology services. This combined with a rich data stream makes the ICU a superb environment in which to explore and develop the capabilities of modeling and simulation methodologies (Kreke et al., 2004).

Description of Discrete Event Simulation of Critical Care Delivery Process

DES (discrete event simulation) is a computer simulation model that studies the behavior of real processes as they advance with time in order to visualize and analyze performance. The model is validated and verified by comparison with real processes, is used to understand the original process and to propose ways in which they may be improved. DES modeling is a very effective analytic mechanism for exploring "what if" scenarios. It is also capable of using various scenarios to cope with changes in conditions and variables. The simulation environment provides the user with an option to perform experiments on the computer and test the likely effectiveness of different solutions before implementation. Figure 1 shows the concept of an event-driven system performance (Hrúz & Zhou, 2007).

During the simulation process, entities wait in a queue before they pass through a series of activities. The order in which activities occur and the conditions that are required for them to take place can be very complex. Each entity can be assigned characteristics which eventually determine what happens to that entity within the system. The duration of these activities are sampled from probability distribution functions. The user has unlimited flexibility regarding the choice of these functions and the logic behind the flow of entities within the system (S.C. Brailsford & Hilton, 2001).

The basic elements of a simulation model are: (Alexander Kolker, 2009)

- Flow chart of the entire process. Here, the flow chart is a diagram that shows the logical flow of entire sepsis resuscitation process from start to finish.
- Entities, defined as items to be processed like patients, x-rays, blood samples, documents, medications, etc.
- Activities, defined as tasks performed on entities for instance medical procedures such as central line insertion, fluid or blood administration, antibiotic administration, review of laboratory results, document approval such as X ray check for line position, customer check-in, etc.
- Resources, which agents are required to perform a particular activity and move an entity through the sepsis resuscitation process
- Entity routings, maps the potential or actual routes and logical condition flow for entities through the system. For example, in order to use a central line for administration of medications, a physician must confirm the position of the line and communicate this to the nurse who can then use the central line. There are several potential routes to this end point such as confirmation using manometry or CXR image.

Discrete event simulation works by tracking entities as they move through systems at distinct points of time. The simulation tracks all process times, waiting times, and entities' statistics associated with its movement and activity at any given time point. A unique feature of DES is that it can track hundreds of individual events that occur during the designed simulation time and can model randomness using a random number generator. Furthermore, it also tracks each event with its own attribute (from different distributions and parameters) and helps to replicate it to the most complex system.

DES models usually use interactive animation and graphics to display results, which can be used to analyze the models output. Also, these simulation models generate a vast range of outputs showing probable outcomes as well as summary of the processes. However, a single iteration of the simulation only represents one possible outcome. So, a highly variable system requires numerous iterations in order to determine possible outcomes in a statistical sense.

In ICU operation analysis, DES models may be used to describe, ICU healthcare delivery behaviors as *different entities* (patient or provider) *utilizing resources* (x-ray machine) to *complete activities* (procedure, exams) within a *specific time period*. Entities and resources can be assigned different variables/attributes (e.g. an average of 3 sepsis patients per day). Logical relationships link the different entities together, e.g. nurse and doctor deliver treatment to the patient entity. Defining logical relationships is a key part of the simulation model; they determine the overall behavior of the model and are informed by local expertise or observational studies of the system. Each logical statement (e.g. "Start the central line if the patient has a diagnosis of sepsis", "Lab test and report will be read by the doctor and they will make a decision about the next treatment") are simple but it is the quantity, variety and the fact that they are widely dispersed throughout the model that increases the model complexity. The interaction of these entities and resources as they perform their various functions are quantified in a framework of "global system behavior." The "system" is defined by system operations (the entities' movement from one activity to another) and events (an event occurs when its associated actions are performed). The "system-state" is the status of the system at a defined moment in time (ICU bed availability, number of total patients, etc.). System performance is then computed from information in a given system trace: e.g. the number of ICU beds available during peak hours. Healthcare delivery system states evolve with the occurrence of enabled events. The occurrence of events often initiates work actions; typically, the time intervals between consecutive events are random (e.g. the time for the next sepsis patient needing an ICU bed is random). The DES can simplify complex systems, enabling providers to understand key issues more clearly without subjective bias. Different "what-if" scenarios can then be carried out in a "prototype" testing environment. There is a growing interest within the healthcare sector to improve complex system dynamics using modeling and simulation (S. C. Brailsford et al., 2009; Eldabi et al., 2002; Eldabi et al., 2007; Fone et al., 2003; Kuljis et al., 2007; Young, 2005; Young et al., 2009). In the next section a DES model of sepsis resuscitation is discussed as an example to demonstrate the potential application of this modeling technique to healthcare.

SEPSIS RESUSCITATION MODEL AS A CASE STUDY

Background

Severe sepsis/sepsis shock accounts for 20% of all admissions to ICUs. It is the leading cause of death in non-cardiac ICUs and the 11th most common cause of death overall. Despite advances in life sustaining interventions, ongoing medical education and quality improvement efforts, a serious gap persists between daily practice and evidence-based guidelines for the treatment of sepsis developed by international organizations under the *Surviving Sepsis Campaign* initiative (Dellinger et al., 2004). Conventional QI approaches have been modestly effective at increasing guideline compliance from a baseline of 5-10% to 30% after their implementation (Ferrer et al., 2008; Levy et al., 2010). Barriers to sepsis guideline implementation are poorly understood but both delayed sepsis recognition and faulty processes of care seem to play a significant role. A deeper understanding of "system factors" affecting resuscitation processes is necessary if interventions to increase guideline compliance, facilitate error prevention and improve patient outcomes are to be developed (Kahn & Bates, 2008; Kahn & Rubenfeld, 2005). A systems engineering approach to sepsis resuscitation begins with the mapping of specific care processes into a computer model to facilitate process modeling and simulation (DES).

Model Building

Sepsis resuscitation team members (including physicians, nurses, pharmacists, respiratory therapists, radiology and laboratory technicians) were interviewed and they identified Sepsis Resuscitation System (SYSTEM) performance functions which were captured by drawing a SYSTEM block diagram of the chronology of patient movement during sepsis resuscitation. Entity variables and time were collected from electronic medical records (EMR), an established ICU DataMart (Herasevich et al., 2010), and hospital administrative databases (admission/discharge). Care processes (provider, process, and time stamp data) that were not available within EMR were collected by field observation (Dong et al., 2010) and provider interviews. An entity (patient)-centric model of sepsis resuscitation was created using Process Simulator Software (ProModel Corporation, Orem, UT). The simulation model is schematically represented in Figure 2) and demonstrates 'entities' (patient or X-ray film) which undergo 'activities' (central line procedure or X-ray film processing) utilizing 'resources' (radiology technician) over a period of time (start and finish time).

Hierarchical modeling enables visualization of sub-system processes at different resolution. The model provides dynamic information and statistics of current processes, entry/exit time

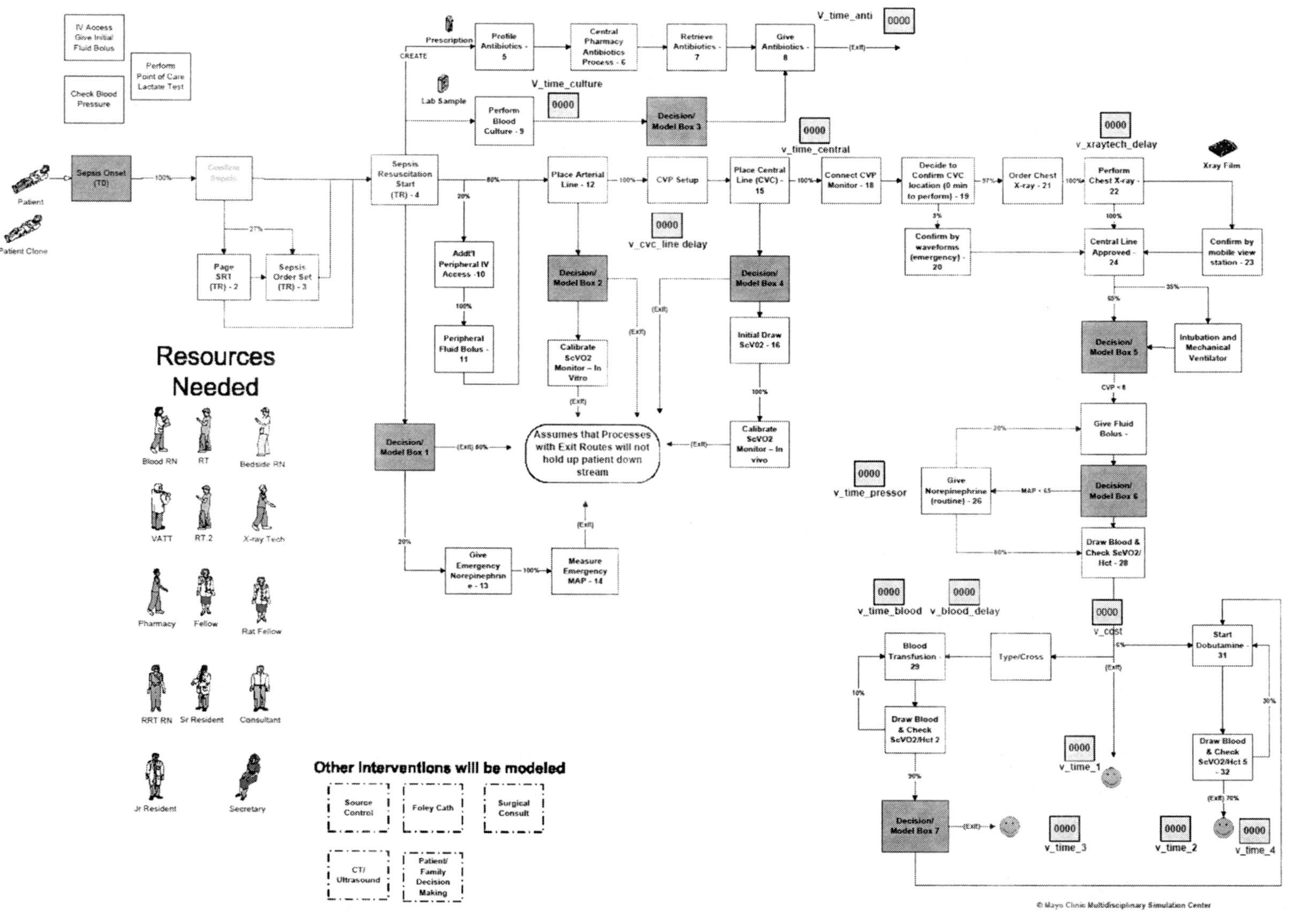

Figure 2. Simulation model of sepsis resuscitation in ICU

Figure 3. The concept of optimization solution search

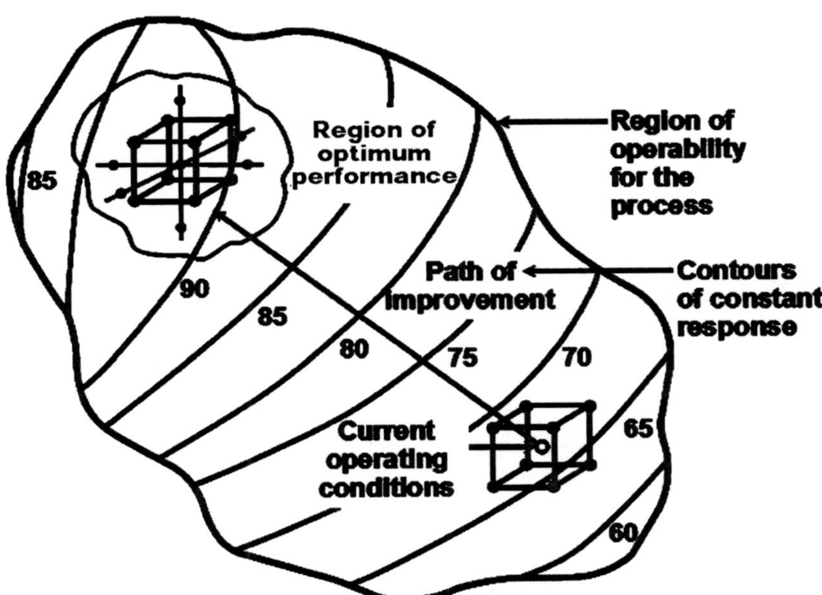

distribution, maximum, minimum and average duration of patient waits at each point of the system, staffing, resource availability and utilization. Because of the complex nature of the sepsis care delivery system, our initial model focused on those high level processes most likely to significantly contribute to a delay of sepsis care (Soliman, 1998). Patient characteristics and provider skill variations were not taken into account in the initial model building.

Model Verification and Validation

The developed DES model simulated 30 days of severe sepsis resuscitation in a medical ICU. Errors were identified and corrected (debugging) during each iteration. Iterative review and testing confirmed the model was programmed correctly and the developed algorithms had been implementing properly (verification). The model outputs were then compared with empirical data to confirm that the model was representative of the actual ICU processes (validation). The average accuracy of the Sepsis Care Cycle Time was within 15% of that recorded in the clinical databases of the host healthcare facility (Dong et al., 2009).

System Model Analysis and Optimization

Performance optimization of the system is a value judgment made by those who design the system, manage the system costs, and use the outputs of the system. In our sepsis resuscitation project, we used Sepsis Care Cycle Time as the primary outcome measure of interest.

The main goal of optimization is to eliminate or minimize "no-value-add" activities. In engineering practice, the analytical solution in a close form is usually not available and substitute-engineering methods are adopted to reach approximate "optimization." The core concept of optimization solution searches are depicted in Figure 3. The goal of solution searching is to define those operation conditions which are associated with optimal system output. The simulation model employs numerical methods, based on random numbers, to "run" the system performance. The observations of the model (output from the model runs) were collected and analyzed for the estimates of actual system performance measured by statistical inferences.

With the objective measure of optimal performance set as decreased Sepsis Care Cycle time, bottlenecks in the care processes were analyzed through system-level investigation with the Lean Six Sigma approach to reduce patient waiting time at each step, taking into consideration resource availability and other constraints. Factors contributing to the operational performance were manipulated within the computer simulation models in order to achieve sepsis resuscitation goals in a timely and cost-effective manner. Optimal or near-optimal solutions (new process or change of old process) were introduced to refine the simulation model of sepsis management. Options for optimization of system performance included change in processes to eliminate unnecessary steps or change of sequential steps to parallel steps. Preliminary simulation results suggested that bundled interventions (early sepsis recognition, streamlined central line placement, blood typing of anemic patients at the onset of resuscitation rather than waiting for before transfusion, and measurement of central venous pressure and venous oxygen saturation before chest x-ray confirmation after central line placement) could reduce sepsis cycle time by 30% compared to baseline. Due to the limitation of the data availability during the initial model building, additional field observation, refinement, validation and optimization are needed to surmount the assumptions used in the preliminary model. While in situ simulation and ultimately clinical testing are necessary prior to implementation of suggested changes, DES methodology provides a critical first step in informing the efficient design of the quality improvement intervention.

ISSUES, CONTROVERSIES, AND PROBLEMS

Acceptance of Systems Thinking Within Heath Care Organizations

The complexity of medical practice, limited resources and increasing demand for quality, safety and efficiency require modification of both the "sharp end" (provider education, etc.) and "blunt end" (organizational optimization, etc.) layers of the healthcare system. (Cook & D.Woods, 1994). There are considerable challenges to introduce the systems concept to healthcare providers who often perceive these efforts as a threat to autonomy and "cookbook medicine". The culture change will require not only a large educational effort but also economic incentives ("Unmet Needs: Teaching Physicians to Provide Safe Patient Care"; Vincent et al., 2004). A pioneer of the Science of Health Care Delivery in the ICU, Dr. Peter Pronovost suggests that there exists a "*need to recognize that standardization offers tremendous benefits, especially when evidence is robust. As medical science matures, we must progress from providing care primarily based on intuition, to a place where this independent approach is properly balanced with care based on collective wisdom and proven scientific evidence.*"(Pronovost & Vohr, 2010).

Limited Access to Process Information

Critical process components which contribute to inadequate sepsis resuscitation such as workflow variation, resource availability, workload, handoffs and communication are seldom accurately recorded, limiting a meaningful understanding of complex system factors responsible for suboptimal performance. Yet without an understanding of such factors and the interdependence of ICU care processes, substantive improvement will be difficult to achieve. In the last ten years, the adoption of the electronic medical record

(EMR) has made patient data (labs, vitals signs, notes, etc) readily available for provider during their practice and related clinical research with various adoption rate between hospitals (*EMR Adoption Model*, 2010). Patient data has been recorded in significant details from continuous monitoring, lab results and treatment plan. But ICU operational data, provider performance and related healthcare delivery process data, are often inaccurate (documentation time does not reflect the intervention/procedure time) or missing (not been captured at all) by current EMR. The data are spread across several system components and require a coordinated approach for gathering and analysis (Herasevich et al., 2010; Pickering et al., 2010). Unlike the "blackbox" used in the aviation industry, healthcare providers can rarely retrospectively reconstruct the healthcare delivery components responsible for the occurrence of an error or complication. Without accurate capture of process data along with patient data, it is extremely difficult to describe the ICU system inputs and outputs quantitatively without subjective assumption and estimation. Along with patient and provider variations, these uncertainties make modeling t health care delivery process in the ICU particularly challenging.

Fragmentation of Care Environment

Although ICU provides the majority of care for sepsis patients in our sepsis resuscitation model, focusing solely on ICU processes may prevent us from understanding the influence of non-ICU environments (delay in transfer to the ICU due to poor recognition of severe sepsis). Other upstream and downstream institutional factors (blood bank, lab, radiology, etc.) might also influence the ICU sepsis resuscitation outcomes. Additional data (from the emergency department and the hospital floor) need to be collected in order to differentiate a micro-system (ICU) from a macro-system (hospital), and determine additional targets for process improvement.

SOLUTIONS AND RECOMMENDATIONS

With the adoption of the EMR, workflow and service centric processes data need to be captured and presented in a meaningful way to facilitate not only system analytics but also the decision making process at the bedside (Zhang & Butler, 2007). Field observation remains the critical component of process modeling with automatic data collection (RFID, video motion capture, etc.) facilitating sustainable process control and analysis (Vankipuram et al., 2010).

A variety of modeling and simulations tools can be used for complex system analysis including Markov modeling, Monte Carlo simulation, system dynamics, supply-chain management, distributed decision making, and agent-based simulation (Chahal & Eldabi, 2010; Kreke et al., 2004). The selection of tools depends on what problems need to be addressed and the investigators perspective (patient, hospital, society, etc.).

The main goal of ICU operation modeling is to improve the quality of patient care. We propose a road map for acute care delivery transformation based on principles of systems engineering (Figure 4, Modified from Kujala (Kujala et al., 2006)). Care delivery process in acute hospitals can be divided into four parts: 1) clinical practices and procedures (value added time for the core business of healthcare service, procedures, physical examination, etc.); 2) hospital business and regulations (charting, billing, etc.); 3) no value added activities (waiting for a computer log on, gathering of disparate information); 4) service time (time providers spend with patient/family members showing compassion, holding hands a key human interaction that can't be replaced by technology). Importantly, optimization of health care delivery does not merely equate to increased productivity by increasing the number of patients each service can "process" in a given time. Rather, the value added time gained by process optimization can be used to enhance the human interaction between

Figure 4. Road map for healthcare delivery transformation

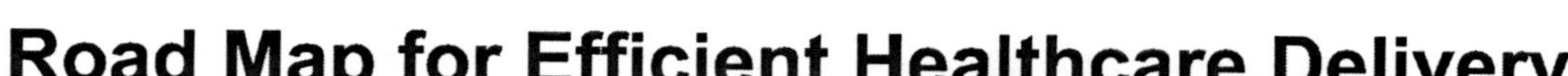

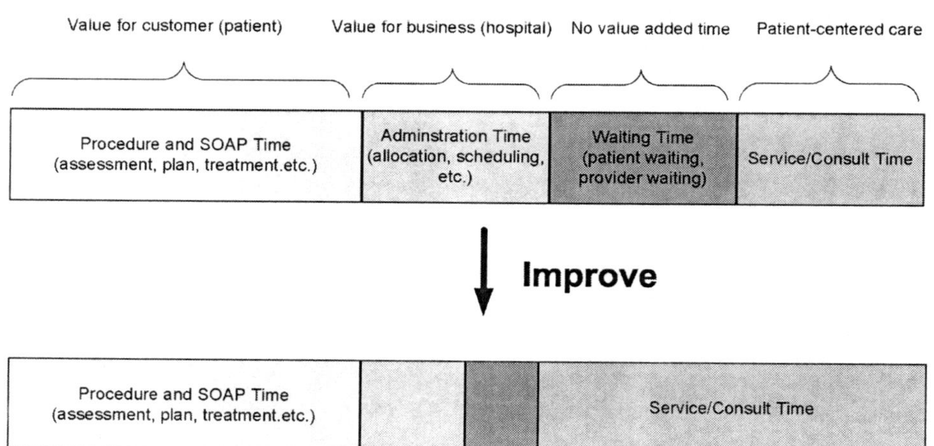

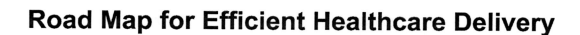

patients, families and providers according to ultimate values of patient center care as proposed by Institute of Medicine (Porter, 2009).

CONCLUSION

With increased demands and limited resources there is a great need to improve safety and efficiency of care delivery and optimize outcome of critically ill patients. Systems engineering and operations research methodology (i.e. computer process modeling) improves "systems" understanding of ICU processes and facilitate safe testing of potential optimization solutions, prior to clinical testing and implementation. The proposed framework is transferable to other complex health care environments (emergency department, operating room) where timely execution of complex processes can greatly influence patient outcome. A clinically relevant, systematic approach requires the development of multidisciplinary collaborations between bedside health care providers and researchers skilled in operational research, biomedical informatics and human factor engineering (Martinez et al., 2010).

REFERENCES

Allenbach, R. L., & Huffman, J. E. (1998). Improving simulation engineering practices I - A capability maturity model for simulation processes improvement. *International Journal of Industrial Engineering: Theory Applications and Practice*, *5*(2), 150–156.

Analytics, H. I. M. S. S. (2010). *EMR adoption model*. Retrieved July 20, 2010, from http://www.himssanalytics.org/ hc_providers/emr_adoption.asp

Baker, D. R., Pronovost, P. J., Morlock, L. L., Geocadin, R. G., & Holzmueller, C. G. (2009). Patient flow variability and unplanned readmissions to an intensive care unit. *Critical Care Medicine*, *37*(11), 2882–2887. doi:10.1097/CCM.0b013e3181b01caf

Barth, T., & Algee, J. (1996). *Proving and improving your processes with simulation.* Paper presented at the International Industrial Engineering Conference, Minneapolis, MN, USA.

Bertsimas, D., & De Boer, S. (2005). Simulation-based booking limits for airline revenue management. *Operations Research, 53*(1), 90–106. doi:10.1287/opre.1040.0164

Blendon, R. J., DesRoches, C. M., Brodie, M., Benson, J. M., Rosen, A. B., & Schneider, E. (2002). Views of practicing physicians and the public on medical errors. *The New England Journal of Medicine, 347*(24), 1933–1940. doi:10.1056/NEJMsa022151

Bracco, D., Favre, J. B., Bissonnette, B., Wasserfallen, J. B., Revelly, J. P., & Ravussin, P. (2001). Human errors in a multidisciplinary intensive care unit: A 1-year prospective study. *Intensive Care Medicine, 27*(1), 137–145. doi:10.1007/s001340000751

Brailsford, S. (2005). Overcoming the barriers to implementation of operations research simulation models in healthcare. *Clinical and Investigative Medicine. Medecine Clinique et Experimentale, 28*(6), 312–315.

Brailsford, S. C., Harper, P. R., Patel, B., & Pitt, M. (2009). An analysis of the academic literature on simulation and modelling in health care. *Journal of Simulation, 3*(3), 130–140. doi:10.1057/jos200910

Brailsford, S. C., & Hilton, N. A. (2001). A comparison of discrete event simulation and system dynamics for modelling health care systems. In Riley, J. (Ed.), *Planning for the future: Health service quality and emergency accessibility. Operational research applied to health services (ORAHS)*. Glasgow Caledonian University.

Cates, G. R., & Mollaghasemi, M. (2005). *Supporting the vision for space with discrete event simulation.* Paper presented at the Winter Simulation Conference.

Chahal, K., & Eldabi, T. (2010). A multi-perspective comparison for selection between system dynamics and discrete event simulation. *International Journal of Business Information Systems, 6*(1), 4–17.

Chantler, C. (1999). The role and education of doctors in the delivery of health care. *Lancet, 353*(9159), 1178–1181. doi:10.1016/S0140-6736(99)01075-2

Cook, R. I., & Woods, D. (1994). Operating at the sharp end: The complexity of human error. In Bogner, M. (Ed.), *Human errors in medicine*. Hillsdale, NJ: Erlbaum.

Dellinger, R. P., Carlet, J. M., Masur, H., Gerlach, H., Calandra, T., & Cohen, J. (2004). Surviving sepsis campaign guidelines for management of severe sepsis and septic shock. *Critical Care Medicine, 32*(3), 858–873. doi:10.1097/01.CCM.0000117317.18092.E4

Dittus, R. S., Klein, R. W., DeBrota, D. J., Dame, M. A., & Fitzgerald, J. F. (1996). Medical resident work schedules: Design and evaluation by simulation modeling. *Management Science, 42*(6), 891–906. doi:10.1287/mnsc.42.6.891

Donchin, Y., Gopher, D., Olin, M., Badihi, Y., Biesky, M., & Sprung, C. L. (2003). A look into the nature and causes of human errors in the intensive care unit. *Quality & Safety in Health Care, 12*(2), 143–147. doi:10.1136/qhc.12.2.143

Dong, Y., Lu, H., Rotz, J., Schieffer, C., Kashyap, R., & Pickering, B. W. (2009). Simulation modeling of healthcare delivery during sepsis resuscitation. *Critical Care Medicine, 37*(Suppl S), 686.

Dong, Y., Suri, H. S., Cook, D. A., Kashani, K. B., Mullon, J. J., & Enders, F. T. (2010). Simulation-based objective assessment discerns clinical proficiency in central line placement: A construct validation. *Chest*, *137*(5). doi:10.1378/chest.09-1451

Eldabi, T., Irani, Z., & Paul, R. J. (2002). A proposed approach for modelling health-care systems for understanding. *Journal of Management in Medicine*, *16*(2-3), 170–187. doi:10.1108/02689230210434916

Eldabi, T., Paul, R. J., & Young, T. (2007). Simulation modelling in healthcare: Reviewing legacies and investigating futures. *The Journal of the Operational Research Society*, *58*(2), 262–270.

Ferrer, R., Artigas, A., Levy, M. M., Blanco, J., Gonzalez-Diaz, G., & Garnacho-Montero, J. (2008). Improvement in process of care and outcome after a multicenter severe sepsis educational program in Spain. *Journal of the American Medical Association*, *299*(19), 2294–2303. doi:10.1001/jama.299.19.2294

Fone, D., Hollinghurst, S., Temple, M., Round, A., Lester, N., & Weightman, A. (2003). Systematic review of the use and value of computer simulation modelling in population health and health care delivery. *Journal of Public Health Medicine*, *25*(4), 325–335. doi:10.1093/pubmed/fdg075

Garrouste-Orgeas, M., Timsit, J. F., Vesin, A., Schwebel, C., Arnodo, P., & Lefrant, J. Y. (2010). Selected medical errors in the intensive care unit: Results of the IATROREF study: Parts I and II. *American Journal of Respiratory and Critical Care Medicine*, *181*(2), 134–142. doi:10.1164/rccm.200812-1820OC

Gawande, A. (2007, December 10). The checklist If something so simple can transform intensive care, what else can it do? *New Yorker (New York, N.Y.)*, 86–101.

Griffiths, J. D., Jones, M., Read, M. S., & Williams, J. E. (2010). A simulation model of bed-occupancy in a critical care unit. *Journal of Simulation*, *4*(1), 52–59. doi:10.1057/jos.2009.22

Grol, R., & Grimshaw, J. (2003). From best evidence to best practice: Effective implementation of change in patients' care. *Lancet*, *362*(9391), 1225–1230. doi:10.1016/S0140-6736(03)14546-1

Halpern, N. A., & Pastores, S. M. (2010). Critical care medicine in the United States 2000-2005: An analysis of bed numbers, occupancy rates, payer mix, and costs. *Critical Care Medicine*, *38*(1), 65–71. doi:10.1097/CCM.0b013e3181b090d0

Haut, E. R., Chang, D. C., Hayanga, A. J., Efron, D. T., Haider, A. H., & Cornwell Iii, E. E. (2009). Surgeon- and system-based influences on trauma mortality. *Archives of Surgery*, *144*(8), 759–764. doi:10.1001/archsurg.2009.100

Haynes, A. B., Weiser, T. G., Berry, W. R., Lipsitz, S. R., Breizat, A. H. S., & Dellinger, E. P. (2009). A surgical safety checklist to reduce morbidity and mortality in a global population. *The New England Journal of Medicine*, *360*(5), 491–499. doi:10.1056/NEJMsa0810119

Herasevich, V., Pickering, B. W., Dong, Y., Peters, S. G., & Gajic, O. (2010). Informatics infrastructure for syndrome surveillance, decision support, reporting, and modeling of critical illness. *Mayo Clinic Proceedings*, *85*(3), 247–254. doi:10.4065/mcp.2009.0479

Hrúz, B., & Zhou, M. (2007). *Modeling and control of discrete-event dynamic systems: With Petri nets and other tools* (1st ed.). Springer.

Institute of Medicine. (2001). *Crossing the quality chasm: A new health system for the 21st century*. Washington, DC: The National Academies Press.

Kahn, J. M., & Bates, D. W. (2008). Improving sepsis care: The road ahead. *JAMA -. Journal of the American Medical Association*, *299*(19), 2322–2323. doi:10.1001/jama.299.19.2322

Kahn, J. M., & Rubenfeld, G. D. (2005). Translating evidence into practice in the intensive care unit: The need for a systems-based approach. *Journal of Critical Care*, *20*(3), 204–206. doi:10.1016/j.jcrc.2005.06.001

Kelley, R. (2009). *Where can $700 billion in waste be cut annually from the U.S. healthcare system?* Retrieved July 27, 2010, from http://thomsonreuters.com/content/ corporate/articles/healthcare_reform

Kolker, A. (2009). Process modeling of ICU patient flow: Effect of daily load leveling of elective surgeries on ICU diversion. *Journal of Medical Systems*, *33*(1), 27–40. doi:10.1007/s10916-008-9161-9

Kolker, A. (2009). Queuing theory and discrete events simulation for health care: From basic processes to complex systems with interdependencies. In Abu-Taieh, E. M. O., & El-Sheikh, A. A. (Eds.), *Handbook of research on discrete event simulation environments: Technologies and applications* (pp. 443–483). Hershey, PA: Information Science Reference. doi:10.4018/978-1-60566-774-4.ch020

Kreke, J. E., Schaefer, A. J., & Roberts, M. S. (2004). Simulation and critical modeling. *Current Opinion in Critical Care*, *10*(5), 395–398. doi:10.1097/01.ccx.0000139361.30327.20

Kujala, J., Lillrank, P., Kronstrom, V., & Peltokorpi, A. (2006). Time-based management of patient processes. *Journal of Health Organization and Management*, *20*(6), 512–524. doi:10.1108/14777260610702262

Kuljis, J., Paul, R. J., & Stergioulas, L. K. (2007). *Can health care benefit from modeling and simulation methods in the same way as business and manufacturing has?* Paper presented at the Winter Simulation Conference.

Kumar, K., Zarychanski, R., Bell, D. D., Manji, R., Zivot, J., & Menkis, A. H. (2009). Impact of 24-hour in-house intensivists on a dedicated cardiac surgery intensive care unit. *The Annals of Thoracic Surgery*, *88*(4), 1153–1161. doi:10.1016/j.athoracsur.2009.04.070

Law, A., & Kelton, W. D. (1999). *Simulation modeling and analysis* (3rd ed.). McGraw-Hill Science/Engineering/Math.

Lawrence, D. (2005). Bridging the quality chasm. In Reid, P. P., Compton, W. D., Grossman, J. H., & Fanjiang, G. (Eds.), *Building a better delivery system: A new engineering/healthcare partnership* (p. 99). Committee on Engineering and the Health Care System, Institute of Medicine and National Academy of Engineering.

Levy, M. M., Dellinger, R. P., Townsend, S. R., Linde-Zwirble, W. T., Marshall, J. C., & Bion, J. (2010). The surviving sepsis campaign: Results of an international guideline-based performance improvement program targeting severe sepsis. *Critical Care Medicine*, *38*(2), 367–374. doi:10.1097/CCM.0b013e3181cb0cdc

Martinez, E. A., Marsteller, J. A., Thompson, D. A., Gurses, A. P., Goeschel, C. A., & Lubomski, L. H. (2010). The society of cardiovascular anesthesiologists' FOCUS initiative: Locating errors through networked surveillance (LENS) project vision. *Anesthesia and Analgesia*, *110*(2), 307–311. doi:10.1213/ANE.0b013e3181c92b9c

National Patient Safety Foundation. (2010). *Unmet needs: Teaching physicians to provide safe patient care*. Report of the Lucian Leape Institute Roundtable On Reforming Medical Education.

Pickering, B., Herasevich, V., Ahmed, A., & Gajic, O. (2010). Novel representation of clinical information in the ICU: Developing user interfaces which reduce information overload. *Applied Clinical Informatic*, *1*(2), 116–131. doi:10.4338/ACI-2009-12-CR-0027

Porter, M. E. (2009). A strategy for health care reform - Toward a value-based system. *The New England Journal of Medicine*, *361*(2), 109–112. doi:10.1056/NEJMp0904131

Pronovost, P., & Vohr, E. (2010). *Safe patients, smart hospitals: How one doctor's checklist can help us change health care from the inside out* (1st ed.). Hudson Street Press.

Reid, P. P., Compton, W. D., Grossman, J. H., & Fanjiang, G. (2005). *Building a better delivery system: A new engineering/health care partnership*. Committee on Engineering and the Health Care System, Institute of Medicine and National Academy of Engineering.

Research, C. f. H. S. (2009). *Federal funding for health services research. Nominal spending increase does not compensate for years of real declines*. Retrieved March 10, 2010, from http://www.chsr.org/ coalitionfunding2008.pdf

Schmidt, J. W., & Taylor, R. E. (1970). *Simulation and analysis of industrial systems*. Homewood, IL: R. D. Irwin.

Schrage, M. (1999). Measure prototyping paybacks. In Schrage, M. (Ed.), *Serious play: How the world's best companies simulate to innovate*. Harvard Business School Press.

Soliman, F. (1998). Optimum level of process mapping and least cost business process reengineering. *International Journal of Operations & Production Management*, *18*(9-10), 810–816. doi:10.1108/01443579810225469

van Sambeek, J. R. C., Cornelissen, F. A., Bakker, P. J. M., & Krabbendam, J. J. (2010). Models as instruments for optimizing hospital processes: A systematic review. *International Journal of Health Care Quality Assurance*, *23*(4), 356–377. doi:10.1108/09526861011037434

Vankipuram, M., Kahol, K., Cohen, T., & Patel, V. L. (2010). Toward automated workflow analysis and visualization in clinical environments. *Journal of Biomedical Informatics*.

Vincent, C., Moorthy, K., Sarker, S. K., Chang, A., & Darzi, A. W. (2004). Systems approaches to surgical quality and safety: From concept to measurement. *Annals of Surgery*, *239*(4), 475–482. doi:10.1097/01.sla.0000118753.22830.41

Westfall, J. M., Mold, J., & Fagnan, L. (2007). Practice-based research-"Blue highways" on the NIH roadmap. *Journal of the American Medical Association*, *297*(4), 403–406. doi:10.1001/jama.297.4.403

Young, T. (2005). An agenda for healthcare and information simulation. *Health Care Management Science*, *8*(3), 189–196. doi:10.1007/s10729-005-2008-8

Young, T., Brailsford, S., Connell, C., Davies, R., Harper, P., & Klein, J. H. (2004). Using industrial processes to improve patient care. *British Medical Journal*, *328*(7432), 162–164. doi:10.1136/bmj.328.7432.162

Young, T., Eatock, J., Jahangirian, M., Naseer, A., & Lilford, R. (2009). *Three critical challenges for modeling and simulation in healthcare*. Paper presented at the Winter Simulation Conference.

Zhang, J., & Butler, K. A. (2007). *UFuRT: A work-centered framework and process for design and evaluation of information systems*. HCI International Proceedings.

KEY TERMS AND DEFINITIONS

Discrete Event: A discrete event is something countable that happens at an instant of simulated time that might change attributes, variables or statistical outputs. A new patient enters the ICU is an event example.

Discrete Event Simulation: Computer simulation of system operations which is presented as a chronological sequence of events. Each event occurs at an instant in time and marks a change of state of the system

Model Analysis and Optimization: Model analysis is to study the relationship between the inputs and outputs of a component or system. The optimization process is to find the inputs and system parameters, under which the system output(s) are optimal or near-optimal.

Model Validation: In discrete event simulation modeling, model validation is the process of ensuring that the model behaves the same as the real system to be simulated. It usually involves the comparison between simulation data and real system data.

Modeling and Simulation (M&S): Modeling is a process to set up the relationship between the system inputs and outputs to study the system performance. For some complex and random system behaviors, computer simulation technology is adopted for modeling study.

Model Verification: In discrete event simulation, model verification is the model debug process to ensure that the simulation model behaves as intended; the inputs, outputs, and main components in the flowchart of the system match the real system to be simulated.

Operational Modeling: Modeling of operations of a system performance, usually the system performance is complicated and involves uncertainties.

Sepsis Resuscitation: A process of taking series of treatments and therapies to treat patients with severe sepsis and septic shock.

Severe Sepsis Bundles: A distillation of the concepts and recommendations found in the practice guidelines published by the Surviving Sepsis Campaign in 2004. The Severe Sepsis Bundles are designed to allow teams to follow the timing, sequence, and goals of the individual elements of care, in order to achieve the goal of a 25 percent reduction in mortality from severe sepsis.

Systems Engineering: Systems engineering is an interdisciplinary field of engineering that focuses on how complex engineering projects should be designed and operated. Some methodologies used in system engineering are adapted from industrial engineering and management science such as operations research, decision theory, queuing theory, computer simulation, etc.

System State: It is a collection of variables in any time that describe the system status in simulation process.

Chapter 7
Human-Centered Systems Engineering:
Managing Stakeholder Dissonance in Healthcare Delivery

GM Samaras
Samaras & Associates, Inc., USA

ABSTRACT

Deploying new tools and technologies often results in creating new problems while solving existing problems. A root cause is the interaction between tool design and organizational deployment. One undesirable result is the creation of stakeholder dissonance (SD). SD is a term for the conflict between the needs, wants, and desires (NWDs) of different stakeholders. In healthcare delivery systems, it is evidenced by errors, workarounds, and threats to patient safety and organizational profitability.

Human-Centered Systems Engineering (HCSE) is the foundational paradigm for managing SD. HCSE emphasizes the criticality of the interfaces between humans, their tools, and their organizations, offering methods to recognize, measure, and control SD. It is complimentary to Lean, Six Sigma, Balanced Scorecard, and Quality Function Deployment approaches.

Managing SD requires recognition of all stakeholders and their NWDs, permitting discovery and mapping of potential conflicts. Prioritizing conflicts for mitigation relies on standard risk analysis and decision analysis methods. HCSE provides methods for measuring only those NWDs involved, once the critical conflicts are chosen. This permits the mitigations to be verified, and the deployment design to be validated in a pilot setting, prior to general release of the new tools and technologies into the organization.

DOI: 10.4018/978-1-60960-872-9.ch007

INTRODUCTION

Effectiveness is the foundation of success –

Efficiency is a minimum condition for survival

after success has been achieved.

Efficiency is concerned with doing things right.

Effectiveness is doing the right things.

Peter F. Drucker (1909 - 2005)

I spend a considerable amount of my time haranguing my clients (the majority of whom are medical device manufacturers) that absent rigorous Design Controls (Samaras, 2010a) their products will have problems, will dissatisfy customers, and be potential sources of adverse events. What I conveniently forget to tell them is that, even though they may do everything perfectly, the way their products are deployed has a profound impact on meaningful use, patient safety, and profitability in the user organization. Why the concern with profitability? Because organizations that are not, by some measure, profitable will wither and die. Meaningful use, patient safety, and profitability in the user organization are three core issues for effective healthcare delivery.

Figure 1 shows two connected Venn diagrams. The upper Venn diagram depicts the interactions of hardware, software, and human factors issues in the design of tools resulting in tool-level problems; the locus of control is the manufacturer of medical devices, information technology systems, etc. The lower Venn diagram depicts the interactions of business, technical and regulatory issues in the user organization resulting in organizational-level problems; the locus of control is the hospital system, the nursing home, the physician's office, etc. In recent years, especially with increased emphasis on human factors engineering, manufacturers have become quite good at identifying

Figure 1. Source of errors from two levels of interaction

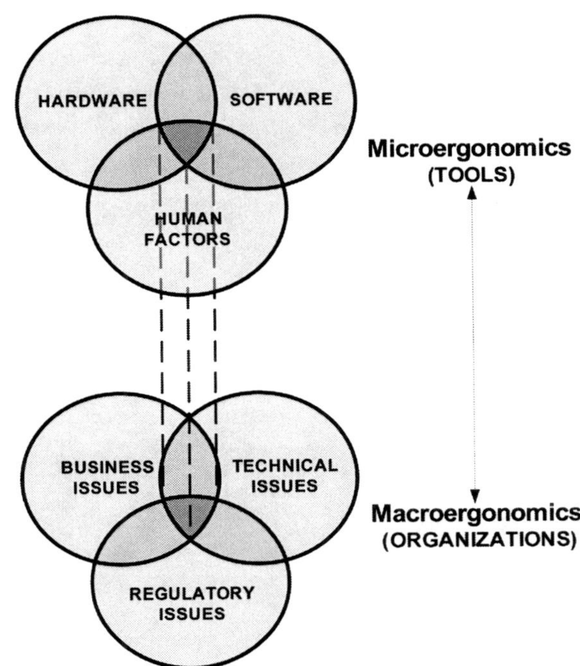

and mitigating tool-level problems. Businesses that deliver healthcare are quite facile at dealing with traditional organizational-level issues common to non-healthcare businesses.

The purpose of Figure 1 is to highlight the multi-level problem of the interaction of tool-use and organizational deployment of these tools in healthcare delivery. This class of problems leads to a phenomenon termed *stakeholder dissonance* (SD) – a lack of agreement, consistency, or harmony among the stakeholders (Samaras & Samaras, 2010). SD in the healthcare delivery system, results in decreased patient safety and decreased organizational profitability. In the jargon of human factors engineering, the two levels in Figure 1 are called *microergonomics* and *macroergonomics*. They are subdisciplines of human factors science and are practiced by different specialists, not unlike industrial versus electrical engineering.

SD is a management concept. It is not the concept of "cognitive dissonance" related to an inconsistency between beliefs and actions. SD is not related to negative drives; it refers to the conflicting needs, wants, and desires (NWDs) among different stakeholders. NWDs are not static; they devolve over time, so that what today may be a Desire tomorrow often devolves to a Want or a Need and is replaced by new Desires. Conflicts between the NWDs of various stakeholders, in the context of healthcare delivery, is evidenced by errors, workarounds, decreased motivation, decreased satisfaction, and even outright rejection of new products, processes, or services. SD is diagnostic for quality deficits.

So, how do we deal with SD in the delivery of healthcare? It is important to realize that SD never can be eliminated totally in any system, including healthcare delivery systems. SD arises from the intentional or unrecognized conflicts between the NWDs of the various system stakeholders. The Venn diagram of Figure 2 depicts the needs of four different stakeholder groups, how they align pair-wise, and how they align for all four stakeholders. It should be self-evident that complete alignment of the NWDs of patients, clinicians, support staff, and management will be very rare, if not impossible.

So, how do we manage SD in the delivery of healthcare? Ask it another way. How do we measure and control SD, to manage it in healthcare delivery? One approach is to use the principles of human-centered systems engineering. This will allow us to characterize, quantify, prioritize, and control conflicts in the NWDs of the various stakeholders. In human-centered systems engineering, we go beyond the "voice of the customer" and recognize that all stakeholders (individuals and their organizations) are critical to safety, effectiveness, efficiency, and satisfaction.

Human-centered systems engineering is the foundational paradigm for addressing SD. Our objective in the application of human-centered systems engineering will be to *satisfice* all the stakeholders, which Simon (1957) defined as to obtain a good result that is good enough, though not necessarily the best, for each stakeholder. The term *satisfice* is presumed to be a contraction of the terms *satisfy* and *suffice*. Nobel Laureate economist and sociologist Herbert Simon first defined the concept of *satisficing* in an attempt to reduce the computational complexity of a linear programming problem for individual and

Figure 2. Alignment of stakeholder needs

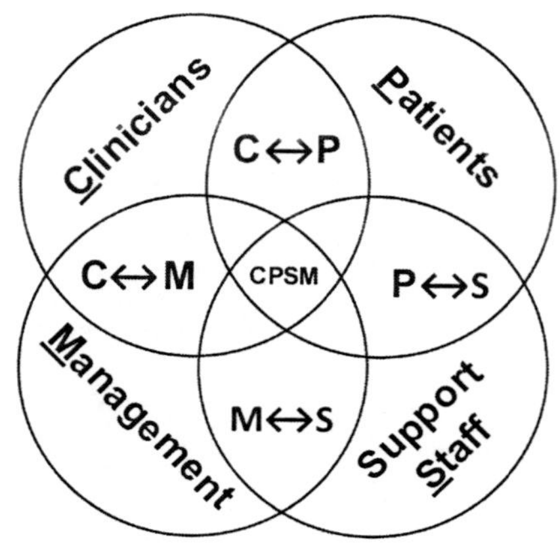

organizational behaviors. This SD reduction strategy is akin to "greasing the skids", thereby reducing known and unknown forces preventing realization of organizational goals. Solving the problems of *satisficing* ALL the stakeholders is a proper endeavor for management engineering,

A HUMAN-CENTERED APPROACH

Human-Centered System Engineering

Products, processes, and services are developed and maintained solely because their use by humans has real or perceived value that is utilitarian and/or esthetic. Even completely automated, unsupervised systems have human users (maintenance personnel) and maintenance is typically a significant portion of the Total Cost of Ownership (TCO). This is the fundamental justification and rationale for human-centered systems engineering (HCSE).

Classical systems engineering is a very powerful mechanism for reducing business and technical risks. It is a structured, systematic approach to the design, development, deployment, and replacement of products, processes, and services. HCSE extends systems engineering to expose the criticality of human actors and their organizations in the engineering process (Samaras & Horst, 2005). The HCSE process has an essential iterative nature (Samaras, 2010a), each new iteration (Figure 3) beginning with the (re-) identification of stakeholders and assessment of their NWDs (**N**eeds - basic needs or "*must haves*", **W**ants - performance needs or "*like to haves*", and **D**esires - latent needs or "*I'll know it when I see it*").

We constantly hear of incidents and accidents that are alleged to be caused by human error, but which human error? *Use* error or *UseR* error? *Use* errors are attributable to the design and/or deployment of the system; they result from the myriad interactions of tool design errors and organizational deployment issues (Figure 1). The major causal factors associated with *Use* error (Samaras,

Figure 3. HCSE iterative deployment paradigm

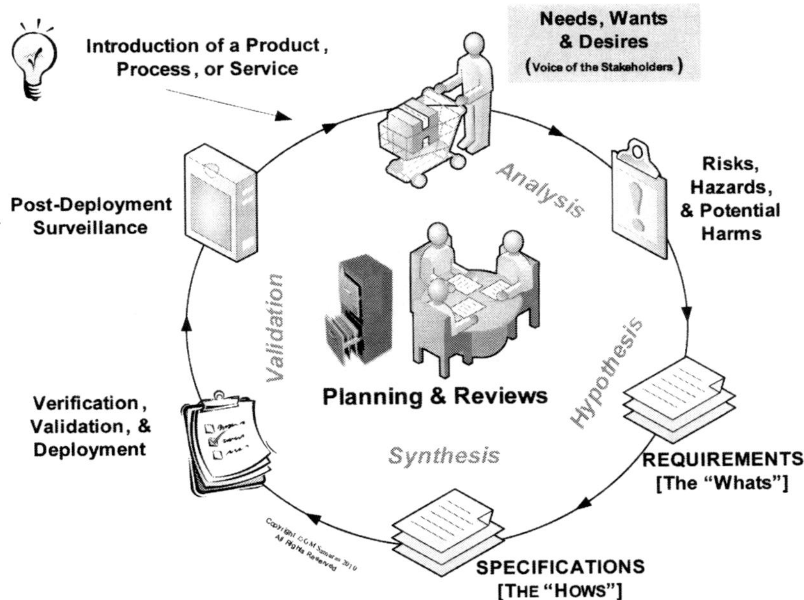

2010b) are improper management controls, improper design controls (at either the technology manufacturer and/or the deploying organization), inadequate non-financial risk management, and inadequate record-keeping controls (Figure 4). *UseR* errors are attributable to the internal or external human user environment, <u>excluding</u> the system itself (Figure 5); these are some of the "human factors" associated with the individual involved with the error (Samaras, 2010b). So, who is at fault? The human operators? Or, the human developers and deployers? Human *Use* errors are largely within the locus of control of system developers and deploying organizations. Even future *UseR* errors may be influenced by the developer and/or deploying organization (e.g., avoid confusing or frustrating the operator, avoid undesirable physical or cognitive exercises, avoid delays and operator attention loss, avoid inappropriate workloads and work schedules).

In the healthcare arena, safe and effective healthcare delivery systems (products, processes, and services) are the goal. However, human stakeholders complicate the process at a myriad of levels from conceptualization through design, development, deployment, and replacement. Great care must be exercised in finding fault with end-users, when design and development, organizational deployment, or a combination (see Figure 1) may actually be the root cause. This is especially important, since from an organizational perspective, we have far less control over daily use by end-users than we do over organizational deployment or tool selection and acquisition

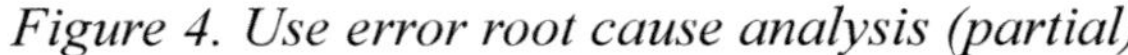

Figure 4. Use error root cause analysis (partial)

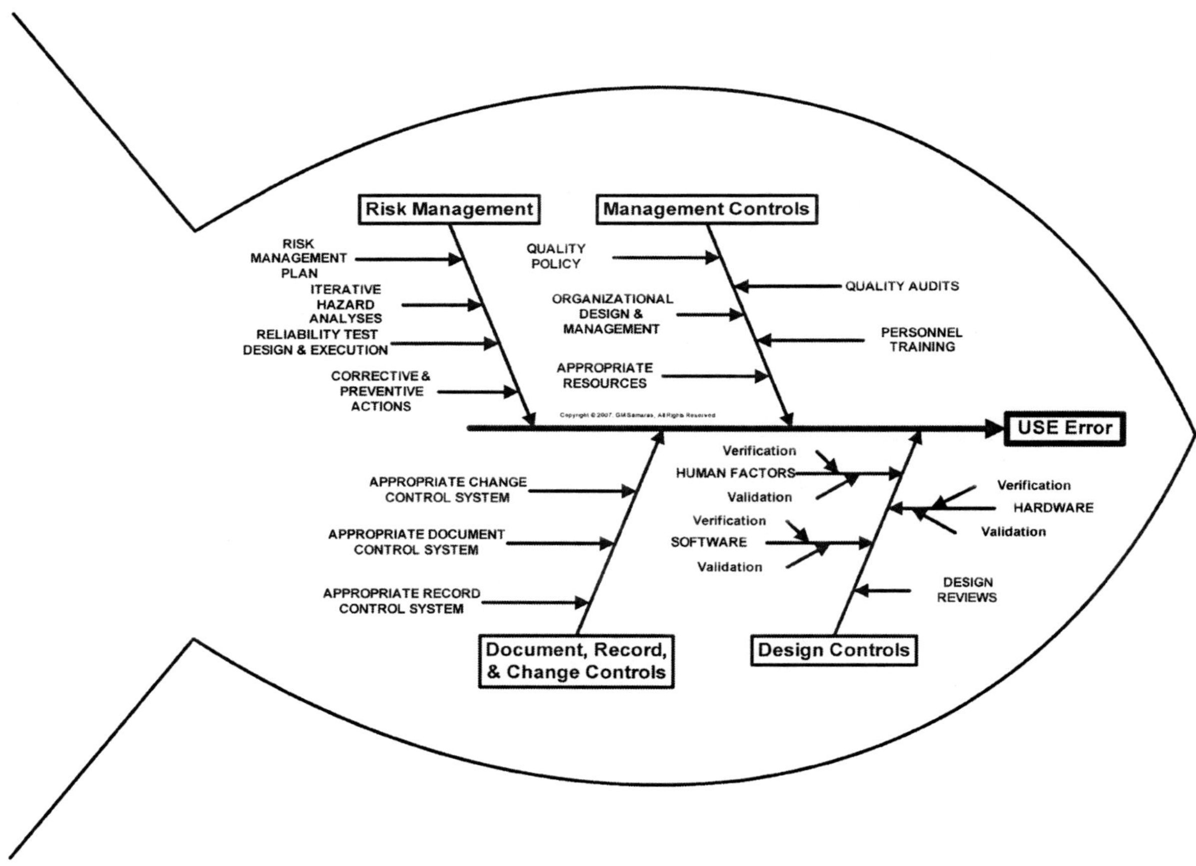

Figure 5. UseR errors root cause analysis (partial)

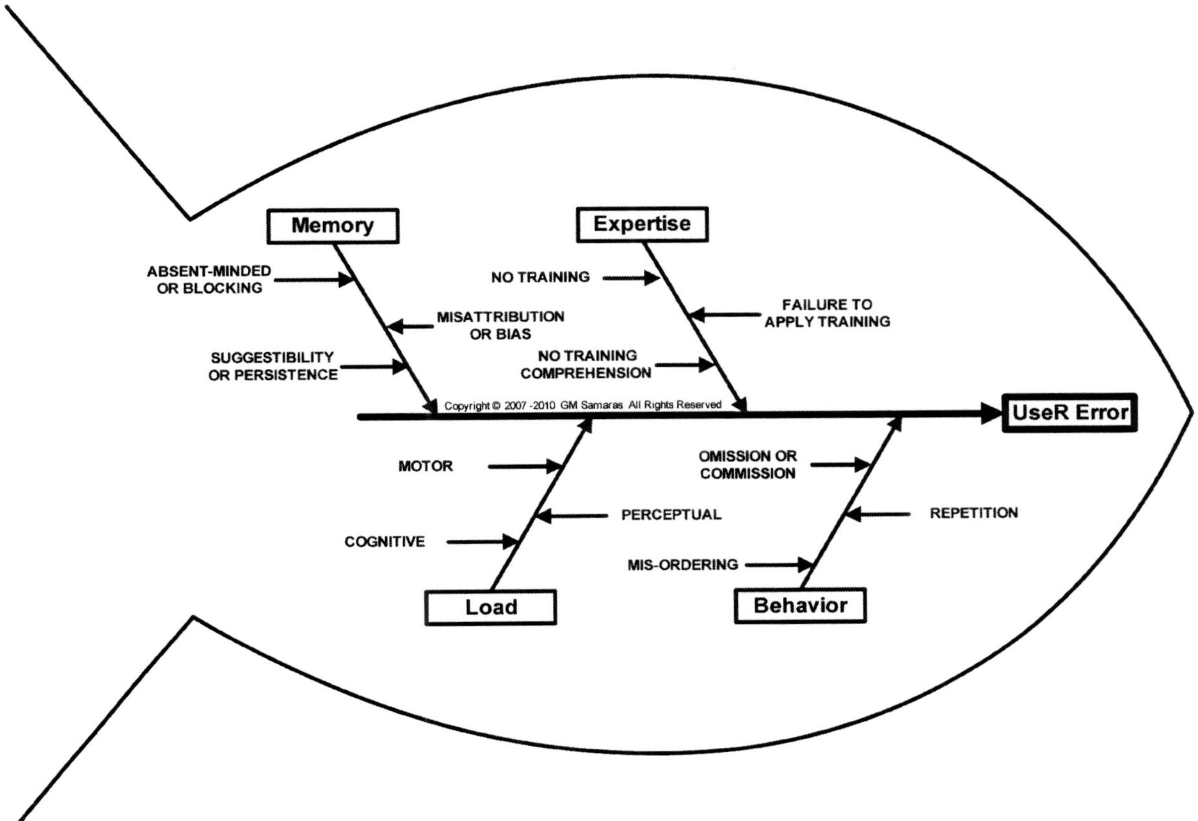

(which ultimately controls design and development).

Human-Centered System Complexity

Introducing human actors (*actor* is a term of art in social science and economics that subsumes *user*) into any endeavor dramatically increases the possible number of incorrect or inappropriate responses of a "simple" hardware/software system. The ratio of "wrong to right" responses often is used to characterize the complexity of tasks; it also imputes the requisite level of expertise (training and experience) to execute a series of such tasks successfully by the operators (or groups of operators and/or their automated aides). Humans dramatically increase system complexity.

Complex systems have *emergent* properties – the result of component interactions at the interfaces – that are not readily predictable without appreciation of the system as a whole. It is now generally recognized that product, process, and service design-induced errors are a serious problem, a critical system safety issue, and an important source of reduced quality. They can rarely be alleviated simply with labeling or user training!

Not fully appreciating human-centered system complexity, especially in risk management, has been an important obstacle in the design and deployment of essential clinical systems (e.g., clinical decision support, medication management, and clinical information exchange). Using technology merely to solve identified problems often creates new, previously unidentified, problems (e.g., see

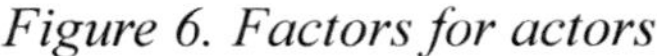

Figure 6. Factors for actors

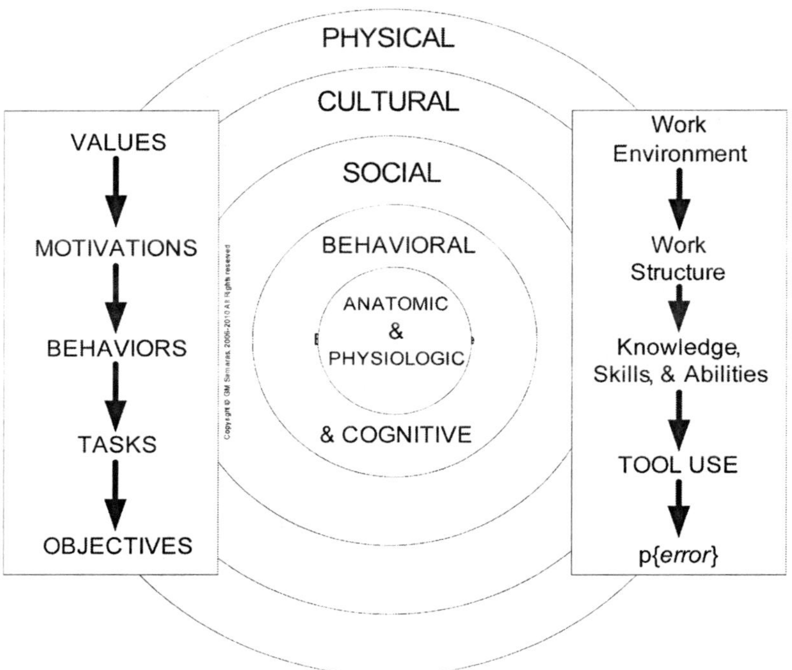

how a decade's difference dramatically altered perspectives of computerized physician order entry [Tierney et al, 1993 vs. Koppel et al, 2005]).

Stakeholders operate in a complex environment (Figure 6) that influences both what they achieve and how they err. Whether they are patients, clinicians, support staff, managers, or other stakeholders (e.g., 3rd party payers, regulators, stockholders, suppliers, manufacturers, competitors, etc.) their behaviors are determined in large part by their disparate values and motivations. How they work and how probable will it be for them to be involved with errors, is influenced not only by training and by experience, but also by the work environment and work structure (e.g., 8-hour shifts versus 12-hour shifts). These all are influenced by individual biological, behavioral, social, cultural, and physical environmental factors – yielding a complex environment and a resulting increase in overall system complexity.

Complexity arises at the interfaces. A human-centered approach requires a detailed appreciation of the interfaces to actors and between actors. Otherwise, we remain unable to predict and control the critical human and organizational influences both on system design parameters and on system sensitivities to external factors.

Our fundamental need to study the system as a whole requires a model of human-centered complexity (Samaras & Samaras, 2009) from which we can derive an operationalization schema, a means of defining what needs to be measured and how it may be measured (Table 1). It offers a way of appreciating both the system components and their potential interactions.

In all cases, the interfaces consist of both overt factors (quantities we can detect with one or more of our five senses) and covert factors (quantities we cannot detect with our five senses). An engineering example would be the externally observed *distance* (an overt factor) a free body traveled versus the externally observed *acceleration* (the second time derivative of distance, a covert factor) of the free body. At the level of *individual* actors

Table 1. The interdisciplinary nature of measuring human-centered system complexity

	HCSE METROLOGY CATEGORIES			
	INDIVIDUAL		GROUP	
FACTORS	PHYSICAL	BEHAVIORAL	SOCIAL	CULTURAL
Overt	Anthropo-morpho-metry	Verbal & Nonverbal Behaviors	Communication & Coordination	Language & Artifacts
Covert	Biomechanical & Sensory Processes	Affective, Cognitive, & Physiological Behaviors	Conventions & Expectations	Beliefs, Customs, Ethics, & Morals

and their tools, the interfaces consist of overt and covert physical and information management behavioral factors. Here we are concerned with the static and dynamic "physical fit" of tools as well as the requisite behaviors involved in the decision-making processes of tool use. At the level of *groups* of actors and their tools, the interfaces consist of overt and covert social and cultural factors. These include communication and coordination, norms and roles, as well as language differences (e.g., the language of clinicians versus the language of engineering or business) and differing value systems (shared beliefs, customs, ethics, and morals that vary among stakeholders). Using this operationalization model supports comprehensive consideration of system, parameter, and tolerance design for engineering human-centered systems – an essential set of tasks in quality engineering.

In HCSE, the emphasis shifts to iterative discovery of stakeholders, iterative identification of their evolving NWDs, and iterative reconciliation of conflicts; the objective is to *satisfice* ALL the stakeholders (concurrent engineering is a subset of this approach). This precedes, and is the basis for, the requirements formulation process in each iteration (Figure 3). This shift in emphasis tends to mitigate errors and omissions early in the system deployment cycle, increasing effectiveness and efficiency. Absent robust HCSE, essential systems (e.g., clinical decision support, medication management, and clinical information exchange) will continue to hinder rather than help, be economically inefficient, and be examples of poor quality. However, to manage this, we must be able to measure and control the interfaces.

Examination of Table 1 indicates the measurement methods belong to a wide range of scientific disciplines – from biomechanics to cultural anthropology. These are well-established measurement techniques in each scientific discipline; therefore, threats to construct validity are minimized, although not eliminated. Physical measurements include essentially static human characteristics as well as dynamic measurements used in biomechanics and sensory physiology. Behavioral measurements use traditional techniques of experimental psychology. Techniques of social anthropology, social psychology, and sociology are used for social measurements. Cultural measurements use techniques of linguistics (for language), archaeology (for tools and other artifacts), and cultural anthropology (for value systems). Some practical examples to illustrate application of this measurement schema are shown in Table 2.

At a workshop related to HCSE that I teach annually, I am invariably asked, either in dismay or cynically, "You don't really expect us to do all these measurements; we do not have the cognitive psychologists, sociologists, and cultural anthropologists on staff!" My answer is invariably, "I do not expect an industrial engineer to program

Table 2. Measurement examples for table 1 metrology categories

INDIVIDUALS	PHYSICAL	**Overt factors** – the static size and fit of an individual (e.g., the range of adjustment of an operating table for the comfort of individual surgeons of different heights and reach)
		Covert factors – biomechanical factors (e.g., the weight and balance of an individual surgeon's tools) and sensory factors (e.g., multiple audible alarms in the operating theater interfering with recognition of a high priority alarm)
	BEHAVIORAL	**Overt factors** – verbal and non-verbal information management behaviors (e.g., verbalization and mouse/trackball operation while using a computerized provider order entry system)
		Covert factors – affective (e.g., a surgeon's frustration with multiple simultaneous alarms), cognitive (e.g., difficulties comprehending which alarm has the highest priority), and physiological behaviors (e.g., increased heart and respiration rate due to time pressures and frustration with discrimination of the alarms)
GROUPS	SOCIAL	**Overt factors** – communication and coordination (e.g., a physician putting medication orders or other directives in an inappropriate location of the computerized provider order entry system)
		Covert factors – conventions and expectations (e.g., the buyer routinely selects the diagnostic radiology device based upon the radiologist's desire for high image quality, erroneously expecting that the technicians and nurses – the actual users, not the readers – will deliver high productivity and profitability, regardless of the choice of device)
	CULTURAL	**Overt factors** – language and artifacts (e.g., clinical users and clinical engineers do not speak exactly the same language and patient safety problems often arise when there are gaps in communication due to language difficulties; what may be obvious to the engineer may not be obvious to the clinician and omission leads to miscommunication)
		Covert factors – shared values, such as beliefs, customs, ethics, and morals (e.g., the classical example of covert cultural factors is the discrepancy between clinical professionals and business professionals, both of whom are well-meaning but neither of whom recognize that they are starting with different assumptions and value systems)

a computer operating system and I do not expect YOU to do all these measurements, but I do expect that you will require some of these types of measurements for any particular deployment". What needs to be measured depends upon the particular circumstances and what needs to be measured should be measured.

If you are deploying a new infusion pump, your primary focus probably will be on individual factors. Are the displays intuitive, are the screens easy to read, or are the manual controls laid out well? If not, what can you do to minimize the impact on workload, how do you reduce the probability of medication errors, and is the TCO of the new infusion pump you are planning to buy consistent with your strategic objectives? Alternatively, if you are deploying a new medical record or provider order entry system, your primary focus will most likely be on group factors. How will this impact communication and coordination among physicians, pharmacists, and nurses? What "normal" conventions might undermine success of the deployment? What are the expectations of these stakeholder groups for the impact of this deployment on their workload, probable medication errors, and the TCO to the organization? In both these cases, TCO can no longer include just initial purchase price or maintenance costs, but also must include the cost of reduced clinician efficiency, increased medication errors, and the cost of not being reimbursed, if the deployment does not satisfy the "meaningful use" criterion.

Managing requires measuring. What gets measured depends specifically on what you are trying to deploy. Who needs to do the measurement is determined by what needs to get measured, not the other way around. The assessment and validation of human interface attributes is a process that is inescapably multi-disciplinary (Samaras, 2006).

Human-Centered Quality

HCSE takes a different approach to quality definition and quality management (including improvement). The definition encompasses, for example, all of Holpp's (1993) eight definitions of quality in healthcare and subsumes all six of Berwick's (2002) dimensions of healthcare performance. HCSE defines quality as *the degree to which the needs, wants, and desires of* *<u>all</u>* *the stakeholders have been satisficed* (Samaras, 2010b). With this quality definition, quality (Q) and SD are related concepts: zero SD corresponds to total quality (Q = 1 - SD). Under this definition, total quality (SD = 0) is unachievable, except in the most trivial cases. Reducing SD is the means to increasing quality. Furthermore, a quality improvement intervention – even if successful in the short term – can never be expected to endure without additional effort, because the system of humans (the organization) is dynamic, not static. Because SD can never be eliminated totally, the *satisficing* task, as first put forth by Simon, is a linear/nonlinear programming question and a classical management engineering problem.

There exist a myriad "definitions of quality" and many believe that the concept of quality is elusive. Holpp (1993) offered eight definitions of quality in healthcare that endure today. He stated that quality is customer satisfaction, meeting requirements, continuous process improvement, teamwork and empowerment, outstanding service, cost control and resource utilization, doing the right things right the first time, and (finally) how we do business.

The HCSE definition of quality encompasses all of Holpp's eight definitions; each of the eight definitions may be derived from the single HCSE definition: Stakeholders include both internal and external customers; *satisficing* their NWDs results in their satisfaction (although not necessarily their delight). Requirements (design inputs) in HCSE are defined as the subset of identified or discovered NWDs that are economically and technologically feasible at a given point in time (Samaras & Horst, 2005; Samaras, 2010a). Continuous process improvement, also called corrective and preventive action (CAPA) or continuous quality improvement (CQI), is a central element of the HCSE lifecycle, whose objective is to *satisfice* stakeholder NWDs. *Satisficing* the NWDs of all the stakeholders promotes teamwork and empowerment, outstanding service (we are *satisficing* the NWDs of both internal and external customers), and cost control and resource utilization (we are *satisficing* the NWDs of managers and business staff). *Satisficing* the NWDs of all the stakeholders moves us closer to doing "the right things right the first time". Finally, if you are *satisficing* the NWDs of all the stakeholders, that is how you do business.

All stakeholders have the same top-level NWDs (Samaras & Samaras, 2009); they are: **S**afety, **E**ffectiveness, **E**fficiency, and **S**atisfaction (SEES). The first three are objective measures (safety, effectiveness, and efficiency). The fourth (satisfaction) is a set of five subjective measures (perceived effectiveness, perceived efficiency, engaging, error tolerant and easy to learn). While these are the top-level NWD categories, their specific meaning varies by stakeholder (by the frame of reference).

Etzioni's (1964) defines "The actual *effectiveness* of a specific organization is determined by the degree to which it realizes its goals. The *efficiency* of an organization is measured by the amount of resources used to produce a unit of output."

Dubin (1976) asserts that effectiveness has a different meaning based on whether the organization is viewed from the inside (efficiency) or from the outside (social utility), which begins to get to the contemporary issue of "meaningful use". As you change the frame of reference from that of a single stakeholder to a stakeholder group, then to multiple stakeholder groups, and then to ALL the stakeholders, the effectiveness criterion is transformed. As you alter the system boundaries, the computation of efficiency is changed, because only resources that cross the system boundary are considered.

Where you decide to draw the system boundary, while always considered arbitrary, has profound consequences. The reference frame is crucial. For the patient, safety may mean that their health status is not degraded further; for the clinician, safety may mean that they are not injured/infected during the course of providing care; and for the healthcare delivery organization, their safety will most likely be expressed in financial terms. Similarly, the clinician and the healthcare delivery organization may disagree on both objective and subjective efficiency: management is satisfied that fewer clinicians are required to service a fixed number of patients, whereas clinicians are dissatisfied that their workload is above the generally accepted professional norm.

Berwick (2002) identifies six dimensions of healthcare performance cited in the IOM report *Crossing the Quality Chasm*: safety, timeliness, effectiveness, efficiency, equity, and patient-centeredness. These IOM's six dimensions or domains translate to only four <u>independent</u> quality dimensions – safety, effectiveness, efficiency, and satisfaction. Safety is not just a matter of avoiding physical, psychological, or socioeconomic injuries to patients, but also avoiding such injuries to other stakeholders including clinicians, support staff, and healthcare delivery organizations. Effectiveness is not only provision of evidence-based "treatment", but also provision of that treatment to all where (location) and when (timeliness) they can benefit; "treatment" needs to be understood in the broadest sense for all stakeholders (not just receiving a pill, but also having your work structure changed, your reimbursement terms altered, etc.). Efficiency is about avoiding waste, but as Dubin indicated, it is totally dependent upon where you draw your system boundary (your frame of reference). Timeliness is not an orthogonal quality dimension; it is an element of effectiveness (providing treatment when there will be benefit), efficiency (not wasting time), and satisfaction (because, as previously stated, satisfaction is a function of perceived effectiveness and perceived efficiency). Patient-centeredness (while the *raison d'être* of healthcare delivery) is not an independent dimension of quality; it is but one of a number of foci of the complete set of stakeholders that must be balanced in the implementation of a rational healthcare delivery system. Finally, equity (providing care invariant over demographic and socioeconomic status) does not survive careful analysis as an independent quality dimension (even though it is very attractive from a social justice perspective). Inequitable distribution of care jeopardizes the safety of some patients, is ineffective from a public health perspective (think of herd immunity), is inefficient from a national economic perspective (think of who is paying for whom to go to the emergency room), and is dissatisfying to many of the stakeholders (not all of whom are merely recipients of the inequitable care).

A basic premise of management engineering is that you *cannot manage what you cannot define*. The HCSE definition of quality is neither *ad hoc* nor "elusive", but contained, constrained, and quantifiable. It is derived from the fundamental principles of human-centered systems engineering and it is susceptible to effective management. Attempting to meet some or all the stakeholder NWDs is the sole purpose for system development <u>and</u> system deployment. The degree to which you are *satisficing* all the stakeholder NWDs is the fundamental measure of quality.

DIFFERENT PERSPECTIVES

Management engineering, like all other engineering disciplines, may be characterized by a set of tools, often borrowed from other scientific disciplines. Some of the more widely used (albeit, less rigorous) tools are identified and compared to HCSE.

Lean Approach

"Lean" got its name from a bestseller (Womack, Jones, & Roos, 1990) discussing how automobile manufacturing moved from craft production to mass production to lean manufacturing. Healthcare delivery is fundamentally a lean engineering problem characterized by the inherent tension between the search for high throughput and the involvement of primarily professional workers. The basic principles of lean engineering process optimization are simple to understand, but often difficult to achieve: (1) add nothing, but value (eliminate waste), (2) organize based upon people who add value, (3) create flow from pull (delay commitment), and (4) reduce barriers by optimizing across organizations. Critical to the lean engineering process is the recognition and analysis of the value stream (the flow of increasing value). Mapping out the value stream facilitates identification of waste and facilitates identification of stakeholders, including not only those who add value, but also those who might add barriers. Adding value and eliminating waste are central NWDs of all stakeholders. While lean engineering practitioners normally focus on adding value that an internal or external customer cares about, there is no reason it cannot be extended to adding value for all stakeholders.

Balanced Scorecard Approach

The first balanced scorecard was created in 1987 at Analog Devices, Inc. (Schneiderman, 2006). It achieved "balance" by adding non-financial measures that characterize progress towards the organization's strategic objectives. It considered five major stakeholder groups (communities, customers, employees, stockholders, and suppliers) focusing on gaps in their satisfaction that could be mapped to internal process improvements. The original balance was achieved by considering four perspectives (financial, customer, internal processes, and innovation & learning). Over time, more rigorous design methods have evolved (Lawrie & Cobbold, 2004) including the strategic linkage model (connecting strategic objectives with scorecard measures and targets to yield strategy maps) and the incorporation of a strategic goal or end-state definition (the "Destination Statement"). These improvements have tended to make the selection of perspectives, measures, and targets more closely linked to the actual organizational strategy designed to serve the stakeholders.

Six Sigma Approach and DMAIC

In 1988, Motorola, Inc. received the Malcolm Baldrige National Quality Award in part for their six sigma program (Pyzdek, 2003). The Six Sigma (6σ) approach is fundamentally about a process quality objective used for defects reduction by reducing process variability. It is now viewed as a method for improving organizational performance through the reduction of variability and elimination of waste. It focuses on control of a process to $\pm$ six standard deviations (6σ) from a target, which translates to about 2 defects per billion opportunities (3.4 defects per million opportunities $=\pm4.5\sigma$, so you must be willing to accept an additional 1.5σ drift). It assumes a "normal" or Gaussian distribution, a frequent simplifying assumption of industrial practitioners, which may or may not always be true, but is often a good first-order approximation. The major impact of Six Sigma is that Motorola and subsequent practitioners fundamentally changed the acceptable quality level discussion - from performance levels measured in percents to performance levels measured at least four orders of magnitude smaller.

Like the Lean approach, Six Sigma is a framework for increasing value, decreasing variability and eliminating waste; Lean focuses on flow, whereas Six Sigma focuses on variability. Both Lean and Six Sigma can benefit from the application of sophisticated mathematical and statistical analyses; both also can be applied with simple arithmetic. The Six Sigma paradigm is based upon on a 5-step process: Define, Measure, Analyze, Improve, and Control (DMAIC). DMAIC refers to a measurement-dependent, data-driven quality strategy for process improvement. Central to the DMAIC approach is defining the "Customer", their "Critical to Quality" issues, and core business processes.

Quality Function Deployment (QFD) Approach

QFD is a key practice in Design for Six Sigma (DFSS). Broadly defined (Akao, 1990), it is a method that "converts user demands into substitute quality characteristics …, determines the design quality of the finished good, and systematically deploys this quality into component quality, individual parts quality, and process elements and their relationships." The QFD lifecycle may be directly mapped on to the classical systems engineering lifecycle (Samaras, 2006). In this schema, the 'Voice of the Customer" (Figure 7) appears as a subset of the "Voice of the Stakeholders" (Figure 8); other than that, everything appears basically the same. A powerful tool of QFD, the "House of Quality" is a mechanism for selecting and verifying the relationship between Design Inputs (Requirements or "Whats") and Design Outputs (Specifications or "Hows").

HCSE Approach

HCSE is a general paradigm that applies to both the development and deployment of products, processes, and services. A wide variety of lifecycle models, published over the last quarter century,

Figure 7. QFD mapped to HCSE lifecycle

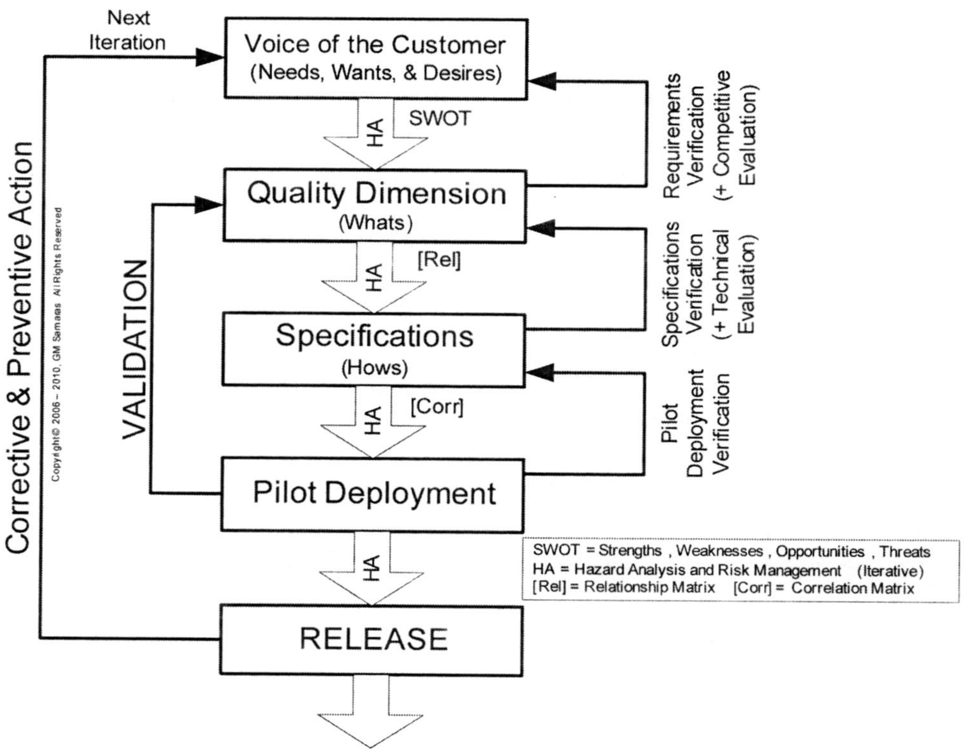

directly map to the classical systems engineering lifecycle model (Samaras & Horst, 2005). The primary difference between the classical systems engineering lifecycle and the HCSE lifecycle is the iterative emphasis on identifying all stakeholders and their NWDs (Figure 8).

Comparing Perspectives

All five approaches share a number of distinct similarities. All focus on increasing value and target process improvement. All focus on some or all of the stakeholders' NWDs. All focus on core business processes to support the particular approach. Some are explicitly iterative, while others are implicitly iterative.

The Lean approach, with its historical roots in reconciling artisanship and mass production, is a good match for healthcare delivery's search for high throughput from highly skilled professionals. Six Sigma can stabilize gains from the Lean approach by reducing variability along the value stream. The Balanced Scorecard approach exposes the connections between organizational strategy and goal(s) with specific process measures and target values. Both the QFD and the HCSE lifecycles map directly to the classical systems engineering lifecycle and support design of products, processes, and services.

A crucial strength of HCSE is the focus on all stakeholders, rather than just a subset (i.e., customers), thus exposing previously unrecognized SD. Other strengths include the definition of quality and procedures for identifying, classifying, and operationalizing stakeholder NWDs. Recognition and quantification are prerequisites for measurement, control, and management.

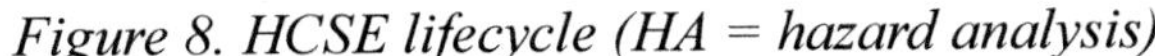

Figure 8. HCSE lifecycle (HA = hazard analysis)

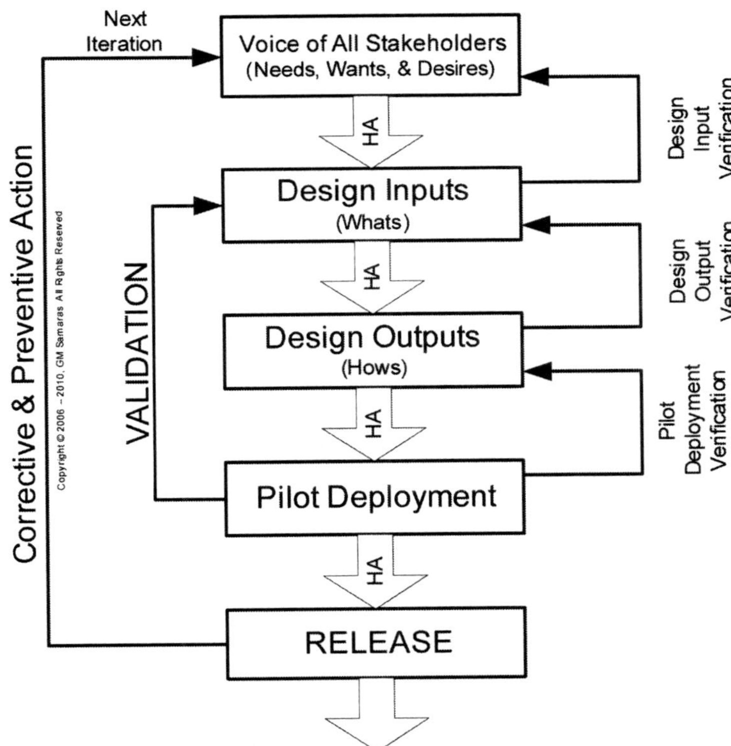

EXPOSING STAKEHOLDERS, THEIR NWDs, AND DISSONANCE

SD in a system never can be eliminated totally; it can only be reduced, except in the most trivial situations. SD arises from the intentional or unrecognized conflicts between the NWDs of the various system stakeholders. In order to manage SD, you must be able to control it. This requires that you are able to measure SD. Increased workload, increased errors, appearance of workarounds, and outright rejection of newly introduced tools are symptomatic of SD in healthcare delivery. While recognizing symptoms is important from a diagnostic perspective, treating (controlling) SD requires recognition and mitigation of the root cause - conflicting NWDs between stakeholders. The objective is SD reduction by reducing NWD conflicts among the stakeholders. Initially, this means identifying the stakeholders, soliciting and classifying their NWDs, and then searching for conflicts.

Identifying and Prioritizing Stakeholders

A stakeholder is any individual or group that potentially can threaten or cooperate in the deployment process (Savage, Nix, Whitehead, & Blair, 1991). Attributes of power, legitimacy, and urgency (Mitchell, Agle & Wood, 1997) are important elements for the identification and prioritization of stakeholders. Visualizing and mapping stakeholder influence (Bourne & Walker, 2005; Walker, Bourne & Shelley, 2008) is a critical step in identifying ALL the stakeholders, to avoid unrecognized NWD conflicts that may lead to SD. The degree to which the identification is more coarse-grained (e.g., clinicians) or fine-grained (e.g., physicians, nurses, pharmacists, occupational/radiation/physical therapists, nurse assistants, pharmacy technicians, aides/orderlies/attendants) will depend in part on the particular deployment and in part on the iteration in the deployment design process. There is little reason to begin in the first iteration with a very fine-grained analysis; however, as SD is mapped, the original course-grained analysis will very likely be expanded in future iterations for particular stakeholder groups.

Defining NWDs

We previously stated that NWDs may be envisioned as: **N**eeds - basic needs or "*must haves*", **W**ants - performance needs or "*like to haves*", and **D**esires - latent needs or "*I'll know it when I see it*". From the work of Kano (1984), we have a simple means of discriminating NWDs based upon stakeholder response (Figure 9). This stakeholder response matrix permits discrimination and identification of basic needs versus performance needs versus latent needs. However, it is not a good mechanism for soliciting NWDs from stakeholders. Most stakeholders do not readily relate to the terms "needs, wants, and desires" and encounter difficulties identifying their NWDs.

Soliciting NWDs

However, all stakeholders seem readily able and willing to discuss and give multiple opinions regarding safety, effectiveness, efficiency, and whether a tool is satisfying to use. This is convenient, because all stakeholders have the same top-level set of NWDs: the product, process, or service should be "Safe, Effective, Efficient, and Satisfying in a Specified Context of Use" (ISO/IEC, 2001). As previously stated (see section on Human-Centered Quality), the first three SEES elements are objective measures, whereas the fourth is a set of subjective measures encompassing perceived effectiveness, perceived efficiency, engaging, error tolerant, and easy to learn.

Figure 10 is an example of a worksheet for soliciting and organizing these across all stakeholder categories. The stakeholders' inputs are solicited in a number of different ways, including

Figure 9. Stakeholder response matrix

	POORLY MET	MET	VERY WELL MET
NEEDS (Basic Needs)	DISGUSTED	UNHAPPY	NEUTRAL
WANTS (Performance Needs)	UNHAPPY	NEUTRAL	HAPPY
DESIRES (Latent Needs)	NEUTRAL	HAPPY	DELIGHTED

Figure 10. Organizing commensurable stakeholder NWDs

			STAKEHOLDER CATEGORIES			
			CLINICIANS	PATIENTS	MANAGEMENT	STAFF
TOP LEVEL NEEDS, WANTS, & DESIRES	OBJECTIVE MEASURES	SAFETY				
		EFFECTIVENESS				
		EFFICIENCY				
	SUBJECTIVE MEASURES	SATISFACTION				
		Perceived Effectiveness				
		Perceived Efficiency				
		Engaging				
		Error Tolerant				
		Easy to Learn				

one-on-one interviews, structured focus groups, questionnaires, technical conferences (where participant stakeholders are invited to comment on relevant presentations), and traditional best practices benchmarking of competitors. No one particular technique appears totally adequate, but since the process is iterative, different techniques may be used in different iterations. Furthermore, an initial analytic effort to forecast stakeholder responses tends to expedite the process.

It is important for engineers to appreciate that subjective measures may be as important as, or even more important than, objective measures. Our natural inclination as engineers is to tend to discount "feelings" and other "human" things we are not trained to measure. However, from the point of view of the individual stakeholder, if they feel the tool is not working for them or if they feel it is increasing their workload, they will perceive it as ineffective or inefficient, regardless of what your objective data may indicate. Their "subjective" perception invariably will lead to workarounds or rejection of the tool, both of which are diagnostic for SD.

A very good example is the work on "ergonomic" versus "non-ergonomic" computer carts (Anderson, et. al., 2009). Nurses overwhelmingly rejected a slick ergonomic design in favor of a generic trolley that had a larger work surface and storage space for medications, papers, and other nursing artifacts. However, it has been my personal observation that a different group of clinicians (physical and occupational therapists), whose professional artifacts are mostly large and immobile, routinely use the modern, ergonomically designed computer on wheels.

Whether or not the ergonomic cart is perceived as effective and efficient is dependent upon the stakeholder group (on their frame of reference), in this case two subgroups of clinicians. In fact, the meaning and priority of each of these top level NWDs vary according to the specific (sub-) category of stakeholder. In our attempt to achieve SD reduction, we are not directly interested is SEES, but in the identification of basic needs, performance needs and latent needs for each specific stakeholder group and how they might conflict. Only a subset of all these NWDs will be translated into the design requirements for the deployment of the product, process, or service.

Classifying NWDs

In any given iteration, once we have a SEES set, it is relatively simple to classify each of the members of the SEES set as Needs, Wants, or Desires. For each given stakeholder group (actually their sampled representatives), we ascertain their response on a scale from addition to elimination of the particular design requirements, couched in terms that permits them to respond based upon whether the putative requirement is poorly met, met or very well met (see Figure 9).

Consistent with good survey and questionnaire practices, once you have constructed the questions based upon the subject matter, you need to randomize their sequence and ensure that you have both a balanced presentation (positive and negative interrogatories, as well as any other internal controls deemed necessary). The responses may be elicited in writing, in group sessions, or in any number of other formats. What is important, as with every other scientifically–based investigation, is that bias is minimized (use multiple representatives, minimize self-selection, avoid leading questions, do not suppress discussions and other interactions among stakeholder representatives in a group setting, etc.)

Since HCSE is inherently an iterative process, it is both unnecessary and inefficient to "get it right the first time"; that definition of quality does not apply here! Trying to complete the effort in a single iteration is usually counterproductive (Samaras, 2010a); the optimal design will usually change with each iteration. Attempting to "finalize" any subsystem will usually constrain future decision-making options and yield suboptimal results. The key, as in any iterative and agile endeavor, is to preserve flexible decision-making, maintain a high tolerance for ambiguity and uncertainty, and enforce short time intervals for each iteration.

Discovering and Mapping Potential Stakeholder Dissonance

SD arises from the intentional or unrecognized conflicts between the NWDs of the various system stakeholders. The best kind of SD is the intentional kind; the very worst kind is the result of unrecognized conflicts – especially with one or more stakeholders being unknown. In order to avoid unintentional or unrecognized SD, we need to analyze and map potential conflicts between different stakeholder NWDs.

I am unaware of any structured, systematic approach for discovering potential SD. At present, it seems that only a tedious, subjective analysis is available. The analysis benefits from visualization by simple mapping of both agonistic and antagonistic NWDs from the different identified stakeholders. While this reveals an important weakness, it is by no means fatal for the approach. Any potential SD that can be discovered or predicted before deployment is one less cause of reduced safety, effectiveness, efficiency, and/or user satisfaction.

Risk Analysis

Once potential sources of SD have been identified, they need to be prioritized for mitigation. Not all SD can or will be mitigated. A well-established initial method for mitigation prioritization is risk analysis. Frequently used is the FMEA (Failure Modes and Effects Analysis); this is a "bottom up" approach that yields a risk prioritization index. However, this inductive analysis relies not on quantitative, historical data, but on subjective, experiential input provided by the analyst. Using this technique alone is dangerous, in that it does not identify nearly all the actual hazards. Wetterneck et al (2006) report data that indicates less than 75% of infusion pump failure modes identified in actual practice were captured, in advance, by their FMEA. When historical, quantitative, failure rate data are not available (this is very often the case), improving the reliability of the risk analysis can be achieved by iteratively combining inductive and deductive analyses (e.g., FMEA and RCA, see Figure 11). The combined use of the "top down" and the "bottom up" analyses usually gives greater coverage, compensates for inherent weaknesses in each of these analytic techniques, and assists the analyst by providing two points of view (not unlike depth perception for a biological visual system).

Prioritizing Stakeholder Dissonance for Mitigation

Prioritizing SD for mitigation initially is based upon risk analysis. However, unless financial

Figure 11. Risk analyses

Analytic Technique	Input Data: Historical, Quantitative	Input Data: Subjective, Experiential
Top Down (Deductive)	Fault Tree Analysis (FTA) Event Tree Analysis (ETA)	Root Cause Analysis (RCA)
Bottom Up (*Inductive*)	Failure Modes , Effects and Criticality Analysis (FMECA)	Failure Modes Effects Analysis (FMEA) Hazard & Operability Studies (HazOp) Hazard Analysis & Critical Control Points (HACCP)

and technical risks are included in the initial analyses, further prioritization based first upon technical feasibility (can we do anything about it?) and then based upon cost-benefit (is it actually worth doing?) is required to arrive at a final prioritization list.

While technical feasibility is always used to eliminate candidates for priority, unless cost is the only optimization criterion, we must then turn to the general category of decision analysis methods. They can be as simple as Pareto, paired comparison, grid, force field, or decision tree analysis (Pyzdek, 2003). When multiple criterion optimization is sought, well-established techniques routinely used in business are of value. These include linear or non-linear programming (depending upon the shape of the constraints) and multiple criteria decision-making (cf., Dyer et. al., 1992; Zeleny, 1998).

QUANTITATIVE DESIGN INPUTS FOR SYSTEM VALIDATION

An un-validated system deployment is a "shot in the dark" and an unknowable risk to the organization. System validation is the demonstration that the deployed system actually conforms to the system design inputs (the system requirements). Requirements in HCSE are defined as the subset of identified or discovered NWDs that are economically and technologically feasible at a given point in time. One critical attribute of system requirements is that they must be measureable, which means they must be unambiguously operationalized, so they can be quantified.

The general outline for managing SD is shown in Figure 12. The approach may be used both for technology deployment as well as for deployment of other processes and services. Figure 12 provides a high-level overview, depicting it as three interlocking process cycles: a technology (re-) development cycle, a deployment (re-) design cycle, and a post-deployment surveillance cycle. These activities are drawn as cycles to emphasize that they represent iterative processes – a key feature of HCSE.

The deployment design cycle, the subject of this chapter, consists of 10 sub-processes (the last of which is deployment validation in a pilot setting prior to general release) and 2 critical decision points (see Figure 12). The first five sub-processes consist of:

a. identifying and mapping all the stakeholders,
b. soliciting stakeholder input on SEES,
c. translating the SEES to NWDs,
d. identifying and mapping dissonance among stakeholders, and
e. conducting risk analyses to help prioritize dissonance mitigations.

At this juncture, if technology is involved, a critical management decision is made whether or not the candidate product is acceptable; if not, technology redesign or selection of a different vendor may be warranted. The last five sub-processes of the deployment design cycle are:

f. prioritizing identified dissonance mitigations,
g. operationalizing and quantifying only the relevant NWDs involved in the selected mitigations,
h. implementing the selected dissonance mitigation(s),
i. verifying in a pilot setting that the selected dissonance was actually reduced, and
j. validating the deployment design in that pilot setting.

At this juncture, the second critical management decision is made whether or not to deploy the product, process, or service throughout the organization.

The seventh step in the process (step g of the deployment design cycle) requires quantification of the relevant NWDs, which we discussed in detail in the section on human centered system complex-

Figure 12. Three interlocking cycles of the SD management process

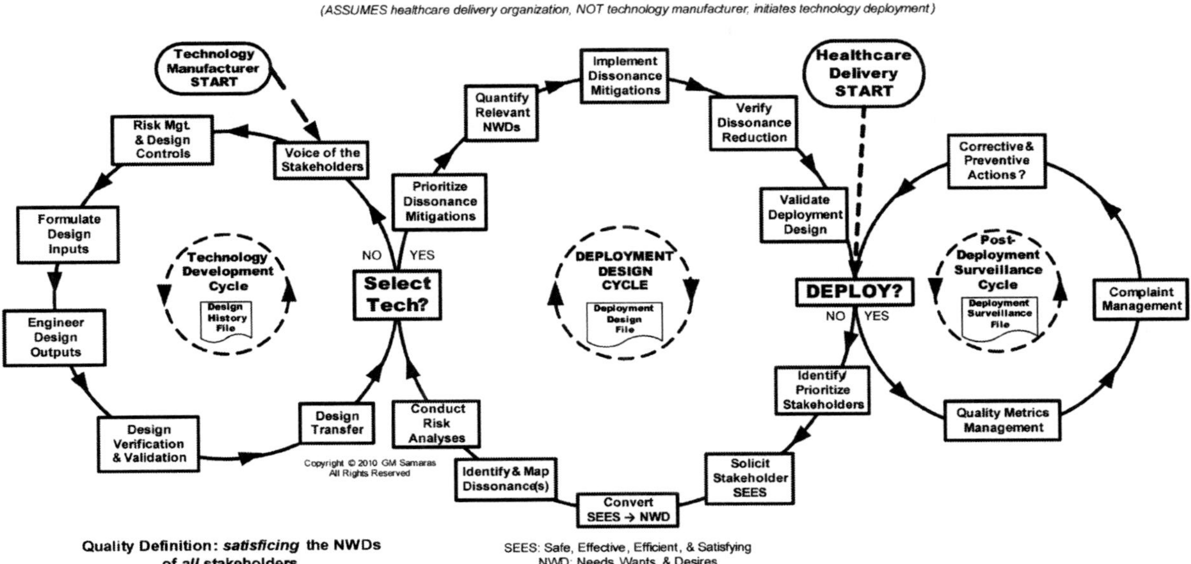

ity. There we identified how various physical, behavioral, social, and cultural (PBSC) factors may be operationalized. The relevant NWDs are those NWDs expected to lead to critical SD and have high priority for reduction or elimination. The reason we need to quantify these particular NWDs is that once we have applied a proposed mitigation, we must have a means to ascertain whether the SD was actually reduced, and then we need to validate that the selected NWDs (those transformed into system requirements) were actually met by the deployment design.

It is at this point that we can answer the question "what do I need to measure" and it is at this point that the measurement techniques in Table 1 (the previously defined PBSC measures) finally are used. Those NWD conflicts identified by prioritization for reduction or elimination are operationalized and quantified using the scientific measurement techniques identified in Table 1. Who (what individuals) will do the measurements depends solely upon what areas of expertise you have in-house; for measurements outside their areas of expertise you will have to turn to academics, consultants, etc.

Consider the deployment of a new infusion pump. NWD conflicts will probably arise among management, purchasing, nursing, and biomedical engineering. Among all four stakeholder groups, we will likely be dealing with covert social factors (conventions and expectations) related to efficiency and effectiveness that require measurement skills from social psychology and sociology. Between purchasing and nursing stakeholders, we will likely be dealing with overt and covert information management behaviors related to workload, safety, and ease of use issues associated with pump programming that require measurement skills from cognitive and physiological psychology. Between nursing and biomedical engineering stakeholders, we will most likely be dealing with overt social and cultural factors related to language differences and safety/risk communication; there may also be conflicts related to differences in shared values between these two stakeholder groups. Prior to full deployment, you will need to demonstrate that some or all of these potential NWD conflicts have been adequately mitigated; if not, validation fails and deployment throughout the organization is ill advised.

In the next section, using 20-20 hindsight, we look back at healthcare delivery system deployment situations (computerized provider order entry and bar coded medication administration) where SD occurred, subsequently became evident, and where some SD might have been avoided by the application of the principles of human-centered systems engineering.

RETROSPECTROSCOPY

Campbell et. al. (2006) have identified nine unintended consequences of computerized provider order entry (CPOE) systems deployment: more or new work for clinicians; unfavorable workflow issues; never-ending system demands; problems related to persistence of paper orders; unfavorable changes in communication patterns and practices; negative feelings toward the new technology; generation of new types of errors; unexpected changes in an institution's power structure, organizational culture, or professional roles; and overdependence on the technology. These correlate well with the findings of Koppel et. al. (2005). With the possible exception of "never-ending system demands", we can be quite confident that the remaining eight issues would have surfaced in structured interviews and structured focus groups of clinicians seeking to solicit stakeholder's SEES opinions. The extent to which SD could have been reduced would depend upon the deploying organization's conclusions regarding their risks. It would also depend upon their ability to delay deployment, until a validated deployment process design was achieved. Weighing the risks of delays versus the risks of failures is a critical management engineering activity.

Patterson, Cook, and Render (2002) identified five negative side effects of deployment of Bar Code Medication Administration (BCMA): nurses confused with automated removal of medications; reduced communication and coordination among physicians and nurses; nurses skipping steps (e.g., wrist band scanning versus entering patient identification) to reduce workload at peak times; increased prioritization of timely medication administration during goal conflicts; and difficulty modifying routine tasks. Koppel et. al. (2008) report a variety of BCMA-related workarounds, including omission of process steps and unauthorized BCMA process steps, all of which appear to have the intent of workload leveling. Bargren & Lu (2009) conducted a detailed case study analysis of altered nursing workflow following introduction of a BCMA system, reporting that the number of steps (a measure of workload) nearly doubled for their inpatient unit. Rothchild & Keohane (2008) assert that unintended consequences of healthcare technologies "more commonly are due to design flaws related to human factors and real world use, unexpected or unaccounted cultural and behavioral interactions, and inadequate training and implementation." While BCMA has the potential to improve patient safety by supporting the five "*rights*": *right* Patient, *right* Drug, *right* Dose, *right* Route, and *right* Time, failure to deploy BCMA systems properly facilitates errors in each of these five parameters. Deploying a system that adversely impacts actual or perceived workflow results in undermined communication & coordination, challenges conventions, expectations, and shared values, and results in stress that compromises covert physical and behavioral factors (see Table 1); clearly, this was never the intent of the deploying organization. Proper application of HCSE would have permitted mitigation of many of these problems.

CONCLUSION: ADDING THE RIGHT VALUE RIGHT AWAY

No matter how well a tool is designed (and there is always room for improvement), how the tool is actually deployed in a particular organization will always be a rate-limiting step in progress towards excellence in healthcare delivery. Value is what each stakeholder cares about, regardless of the views of all other stakeholders. *Satisficing* the NWDs of all the stakeholders provides a balanced local definition of value objectives. SD is "waste" and we attempt to reduce it to minimize its adverse effects on the value stream. Pre-deployment SD recognition and mitigation offers an opportunity to improve healthcare delivery by supporting **S**afe, **E**ffective, **E**fficient, and **S**atisfying organizational operations. The focus on identifying all the stakeholders and satisficing their NWDs provides a powerful mechanism for adding the right value right away. As healthcare delivery cost constraints intensify and sensitivity to TCO increases, avoiding costly errors, misjudgments, threats to patient safety, and threats to organizational profitability will require increasingly rigorous approaches for development and deployment of new technology. Human-centered systems engineering offers a powerful tool for management engineers.

REFERENCES

Akao, Y. (1990). *History of quality function deployment in Japan* (vol. 3, pp. 183-196). International Academy for Quality: IAQ Book Series.

Anderson, P., Lingaard, A.-M., Prgomet, M., Creswick, N., & Westbrook, J. I. (2009). Mobile and fixed computer use by doctors and nurses on hospital wards: Multi-method study on relationships between clinician role, clinical task and device choice. *Journal of Medical Internet Research, 11*(3), 32. doi:.doi:10.2196/jmir.1221

Bargren, M., & Lu, D.-F. (2009). An evaluation process for an electronic bar code medication administration Information System in an acute care unit. *Urologic Nursing, 29*(5), 355–368.

Berwick, D. M. (2002). A user's manual for the IOM's "quality chasm" report. *Health Affairs, 21*(3), 80–90. doi:10.1377/hlthaff.21.3.80

Bourne, L. M., & Walker, D. H. T. (2005). Visualising and mapping stakeholder influence. *Management Decision, 43*(5), 649–660. doi:10.1108/00251740510597680

Campbell, E. M., Sittig, D. F., Ash, J. S., Guappone, K. P., & Dykstra, R. H. (2006). Types of unintended consequences related to computerized provider order entry. *Journal of the American Medical Informatics Association, 13*, 547–556. doi:10.1197/jamia.M2042

Dubin, R. (1976). Organizational effectiveness: Some dilemmas of perspective. In Lee, S. (Ed.), *Organizational effectiveness: Theory-research-utilization* (p. 7). Kent, OH: Kent State University Press.

Dyer, J. S., Fishburn, R. E., Wallenius, J., & Zionts, S. (1992). Multiple criteria decision making, multiattribute utility theory: The next ten years. *Management Science, 38*(5), 645–654. doi:10.1287/mnsc.38.5.645

Etzioni, A. (1964). *Modern organizations*. Englewood Cliffs, NJ: Prentice-Hall.

Holpp, L. (1993). Eight definitions of quality in healthcare. *Journal for Quality and Participation, 16*(3), 18–26.

ISO/IEC DTR 9126-4. (2001). *Software engineering- Product quality – Part 4: Quality in use metrics*. International Standards Organization.

Kano, N. (1984, April). Attractive quality and must-be quality. *Journal of the Japanese Society for Quality Control, 14*(2), 39–48.

Koppel, R., Metlay, J. P., Cohen, A., Abaluck, B., Localio, A. R., Kimmel, S. E., & Strom, B. L. (2005). Role of computerized physician order entry systems in facilitating medication errors. *Journal of the American Medical Association*, *293*(10), 1197–1203. doi:10.1001/jama.293.10.1197

Koppel, R., Wetterneck, T., Telles, J. L., & Karsh, B. (2008). Workarounds to barcode medication administration systems: their occurrences, causes, and threats to patient safety. *Journal of the American Medical Informatics Association*, *15*(4), 408–423. doi:10.1197/jamia.M2616

Lawrie, G. J. G., & Cobbold, I. C. (2004). Third-generation balanced scorecard: Evolution of an effective strategic control tool. *International Journal of Productivity and Performance Management*, *5*(7), 611–623. doi:10.1108/17410400410561231

Mitchell, R. K., Agle, B. R., & Wood, D. (1997). Toward a theory of stakeholder identification and salience: Defining the principle of who and what really counts. *Academy of Management Review*, *22*(4), 853–888.

Patterson, E. S., Cook, R. I., & Render, M. L. (2002). Improving patient safety by identifying side effects from introducing bar coding in medication administration. *Journal of the American Medical Informatics Association*, *9*, 540–553. doi:10.1197/jamia.M1061

Pyzdek, T. (2003). *Quality engineering handbook*. Tucson, AZ: Quality Publishing.

Rothchild, J. M., & Keohane, C. (2008). *The role of barcoding and smart pump safety: Perspective*. Agency for Healthcare Research and Quality Web Morbility and Mortality Rounds. Retrieved on July 19, 2010, from http://www.webmm.ahrq.gov/ perspective.aspx? perspectiveID=64

Samaras, E. A., & Samaras, G. M. (2010). Using Human-Centered Systems Engineering to Reduce Nurse Stakeholder Dissonance. *Biomedical Instrumentation & Technology*, *44*(s1), 25–32. doi:10.2345/0899-8205-44.s1.25

Samaras, G. M. (2006). An approach to human factors validation. *Journal of Validation Technology*, *12*(3), 190–201.

Samaras, G. M. (2010a). The use, misuse, and abuse of design controls. *IEEE Engineering in Medicine and Biology Magazine*, *29*(3), 12–18. doi:10.1109/MEMB.2010.936551

Samaras, G. M. (2010b). Human-centered systems engineering: Building products, processes, and services. *Proc. 2010 SHS/ASQ Joint Conference*. February 25-28. Atlanta, Georgia USA.

Samaras, G. M., & Horst, R. L. (2005). A systems engineering perspective on the human-centered design of health information systems. *Journal of Biomedical Informatics*, *38*(1), 61–74. doi:10.1016/j.jbi.2004.11.013

Samaras, G. M., & Samaras, E. A. (2009). Feasibility of an e-health initiative: Information NWDs of cancer survivor stakeholders. *Proceedings of IEA 2009*. Beijing. *China*, (August): 9–14.

Savage, G. T., Nix, T. W., Whitehead, C., & Blair, J. (1991). Strategies for assessing and managing organizational stakeholders. *The Academy of Management Executive*, *5*(2), 61–76.

Schneiderman, A. M. (2006). *The first Balanced Scorecard*. Retrieved on July 19, 2010, from www.Schneiderman.com/ Concepts/ The_First_Balanced_Scorecard/ BSC_INTRO AND CONTENTS.htm

Simon, H. A. (1957). *Models of man: Social and rational*. New York, NY: Wiley.

Suneja, A., & Suneja, C. (2010). *Lean doctors*. Milwaukee, WI: ASQ Quality Press.

Tierney, W. M., Miller, M. E., Overhage, J. M., & McDonald, C. J. (1993). Physician inpatient order writing on microcomputer workstations. Effects on resource utilization. *Journal of the American Medical Association*, *269*(3), 379–383. doi:10.1001/jama.269.3.379

Walker, D. H. T., Bourne, L. M., & Shelley, A. (2008). Influence, stakeholder mapping and visualization. *Construction Management and Economics*, *26*(6), 645–658. doi:10.1080/01446190701882390

Wetterneck, T. B., Skibinski, K. A., Roberts, T. L., Kleppin, S. M., Schroeder, M. E., & Enloe, M. (2006). Using failure mode and effects analysis to plan implementation of smart i.v. pump technology. *American Journal of Health-System Pharmacy*, *63*, 1528–1538. doi:10.2146/ajhp050515

Womack, J. P., Jones, D. T., & Roos, D. (1990). *The machine that changed the world: The story of lean production-- Toyota's secret weapon in the global car wars that is now revolutionizing world industry*. New York, NY: Free Press.

Zeleny, M. (1998). Multiple criteria decision making: Eight concepts of optimality. *Human Systems Management*, *17*, 97–107.

Chapter 8
Enabling Real-Time Management and Visibility with RFID

Peter J. Hawrylak
The University of Tulsa, USA

Ajay Ogirala
University of Pittsburgh, USA

Bryan A. Norman
University of Pittsburgh, USA

Jayant Rajgopal
University of Pittsburgh, USA

Marlin H. Mickle
University of Pittsburgh, USA

ABSTRACT

Radio frequency identification (RFID) and Real Time Location Systems (RTLS) provide a wireless means to identify, locate, monitor, and track assets and people. RFID technology can be used for resource and patient location, to reduce costs, improve inventory accuracy, and improve patient safety. A number of pilot deployments of RFID and RTLS technology have yielded promising results, reduced costs, and improved patient care. However, there are three major issues facing RFID and RTLS systems, privacy, security, and location accuracy. As described in this chapter the privacy and security issues can be easily addressed by employing standard security measures. Location accuracy issues are physics-related and new advances continue to improve this accuracy. However, in hospital applications accuracy to the room level is sufficient.

DOI: 10.4018/978-1-60960-872-9.ch008

INTRODUCTION

While radio frequency identification (RFID) technology has a long history of providing efficiency and savings in the consumer goods and supply chain areas, it is now also moving into a number of other application domains. This chapter will examine how Radio Frequency Identification (RFID) technology can be used to improve resource management and quality of care, and reduce costs in healthcare. The issues of security, privacy, and location accuracy with respect to hospital management and RFID/RTLS will be investigated. Solutions to these issues and future research directions in this area will be presented in this chapter.

BACKGROUND

RFID Background

Radio frequency identification (RFID) systems are composed of three types of components: tags, readers, and application software. Hawrylak, Cain, and Mickle provide a detailed overview of RFID and its history (Hawrylak, Cain, Mickle, 2008). Tags are attached to assets, items, or people that are being tracked or inventoried. RFID tags contain a unique identifier (UID) that links a tag to a particular asset, item, or person in the application software database. Modern tags have varying amounts of memory for data in addition to the simple UID. An expiration date or manufacturer lot number are two examples of the data that are stored in the tag's memory. Readers, sometimes called interrogators, communicate with the RFID tags and provide the link between the tags and the application software. One common use of RFID readers is to read the RFID tags attached to items on a pallet as it is loaded onto a tractor-trailer. Unlike bar codes and other printed labels, RFID does not need a visual line of sight between the reader and tag to be read. RFID tags can be read through cardboard, packaging, water, and even people. RFID tags can typically be read even if they are dirty or wrinkled; currently these cause problems for bar codes. Finally, the application software provides information to the user and allows the user to interact with a larger information system. The application software can perform complex analysis based on the collected data to infer a number of conditions (including maintenance information) beyond simply reading a tag.

An example RFID system with one reader and three tags is illustrated in Figure 1. Such a system could be used for many purposes, including inventory control for a hospital. For example, if the hospital manager is required to take an inventory because a particular batch of medication has been recalled based on a list of lot numbers and manufacture dates provided by the pharmaceutical company. With RFID tags linked to the lot number and date of manufacture in the database attached to the medication containers, this is a simple task. First, the hospital manager would instruct the backend software to take the inventory. The backend software would then issue the inventory command to the RFID reader. The RFID reader would then proceed to collect an inventory of all the tags within range and report the unique identification number of each tag to the backend software. The backend software would then use each tag unique identifier to search the database for that unique identifier to retrieve the lot number and manufacture date. The backend software would provide this information to the hospital manager or could even check the retrieved information for matches against a list if the list was in electronic format. This is one example of how RFID technology can improve hospital management.

RFID tags can be grouped into three general categories, passive, battery assisted passive (BAP), and active. How the tag is powered determines the category it falls into. Passive tags have no on-board power source (e.g. a battery) and must

Figure 1. Overview of RFID system and associated backend software and database

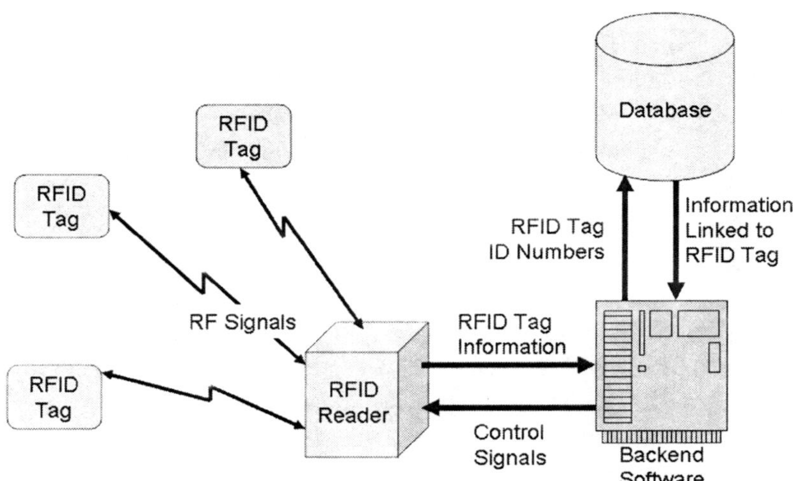

harvest energy from the reader's radio frequency (RF) transmission for operation.

Passive tags communicate with the reader using *backscatter*. Backscatter communication uses the fact that all objects reflect radio waves in order to transmit data from the tag to the reader. Radar is based on backscatter. The impedance matching between the antenna and the tag integrated circuit (IC) determines whether a lot or a little energy is reflected back to the reader. The tag controls this matching and uses it to transmit data back to the reader (similar to a Morse code message). Passive tags are the most popular type of tag. Two early and continuing uses of passive tags are in public transportation fare cards and in monitoring consumer goods. RFID tags designed to the EPCglobal Gen-2 specification are one of the most common types of passive RFID tags. Hawrylak and Mickle (Hawrylak and Mickle, 2009) provide an overview of the EPCglobal Gen-2 specification. Taking the inventory of the tags within the reader's field is a feature found in nearly all RFID protocols. The Gen-2 protocol uses a slotted Aloha anti-collision system where the number of response slots is controlled by the reader. Maillart, et. al. describe a method to obtain the optimal policy for controlling the inventory parameters to read the most tags in the smallest possible time (Maillart, Kamrani, Norman, Rajgopal & Hawrylak 2010).

BAP tags contain a battery that is used to power a microprocessor (some intelligence) and potentially a sensor on the tag. The BAP tag still uses backscatter to communicate, but the added battery allows sensor readings to be obtained when the tag is not being read, e.g. to monitor the temperature of a shipment of pharmaceuticals or food. Because BAP tags do not need to use part of the received energy to power the entire tag, all the received energy can be used for backscatter communication resulting in greater communication range than passive tags.

Active tags are entirely battery operated having a powered transmitter and receiver. They can communicate at much larger distances (100 to 300 meters) than BAP or passive tags (approximately 1 to 5 meters). Because active tags are battery powered, energy consumption is critical. Hawrylak, Cain, and Mickle describe a framework to model the energy consumption of an active RFID network (Hawrylak, Cain, & Mickle, 2007). This method can be applied to any active RFID net-

Figure 2. Passive tag (a) and an active tag (b)

work to determine how long a tag's battery will last under a given set of conditions. Replacing batteries must be done manually and hence, it is expensive. Hawrylak, Mats, Cain, Jones, Tung, and Mickle describe a method that dramatically increases device lifetime by minimizing energy consumption while listening for incoming messages (Hawrylak, Mats, Cain, Jones, Tung, & Mickle, 2006). Active tags are often employed in harsh radio frequency (RF) environments having significant interference or RF-unfriendly materials. The United States Department of Defense uses active RFID tags to monitor and track cargo containers. Figure 2 shows examples of a passive RFID tag Figure 2(a) and an active RFID tag Figure 2(b).

RFID in Healthcare

RFID technology can be used to reduce costs in hospitals and improve the quality of care of patients (Revere, Black & Zalila, 2010; Wicks, Visich & Li, 2006). RFID technology provides the ability to remotely identify a patient or asset (Lahtela, 2009; Roark & Miguel, 2006; Nursing, 2006). This can assist in preventing medical errors such as giving Patient A the medication intended for Patient B (Lai, Chien, Chang, Chen, & Fang, 2007). Kim and Jo present a system using RFID to identify a patient and then display that patient's medical record on a monitor screen or PDA for use by hospital staff or the patient to review and correct any incorrect information (Kim and Jo, 2009). Presently, in addition to simple identification, sensors are being combined with RFID tags to monitor things such as the tag's battery level as well as to provide application data such as the patient's temperature. Such information allows the user to infer the state or condition of the asset or person to which the tag is attached. Chen, et. al. (Chen, Gonzalez, Leung, Zhang, & Li, 2010) describe a system that uses RFID tags to identify a patient and link that patient to a database with a set of rules that monitor a patient's health and/or behavior. Another example of using RFID to monitor a patient's adherence to the medication policy prescribed by their doctor (compliance) is presented by Pang, et. al. (Pang, Chen, & Zheng, 2009). Such systems can provide a patient with independence while providing increased monitoring of their medical condition. RFID technology has been employed by Covidien Ltd. and Bayer HealthCare Pharmaceuticals Inc. to identify and track contrast die used for medical imaging to link the correct contrast to the patient (Lavine, 2008).

RFID is often used in supply chain management and can be used to track inventories for billing and safety purposes. In one system, developed by Mobile Aspects, RFID tags are affixed to medical supplies stored in special cabinets. A nurse gains access with an ID card and enters information on the patient for whom the supplies are needed. The cabinet contains RFID readers that record the supplies that are removed and automatically bills the patient for those supplies. This system reduces billing errors. It also provides better inventory control for the hospital by reducing the amount of extra/unnecessary supplies that are ordered. As a result, hospitals can better employ more of a just-in-time type of inventory system.

Another RFID application affixes RFID tags to orthopedic implants. These implants typically come in kits with several different sizes for each part because every person is different and the surgeon typically does not know what size implant best fits the patient until the surgery has started. The surgeon receives the orthopedic implant kit and then selects the appropriate size parts and completes the surgery. Unused parts are returned to the manufacturer, and the hospital and patient are only billed for the parts used. The manufacturer then replaces the used parts and sends the kit to the next hospital. One manufacturer of the orthopedic implants affixes RFID tags to the bags containing the parts and one RFID tag to the kit itself. The bags of the used parts are discarded by the surgeon and not placed back in the kit being returned. When the kit arrives, it is scanned with an RFID reader, which takes an inventory of the kit and also identifies the kit itself. The tag on the kit identifies the inventory the kit contained when it was sent to the hospital. The system then compares the present inventory to the inventory of the kit before it was sent. With the information, the used and thus missing parts are identified. This simplifies billing while quickly and automatically generating a list of items that must be replaced in the kit. In this application, the use of RFID saves significant time at the manufacturer's facility in restocking the kits.

RFID combined with other management systems provides greater visibility within the supply chain. One example reported by RFID Journal is the combination of RFID and scales to determine which tools are missing from an orthopedic implant kit (Swedberg, 2010e). The scale weighs the full kit before it is sent to the hospital and then weighs the kit when it is returned. Distinct differences in weights indicate that tools have been removed or added to the kit. The kits are then restocked and hospitals billed for the missing parts. This reduces the time needed to identify missing parts and helps verify that all components are present in the kit before it is sent to the hospital.

The lack of the need of a visual line-of-sight between the RFID tag and reader provides numerous opportunities for RFID technology to be employed to improve safety. One example is accounting for surgical sponges during a surgery. If a sponge is left inside a patient it will decay and most likely cause an infection. Such an infection can quickly spread throughout the patient's system and in some cases lead to the patient's death. In practice, sponges must be manually counted to ensure that the number of sponges discarded is equal to the number of sponges issued for the operation. RFID can help provide a superior solution to this problem. ClearCount Medical Solutions has developed a system for counting surgical sponges during a surgery. RFID tags are placed into each surgical sponge. Surgical sponges are entered into the system when they are introduced into the operating room. This gives a count of all sponges used during the surgery. As one element, a specially equipped waste can is used to collect the used surgical sponges. An RFID reader is incorporated into the waste can, and the reader records each surgical sponge as it is deposited in the waste can. This system provides a count of the number of surgical sponges discarded. If the two counts match, no surgical sponges are remaining in the patient or the vicinity. If the counts do not match, a specially designed wand can be used to check if there is a surgical sponge inside the patient. This wand is a specialized RFID reader antenna that simply reads the RFID tag attached to the surgical sponge. This system helps medical staff locate missing sponges and reduces the time the patient is opened during surgery as well as the time to clear the operating room.

RFID in Hospital Management

RFID technology can be employed to fill the *last mile* gap between the decision makers and the patients and staff. With this information, more informed decisions can be made resulting in improved quality of care, increased efficiency, and decreased item costs. The last mile refers to the common business case that the final connection between the larger business process, industry, or system and the end user often requires the lion's share of the effort and cost of development and implementation.

The following are examples of how RFID can be used to provide that last mile connection for hospital management. First, RFID can be used to track the location of assets and equipment. This enables staff to quickly find equipment when it is needed. As a result, hospitals can reduce the amount of surplus equipment they maintain. For equipment such as crash carts, this can result in significant savings. Second, RFID can provide a platform for remote patient monitoring. It can be used to identify a particular patient, locate and track patients, and when coupled with a sensor, it can monitor the patient. Finally, the data collected from the RFID systems can be used for patient volume forecasting and to improve patient throughput.

Several issues must be considered with RFID use in asset tracking. The cost and effort of deploying an RFID system are important. Tags to be placed on assets must not interfere with normal operation of the asset and should be unobtrusive. Readers must also be unobtrusive. The need for additional data or power connections to the readers, or for installation must be considered when comparing systems. Ideally, the readers should work with and be integrated into the existing hospital information technology (IT) infrastructure. This greatly simplifies and reduces the cost of the installation. One such example is RFID readers that use the existing Wi-Fi network to communicate with the application software or central database.

For medical equipment that must be sterilized, the tags used must be able to withstand the sterilization process. Heat based sterilization can be particularly problematic for tags. The primary issue with heat sterilization is that the heating can cause the materials making up the tag to expand at different rates. This generates stress on the connections between these materials. One common area of failure is the connection between the tag IC (chip) and the antenna. This connection can be weakened (altered) or even broken entirely. When the connection is weakened the impedance matching between the tag IC and antenna degrades, causing less power to be transferred to the tag IC from the antenna. This in turn reduces the range at which the tag can be read. If the connection is broken, the range at which the tag can be read is limited to a few millimeters at best. Ethylene oxide is one alternative to sterilize medical equipment that cannot withstand heat sterilization. Ethylene oxide based sterilization is less problematic as a tag can be encased with a protective coating that allows RF signals to pass through but keeps out ethylene oxide. However, ethylene oxide is toxic and appropriate safety measures must thus be taken.

Gamma radiation is frequently used for sterilization. For most RFID chips, this radiation is problematic. Recently, a few tags have been introduced that are reported to survive sterilization that uses gamma radiation (Bacheldor, 2006; RFID Journal, 2010b).

The spread of infectious diseases within the hospital is a major concern. RFID can help solve this problem by enabling improved asset and patient tracking (Reiner & Sullivan, 2005). Herman et. al. describe a method to model the number of individuals that an infected individual could spread an infection too (Herman, et. al., 2009). The method proposed by Herman, et. al. requires information about where the infected person was over time. RFID can provide this information by assuming that the infected person is in a room if their RFID tag is read by a reader in that room.

With this information preventative measures can be taken to treat and stop the further spread of the infection.

RFID can be employed to track compliance with hand washing guidelines. Each year a significant number of infections are caused by lack of hand washing by medical staff. Often, the hospital must cover the cost for additional treatment for an infection caused by lack of proper hand washing. RFID readers can be placed in soap dispensers and medical staff provided with an RFID tag (Swedberg, 2010j). Such a system has been deployed in Princeton Baptist Medical Center (Birmingham, AL). This system provides a display above the hand washing station to display lab results or current news and sports events. The Princeton Baptist Medical Center uses the system to reward staff and has reportedly generated friendly competition to obtain the highest hand washing compliance percentage. Increasing hand washing compliance reduces the risk of transmitting infections and lowers the overall cost of a hospital stay both for the patient and hospital.

Combining RFID with sensor technology enables monitoring of the state of the asset in addition to simply identifying the asset. Mission Hospital in Mission Viejo, California has installed an RTLS to track medication and blood bags among other items, patients, and personnel (RFID Journal, 2010a). A derivative of RFID technology, termed *real-time location system* (RTLS) technology provides the ability to locate and track assets and patients in real-time. In this application, temperature sensors are combined with RFID tags to monitor the temperature of medication and blood bags. Here the addition of sensors enables monitoring of these assets efficiently from a centralized location. In another application, Hospital Israelita Albert Einstein in Brazil employed RTLS tags equipped with a temperature sensor to monitor the temperature of coolers containing blood, medicine, and tissue samples (Swedberg, 2010g). The system was also employed to track assets as well. Both systems enable continuous monitoring of the asset and allow hospitals to quickly identify defective assets. These systems enable the hospital to also monitor the health of equipment. For instance, a continued increase in the temperature inside a cooler over one day indicates that the cooler is beginning to fail and preventive action can be taken before any assets are damaged from the rising temperature.

Passive RFID tags are typically employed to identify a specific asset from among many assets. One example of this being used in a hospital is to locate a particular bag of blood plasma in the freezer. The Blood and Tissue Bank of the Balearic Islands is testing a system using passive UHF Gen-2 RFID tags to track which bags of blood plasma are in which cooler (Swedberg, 2010h). The RFID tag not only simplifies the process of finding the needed bag in the freezer, but also the processing of the blood from the donor to the patient.

RFID can provide hospital staff with the ability to quickly locate required assets. At Kaiser Permanente San Jose Medical Center, an RTLS is used to locate equipment providing significant savings in the time required to find equipment and produced significant cost savings by eliminating the need for redundant equipment (Swedberg, 2010b). This system employed ZigBee based readers and tags. The RFID readers were designed to plug into standard electrical outlets, thus simplifying the installation. RFID is being employed inside the operating room to identify and track assets (Agarwal, Joshi, Finin, Yesha, & Ganous, 2007).

RFID can be used beyond the hospital to improve patient care. A common problem for patients is taking the medications prescribed by a doctor at the correct times and taking all the doses. RFID systems can be used to monitor a patient's compliance with the prescribed treatment. In one example, RFID tags are affixed to medication bottles indicating the type of medication, and an RFID reader is attached to a special drawer where the medications are stored by the patient (Becker et. al., 2009). The system uses RFID tag reads to determine which medications were removed from the drawer and presumably taken by the patient. The caregiver can then access a record of the patient's medication activities to verify that the prescribed treatment plan was being followed. Recently sensors were incorporated into this design to measure the weight of each pill bottle in order to track how many pills were removed by the patient (Vinjumur, Becker, Ferdous, Galatas, & Makedon, 2010). Another system links RFID and a cell phone to assist patients in taking the medications properly and to record symptoms and side effects patients might be experiencing (Swedberg, 2010i). In this system, the patient is called on the cell phone when they are scheduled to take the medication. The cell phones are equipped with a touch screen and the system asks the patient questions about any symptoms or side effects they may be experiencing. The patient selects an answer from a list of selections using the touch screen capability of the cell phone. The cell phone is equipped with a short-range RFID reader that allows the patient to scan the medication before they take it. This allows the doctor to maintain a list of times when the medication was taken along with a list of any symptoms or side effects the patient may have experienced. This detailed history of the patient assists the doctor in treating the patient in the event they experience side effects or need to have their medication changed.

Locating Patients and Assets

Locating patients and assets is critical for any hospital. For instance, critical equipment (e.g. a crash cart) must be located quickly, and at-risk patients (e.g. a patient suffering from Alzheimer's disease) must be monitored. RTLS technology couples the ability of RFID to identify an object or person with a system to determine the approximate location of that object or person. An RTLS can provide significant improvement for monitoring situations, patient monitoring, and process improvement (Sanders, et. al., 2008; Hanser, Gruenerbl, Rodegast, & Lukowicz, 2008; Lee & Cho, 2007; Swedberg, 2010; Cangialosi, Monaly, & Yang, 2007; Xiong, Seet, & Symonds, 2009). Wang, et. al., (Wang, Chen, Ong, Liu, & Chuang) describe how an RFID system was used to implement an RTLS system in the Taipei Medical University Hospital to contain the SARS virus.

RTLS can also be used to monitor activities and to increase security. One example is the U.S. Department of Homeland Security Customs and Border Protection agency's use of an RTLS system to track when and who enters a secure area (Swedberg, 2010f). This system incorporates sensors with the RTLS system to identify unauthorized persons in the restricted area. There are similar needs within the hospital, such as securing a pharmaceutical storage room. In this application, there is no physical barrier to entry into the secured area of the warehouse.

In an RF-based RTLS, location is determined based on the characteristics of radio messages sent and received by devices in the system. The two most common techniques are based on received signal strength (RSS) measurements and on the time of arrival (TOA) of messages. Accuracy and precision can be improved by combining the RSS and TOA methods. All three methods depend on the RF transmission characteristics that exist in the current environment. Errors are introduced into these measurements because the RF environment is dynamic and changes over time. Over time these errors can accumulate, causing significant errors in reported location. Frequently recalibrating the RTLS system to account for such changes is recommended. The ease and cost effectiveness of recalibration of an RTLS system are critical factors in selection. Ideally, a system with an automatic update feature is preferable.

Location determination algorithms based on RSS measure the strength of the received RF signal. Generally, the signal strength increases as the tag (receiver) moves closer to the reader (transmitter). Scattering and multipath effects cause hotspots of strong signals and weak signals irrespective of the distance between the tag (receiver) and reader (transmitter). These hotspots introduce error into RSS based methods. Over time, these hotspots can move or disappear, and new hotspots can appear due to the changing RF environment. There are a number of methods that attempt to minimize such errors.

Location determination algorithms based on TOA use the arrival time of messages to estimate distance between the transmitter and receiver. RF waves travel at essentially fixed velocity. A simple implementation includes the time a message is transmitted (as a timestamp) as part of the message data and the receiver records the time it receives the message. The receiver knows the time the message was sent based on the time-stamp in the data portion of the message. Thus it can compute the time the message took to travel from the transmitter to the receiver. Based on this knowledge, the distance between the transmitter and receiver can be estimated. Another method uses a round-trip time where the receiver adds to the message the time it received the message and then sends the message back to the transmitter. This allows both the receiver and transmitter to compute the distance to each other. However, this requires the receiver to minimize the time spent processing the message between reception and retransmission. This can be difficult in a device tasked with multiple responsibilities. However, this distance gives only a circular ring of locations for the device being located. The distance from at least three transmitters must be obtained to get a single location estimation for the device being located. This process is termed *triangulation*. Multipath and scattering affect TOA because the path that the message takes is not the shortest distance from the transmitter to the receiver. The message traveling the shortest path (shortest distance) will yield the correct time, other paths will yield a longer time. As with RSS, most algorithms attempt to minimize such errors.

Several RTLSs combine RF location determination with another location determination technology, such as infrared (IR). IR communication is used in remote controls, e.g. TV, and is typically limited to a single room. IR cannot penetrate walls or opaque surfaces, but can bounce off such surfaces or be reflected by mirror-like surfaces. Here, IR is used to determine which room a tag is in and then RF provides the long-haul communication link to the central system (Swedberg, 2010k; Swedberg, 2010l). Such a technology is applicable to locating and tracking equipment but not for patient tracking.

In the hospital environment there are several levels of patient tracking and identification. In the simplest case, an RFID tag is used to replace the wristband with the patient's information. Often this information is encoded on a bar-code for easy access and entry into a computerized identification system. The wristband provides a check against the wrong patient file being placed on the bed. Both the printed information and the bar-code require a visual line of sight to read and this is problematic if the patient is sleeping and the wristband is not easily accessible. Neither RFID or RTLS requires a visual line of sight to be read patients can be identified without being disturbed. The information on the wristband provides a check against the information in the chart. Thus for example, one could use this to prevent a patient from receiving the wrong set of medications.

Patient Forecasting and Workforce Allocation

Patient forecasting and workforce allocation are critical components to an efficient hospital. To maintain optimal throughput and control costs, the appropriate workforce must be allocated to meet the current patient volume. This requires estimation of future patient volume and the accuracy of such estimates directly relates to the effectiveness of any planning method. With accurate estimates, the appropriate resources, personnel and equipment, can be allocated to address that demand. RFID and RTLS technology can provide accurate and detailed information about the current patient state. Actions can then be taken to address any issues that might arise. This information can then be used to forecast future patient demand.

If patient locations are tracked using RFID, then it may be possible to determine where bottlenecks are arising in the treatment process by determining where queues of patients are building. These bottlenecks may be an indication that more staff and/or equipment are necessary to provide services to patients.

Tracking of hospital assets and personnel involved in linen distribution, replenishment of supplies, pharmaceutical delivery, patient transport, etc., provides an opportunity to see if the delivery patterns and routes currently in use are effective. Optimizing the routing of deliveries provides an opportunity to better utilize resources. Package delivery companies such as FedEx Ground and UPS use GPS systems to conduct similar types of routing optimization on their larger scale systems (Larsen, 2008).

Tracking the availability of patient beds is important for hospitals. With such information, nurses do not need to search for an available room for each patient. Instead, beds can be scheduled from a central location avoiding confusion between and among different departments. This reduces the time spent transporting each patient and increases patient throughput. Trident Health System in South Carolina has deployed an RTLS system to track the status of patient beds, particularly for moving patients from the intensive case unit (ICU) to regular units (Claire Swedberg 2010c). This system interacts with the cleaning staff and indicates when a bed is being cleaned and then when the bed is ready for the next patient. Trident Health System is looking into using wristbands with RFID tags to track when a patient is discharged and to then immediately flag their bed as needing to be cleaned (Swedberg 2010c).

CURRENT CHALLENGES RELATED TO RFID IN THE HOSPITAL

Patient Privacy

Privacy is a key issue in any identification system. Counterfeit pharmaceutical drugs are a growing concern worldwide (The Economist, 2010). One use of RFID is to assist in authenticating pharmaceuticals in order to identify and remove counterfeits (Mickle, Mats, & Hawrylak, 2008). Identity theft (Thompson and Thompson, 2007) and release of private information are two major privacy concerns. In the context of monitoring patient privacy, this normally means that only authorized personnel can access the patient's information. Because RFID is a wireless technology, the number of potential privacy threats increases. Attacks such as snooping or monitoring of the over-the-air transmissions and rogue RFID equipment could be employed to read a patient's personal information. Several solutions have been proposed (Garfinkel, Juels, & Pappu, 2005; Xiao, Shen, Sun, & Cai, 2006; Liu, & Bailey, 2008) but do not fit well within the hospital environment because they negatively impact legitimate use of RFID. However, one could argue that other low-tech methods such a reading the patient's chart or following a patient are equally problematic. Juels (Juels, 2006) presents an excellent technical overview of privacy and security issues relating to RFID systems.

Typical RFID tags contain a unique identifier (UID) and memory to store data, e.g. lot number or expiration date. The VeriMed system produced by VeriChip Corp. uses an implantable RFID tag that links a UID (16-bit number) to a particular individual and their medical information (O'Connor, 2006). Typically, information such as a patient's name, age, or medical condition would not be stored in an RFID tag. However, there are cases where such information can be useful, e.g., to alert medical personnel to a known condition or to drug allergies. With the VeriMed system, the 16-bit number is meaningless to anyone who does not have access to the appropriate patient information database. Conversely, until patient information can be shared among all medical facilities, the effectiveness of this system will be limited to only those hospitals that have access to the appropriate database. Further, the UID must include information as to which database to search for the patient, as one number could represent a different patient in databases for different hospital systems. This requires breaking the UID into a set of fields with one field identifying a hospital and the remainder a unique patient ID within that hospital. This has been achieved with the electronic product code (EPC) to identify the product manufacturer or owner, the product type, and a unique serial number for that product (EPCglobal 2007). Knowing the UID will not provide an attacker with any information about a patient's medical history. The attacker would need to have access to the patient information database to retrieve the patient's medical history. Existing security measures can prevent such unauthorized database access.

Privacy is an important concern and mechanisms to protect privacy have been incorporated into RFID systems. In the medical environment, the privacy of the patient's medical data is the most critical privacy aspect. Eavesdropping of the over-the-air messages or introduction of a rogue RFID reader are the simplest ways to collect a patient's medical data. Encrypting the data stored in the RFID tag is an effective counter to this attack. The attacker cannot decrypt the data to obtain the patient's medical history without the appropriate key. Public key encryption techniques are widely used on the Internet and could be employed. Existing key management systems can be employed to manage, store, and distribute keys to legitimate RFID readers.

Typical passive RFID tags do not provide the computational power necessary to perform advanced encryption, e.g., AES, elliptic curve, or RSA encryption. Thus, data would have to be encrypted on the legitimate RFID reader (handheld or fixed) prior to being transmitted to the tag. Active RFID tags can support advanced encryption procedures, but in a hospital application, it appears that having the reader encrypt the data adequately protects patient privacy. This has the benefit of reducing the power draw of the active tag on its battery, thus extending its lifetime and simplifying its design.

The RFID communication protocols include mechanisms to protect privacy. For example, in ISO 18000-6, the protocol for UHF (ultra-high frequency) passive RFID systems (operating between 860 MHz and 960 MHz), includes a password feature to read and write memory on the tag. Without the correct password, both read and write access to the data are prevented. A similar mechanism is also used in ISO 18000-7, the standard defining the operation of active RFID systems operating at 433 MHz. In both cases, the passwords are transmitted in plain text and as such, they are highly susceptible to snooping and replay attacks. However, when coupled with data encryption, the password feature provides an extra layer of security increasing the difficulty that an attacker must overcome to compromise a patient's security.

Security Concerns

Maliciously reading patient data compromises the patient's privacy but does not impact their security while in the hospital. Trček and Jäppinen (Trček & Jäppinen, 2008) provide an overview of some of the physical attacks against RFID tags. Introduction of false data, modification of existing data, and erasure of existing data are three other security concerns that directly impact the patient while he or she is in the hospital. Grave physical harm could result from all three cases. For instance, an attacker altering a patient's drug allergies could result in that patient being given a drug to which the patient is allergic. The password described in the previous section provides minimal protection against such attacks. However, the tag UID can be used as a safeguard against such an attack. The tag UID links the tag to a particular patient entry in the hospital database. This database would contain all of the patient's medical information. If the tag contained key patient information, such as drug allergies, the two sets of information could be synchronized and checked against each other. Any discrepancy between the tag data and database record would alert the medical provider that something is wrong. Using existing security procedures, the database will have a higher level of security than the RFID tag. The tag UID can be stored in a read-only-memory (ROM) which can be programmed only one time. The RFID tag UID would be written to the ROM during tag manufacture and that UID cannot be modified or overwritten.

Cloning an RFID tag is a common concern due to the use of RFID tags for public transit fare payment. By cloning a tag, a thief would be able to charge rides to a legitimate customer. From the patient's point of view, in the hospital environment, cloning is not a major concern as the attacker would simply appear to be the patient. Conversely, from a staff member's point of view, cloning could be a significant problem because an attacker who has cloned a staff member's ID card could gain access to restricted areas. Linking the RFID enabled ID badge to an RTLS would help address this problem. With the RTLS information, the system could instantly determine if the real staff member and the imposter are both present in the hospital. If so, security could be alerted to investigate both staff members, and the imposter would be identified. Additionally, the RTLS could be linked to a work schedule database which could alert security if a staff member is detected in the hospital when they are not scheduled to be working. In this case, security personnel could investigate to determine if the member's presence is legitimate, e.g., the staff member is filling in for a colleague or assisting other staff in an emergency. Conventional security measures, such as two-way identification (e.g. RFID ID badge and fingerprint recognition) can be employed to secure areas such as the pharmacy dispensary.

Location Accuracy

The accuracy of any RTLS is a critical metric. The required accuracy is determined based on the requirements of each application. For example, for an RTLS focusing on tracking wheelchairs, room level accuracy is usually sufficient; however, for a patient monitoring system finer resolution is required to provide additional information about the patient's status. Researchers are developing an RTLS to monitor a patient's location as well as the elevation of the tag (Swedberg, 2010d). Monitoring elevation as well as location provides additional information such as an alert when a patient falls. By incorporating additional sensors into the system the patient's behavior can be tracked. This alerts medical professionals to changes in a patient's behavior that could be related to health problems.

In terms of radio frequency, hospitals are very noisy and complicated environments. X-rays, magnetic resonance scanners (MRIs), shielded walls, and medical equipment (made of metal) present significant problems for RFID communication. The X-rays and MRIs emit electromagnetic (EM) radiation that interferes with communication between RFID tags and readers. Shielded walls used to contain X-rays, and medical equipment affect the radio signal propagation, thus reducing the range at which a RFID tag and RFID reader can communicate, or cause RFID *dead zones*. RFID dead zones are areas where tags cannot be read. The primary problem is multipath and scattering which negatively impacts the accuracy of RSS based location systems. Shielded walls can lead to the creation of RF dead-zones. Scattering occurs when an RF signal reflects off of a surface. Metal is one such surface. Because the RF signal travels to more than one point in space with scattering, it is possible for a fixed receiver to receive the same signal multiple times within a short time. These copies of the transmission produce false RSS readings (usually higher RSS measurements) at the receiver. As a result, the receiver will calculate a larger or smaller RSS depending on whether the signals add constructively or destructively. In either case, the accuracy of the estimated location will be reduced. Medical equipment introduces a multitude of scattering opportunities causing significant accuracy degradation due to multipath.

The RSS multipath problem can be addressed to some extent by including timestamps within the message and employing TOA techniques with RSS techniques. The message having the shortest round-trip time corresponds to the message that took the most direct path between the RFID tag and RFID reader. The RFID reader can measure the RSS of each message independently provided the messages are separated in time. The RSS technique can then be applied using the RSS of the message with the shortest round-trip. This will eliminate some of the multipath and scattering concerns.

Combining TOA and RSS measurements can further improve the accuracy. However, more research is required to determine how best to combine the two measurements. Unfortunately, the RF communication link is dynamic and changes over time, affecting the RSS and TOA measurements in different ways. Accurate modeling of the RF communication link (channel) is difficult and must be customized for each case, but this is necessary in order to achieve precise locations.

Alternatively, RFID can be used for long-range and data intensive operations while other technologies, e.g., infrared (IR) and ultrasound, are used for locating a tag within a short distance. Both IR and ultrasound are effective technologies to locate a tag to a particular room because a typical wall will absorb (stop) both types of signals. Any tag seen by an IR or ultra-sound reader is most likely in the same room. RFID provides the bandwidth (data rate) and long-range necessary to transmit the tag's UID and other information to the reader. Such a system can reduce the number of RFID readers, but still requires at least one IR or ultrasound reader in each room.

Solutions and Recommendations

RFID can provide a number of benefits to hospital management. This chapter has examined how RFID can assist with patent and asset location and tracking, improving patient safety, and reducing costs. While the technology is promising, some obstacles exist that must be addressed. These are the accuracy of a location determination system, a means to protect patient privacy, and the integration of security into RFID systems.

Improving Location Accuracy

Location accuracy and throughput are the two major areas of research in RTLS development. As the location accuracy of RTLSs improves, the number of assets and patients tracked will increase. The RTLS must be designed to support a large number of tags (patients and assets) in a small area. It must be able to read all tags quickly in order to provide tracking information to the central system. It must also adapt to changing RF environments, which introduce errors into the location determination algorithm. The RTLS must update itself quickly to minimize downtime while maintaining high location accuracy.

The ability to identify all tags quickly and correctly is imperative. Therefore, the location determination algorithms must be computationally simple, while providing accurate results. If the location determination algorithm requires complex computations that take too much time to locate a tag, then the ability to track many tags is impaired. In such situations, the RTLS might not be able to adequately track tags. Some tags may be momentarily lost, resulting in a reduction in the value of the information. The RTLS must adapt to changing RF environmental conditions because the RF environment is dynamic. The RTLS should be capable of performing this process by itself without outside assistance. This lowers the operating cost of the RTLS and ensures that updates can be performed as frequently as needed. Updates should be quick so as to minimize the impact on system performance. In many systems, updates are scheduled for the slow times such as at night in office buildings. Because a hospital operates around the clock there are relatively few slow times, and therefore a quick update is required. Performing this update in a distributed fashion is easier from a logistical standpoint but involves additional technical challenges. A distributed system enables updating individual zones when they are experiencing a slow or stable time. How these partial updates are integrated is a critical step as accuracy must be maintained when aggregating multiple updates.

Addressing Privacy Concerns

Privacy can be addressed by using a meaningless ID number for each patient. In the central database this ID number is linked to a particular patient or medical record. Only with access to this central database could an attacker determine the identity or medical history of the patient. From a tracking standpoint, while RFID enables tracking, this would require compromising legitimate RFID readers or planting rogue RFID readers. Both of these issues are easily deterred with proper security measures. Most of the privacy concerns relating to RFID are solved by simply enforcing proper security measures that most hospitals and doctor's offices already have in place.

Addressing Security Concerns

As RFID systems become ubiquitous and take on more responsibility in the medical environment, the need to secure these systems is paramount. Security must be built into the RFID system to prevent unauthorized users from gaining access to the larger systems that employ RFID. For example, an RFID system that is part of a heart monitor must not be a means by which an attacker could gain access to the heart monitor to change the settings or falsify the readings. Authentication of the RFID tag and RFID reader addresses this problem. Because each hospital can be viewed as a closed system, it is possible to employ security solutions that require a centralized repository of passwords and encryption keys. Standard security solutions such as shared secrets or challenge-response can be used for this authentication. The central repository would be secured by the hospital using similar means that are used to protect electronic medical records.

FUTURE RESEARCH DIRECTIONS

RFID is a tool that can be used to identify and monitor assets and/or patients. Larger software systems can use this information to track assets and patients, or as input into workflow and resource scheduling algorithms. Future work with respect to RFID includes increasing the range over which a tag can be reliably read, improving location accuracy, ensuring privacy, and safeguarding wireless systems.

Increasing read range addresses two problems. First, it reduces the number of RFID readers required for a given deployment because tags can be read from farther away. This lowers the cost of deployment of a RFID system. Second, for a given distance between tag and reader, the RF signal can cut through larger amounts of RF noise. This is particularly true in hospitals where X-rays, reinforced walls, and other wireless signals often interfere with RFID. Longer read range may allow passive RFID systems to be used where active RFID systems are required today because of the high RF noise levels. Switching to passive RFID will save on the tag cost and avoid the battery maintenance required with active RFID tags.

Location accuracy is paramount to any asset or patient tracking system because inaccuracy leads to wasted time searching for the asset or patient. A number of solutions exist for room level location. However, providing detailed location accuracy (e.g., "in the far left corner of the room") will enable many new applications for RFID. For example, with this level of location accuracy RFID can be used to monitor patient behavior in real-time. Thus, abnormal conditions are more easily spotted and addressed in a timely manner. Patient privacy is important regardless of what technology is used. Most RFID systems today contain simply a UID and limited information such as an expiration date. The UID is used to access a database containing the detailed information about the item to which the tag is attached. Thus, without access to this database, tracking is the most significant privacy concern. However, as RFID continues to evolve and includes sensors and larger memories, more sensitive information may be stored on the RFID tag. For example, RFID tags could be used to store portions of, or even entire patient medical records. Encryption is the best solution because without the correct key the attacker cannot decode and use this information. Current encryption methods, such as those used on the Internet, consume too much power and require too much circuitry to be economically executed on the RFID tag. High strength encryption techniques and circuitry that are low power and small in terms of circuitry would enable some of the encryption tasks to be moved from the reader to the tag.

CONCLUSION

Radio frequency identification (RFID) technology will provide significant cost savings, process improvement, and increased quality of care in a medical environment. RFID provides a means to collect significant amounts of data about patients, personnel, and assets in an efficient manner. This information can then be used by larger software systems to allocate resources, locate assets and patients, monitor a patient's condition, and collect a more detailed medical history of a patient. All of these allow the hospital to offer a higher quality of care and operate more efficiently.

From a technology standpoint, location accuracy, privacy, and security concerns must be addressed in RFID and real-time location systems (RTLSs). The changing RF environment negatively affects the location accuracy of an RTLS, but frequent recalibrations and modified location estimation techniques address this issue. In a hospital setting, patient privacy can be addressed using surrogate ID numbers, with encryption of sensitive data, and by requiring authentication of RFID readers and tags. Existing technology and security practices exist that address each of these issues. With respect to security in RFID systems, robust authentication addresses these concerns.

From a systems perspective, how the data gathered from RFID and RTLS are used is critical. How the data are processed opens up a number of fields for future development. Based on the data, medical personnel can infer information about a patient's condition and remotely monitor the patient. This allows preventive action to be taken to mitigate the risk of a patient having to reenter to the hospital.

RFID and RTLS technology provide a means to collect large and detailed sets of data about patients, assets, and personnel. With adequate security measures in place to protect patient privacy and security and improved location accuracy, RFID and RTLS technologies can provide data that are safe and reliable. Hospital medical management can then process this data in a number of ways to improve workflow, resource allocation, patient quality of care and cost reimbursement.

REFERENCES

Agarwal, S., Joshi, A., Finin, T., Yesha, Y., & Ganous, T. (2007, March). A pervasive computing system for the operating room of the future. *Mobile Networks and Applications*, *12*(2-3), 215–228. doi:10.1007/s11036-007-0010-8

Bacheldor, B. (2006, December 11). RFID tag built to survive gamma rays. *RFID Journal*. Retrieved October 29, 2010, from http://www.rfidjournal.com/ article/print/2884

Becker, E., Metsis, V., Arora, R., Vinjumur, J., Xu, Y., & Makedon, F. (2009, June). SmartDrawer: RFID-based smart medicine drawer for assistive environments. *Proceedings of the 2nd International Conference on Pervasive Technologies Related To Assistive Environments* (PETRA '09), (pp. 1-9). New York, NY: ACM. DOI= http://doi.acm.org/10.1145/ 1579114.1579163

Cangialosi, A., Monaly, J. E., & Yang, S. C. (2007, September). Leveraging RFID in hospitals: Patient life cycle and mobility perspectives. *IEEE Communications Magazine*, *45*(9), 18–23. doi:10.1109/MCOM.2007.4342874

Chen, M., Gonzalez, S., Leung, V., Zhang, Q., & Li, M. (2010). A 2G-RFID-based e-healthcare system. *IEEE Wireless Communications*, *17*(1), 37–43. doi:10.1109/MWC.2010.5416348

EPCglobal. (2007). *Tag data standards version 1.3.1*. EPCglobal Inc

Garfinkel, S. L., Juels, A., & Pappu, R. (2005, May-June). RFID privacy: An overview of problems and proposed solutions. *IEEE Security & Privacy*, *3*(3), 34–43. doi:10.1109/MSP.2005.78

Hanser, F., Gruenerbl, A., Rodegast, C., & Lukowicz, P. (2008, February). *Design and real life deployment of a pervasive monitoring system for dementia patients*. Second International Conference on Pervasive Computing Technologies for Healthcare, (pp. 279-280).

Hawrylak, P. J., Cain, J. T., & Mickle, M. H. (2007). Analytic modeling methodology for analysis of energy consumption for ISO 18000-7 RFID networks. *International Journal of Radio Frequency Identification Technology and Applications*, *1*(4), 371–400. doi:10.1504/IJRFITA.2007.017748

Hawrylak, P. J., Cain, J. T., & Mickle, M. H. (2008). RFID tags. In Yan, L., Zhang, Y., Yang, L. T., & Ning, H. (Eds.), *The Internet of things: From RFID to pervasive networked systems*. Boca Raton, FL: Auerbach Publications, Taylor & Francis Group. doi:10.1201/9781420052824.ch1

Hawrylak, P. J., Mats, L., Cain, J. T., Jones, A. K., Tung, S., & Mickle, M. H. (2006, July). Ultra low-power computing systems for wireless devices. *International Review on Computers and Software*, *1*(1), 1–10.

Hawrylak, P. J., & Mickle, M. H. (2009). EPC Gen-2 standard for RFID. In Y. Zhang, L. T. Yang & J. Chen (Eds.), *RFID and sensor networks: Architectures, protocols, security and integrations* (pp. 97-124), Boca Raton, FL: Taylor & Francis Group, CRC Press.

Herman, T., Pemmaraju, S. V., Segre, A. M., Polgreen, P. M., Curtis, D. E., & Fries, J. … Severson, M. (2009, May). Wireless applications for hospital epidemiology. In *Proceedings of the 1st ACM International Workshop on Medical-Grade Wireless Networks*, (pp. 45-50). New York, NY: ACM.

Journal, R. F. I. D. (2010a, April 29). RFID news roundup – April 29, 2010. *RFID Journal*. Retrieved April 30, 2010, from http://www.rfidjournal.com/ article/view/7564

Journal, R. F. I. D. (2010b, July 8). RFID news roundup – July 8, 2010. *RFID Journal*. Retrieved October 29, 2010, form http://www.rfidjournal.com/ article/view/7712

Juels, A. (2006, February). RFID security and privacy: A research survey. *IEEE Journal on Selected Areas in Communications*, *24*(2). doi:10.1109/JSAC.2005.861395

Kim, Y., & Jo, H. (2009, August). Patient information display system in hospital using RFID. In *Proceedings of the 2009 International Conference on Hybrid Information Technology*, (pp. 397-400). New York, NY: ACM. Aug. 27 - 29, 2009.

Lahtela, A. (2009, September) *A short overview of the RFID technology in healthcare*. Paper presented at the Fourth International Conference on Systems and Networks Communications, (pp. 165-169). Sept. 20-25, 2009.

Lai, C.-H., Chien, S.-W., Chang, L.-H., Chen, S.-C., & Fang, K. (2007, August). *Enhancing medication safety and healthcare for inpatients using RFID*. Paper presented at Portland International Center for Management of Engineering and Technology, (pp. 2783-2790). August 5-9, 2007.

Larsen, A., Madsen, O. B. G., & Solomon, M. M. (2008). Recent developments in dynamic vehicle routing systems. In Golden, B., Raghavan, S., & Wasil, E. (Eds.), *The vehicle routing problem: Latest advances and new challenges* (*Vol. 43*, pp. 199–218). Operations Research/Computer Science Interfaces Series. doi:10.1007/978-0-387-77778-8_9

Lavine, G. (2008, August). RFID technology may improve contrast agent safety. *American Journal of Health-System Pharmacy*, *65*(15), 1400–1403. doi:10.2146/news080064

Lee, S.-Y., & Cho, G.-S. (2007, September). *A simulation study for the operations analysis of dynamic planning in container terminals considering RTLS*. Paper presented at Second International Conference on Innovative Computing, Information and Control (ICICIC '07), (p. 116).

Liu, A. X., & Bailey, L. A. (2008). RFID authentication and privacy. In Yan, L., Zhang, Y., Yang, L. T., & Ning, H. (Eds.), *The Internet of things: From RFID to pervasive networked systems*. Boca Raton, FL: Auerbach Publications, Taylor & Francis Group.

Maillart, L. M., Kamrani, A., Norman, B. A., Rajgopal, J., & Hawrylak, P. J. (2010). Optimizing RFID tag-inventorying algorithms. *IIE Transactions*, *42*(9), 690–702. doi:10.1080/07408171003705714

Mickle, M. H., Mats, L., & Hawrylak, P. J. (2008). Resolution and integration of HF and UHF. In Miles, S. B., Sarma, S. E., & Williams, J. R. (Eds.), *RFID technology and applications* (pp. 47–60). New York, NY: Cambridge University Press. doi:10.1017/CBO9780511541155.005

Nursing. (2006, December). Replacing bar coding: Radio frequency identification. *Nursing*, *36*(12), 30.

O'Connor, M. C. (2006). Insurer running VeriChip trial. *RFID Journal*. Retrieved April 22, 2010, from http://www.rfidjournal.com/ article/articleview/2496/1/1/

Pang, Z., Chen, Q., & Zheng, L. (2009, November). *A pervasive and preventive healthcare solution for medication noncompliance and daily monitoring*. Paper presented at the 2nd International Symposium on Applied Sciences in Biomedical and Communication Technologies (pp. 1-6). November 24-27, 2009.

Reiner, J., & Sullivan, M. (2005, June). RFID in healthcare: A panacea for the regulations and issues affecting the industry? *Healthcare Purchasing News*, *29*(6), 74–76.

Revere, L., Black, K., & Zalila, F. (2010). RFIDs can improve the patient care supply chain. *Hospital Topics*, *88*(1), 26–31. doi:10.1080/00185860903534315

Roark, D. C., & Miguel, K. (2006, February). RFID: Bar coding's replacement? *Nursing Management*, *37*(2), 28–31. doi:10.1097/00006247-200602000-00009

Sanders, D., Mukhi, S., Laskowski, M., Khan, M., Podaima, B. W., & McLeod, R. D. (2008, August). *A network-enabled platform for reducing hospital emergency department waiting times using an RFID proximity location system*. Paper presented at International Conference on Systems Engineering, 2008 (ICSENG '08), (pp. 538-543).

Swedberg, C. (2010a). Byrne Group automates asset management, orders. *RFID Journal*. Retrieved April 2, 2010, from http://www.rfidjournal.com/ article/articleview/7508

Swedberg, C. (2010b). San Jose Medical Center installs ZigBee-based RTLS across 10 buildings. *RFID Journal*. Retrieved April 1, 2010, form http:// www.rfidjournal.com/ article/view/7470

Swedberg, C. (2010c). Trident health system boosts patient throughput, asset utilization. *RFID Journal*. Retrieved April 22, 2010, from http:// www.rfidjournal.com/ article/view/7547

Swedberg, C. (2010d). Wright University researchers test RFID and ultrasound for 3-D RTLS. *RFID Journa*l. Retrieved April 23, 2010, from http://www.rfidjournal.com/ article/view/7546

Swedberg, C. (2010e). Zimmer Ohio to use RFID to manage orthopedic products. *RFID Journal*. Retrieved May 13, 2010, from http://www.rfidjournal.com/ article/view/7588

Swedberg, C. (2010f). U.S. customs' bonded warehouse deploys virtual perimeter. *RFID Journal*. Retrieved May 13, 2010, from http://www. rfidjournal.com/ article/view/7591

Swedberg, C. (2010g). Israelita Albert Einstein hospital uses RFID to track temperatures, assets. *RFID Journal*. Retrieved June 2, 2010, from http:// www.rfidjournal.com/ article/view/7639

Swedberg, C. (2010h). RFID to take the chill out of frozen plasma tracking. *RFID Journal*. Retrieved June 2, 2010, from http://www.rfidjournal.com/ article/view/7632

Swedberg, C. (2010i). Nyack Hospital tracks medication compliance. *RFID Journal*. Retrieved June 2, 2010, from http://www.rfidjournal.com/ article/view/7631

Swedberg, C. (2010j). RFID-based hand-hygiene system prevents health-care acquired infections. *RFID Journal*. Retrieved June 11, 2010, from http://www.rfidjournal.com/ article/view/7660

Swedberg, C. (2010k). Mobile RTLS tracks health-care efficiency. *RFID Journal*. Retrieved June 16, 2010, from http://www.rfidjournal.com/ article/view/7668

Swedberg, C. (2010l). New Oregon hospital adopts IR-RFID hybrid system. *RFID Journal*. Retrieved June 16, 2010, from http://www.rfidjournal.com/ article/view/4846

The Economist. (September 4, 2010). Poison pills. *The Economist*.

Thompson, C. W., & Thompson, D. R. (2007, May-June). Identity management. *Internet IEEE Computing*, *11*(3), 82–85. doi:10.1109/MIC.2007.60

Trček, D., & Jäppinen, P. (2008). RFID security. In Yan, L., Zhang, Y., Yang, L. T., & Ning, H. (Eds.), *The Internet of things: From RFID to pervasive networked systems*. Boca Raton, FL: Auerbach Publications, Taylor & Francis Group.

Vinjumur, J. K., Becker, E., Ferdous, S., Galatas, G., & Makedon, F. (2010). Web based medicine intake tracking application. In *Proceedings of the 3rd International Conference on Pervasive Technologies Related To Assistive Environments*. June 23 - 25, 2010.

Wang, S.-W., Chen, W.-H., Ong, C.-S., Liu, L., & Chuang, Y.-W. (2006, January). RFID application in hospitals: A case study on a demonstration RFID project in a Taiwan hospital. In the *Proceedings of the 39th Annual Hawaii International Conference on System Sciences* (vol. 8, p. 184a).

Wicks, A. M., Visich, J. K., & Li, S. (2006). Radio frequency identification applications in hospital environments. *Hospital Topics*, *84*(3), 3–8. doi:10.3200/HTPS.84.3.3-9

Xiao, Y., Shen, X., Sun, B., & Cai, L. (2006, April). Security and privacy in RFID and applications in telemedicine. *IEEE Communications Magazine*, *44*(4), 64–72. doi:10.1109/MCOM.2006.1632651

Xiong, J., Seet, B.-C., & Symonds, J. (2009, July). *Human activity inference for ubiquitous RFID-based applications*. Paper presented at the 2009 Symposia and Workshops on Ubiquitous, Autonomic and Trusted Computing, (pp. 304-309). July 7-9, 2009.

KEY TERMS AND DEFINITIONS

Application Software: This is the system, usually all software, which controls the RFID Readers and interprets the data received from the RFID Readers. The Application Software can use the collected data to infer information about a patient or asset.

Received Signal Strength (RSS): A method that calculates the distance between two devices by measuring the power level of a received wireless message transmitted from the other device. This method suffers from false RSS reading due to multipath propagation, causing artificially high or low readings that can lead to an incorrect distance estimate.

RFID Reader: A device that communicates with RFID tags wirelessly. The RFID Reader provides the link between the RFID Tag and the application software. It is sometimes called an RFID Interrogator.

RFID Tag: A device that is attached to a person or asset, and that communicates wirelessly with an RFID reader.

RFID: RFID stands for Radio Frequency Identification and is a system of tags and readers used to monitor and identify people and assets.

RTLS: RTLS stands for Real Time Location System and is a derivative of RFID that enables the Application Software to identify the location of a RFID tag.

Time of Arrival (TOA): A method to determine the distance between two wireless transmitters by measuring the time required for a message to travel from the source to the destination and back to the source. This method suffers from signal propagation issues because it is not always possible for the signal to travel along the shortest path.

Chapter 9
Healthcare Delivery as a Service System:
Barriers to Co-Production and Implications of Healthcare Reform

Arjun Parasher
Leonard M. Miller School of Medicine, USA

Pascal J. Goldschmidt-Clermont
Leonard M. Miller School of Medicine, USA

James M. Tien
University of Miami, USA

ABSTRACT

Both during and after the recent reform efforts, healthcare delivery has been identified as the key to transforming the U.S. healthcare system. In light of this background, we borrow from systems engineering and business management to present the concept of service co-production as a new paradigm for healthcare delivery and, using the foresight afforded by this model, to systematically identify the barriers to healthcare delivery functioning as a service system. The service co-production model requires for patient, provider, insurer, administrator, and all the related healthcare individuals to collaborate at all stages – prevention, triage, diagnosis, treatment, and follow-up – of the healthcare delivery system in order to produce optimal health outcomes. Our analysis reveals that the barriers to co-production – the misalignment of financial and legal incentives, limited incorporation of collaborative point of care systems, and poor access to care – also serve as the source of many of the systemic failings of the U.S. healthcare system. The Patient Protection and Affordable Care Act takes steps to reduce these barriers, but leaves work to be done. Future research and policy reform is needed to enable effective and efficient co-production in the twenty-first century. With this review, we assess the state of service co-production in the U.S. healthcare system, and propose solutions for improvement.

DOI: 10.4018/978-1-60960-872-9.ch009

INTRODUCTION

Even with the passage of the Patient Protection and Affordable Care Act (hereafter referred to as PPACA), the U.S. healthcare system faces the enduring challenges of increasing access, improving quality, and lowering cost. By 2020, 23 million Americans are estimated to still lack health insurance coverage (Congressional Budget Office [CBO], 2010) and healthcare costs are expected to rise to 21.1 percent of gross domestic product (Center for Medicare and Medicaid Services [CMS], 2010). From 2000 to 2008, U.S. per capita healthcare expenditures grew annually by 3.5 percent, somewhat less than a 4.2 percent average annual growth rate for the 30 industrialized nations included in the Organization for Economic Cooperation and Development (OECD) database (OECD, 2010). These rising healthcare costs, while part of a larger global trend (see Table 1), hold significant consequences for employees, business, and government alike.

In the United States, between 2000 and 2008, health insurance premiums grew by 119 percent - three to four times faster than wages or inflation (Rowland, Hoffman, & McGinn-Shapiro, 2009). With rising healthcare costs and an aging population, the Congressional Budget Office (2009) anticipates future fiscal deficits to be directly linked to increased Medicare and Medicaid spending. Many experts question whether this increased expenditure has provided concomitant improvements in quality, raising questions of value. In addition to these challenges, preventive health and public health initiatives to stem future disease burdens have not received the required attention. Chronic diseases, such as diabetes, heart disease, and renal failure, currently account for 70 percent of healthcare costs and are expected to continue to dominate future U.S. disease profiles, particularly with childhood obesity rates reaching all-time highs (Agency for Health Research and Quality [AHRQ], 2002). Given the cost associated with the increased incidence of chronic disease and neuropsychiatric disorders affecting the elderly, the increasingly aging population will further aggravate the problem.

In light of these systemic failings, the healthcare delivery system has been identified as the key to transforming U.S. healthcare. At present, ideas, rather than precise models, for redesigning the healthcare delivery system exist; as a result, the Patient Protection and Affordable Care Act authorizes demonstration projects and pilot programs to experiment with delivery reform, laying the foundation for another round of healthcare reform. With this background, this chapter builds upon our previous work and borrows from systems engineering and business management to present the concept of service co-production as a paradigm to analyze the current U.S. healthcare system, evaluate demonstration projects, and provide a comprehensive and consistent approach to future reform efforts (Parasher, Tien, & Goldschmidt-Clermont, 2010a; Parasher, Tien, & Goldschmidt-Clermont, 2010b).

Unlike the "goods" sector, service industries, like healthcare delivery, require producers and consumers to collaborate at the point of production and delivery to jointly produce an outcome, i.e., co-production (Tien and Goldschmidt-Clermont, 2009). In healthcare, service co-production requires patient, provider, insurer, administrator and all the related healthcare individuals to collaborate at all stages – prevention, triage, diagnosis, treatment and follow-up – of the healthcare delivery system in order to produce optimal health outcomes and to ensure sustainability of the delivery system. Yet, healthcare delivery has traditionally failed to optimize this collaboration, even though healthcare outcomes have increasingly been linked to a number of patient-dependent factors such as healthcare literacy, socioeconomic status, and education level (Pappas, Queen, Hadden, & Fisher, 1993; Pamuk, Makuc, Heck, Reuben, & Lochner, 1998; Wolfson, Kaplan, Lynch, Ross & Backlund, 1999).

Table 1. Growth in healthcare expenditure for OECD nations (2000-2008)

	2000-2001	2001-2002	2002-2003	2003-2004	2004-2005	2005-2006	2006-2007	2007-2008	2000-2008 Avg.
OECD countries									
Australia	3.5	4.9	2.0	4.8	0.4	2.6	2.5		3.0
Austria	1.6	1.4	2.1	3.0	1.7	1.8	3.3	3.5	2.3
Belgium	1.9	3.0	3.8	7.0	-0.8	-1.0	7.0	4.9	3.2
Canada	6.1	5.1	2.9	2.0	2.7	3.4	1.9	3.3	3.4
Chile	4.2	0.7	-0.4	1.1	1.8	0.3	8.6	13.0	3.7
Czech Republic	5.1	8.2	8.8	0.9	6.9	2.4	2.4	8.5	5.4
Denmark	4.0	2.4	6.3	3.7	2.6	4.3	2.7		3.7
Finland	4.7	6.7	6.6	4.7	5.1	3.3	2.3	3.1	4.6
France	2.4	3.5	3.9	2.8	2.0	1.3	1.2	0.8	2.2
Germany	2.3	2.0	1.2	-0.8	1.9	1.9	1.5	2.5	1.6
Greece	16.1	6.5	3.7	1.0	12.3	5.4	4.1		7.0
Hungary	6.1	10.5	15.4	1.0	7.9	1.2	-7.1	-1.3	4.2
Iceland	0.8	7.9	4.1	1.5	1.3	-1.6	3.1	-1.7	1.9
Ireland	14.9	9.6	7.2	5.8	2.9	2.0	4.4	14.8	7.7
Italy	3.6	1.7	-0.7	4.2	3.2	2.3	-2.7	3.5	1.9
Japan	3.3	0.4	2.8	2.1	3.4	1.0	2.8		2.3
Korea	14.4	3.4	6.9	4.4	10.3	11.4	9.1	4.7	8.1
Luxembourg	7.9	8.7	10.4	9.6	-2.6	-3.7			5.1
Mexico	6.1	2.7	3.1	6.5	0.5	0.6	5.3	1.4	3.3
Netherlands	5.5	6.3	10.0	3.9	0.4	2.1	3.3	3.5	4.4
New Zealand	4.4	7.4	0.0	8.1	6.9	5.4	-0.3	6.3	4.8
Norway	6.1	12.3	2.7	-0.5	-3.9	-3.5	5.0	-3.9	1.8
Poland	7.4	9.8	2.4	4.7	3.8	6.1	10.8	14.5	7.4
Portugal	1.0	2.0	6.3	3.8	2.4	-1.3			2.4
Slovak Republic	4.0	7.0	8.3	30.1	4.1	12.9	16.5	7.4	11.3
Spain	2.9	1.4	14.0	2.1	3.1	3.3	2.8	8.4	4.8
Sweden	9.7	5.9	2.7	1.4	2.5	2.6	2.2	2.2	3.7
Switzerland	4.9	2.7	2.2	2.2	1.3	-1.3	1.1	1.7	1.9
Turkey	-3.1	8.7	3.5	8.6	8.6	12.6	7.4		6.6
United Kingdom	5.3	6.2	5.1	5.5	4.5	4.8	3.0	2.6	4.6
United States	5.0	6.2	5.1	3.0	2.5	2.3	2.2	1.3	3.5
								Average: 4.2	

Source: OECD Health Data, 2010

By failing to emphasize the co-production approach to healthcare delivery, the U.S. healthcare system cannot act as an effective and efficient system, and thus, will continue to fall short of its potential. Optimization of service co-production is vital to the evolution of the U.S. healthcare

Table 2. Scope and size of U.S. employment

Industries	Employment (M)	Percent
Trade, Transportation & Utilities	26.1M	19.0%
Professional & Business	17.2	12.6
Healthcare	14.8	10.8
Leisure & Hospitality	13.0	9.5
Education	13.0	9.5
Government (Except Education)	11.7	8.5
Finance, Insurance & Real Estate	8.3	6.1
Information & Telecommunication	3.1	2.2
Other	5.4	3.9
SERVICES SECTOR	**112.6**	**82.1**
Manufacturing	14.3	10.3
Construction	7.5	5.5
Agriculture	2.2	1.6
Mining	0.7	0.5
GOODS SECTOR	**24.7**	**17.9**
TOTAL	**137.3**	**100.0**

Source: *Bureau of Labor Statistics, Employment Statistics*, April 2006.

delivery system – an evolution necessary to address the current systemic failures of access, cost, and quality. Accordingly, this chapter will first highlight the importance of healthcare within the service sector and define and position service co-production as it relates to healthcare delivery. Then, utilizing this paradigm, we examine the barriers to co-production which prevent effective patient and provider collaboration. Finally, we evaluate the provisions of the healthcare reform legislation, as embodied by the PPACA (Public Law No: 111-148, 2010), and its associated reconciliation bill, the Healthcare and Education Affordability Reconciliation Act (Public Law No: 111-152, 2010), that specifically impact these barriers to co-production. For healthcare providers, policymakers, academics, and patients, this chapter provides an understanding of the present day status of U.S. healthcare delivery, the potential impact of service co-production, and the future work ahead.

THE CONCEPT AND CHARACTERISTICS OF SERVICE CO-PRODUCTION

The importance of the services sector cannot be overstated; it employs a large and growing proportion of workers in the developed nations. As reflected in Table 2 below, the services sector includes a number of large industries and employs 82.1 percent of the U.S. work force, while the remaining four economic sectors (i.e., manufacturing, agriculture, construction, and mining), which together can be considered to be the physical "goods" sector, employ the remaining 17.9 percent. Healthcare – which employs 10.8% of the U. S. workforce – is, of course, one of the largest industries in the services sector.

As indicated earlier, the concept of co-production is central to the delivery of services, and to the service industry in general. Unlike the "goods" sector, service industries (i.e., healthcare delivery) require co-production: in the simple model of a

Figure 1. Healthcare co-production: A predictable information and knowledge exchange

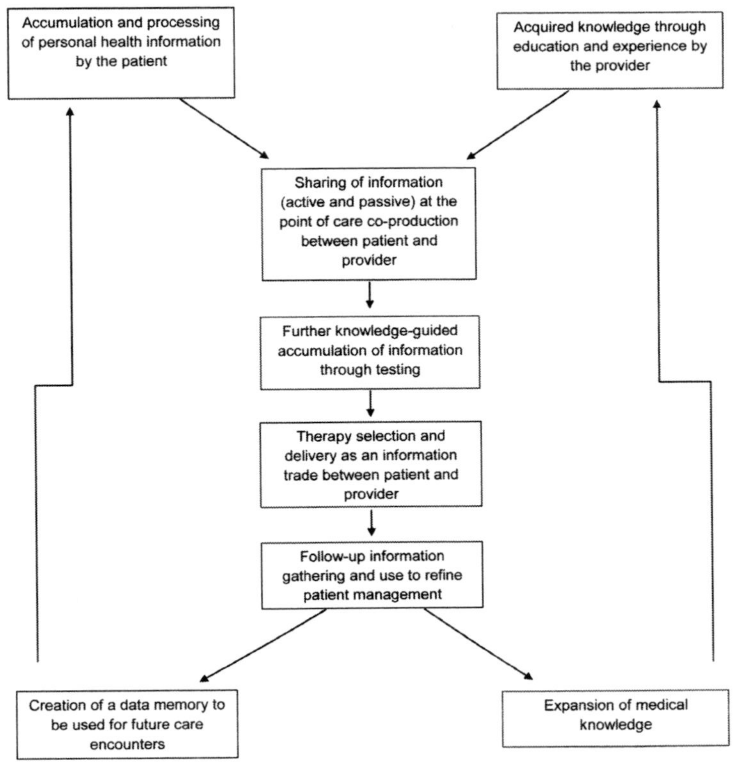

producer and a consumer, both the producer (provider) and consumer (patient) must collaborate at the production and delivery stages in order to jointly produce an effective outcome. As reflected in Figure 1, the need for effective information sharing and knowledge transfer within healthcare necessitates co-production. At a systems level, as indicated in Figure 1, this co-production enables feedback to improve future patient care and enhance knowledge acquisition. Optimizing this collaboration and utilizing the service co-production model in healthcare would, at once, enable U.S. healthcare delivery to function more effectively as a service system and to maximize the abilities of the patient and provider to achieve a common goal: improved health and, to a certain extent, sustainability of the delivery system.

In addition to improving the outcome of treatment provisions, the co-production model has the capacity to re-focus the essence of a healthcare system by systematically incorporating patient inputs. Clinically, the role of the patient in improving outcomes has been demonstrated through symptom recognition, personal health information gathering and sharing, treatment compliance, follow-up adherence, preventive care pursuance, and lifestyle modification. As evidenced by the examples in Table 3, patients and providers must co-produce at each stage within healthcare delivery.

By emphasizing patient centricity, co-production reinforces increasing trends to highlight patient factors and experience – a prime example being the use of patient satisfaction measures (Press Gainey Associates ranking system) as performance indicators for healthcare. Again, improving patient satisfaction requires an active exchange of knowledge and information to man-

Table 3. Examples of co-production in healthcare

Stage	Role of Patient	Role of Provider
Symptom Recognition	A congestive heart failures patient recognizes weight gain through daily weight measurement and seeks early intervention.	Patient education on acute exacerbation symptoms.
Lifestyle modification	A patient with chronic obstructive pulmonary disease makes decision to quit smoking.	Initial assessment, patient education on adverse health consequences, prescription for pharmacological agents and nicotine supplementation, and follow-up.
Preventive Care	A patient seeks routine screening colonoscopy and has pre-cancerous polyps removed.	Service provision and patient education on future follow-up.

age expectations and co-produce a positive emotion for the patient.

Beyond the infrastructure of healthcare delivery systems, the service co-production paradigm has many applications. For health services research, it empowers an expanded scope of research to readily include patient-centered factors in addition to traditional provider-related factors. For public health, the paradigm re-centers healthcare system objectives around the patient-centered concept of wellness. More specifically, Tien and Goldschmidt-Clermont (2009) elaborate on three overarching characteristics of the service sector (i.e., electronic services, relationship to manufacturing, and mass customization) that enable a better understanding of co-production, and more specifically, how the healthcare delivery system could function more effectively as a service system.

Electronic Services

Electronic or information technology services interact or "co-produce" with their customers in a digital (including e-mail and Internet) medium, as compared to the physical environment in which traditional or bricks-and-mortar service enterprises interact with their customers. Similarly, in contrast to traditional services which include low-wage "hamburger flippers", electronic services typically employ high-wage earners and services that are more demanding in their requirements for self-service, transaction speed, and computation. In regard to data input that could be processed to produce information that, in turn, could be used to help make informed service decisions, it should be noted that both sets of services rely on multiple data sources; however, traditional services typically require homogeneous (mostly quantitative) data input, while electronic services increasingly require non-homogeneous (i.e., both quantitative and qualitative) data input. Paradoxically, the traditional service enterprises have been driven by data, although data availability and accuracy have been limited (especially before the pervasive use of the Universal Product Code – UPC – and the more recent deployment of radio frequency location and identification – RFLID – tags). Likewise, the emerging electronic service enterprises have been driven by information (i.e., processed data), although information availability and accuracy have been limited, due to a data rich, information poor (DRIP) conundrum (Tien, 2003).

Consequently, while traditional services – like traditional manufacturing – are based on economies of scale and a standardized approach, electronic services – like electronic manufacturing – emphasize economies of expertise or knowledge and an adaptive approach. Another critical distinction between traditional and electronic services is that, although all services require decisions to be made, traditional services are typically based on predetermined decision rules, while electronic services require real-time, adaptive decision making; that is why Tien (2003) has advanced a decision informatics paradigm, one that relies on both information and decision technologies from a real-time perspective. High-speed Internet access, low-cost computing, wireless networks, electronic sensors and ever-smarter software are the tools for building a global services economy.

In services, automation-driven software algorithms have transformed human resource-laden, co-producing service systems to software algorithm-laden, self-producing services. Thus, extensive manpower would be required to manually co-produce the services if automation were not available. Although automation has certainly improved productivity and decreased costs in some services (e.g., telecommunications, Internet commerce, etc.), it has not yet had a similar impact on other labor-intensive services like healthcare. However, with new multimedia and broadband technologies and the recently enacted healthcare information technology (HIT) initiative, hospitals are beginning to share electronic records with their patients. In this manner, patients can take increased responsibility for the co-production of their own healthcare. Additionally, while electronic-driven, robotic surgery is quite helpful in the repair of small nerves and blood vessels, its overall efficacy is still under debate – nevertheless, as robotic surgery is further refined, it will undoubtedly become a standard technique in the surgeon's arsenal of tools.

Relationship to Manufacturing

The interdependences, similarities and complementarities of services and manufacturing are significant. Indeed, many of the recent innovations in manufacturing are relevant to the service industries. Concepts and processes such as cycle time, total quality management, quality circles, six-sigma, design-for-assembly, design-for-manufacturability, design-for-recycling, small-batch production, concurrent engineering, just-in-time manufacturing, rapid prototyping, flexible manufacturing, agile manufacturing, distributed manufacturing, and environmentally-sound manufacturing can, for the most part, be recast in services-related terms. Thus, many of the engineering and management concepts and processes employed in manufacturing can likewise be employed to deal with problems and issues arising in the services sector, like healthcare.

Nonetheless, there are considerable differences between goods and services. The goods sector requires material as input, is physical in nature, involves the customer at the design stage, and employs mostly quantitative measures to assess its performance. On the other hand, the services sector requires information as input, is virtual in nature, involves the customer – or, in the case of healthcare, the patient – at both the production and delivery stages, and employs mostly qualitative measures to assess its performance. Actually, co-production is a key difference be-

Table 4. Services versus manufactured goods

FOCUS	SERVICES	MANUFACTURED GOODS
Production	Co-Produced	Pre-Produced
Variability	Heterogeneous	Identical
Physicality	Intangible	Tangible
Product	Perishable	"Inventory-able"
Objective	Personalized	Reliable
Satisfaction	Expectation-Related	Utility-Related
Life Cycle	Reusable	Recyclable

tween services and manufactured goods. Indeed, as indicated in Table 4 (Tien and Berg, 2003), services are, by definition, co-produced; quite variable or heterogeneous in their production and delivery; physically intangible; perishable if not consumed as it is being produced or by a certain time (e.g., before a flight's departure); focused on being personalized; expectation-related in terms of customer satisfaction; and reusable in its entirety. On the other hand, manufactured goods are pre-produced; quite identical or standardized in their production and use; physically tangible; "inventory-able" if not consumed; focused on being reliable; utility-related in terms of customer satisfaction; and recyclable in regard to its parts.

Perhaps a revealing difference between goods and services is highlighted when a presentation is made with the aid of a laptop-based, power point display. The laptop hardware and power point software are, of course, pre-produced goods. The presenter is actually delivering a service, one that requires the co-production of an alert audience; otherwise, if the audience were all asleep then no service could be delivered. Of course, even when there are similarities, it is critical that the co-producing nature of services be carefully taken into consideration. For example, in manufacturing, physical parameters, statistics of production and quality can be more precisely quantified; in contrast, since a services operation depends on an interaction between the recipient and the process of producing and delivering, the characterization is necessarily more subjective and different. Nevertheless, healthcare must adopt some of the same methods that have enabled manufacturing to be efficient (e.g., reduced cycle time, improved quality, etc.), while focusing on service effectiveness (e.g., maintaining a high standard of co-production, meeting consumer expectation, etc.).

Although the comparison between services and manufacturing highlights some obvious methodological differences, it is interesting to note that the physical manufactured assets depreciate with use and time, while the virtual service assets are generally reusable, and may in fact increase in value with repeated use and over time. The latter assets are predominantly processes and associated human resources that build on the skill and knowledge base accumulated by repeated interactions with the service receiver, who is involved in the co-production of the service. Thus, for example, a surgeon should get better over time, especially if the same type of surgery is repeatedly undertaken. Indeed, clinical productivity increases for an average physician, from the dawn of a career to almost the end of a career, with a slight slowing down towards the end. Likewise, most physicians' financial productivity improves over time.

Mass Customization

A third critical influence on services is the computational-driven move towards mass customization. "Customization" implies meeting the needs of a customer market that is partitioned into an appropriate number of segments, each with similar needs (e.g., Amazon.com targets their marketing of a new book to an entire market segment if several members of the segment act to acquire the book). "Mass customization" implies meeting the needs of a segmented customer market, with each segment being a single individual (e.g., a tailor who laser scans an individual's upper torso and then delivers a uniquely fitted jacket). And "real-time mass customization" implies meeting the needs of an individualized customer market on a real-time basis (e.g., a tailor who laser scans an individual's upper torso and then delivers a uniquely fitted jacket within a reasonable period, while the individual is waiting).

It is interesting to note that in regard to customization and in relation to the late 1700s, the U.S. is in some respects going "back-to-the-future"; thus, advanced technologies are not only empowering the individual but are also allowing for individualized or customized goods and services. For example, electronic education reflects a return to individual-centered learning, much like home schooling in a previous century. Moreover, when mass customization occurs, it is difficult to say whether a service or a good is being delivered; that is, a uniquely fitted jacket can be considered to be a co-produced service/good or "servgood". The implication of real-time mass customization, then, is that the resultant, co-produced "servgood" must be carried out locally, although the intelligence underpinning the co-production could be residing at a distant server (located, perhaps, in the "cloud") and delivered like a utility. Thus, while manufacturing jobs have already been mostly relocated overseas (with only about 10.3 percent of all U.S. employees still involved in manufacturing) and service jobs (which now comprise about 82.1 percent of all U. S. jobs) are beginning to be relocated overseas, real-time mass customization should help stem job outflow, if not reverse the trend. In this regard, real-time mass customization should be regarded as a matter of national priority.

Most importantly, healthcare providers must increasingly be more adaptive and must customize their treatments to the needs of their patients, ranging from evidence-based protocols to "servgood" or personalized medications.

THE BARRIERS TO CO-PRODUCTION

As shown in Table 5, in healthcare, co-production requires patients to have timely access to care to enter the healthcare system; once accessing care, collaborative systems must be in place at the point of care to encourage effective patient and provider cooperation; and finally, incentives must empower shared end-points to cement and sustain this partnership. The current U.S. healthcare delivery model fails, to varying degrees, to provide these fundamental requirements for patient and provider collaboration. And as a result, these barriers hinder healthcare delivery functioning as an effective service system. This section will further examine the barriers to co-production in order to provide a comprehensive understanding of their implications to the U.S. healthcare system.

Access to Care

Under the current system of comprehensive insurance, insurance coverage is customarily expected to reimburse for catastrophic and routine healthcare expenditures, minimizing the role of consumerism in healthcare, particularly for individuals receiving employer-based or public insurance coverage. This model of healthcare financing has minimized price transparency and

Table 5. The requirements for enabling healthcare co-production

Requirement	Strategy	Rationale	Intervention
Patient and provider interaction must be optimized.	Access to Care	Enables patients to enter the system to engage providers and enable co-production.	Insurance status Language Socioeconomic factors (income, transportation, etc.) Health Literacy Provider Availability
	Collaborative Point of Care Systems	Encourages collaboration and information sharing through the incorporation of technology.	Electronic Medical Records Tele-health Automated Systems
Patient and provider must have mutual goals.	Alignment of Incentives	Incentivizes co-producers to work towards shared end-point.	Payer Structure Reimbursement mechanisms Medical liability systems

enabled price distortion, ultimately resulting in exorbitant out-of-pocket expenses for the uninsured, while subtly reinforcing the notion of insurance coverage as synonymous with access to care. The issue of access to care, however, moves beyond the problem of the uninsured. As Sen (1999) utilized the capabilities approach to transition the concept of development beyond purely economic indicators, similarly it can serve as a vehicle to move the issue of access to care beyond the current modicum of insurance status. Within healthcare, insurance coverage represents a single component of the capability to access care. An insured individual, for example, may lack the health literacy skills for early symptom recognition, the transportation to visit a primary care physician, or the resources to take a leave from employment. As these examples highlight, preparedness rather than insurance coverage must be the baseline for access to care. Accordingly, appropriate and timely access to care centers on, but is not limited to, insurance status, healthcare literacy, socioeconomic factors, and provider availability.

Insurance Status

Through the service co-production model, effective healthcare requires collaboration among all affected individuals. Without insurance coverage and the previously cited price distortions which limit the feasibility of out-of-pocket payment, many Americans lack viable entry into the healthcare delivery system. While emergency care and federally-funded community health clinics attempt to create access-points for these underserved populations, demand often outstrips supply.

In 2010, 52 million Americans, or nearly 20% of the U.S. population, are uninsured (Gilmer & Kronick, 2009). An Urban Institute (2005) study estimated that the majority, 56%, of the uninsured earned less than 300% of the federal poverty limit (FPL) and were not eligible for public insurance programs. The uninsured are predominately parents and childless adults, American citizens, and from households with one or more full-time worker. Lack of insurance coverage can serve as a significant barrier to accessing healthcare services. 52% of the uninsured lack a usual source of care, 29% postponed seeking care due to cost, and 27% could not afford medications in the past 12 months (Kaiser Family Foundation, 2009).

The uninsured, however, are not the only population affected by insurance status. The "opportunity cost" of caring for patients with public insurance drives many providers to limiting access for patients, thus stifling co-production. The Physician Office Acceptance of Government Insurance Programs Report released in 2009 highlighted that only 83% of U.S. medical offices accept Medicare and 65% accept Medicaid (SK&A, 2009). The conflicting pressures of increasing federal deficits and widening reimbursement gaps between private and public payers converge to create a potentially problematic scenario for the 87.4 million Americans insured by government plans (U.S. Census Bureau, 2002).

Health Literacy

Health literacy, as defined by the American Medical Association (1999), is a skill set that enables an individual to perform basic reading and computation tasks for adequate functioning in the healthcare environment and for acting on healthcare information Health literacy is an essential component of preparedness to accessing healthcare services successfully and functioning as a co-producer. Research indicates that inadequate health literacy levels have been associated with reduced utilization of preventive services such as immunizations, mammograms, pap smears and STD screenings, while concomitantly resulting in increased rates of hospitalization (Agency for Health Research and Quality, 2004); yet, no single measure of health literacy exists – instead, most of the tests currently utilized focus on reading ability.

Low literacy levels are a common occurrence in the United States. Ninety million Americans scored one or two out of five on the National Adult Literacy Survey, indicating a difficulty in identifying pieces of information in a lengthy text, integrating multiple pieces of information, or finding two or more numbers in a chart and performing a calculation (Kirsch, Jungeblut, Jenkins, & Kolstad, 2002). As a result, individuals with low literacy may have limited understanding of medical instructions, worse health outcomes, impaired healthcare functioning, and access to sub-standard medical care (Agency for Health Research and Quality, 2004). Low literacy levels are increasingly prevalent in populations who have completed fewer years of education, have discontinued any form of education following school/college years, and are the elderly, the chronically ill, and individuals at poor or near poor income status (Agency for Health Research and Quality, 2004; Kirsch et al., 2002).

The low literacy level problem is aggravated by the fact that it is often difficult for a patient to really understand the menu of care opportunities available for a given condition. For example, a patient experiencing chest pain related to coronary artery disease may or may not be presented with the choice of "medical management" (use of life-style change and drugs) or a "more invasive management" (performance of a procedure –catheterization of the coronary vessels, with injection of contrast within the coronaries and acquisition of X-ray images of the coronary vessels--, followed, or not, by an angioplasty –remodeling of a narrowed coronary vessel with the use of a specifically designed inflatable balloon, with or without the placement of a metallic device to preserve the remodeling or the coronary artery [stent] and the delivery of a drug by the device [drug-eluting stent]— or by bypass surgery). Depending on the severity and acuteness of symptoms, one of these approaches may be preferentially indicated. However, the reimbursement of a procedure (high) versus medical therapy (lower) may create a bias in the way risk and benefit are being presented to the patient (cost is rarely addressed), hence making it difficult for the patient to make an informed decision. Educated choice may be further challenged by the risk of liability for the provider in the situation where a procedure is not performed and the outcome is complicated by an event (coronary thrombosis resulting in heart attack or death). Hence, misaligned incentives in our current system may compromise the opportunity for improved health literacy (see below for additional information on misalignment of incentives in healthcare delivery).

Nevertheless, as electronic services permeate the healthcare field, with the proactive finding and support of the federal government, health literacy should improve. Patients should be able to not only access medical websites, but also their own medical records; thus, they should be better informed to help their providers in co-producing an effective care plan.

Socioeconomic Factors

Socioeconomic factors, including income status, racial or ethnic background, immigration status, and language, among others, can significantly undermine collaboration, resulting in poorer health outcomes. For example, socioeconomic factors can limit transportation to care, the ability to communicate with providers, or opportunities for employer and public insurance coverage due to immigration status. According to the U.S. Census Bureau (2002), 39.5% of individuals with a family income over 250% of the federal poverty line (FPL) viewed their health status as excellent compared to 29.1% for families earning less than 100% of the FPL. And only 10% of the uninsured have family incomes above 400% of the FPL (Kaiser Family Foundation, 2009).

In addition, disparities between racial and ethnic groups remain prevalent in the United States. 34% of Latino adults and 31% of African-American adults are uninsured, compared to 28%

for non-Hispanic whites (Ku & Waidmann, 2003). Immigration status further alters access to care. For non-citizens, the uninsured rate increases to 70% for Latinos and 54% for African-Americans compared to 30% for whites (Ku & Waidmann, 2003). For individuals who speak a primary language other than English, language can serve as a barrier to healthcare services and lead to communication problems with providers. While 67% of white, English-speaking citizens were likely to have visited a primary care physician, only 48% of Spanish-speaking citizens were likely to do the same (Ku & Waidmann, 2003).

These socioeconomic barriers to co-production highlight the need to enhance the customization of care, taking into consideration, as examples, a patient's income status, race, cultural background, and language. The goal is, of course, to mass customize healthcare.

Provider Shortage

While discussion of access to care has predominately focused on patient-centered factors, provider availability for primary, specialist, and nursing care remains an issue often overlooked. Provider shortages limit access to care, and thus, co-production. Primary care health professional shortage areas (HSPAs), for example, are defined by the U.S. Department of Health and Human Services as areas with population-to-primary care physician ratio of at least 3,500:1 and inaccessible or over-utilized providers in the surrounding areas. As such, the U.S. Department of Health and Human Services (2009) currently identifies 6,204 primary care HSPAs, affecting 65 million Americans and requiring 16, 643 providers to yield a population to provider ratio of 2,000:1.

The Association of American Medical Colleges (2008) predicts a physician shortage of up to 159,300 by 2025. These shortages have a significant impact on access to care, particularly in rural areas. Such limitations are particularly pronounced in regions where primary care is exclusively delivered by physicians, as opposed to medical teams that include nurses and other providers. Interestingly, the provider shortage can and should be addressed as a supply chain problem. More specifically, the manufacturing techniques of supply and demand chain management can help mitigate the looming shortage.

In addition, it is important to consider the appropriateness of healthcare training in producing providers capable of managing the co-production of care for the twenty first century. As examples, it is unlikely that health services research, comparative medical research, and personalized medicine can be effectively employed unless medical education is altered to create a diversified workforce capable of managing these activities. At a time when the cost of education is itself a barrier to some medical activities (primary care, for example), modifying curricula to produce more diverse physician and nurse cohorts, such that trainees can acquire the relevant expertise over a four-year medical school period and two- to three-year nursing school period, without adding the unnecessary cost of supplemental years, and while protecting the quality of the clinical education that involves substantial patient contact.

Collaborative Point of Care Systems

Once accessing the system, patients and providers must be empowered to engage in a collaborative approach to health promotion. A collaborative approach at the point of care requires technologies to lower communication costs, expedite information exchanges, and automate care provision. Unlike other major service industries (banking, transportation, etc.), healthcare delivery has largely remained untouched by the recent technological revolution. From online bill payment to email updates for flight status, the cost of customized interaction between customer and service provider have been drastically reduced. The relatively high communication costs within healthcare, which are empirically exemplified by a patient's return to a hospital records department and by repeated lab tests and imaging, create a barrier to patient and provider collaboration.

Electronic Medical Records

Only 17% of hospitals, and even fewer physician offices, utilize electronic medical records (EMR) (Des Roches et al., 2008). Paper records limit information sharing between patient and provider, among providers, and even between visits for a single provider. EMR may enable a unified patient database utilized by all service providers with access controlled by the patient. As such, EMR has the potential to limit duplication, serve as a health education tool for patients, reinforce evidence-based practice, and enhance quality reporting. Hence, the power of EMR to overcome information gaps in healthcare, increase patient involvement in their own care, and equalize knowledge deficits hold substantial promise for the service co-production model, but unfortunately not for all patients.

Desroches et. al. (2008) reveal that physicians with fully-functional EMR systems reported improved quality of clinical decisions (82%), better communication with other providers (92%) and patients (72%), timely access to medical records (97%), avoidance of medication errors (86%), and increased delivery of guideline-based long-term and preventive care (82-85%). Capital requirements and high maintenance costs, however, were often cited by providers as reasons for not adopting EMR (Jha et al., 2009). Interoperability standards, necessary to ensure that records can be efficiently accessed and utilized by all service providers and patients, also remain ill-defined. Furthermore, not all patients have the ability or capacity to access, use, or benefit from the new IT tools. These challenges continue to limit the expansion of EMR within the U.S. healthcare system, despite the fact that, as mentioned earlier, EMR can greatly enhance the status of health literacy.

Digital Communication Tools

The current payer systems, both public and private, continue to finance patient-provider interaction and communication primarily through one medium: direct contact. Alternate mediums of communication - telephone, email, text message, or teleconference - embodied by tele-health lack comprehensive reimbursement policies and consequently remain under-utilized (Center for Telemedicine Law, 2003). These financing mechanisms impede the assimilation of new technologies into healthcare delivery, restrict patient-provider communication opportunities, and discourage multidisciplinary communication between providers. As a result, potential patient-provider collaboration opportunities are missed.

Automated Processes

Although automation has certainly improved productivity and decreased costs in some services (e.g., telecommunications, Internet commerce, etc.), it has not yet had a similar impact on other labor-intensive services like healthcare. At the point of care, service co-production requires highly specialized and comprehensive collaboration between patients and providers. Current delivery systems in hospital settings identify a primary provider responsible for the patient. While primary providers may utilize consultation services to address the patient's medical, social, and psychological problems, these collaborations often result in a primary focus of care with other issues being marginalized, particularly in a context of capped reimbursement for hospital stay. Under this model, patient concerns and co-morbidities remain un-addressed or under-addressed and providers often encounter issues outside their expertise. With automated systems of care, however, prioritized problem lists could be generated and notification reminders could activate problem-based teams to provide customized care (Goldschmidt-Clermont et al., 2009).

Similarly, automated processes can greatly assist in outpatient settings as well. Automated processes such as appointment reminders have entered traditional medical offices. Yet, the use of automated processes for follow-up care, symptom recognition, and treatment compliance represent potential future applications that can greatly enhance service co-production.

The Misalignment of Incentives in Healthcare Delivery

In the service co-production model, as with any collaboration, parties must be properly incentivized to achieve a shared end-point. The current service delivery approach promotes a misalignment of incentives that fosters incongruent goals and corresponding sub-optimal results.

Healthcare Finance Systems

The current healthcare finance system, often summarized as fee-for-service, has been faulted for limiting provider incentive to supply appropriate levels of information (see paragraph on healthcare literacy) and care – an incentive which may counter a patient's overall objective for improved health, particularly in light of recent research revealing that unnecessary care is associated with increased iatrogenic complications. To many, the fee-for-service description underscores a U.S. healthcare system that is solely financed by retrospective payment models which are based on volume of care. In reality, payment models, such as the diagnosis related group (DRG) utilized by Medicare for hospital admissions, are often a combination of prospective and retrospective reimbursement (Robinson, 2001). Regardless, current payment models can be improved to align provider incentives with patient goals of holistic care, wellness promotion, preventive care, coordinated delivery, improved quality, and minimized waste.

Although developed in the hopes of equalizing pay discrepancies between primary care physicians (often with non-procedural skills) and specialists (often with interventional skill), the relative value unit system, utilized by Medicare and private insurers, has extended the discrepancy in hourly payment between these groups of providers (Vladeck, 2010). Healthcare systems, unsurprisingly, are organized with growth strategies that promote reaction over prevention, intervention over wellness, inpatient care over outpatient services, and specialty over systemic care.

In addition, the current system fails to create a viable system of patient incentives that promote treatment compliance, lifestyle modification, self-education, wellness, optimal healthcare decision-making, or follow-up adherence – many of the essential components of forging a collaborative partnership with providers. Under public and private employer-based insurance schemes, which provide the majority of insurance coverage in the United States, beneficiaries pay a percentage of total healthcare expenditures in the form of premiums, deductibles, and cost-sharing schemes (co-payment or co-insurance). These public and private-employer based insurance plans offer minimal out-of-pocket cost savings to the patient for co-productive behavior (smoking cessation, regular exercise, treatment compliance, etc.), limiting incentives for collaboration.

Finally, the role of third-party payers can often create significant challenges for providers. First, reimbursement schemes often fail to accurately account for the time and skill necessary to provide specific services. In addition, rates depend more on the size of provider network and the competition within provider markets rather than the quality of the service provided. Finally, the high administrative costs related to the incongruent billing practices of multiple payers unnecessarily increases healthcare costs.

Medical Liability Systems

Medical liability models in the United States, often characterized as "regulation by litigation," have focused on adversarial approaches that often stifle collaboration between patients and providers (Viscusi, 2002). Both patients and providers seek a system that improves quality, ensures safety, encourages reporting, and provides appropriate and timely compensation. The current three-pronged regulatory system - legal system, liability insurance issuers, and healthcare providers - falls short on many of these ideals (Sage, 2003). The medical liability system, at present, remains uncoupled to quality improvement, generates sporadic claims, punishes unpredictable complications, compensates inconsistently, encourages under-reporting, promotes defensive medicine, and charges malpractice insurance premiums without experience-rating (Sage, 2003). In aggregate, the adversarial system creates divisions between patients and providers, which is, of course, counter to focused co-production.

A 1999 study from the Institute of Medicine revealed that up to 98,000 Americans were killed every year by preventable medical errors (Kohn, Lorrigan, & Donaldson, 2000). Yet, studies approximate that only 2 percent of victims file claims (Thomas et al., 2000; Brennan et al., 1991) and compensation payments take five years on average (Nordman, Cermak, & McDaniel, 2004). Equally disturbing, the current liability system has limited evidence to support its deterrent effect (Mello & Brennan, 2002) and may actually counter patient safety initiatives such as adverse event reporting (Liang, 2000).

For providers, the system fails to adequately account for systemic factors. In addition, a 2006 Harvard study found 40 percent of malpractice lawsuits to be unfounded (Studdert et al, 2006). While complications for commonly performed surgeries do not differ in frequencies between best (lowest mortality) and worse (highest mortality) hospitals (Ghaferi, Birkmeyer, & Dimick, 2009), lawsuits are quite variable and inconsistent. Recent emphasis on patient safety and evidence from other industries have illustrated that approaches built on collaboration, cultures of improvement, communication, less adversarial forms of dispute resolution, and "non-judicial compensation mechanisms" may provide the needed alternative (Sage, 2003).

THE IMPACT OF HEALTHCARE REFORM ON CO-PRODUCTION

The Patient Protection and Affordable Care Act and its accompanying reconciliation bill (hereafter referred to as PPACA), hailed as the most significant overhaul since the Social Security Act of 1965, have drastically altered the U.S. health insurance landscape (Gruber, 2009). From the outset, the healthcare reform legislation was promoted as a means to expand access, improve quality, and lower costs. While an analysis of the legislation's effectiveness in achieving these objectives remains outside the scope of this work, this section will examine the specific provisions which affect the barriers to service co-production addressed earlier, thus enabling the patient and provider collaboration that is necessary to produce optimal health outcomes.

Access to Care

Access to care – the first step towards collaboration – is, in part, determined by insurance status, health literacy, socioeconomic factors, and provider availability. The CBO (2010) estimates that 50 million Americans lack health insurance in 2010. PPACA will provide health insurance coverage to 32 million previously uninsured Americans by 2019. Half of these newly insured Americans – 16 million – will be covered by an expansion of Medicaid up to 133% of the federal poverty level (FPL) for all individuals, including the often currently excluded subgroups of parents and childless adults (CBO, 2010). The remaining 16 million Americans will gain coverage through the private individual insurance markets bolstered by the formation of state-based health insurance exchanges, federal premium and cost-sharing subsidies for families up to 400% of the FPL, individual mandates to improve risk-distribution, and small-business tax credits for firms with fewer than 25 employees (P.L. 111-148, 2010; P.L. 111-152, 2010).

In addition to the insurance expansion, PPACA authorizes a number of consumer protections to regulate the insurance industry and expand access. To ensure coverage for patients with pre-existing conditions in the individual and small group markets, PPACA encourages the formation of high-risk insurance pools until 2014. Private insurance plans must also provide a minimum set of "essential benefits" to be defined by the Secretary of Health and Human Services, eliminate annual or lifetime coverage limits, abolish cost-sharing for preventive services, and prohibit premium variation based on health status (P.L. 111-148, 2010; P.L. 111-152, 2010). Each of these measures either expands the covered benefits of insurance or the insurance coverage itself, thus, enabling more Americans to readily access needed healthcare services.

The reform bill, in expanding health insurance coverage to 94% of Americans, takes a significant step towards expanding access to care. Despite these efforts, the Lewin Group and Ingenix Consulting (2010) estimate that 15.4 million Americans, will remain uninsured, limiting the opportunity of these populations to access care and engage in co-production.

In addition, serious questions remain for those newly insured. First, public insurance may not necessarily correlate to healthcare access: only 83 and 65 percent of physicians currently accept Medicare and Medicaid, respectively (SK&A, 2009). Given the anticipated cuts to Medicare provider payments, estimated at $195.4 billion through 2019, and reductions in Medicare and Medicaid disproportionate share hospital funding, estimated at $36.1 billion through 2023, included in PPACA, access to care for public insurance beneficiaries may become more tenuous in the future (Lewin Group & Ingenix Consulting, 2010). Second, as evidenced by health reform efforts in Massachusetts earlier this decade, a new influx of insured patients can often overwhelm already overly-stretched provider networks, resulting in increased wait times and restrictions on acceptance of new patients. Finally, the combination of employer mandates, a 40% excise tax on high-cost insurance indexed to inflation, and health insurance exchanges requiring only 60% actuarial value (defined in key terms) for bronze level plans may result in the purchase of lower-cost insurance plans in both the individual and the employer-based markets. With healthcare costs expected to surge above the rate of inflation, lower cost insurance plans will inevitably require increased beneficiary cost-sharing or restricted provider choice. These cost-sharing levels, potentially limited by the possibility of ever-increasing federal subsidies, may serve as a barrier to care for lower income families.

PPACA attempts to address the other barriers to access – health literacy, socioeconomic status, and primary care shortage – through a number of proposals. First, to improve health literacy, PPACA creates a National Prevention, Health Promotion, and Public Health Council and a Prevention and Public Health Investment Fund to improve public health efforts. Moreover, the availability of increased provider quality data (explained in detail later) and the establishment of a Patient Centered Outcomes Research Institute are examples of information transparency initiatives designed to empower patients as more-prepared healthcare consumers. PPACA also authorizes an additional $11 billion in funding over five years for community health centers, effective 2010 – an attempt to expand the public safety net of providers, reduce health disparities, and serve the underprivileged (P.L. 111-148, 2010; P.L. 111-152, 2010). The impact of these reforms in meeting the challenge of poor health literacy and socioeconomic factors cannot be fully ascertained at this time. Yet, even with these proposals, it is almost certain that significant barriers to service co-production will undoubtedly remain.

To address concerns of provider shortages, PPACA endorses a 10 percent Medicare bonus payment for all primary care providers and for general surgeons in health professional shortage areas from 2011 to 2016. Medicaid payments for primary care services will be increased to at least Medicare rates for 2013 and 2014 (P.L. 111-148, 2010; P.L. 111-152, 2010). In addition, 65% of unused residency spots will be redistributed with at least 75% used for primary care and general surgery for at least 5 years. The impact of the residency redistribution, given that many of the unused residency spots are primary care spots initially, remains a matter of debate. Finally, in addition to the establishment of a National Healthcare Work Force Commission, PPACA enhances low-interest loan and scholarship programs for health students and professionals (P.L. 111-148, 2010).

Despite these bonus payments, the reimbursement imbalance for primary care providers, although abated to some degree, will continue. Given the political challenges in altering these disparities via a zero-sum game, Vladeck argues that reimbursement rates for primary care will require future increases to enhance the specialty's appeal to medical school graduates (2010). Moreover, PPACA's proposal for graduate medical education falls short of the Association of American Medical Colleges (AAMC, 2008) recommendation for an expansion of residency positions to address the expected future physician shortage. Combined, these reforms make strides towards expanding access to healthcare required for patient and provider collaboration, but work remains to insure all Americans, improve health literacy, decrease socioeconomic burdens, and increase provider supply.

Collaborative Point of Care Systems

At the point of care, collaboration can be enhanced by systems to encourage information sharing, lower the costs of communication, and promote automated processes for interconnection. Healthcare information technology (HIT) can play a significant role. The American Recovery and Reinvestment Act of 2009 (2009), widely known as the stimulus bill, contained $20 billion in incentive payments for HIT adoption; health professionals who fail to adopt "meaningful use" of HIT by 2016 will face 1% Medicare payment cuts, phased up to 3% by 2018. However, definition of meaningful use and interoperability standards remain areas of ambiguity.

To encourage communication within healthcare, PPACA authorizes demonstration projects for Medicaid global payments from 2010 to 2012, Medicaid bundle payments from 2012 to 2016, and a Medicare bundle payment pilot program for five years starting in 2014 (P.L. 111-148, 2010). Another key element in encouraging collaboration is the expansion of digital communication tools, embodied by tele-health, within the healthcare delivery system. According to the American Telemedicine Association (2010), PPACA empowers the Center for Medicare and Medicaid Innovation to examine the use of patient-based remote monitoring systems and permits an annual comprehensive medication review for Medicare beneficiaries to be conducted via telemedicine.

While PPACA contains few specific provisions for incorporation of technology to assist in communication or for the use of automated systems, these systems may be encouraged by the new financial pressures introduced by value-based purchasing and public insurance reimbursement cuts.

Alignment of Incentives

The current healthcare finance and medical liability systems fail to optimize co-production. As a result, PPACA, at extended lengths, attempts to alter provider payment structures and appropriates funding for numerous demonstration projects under the authority of the Secretary of Health and Human Services, in an attempt to reshape financial incentives for providers and payers. These payment provisions seek to align provider reimbursement with patient goals of increased quality, enhanced transparency, improved outcomes, and decreased cost, thus, encouraging co-production by creating shared end-points. An example of these projects include further support for the development of Accountable Care Organizations (ACOs), public or private, where health of a population segment is reimbursed as covered lives. ACOs attempt to emphasize quality outcomes and reduce costs by making a single system in charge of a patient's total well-being. However, ACOs have also raised the challenge of anti-trust regulations, as opponents fear provider consolidation may reduce competition and shared savings may encourage decreased care provision.

For physicians, a value-based purchasing program consisting of fee modifier based on quality and cost data, the specifics of which are yet to be defined, will begin in 2015. To further encourage transparency, 1 percent incentive payments in 2011 and 0.5 percent from 2012–2014 will be provided for voluntary participation in Medicare's Physician Quality Reporting Initiative (PQRI). Non-participating physicians will be penalized by 1.5% in 2014 and 2% in 2016 and beyond. Providers also will be eligible for an additional 0.5 percent incentive payment for participation in a qualified Maintenance of Certification Program (quality practice-based learning programs through specialty boards) (P.L. 111-148, 2010). A Physician Compare website, modeled on the already established Hospital Compare, will be created to provide patients with quality, cost, and efficiency data on their providers. In addition, a physician feedback program, linked to the value-based purchasing fee modifier, will compare individual physician's patterns of resource use with others. Physicians often encounter paperwork and third party payer interactions as significant obstacles to patient care, and thus, co-production. As a result, between 2013 and 2016, administrative simplification rules will be implemented to streamline health insurance claims processing (P.L. 111-148, 2010). These simplified processes can empower service co-production by limiting physician non-clinical duties and increasing time available for patient interaction.

By requiring transparency and linking payment modifiers to both participation in quality reporting programs and health outcomes, PPACA attempts to align the incentives of patient and physicians to encourage service co-production. Yet, this approach has its limitations which will be elaborated further after examining the incentive alignment proposals applicable to hospitals and patients.

For hospitals, PPACA takes significant steps towards encouraging increased coordination, improved outcomes, and the adoption of data systems infrastructure. First, starting in 2013, Medicare will implement a budget-neutral, value-based purchasing program that will reward hospitals with bonus payments for attainment and improvement in their quality measures and efficiency level (defined as risk-adjusted Medicare spending per beneficiary). The program, financed by payment cuts to all hospitals, will start with a focus on myocardial infarction, pneumonia, congestive heart failure, hospital-acquired infections, and surgical complications. The payment cuts will proceed as follows: 1% (2013), 1.25% (2014), 1.5% (2015), 1.75% (2016), and 2% (2017 and beyond) (P.L. 111-148, 2010).

In an attempt to increase efficiency pressures on hospitals, PPACA calls for market basket update reductions for inpatient and outpatient hospitals by 0.25% in 2010 and 2011, 0.1% in 2012 and 2013, 0.3% in 2014, and 0.75% in 2017 through 2019. In addition, reimbursements will be further reduced by a productivity adjustment starting in 2014 through 2019. And as previously mentioned, starting in 2014, Medicare and Medicaid Disproportionate Share Hospital funding will be reduced by $22.1 billion and $14 billion, respectively, over 10 years (P.L. 111-148, 2010; P.L. 111-152, 2010).

These reimbursement cuts attempt to encourage efficiency, while financing healthcare reform and "bending the cost curve." However, the CMMS Actuaries (2010) report questions the feasibility of enacting these future cuts, given the political ramifications and potential impact on access to care for public insurance beneficiaries.

Furthermore, PPACA creates incentives for specific patient initiatives such as decreased hospital-acquired conditions and reduced readmission rates. For hospital-acquired conditions, which are responsible for considerable morbidity, increased costs, and lengthy hospitalizations, PPACA provides for a 1 percent reduction in Medicare payments to hospitals in the top quartile for highest rates of hospital-acquired conditions beginning in 2015. In addition, Medicaid will no longer reimburse care provided for hospital-acquired conditions starting in 2011 (P.L. 111-148, 2010). For readmission rates, PPACA incorporates payment reductions, starting in 2013, for congestive heart failure, myocardial infarction, and pneumonia. In 2014, the program will be expanded to include coronary artery bypass graft (CABG), chronic obstructive pulmonary disease, percutaneous transluminal coronary angioplasty, and other vascular diagnoses. The reductions, which start at 1% in 2013, will increase by 1% each year until reaching a cap of 3% reduction in payments across all diagnosis-related groups (DRGs) (P.L. 111-148, 2010).

While this section does not cover the full list of demonstration projects or proposals directed at reforming the healthcare finance and delivery systems, it highlights those believed to be most pertinent to service co-production. The proposals included in the bill, however, are not without limitation in their ability to produce the desired effect of optimizing co-production for wellness and health. In particular, many details including the quality and efficiency indicators, the methodology for Medicaid DSH payment cuts, and the implementation of physician fee modifiers remain undefined and under the purview of the Secretary of HHS. As a result, the final impact of this legislation in reducing the barriers to service co-production cannot be precisely evaluated at this time. In addition, a number of reforms are rooted in demonstration projects, which typically take 8-10 years to progress from concept to full-scale implementation. This process is complicated by contracts between HHS, state and local officials, private payers, and providers. As a result, McClellan (2010) argues that a national standard of quality, efficiency, and cost measures with real-time registries could shave years off the demonstration projects timeline.

In regard to service co-production incentives for patients, the health reform bill allows employers to offer premium discounts up to 30% to employees for participation in wellness programs (P.L. 111-148, 2010). Medicare and Medicaid beneficiaries will be provided incentives to complete behavior modification programs. By eliminating cost-sharing for preventive services rated as A or B by the U.S. Preventive Services Task Force, immunizations, and screenings, PPACA reduces economic barriers to necessary healthcare services that may mitigate patient morbidity. While these measures begin to address the misalignment in incentives for patients to act as service co-producers, they are currently limited in scope and evidence-base.

Moving away from the financial incentives, PPACA issues a far more limited approach to solving the barrier to service co-production, represented by the current medical liability system and its adversarial approach to dispute resolution. In addition to the $25 million grant program authorized by the administration in September 2009, PPACA appropriates another $50 million for state-based demonstration projects for innovative medical liability reforms (P.L. 111-148, 2010). The limited funding and unknown infrastructure for expansion of these demonstration projects constitute another barrier to the potential success of reforming the complex medical liability problem.

CONCLUSION

At a time when the proportion of individuals older than 65 is growing steadily (thus, expanding the chronic disease burden, and in particular neuropsychiatric disorders), rising federal deficits threaten to restrict safety net provisions, and systemic inefficiencies limit quality advances, improved healthcare delivery models are urgently required. Moreover, effective healthcare investments extend the preservation of human capital, thus, impacting positively the pace of economic growth (Manton et al., 2009). Given these realities, the U.S. healthcare system must develop a means to shelter patients from morbidities and disabilities through healthcare that promotes co-production.

Service co-production holds the potential to transform U.S. healthcare delivery – enabling it to function more effectively as a service system. Using this model, the challenges to and opportunities for increased access, improved quality, and lower costs are clearly highlighted, providing a paradigm from which to shape future reform efforts and evaluate demonstration projects. As previously described, service co-production in the U.S. healthcare system is frequently obstructed by the lack of appropriate and timely access to care, underdeveloped collaborative point of care systems, and the misalignment of patient and provider incentives.

Yet, too often, patients cannot access necessary care due to lack of insurance coverage, poor health literacy skills, socioeconomic hurdles, and provider shortages. Once accessing care, healthcare delivery systems fail to promote collaborative infrastructures that encourage information sharing, lower costs of communication, and promote automated processes. Furthermore, the U.S. healthcare system must address the current structure of financial incentives for patients and providers and the medical liability system that have limited collaborative approaches in healthcare.

The Patient Protection and Affordable Care Act and its corresponding reconciliation bill attempt to address a number of these challenges. However, despite the steps made toward overcoming these barriers to service co-production, more work is needed. In particular, patient and provider collaboration could be increased by attempts to expand insurance coverage to all Americans, improve health literacy education within schools, increase financing for public health campaigns, reward public insurance providers, increase the use of alternative providers, reform reimbursement structures to appropriately reward time and skill of services rendered, and increase residency training allotments. Moving forward, co-production can be significantly enhanced through the development of a national real-time quality and cost data infrastructure, the establishment of a National Institute for Health Services Research capable of evaluating new delivery and finance models, and the encouragement of public-private experimentation partnership through the Center of Medicare and Medicaid Innovation. Opportunities for future research, particularly within health services, remain abundant.

Creating a 21st century healthcare delivery system will require new innovative technologies, a renewed focus on health services research, a revitalized engagement by patients and healthcare providers, and a focused commitment from government, all to enhancing the co-production of an effective and efficient healthcare system.

REFERENCES

Agency for Health Research and Quality. (2004). Literacy and health outcomes. Retrieved from http://www.ahrq.gov/ downloads/ pub/ evidence/ pdf/ literacy/ literacy.pdf

Agency for Healthcare Research and Quality. (2002). *Healthcare costs fact sheet.* (AHRQ Publication No. 02-P033). Rockville, MD: Author. Retrieved from http://www.ahrq.gov/ news/ costsfact.htm

American Medical Association. (1999). Ad hoc committee on health literacy for the council on scientific affairs. *Journal of the American Medical Association, 281*, 552–557. doi:10.1001/ jama.281.6.552

American Recovery and Reinvestment Act of 2009.P.L. 111-5. Washington, DC: GPO, 2009.

American Telemedicine Association. (2010). *Telemedicine in U.S. healthcare reform.* Retrieved from http://www.americantelemed.org/ files/ public/ policy/ Telemedicine%20in% 20National%20 Health% 20Reform.pdf

Association of American Medical Colleges. (2008). *The complexities of physician supply and demand: Projections through 2025.* Retrieved from http://www.tht.org/ education/ resources/ AAMC.pdf

Brennan, T. A., Leape, L. L., Laird, N. M., Hebert, L., Localio, A. R., & Lawthers, A. G. (1991). Incidence of adverse events and negligence in hospitalized patients. Results of the Harvard medical practice study I. *The New England Journal of Medicine, 324*(6). doi:10.1056/ NEJM199102073240604

Center for Medicare and Medicaid Services, Office of the Actuaries. (2010). *Estimated financial effects of the Patient Protection and Affordable Care Act as amended.* Washington, DC: U.S. Government Printing Office. Retrieved from https:// www.cms.gov/ ActuarialStudies/ Downloads/ PPACA_2010-04-22.pdf

Center for Telemedicine Law. (2003). *Telemedicine reimbursement report.* Prepared for the Office of Advancement of Telehealth, Health Resources and Services Administration. Washington, DC: Center for Telemedicine Law. Retrieved from ftp://ftp.hrsa.gov/ telehealth/ licen.pdf

Congressional Budget Office. (2009). *The long-term budget outlook.* (Publication No. 3216). Washington DC: Author. Retrieved from http:// www.cbo.gov/ ftpdocs/ 102xx/ doc10297/ 06-25-LTBO.pdf

Congressional Budget Office. H.R. 4872, Reconciliation Act of 2010. Washington, DC. March 18, 2010. Retrieved from http://www.cbo.gov/ ftpdocs/ 113xx/ doc11355/ hr4872.pdf

DesRoches, C. M., Campbell, E. G., Rao, S. R., Donelan, K., Ferris, T. G., & Jha, A. (2008). Electronic health records in ambulatory care—A national survey of physicians. *The New England Journal of Medicine, 359*, 50–60. doi:10.1056/ NEJMsa0802005

Ghaferi, A. A., Birkmeyer, J. D., & Dimick, J. B. (2009). Variation in hospital mortality associated with inpatient surgery. *The New England Journal of Medicine, 361*, 1368–1375. doi:10.1056/ NEJMsa0903048

Gilmer, T. P., & Kronick, R. G. (2010). Hard times and health insurance: How many Americans will be uninsured by 2010? *Health Affairs, 28*(4), w573–w577. doi:10.1377/hlthaff.28.4.w573

Goldschmidt-Clermont, P. J., Dong, C., Rhodes, N. M., McNeill, D. B., Adams, M. B., & Gilliss, C. L. (2009). Autonomic care systems for hospitalized patients. *Academic Medicine, 84*, 1727–1731. doi:10.1097/ACM.0b013e3181bf9bfd

Gruber, J. (2009). Getting the facts straight on healthcare reform. *The New England Journal of Medicine, 361*, 2497–2499. doi:10.1056/ NEJMp0911715

Healthcare and Education Reconciliation Act of 2010. P.L. 111-152. Washington, DC: GPO, 2010.

Jha, A. K., DesRoches, C. M., Campbell, E. G., Donelan, K., Rao, S. R., & Ferris, T. G. (2009). Use of electronic health records in U.S. hospitals. *The New England Journal of Medicine*, *360*, 1628–1638. doi:10.1056/NEJMsa0900592

Kaiser Family Foundation. (2009). *The uninsured and the difference health insurance makes*. Retrieved from http://www.kff.org/ uninsured/ upload/ 1420-11-2.pdf

Kirsch, I., Jungeblut, A., Jenkins, L., & Kolstad, A. (2002). *Adult literacy in America: A first look at the findings of the national adult literacy survey*, 3rd edition, vol. 201. Washington, DC: National Center for Education, U.S. Department of Education, 2002.

Kohn, L. T., Corrigan, J. M., & Donaldson, M. S. (Eds.). (2000). *To err is human: Building a safer health system. Committee on Quality of Healthcare in America, Institute of Medicine*. Washington: National Academy Press.

Ku, L., & Waidmann, T. (2003). *How race/ethnicity, immigration status and language affect health insurance coverage, access to care and quality of care among the low-income population*. Prepared for the Kaiser Commission on Medicaid and the Uninsured, August 2003.

Lewin Group and Ingeinx Consulting. (2010). *Brave new world: Healthcare reform - An update on the impact on government and commercial payers and providers*. April 1, 2010. Retrieved from http://www.lewin.com/ healthreformwebinars/

Liang, B. A. (2000). Risks of reporting sentinel events. *Health Affairs*, *19*(5). doi:10.1377/ hlthaff.19.5.112

Manton, K. G., Gu, X. L., Ullian, A., Tolley, H. D., Headen, A. E. Jr, & Lowrimore, G. (2009). Long-term economic growth stimulus of human capital preservation in the elderly. *Proceedings of the National Academy of Sciences of the United States of America*, *106*(50), 21080–21085. doi:10.1073/pnas.0911626106

McClellan, M. (2010). *Reforming provider payment to promote models of integrated delivery.* Presented at National Health Policy Conference. Washington, DC. February 8, 2010.

Mello, M. M., & Brennan, T. A. (2002). Deterrence of medical errors: Theory and evidence for malpractice reform. *Texas Law Review*, 80.

Nordman, E., Cermak, D., & McDaniel, K. (2004). *Medical malpractice insurance report: A study of market conditions and potential solutions to the recent crisis*. Kansas City, MO: National Association of Insurance Commissioners.

Organization of Economic Cooperation and Development. (2010). *OECD health data 2010*. Retrieved from http://www.oecd.org/ document/ 16/ 0,3343,en_2649_34631 _2085200_1_1 _1_37407,00.html

Pamuk, E., Makuc, D., Heck, K., Reuben, C., & Lochner, K. (1998). *Socioeconomic status and health chartbook: United States, 1998*. Hyattsville, MD: National Center for Health Statistics.

Pappas, G., Queen, S., Hadden, W., & Fisher, G. (1993). The increasing disparity between socioeconomic groups in the United States, 1990 and 1996. *The New England Journal of Medicine*, *329*, 103–109. doi:10.1056/NEJM199307083290207

Parasher, A. K., Tien, J. M., & Goldschmidt-Clermont, P. J. (2010a). *Healthcare delivery as a service system: The barriers to co-production*. Manuscript Submitted for Publication.

Parasher, A. K., Tien, J. M., & Goldschmidt-Clermont, P. J. (2010b). *The Patient Protection and Affordable Care Act: The implications for healthcare reform for service co-production*. Manuscript Submitted for Publication.

Patient Protection and Affordable Care Act. P.L. 111-148. Washington, DC: GPO, 2010.

Robinson, J. C. (2001). Theory and practice in the design of physician payment incentives. *The Milbank Quarterly*, *79*(2). doi:10.1111/1468-0009.00202

Rowland, D., Hoffman, C., & McGinn-Shapiro, M. (2009). *Healthcare and the middle class: More costs and less coverage*. Washington, DC: Kaiser Family Foundation.

Sage, W. (2003). Medical liability and patient safety. *Health Affairs*, *22*(4), 26–36. doi:10.1377/hlthaff.22.4.26

Sen, A. K. (1999). *Development as freedom*. New York, NY: Alfred A. Knopf.

SK&A. (2009). *Physician office acceptance of government insurance programs report*. October 2009.

Studdert, D. M., Mello, M. M., Gawande, A. A., Gandhi, T. K., Kachalia, A., & Yoon, C. (2006). Claims, errors, and compensation payments in medical malpractice litigation. *The New England Journal of Medicine*, *354*, 2024–2033. doi:10.1056/NEJMsa054479

Thomas, E. J., Studdert, D. M., Burstin, H. R., Orav, E. J., Zeena, T., & Williams, E. J. (n.d.). … Brennan, T. A. Incidence and types of adverse events and negligent care in Utah and Colorado. *Medical Care*, *38*(3).

Tien, J. M. (2003). Towards a decision informatics paradigm: A real-time, information-based approach to decision making. *IEEE Transactions on Systems, Man, and Cybernetics, Special Issue*, *33*(1), 102–113. doi:10.1109/TSMCC.2003.809345

Tien, J. M., & Berg, D. (2003). A case for service systems engineering. *Journal of Systems Science and Systems Engineering*, *12*(1), 13–38. doi:10.1007/s11518-006-0118-6

Tien, J. M., & Goldschmidt-Clermont, P. J. (2009). Healthcare: A complex service system. *Journal of Systems Science and Systems Engineering*, *18*(4), 285–310.

U. S. Department of Health and Human Services. (2009). *Shortage designation: HPSAs, MUAs & MUPs*. Washington, DC. Retrieved from http:// bhpr.hrsa.gov/ shortage/ index.htm

Urban Institute. (2005). *Analysis of the 2005 annual and social economic supplement to the current population survey for the Kaiser Commission on Medicaid and the uninsured*. Washington, DC: Kaiser Family Foundation.

U.S. Bureau of Labor Statistics. (2006). *Employment statistics*. Retrieved from http://www.bls.gov/ bls/ employment.htm

U.S. Census Bureau. (2006). *Survey of income and program participation, October 2001−January 2002*. Retrieved from http://www.census.gov/ prod/ 006pubs/ p70-106.pdf

Viscusi, W. K. (Ed.). (2002). *Regulation through litigation*. Washington, DC: AEI-Brookings Joint Center for Regulatory Studies.

Vladeck, B. C. (2010). Fixing Medicare's physician payment system. *New England Journal of Medicine*. Retrieved from http://content.nejm.org/ cgi/ content/ short/ NEJMp1004709v1?rss=1&query=current

Wolfson, M., Kaplan, G., Lynch, J., Ross, N., & Backlund, E. (1999). Relation between income inequality and mortality: Empirical demonstration. *British Medical Journal*, *319*, 953–957.

ADDITIONAL READING

Gerdtham, U.-G., & Jönsson, B. (2000). International Comparisons of Health Expenditure. In Culyer, A. J., & Newhouse, J. P. (Eds.), *Handbook of Health Economics, vol. 1A* (pp. 11–53). New York: Elsevier.

Pearson, M. (2009). Disparities in health expenditure across OECD countries:

Why does the United States spend so much more than other countries? Written Statement to Senate Special Committee on Aging, 111th Congress. Retrieved at http://www.oecd.org/ dataoecd/ 5/ 34/ 43800977.pdf

KEY TERMS AND DEFINTIONS

Actuarial Value: Actuarial value is the percentage of medical claims paid by a health insurance plan. The figure is calculated by taking into account a health insurance plans cost-sharing provisions for claims of a standard population.

Co-Production: A key component of the service sector, co-production requires collaboration between the producer and the consumer at both the production and delivery stages in order to produce a joint, effective outcome or service.

Patient Protection and Affordable Care Act (PPACA): The Patient Protection and Affordable Care Act, as amended by the reconciliation bill, Healthcare and Education Reconciliation Act of 2010, refers to the healthcare reform legislation passed in March 2010 under the 111th Congress.

Section 2

Outpatient Clinic Management and Scheduling

Chapter 10
Using Simulation to Design and Improve an Outpatient Procedure Center

Todd R. Huschka
Mayo Clinic, USA

Thomas R. Rohleder
Mayo Clinic, USA

Brian T. Denton
North Carolina State University, USA

ABSTRACT

Discrete-event simulation (DES) is an effective tool to for analyzing and improving healthcare processes. In this chapter we discuss the use of simulation to improve patient flow at an outpatient procedure center (OPC) at Mayo Clinic. The OPC addressed is the Pain Clinic, which was faced with high patient volumes in a new, untested facility. Simulation was particularly useful due to the uncertain patient procedure and recovery times. We discuss the simulation process and show how it helped reduce patient waiting time while ensuring the clinic could meet its target patient volumes.

INTRODUCTION

Effective patient flow through treatment processes is an increasingly important issue for healthcare organizations. Economic pressures are putting a growing importance on treating more and more patients without corresponding increases in staff and other healthcare resources. Expensive resources such as operating rooms and sophisticated diagnostic imaging equipment drive organizations to maximize their utilization. Further, with an increasing array of procedures, equipment, and specialized staff, the complexity of managing patient flow is growing. Add to this, the desire to improve patient satisfaction (i.e., limit patient waiting time) and it is clear that health care organizations have a very challenging problem in managing patient flow.

DOI: 10.4018/978-1-60960-872-9.ch010

To design and manage patient flow processes, healthcare organizations can use a variety of techniques. Often, the treatment processes evolve over time with trial and error. Sometimes, more structured methods like Lean and Plan-Do-Study-Act (PDSA) techniques are applied that help the processes evolve more quickly (Fischman, 2010). However, given the previously discussed complex interaction of people and equipment along with the highly variable nature of treatment times for diverse patients and it appears sensible that sophisticated quantitative methods like discrete-event simulation (DES) may be more appropriate analysis and improvement tools. DES can directly incorporate the uncertainties in the process and provide a more process-wide versus localized analysis approach.

In this chapter we discuss the use of computer simulation modeling applied to the design and operational improvement of an outpatient procedure center (OPC) at the Mayo Clinic. The specific application is for interventional procedures in Pain Medicine – the Pain Clinic. This Clinic was faced with growing demand for its services and desired to optimize patient flow as it moved to new facilities.

Our primary objectives in this chapter are to discuss the modeling process and how it answered the specific questions regarding the design of the new Pain Clinic practice (Huschka et al., 2008). These questions included:

- How many recovery rooms would be sufficient to accommodate the anticipated demand and adequately serve the procedure rooms?
- How could patient waiting time for recovery rooms be minimized?
- When should patients be released at various treatment stages to minimize waiting times?
- Could the desired daily patient volume be achieved and if not, what process improvements were required to achieve this volume?

In addition to addressing these design questions, the DES model was also used to address process flow issues related to nurse staffing. These issues arose subsequent to the initial study as the Pain Clinic approached the desired volume levels. Thus, the simulation model continues to be a useful analysis and improvement tool as the Mayo Clinic strives to maximize value for its patients.

A REVIEW OF PATIENT FLOW SIMULATION LITERATURE

In this section we provide an overview of some of the literature regarding the use of DES to address patient flow problems, in general, and flow issues in outpatient (and similar) clinics, specifically.

Discrete-Event Simulation Applied to Patient Flow

As discussed in Chapter 8 of Hall (2006) the application of discrete-event simulation to study the design and operation of health care delivery systems is steadily increasing. One of the reasons for this, as pointed out by Jun et al. (1999) in their DES literature review article, is that increasing health care costs is driving many health care organizations to consider more sophisticated improvement tools like DES. As the authors state, discrete-event simulation "...allows managers to select management alternatives that can be used to reconfigure existing systems, to improve system performance or design, and to plan new systems, without altering the present system." This what-if analysis capability is a key given the high cost of designing and making changes to health care operations.

Difficulties in managing patient flow are exasperated by the high degree of innate uncertainty in healthcare. In their overview article, Noon et al. (2003) note the sources of variability and the corresponding queuing effects that restrict easy patient flow. This variability due to the way patients and diseases present themselves is termed *natural variation* in Haraden and Resar (2004). These authors contrast this to what they call *artificial variation* that is due to preferences and beliefs of clinicians and administrators. Effectively managing patient flow requires addressing both of these, and suggests that decision support models need to include both to be most useful.

Another issue with modeling in healthcare is the interconnectedness of the patient treatment process. Chapter 1 in Hall (2006) clearly makes this point in considering patient flow in a hospital. As pointed out in Lane et al. (2000) increasing (or decreasing) resources that a particular patient group uses may not have the intended results because other patients are also using those resources. This systems perspective is important and supports the use of tools like DES that are designed to broadly look at processes. However, effective decision-making models also need to be as simple as possible. Thus, most DES research is done at the department, clinic, or provider/resource level.

An example hospital department where DES is frequently applied is surgery. Van Berkel and Blake (2007) show the use of DES to consider wait list time for a general surgery department. Their model highlights the need to consider multiple types of resources because it identified that increasing hospital beds was more important than increasing operating room (OR) time to reduce patient waits. Davies (1994) identified a similar issue for coronary patients at a London hospital.

Another common hospital department where simulation is used to examine patient flow is the emergency room (ER). Blake et al. (1996) use simulation to diagnose the causes for ER delays and identify the availability of staff physicians and training activities as primary issues. Sinreich and Marmor (2005) discuss an overall process for building ER simulation models as well as emphasizing the need to involve ER physicians and administrative staff in model development. This can be viewed as a key success factor for any applied simulation project in healthcare.

Simulating Outpatient Clinics

The previous section identified that DES is prevalent as a tool to model and improve patient flow. In this section we highlight some of the DES literature focusing on patient flow in outpatient clinics.

An aspect that significantly affects flow in outpatient settings is how patients arrive for treatment. A major determinant of patient arrival is the scheduling of patients via appointments. Therefore, there is a large and growing body of research related to appointment scheduling. There are several good overview and literature review articles on appointment scheduling. Gupta and Denton (2008) provides a categorization of appointment scheduling problems including a section on scheduling patients in specialty clinics. They also highlight existing research and opportunities in each category. Cayirli and Veral (2003) present a comprehensive review of research specific to outpatient appointment scheduling, citing 80 references. Here we will focus on some of the research that uses DES to model appointment scheduling systems.

Modeling of appointment scheduling has been studied for decades going back to Bailey (1952). He studied several different scheduling rules, identifying tradeoffs between patient waiting and provider idleness when booking multiple patients at the same time. The value of using arrival information of patients is shown by Rising et al. (1973) who report that increasing the number of patient slots on days with fewer walk-in patients increased patient throughput and reduced clinic overtime. Ho and Lau (1991) test many difference appointment scheduling rules and report that varying the appointment interval length can effectively reduce patient waiting time and provider idle time. Klassen and Rohleder (1996) found that when sequencing patients, using information about their expected treatment time distributions leads to improved performance.

The issue of patients who fail to show up for their appointments ("no shows") is an important consideration when scheduling outpatient clinics. Lawrence and Laganga (2007) effectively present an overview of the issue and show that, when done properly, overbooking can increase patient access and provider productivity but with some negative affect on patient waiting time in the clinic. In their case study article, Kros et al. (2009) show the increased economic and patient access value at an outpatient clinic. The authors used DES to support the changes to the clinic's operations. Kopach et al. (2007) use DES to evaluate Open Access scheduling and its affect on no-show rates in a large inner-city outpatient clinic.

Beyond patient scheduling aspects, simulation has proved an effective tool to more comprehensively study improvement options in outpatient settings. In addition to appointment scheduling changes, Clague et al. (1997) suggested expanding the role of nurses in the outpatient clinic they studied via simulation. Merkle (2002) found similar results in his study of a primary care clinic. This study focused on different ways to allocate clinic activities and resources levels to maximize throughput and reduce patient waiting time. Harper and Gamlin (2003) used simulation to show the importance of prompt arrival of staff at clinic start times as well as improved patient scheduling in their study of patient waiting time at an Ear, Nose, and Throat clinic. Finally, Chand et al. (2009) study an outpatient clinic and identify such improvement options as not batching work (e.g., patient records) and pooling separate patient queues together to reduce processing variability. Reducing these sources of variability served to improve patient waiting time in the clinic.

In the next section we will provide an overview of the Mayo Pain Clinic's operations. After that we will show how DES was applied to the Pain Clinic in similar ways as the research just discussed.

OVERVIEW OF THE PAIN CLINIC AT MAYO CLINIC

Pain disorders in patients are typically complex and multisystemic. Therefore, the practice of Pain Medicine requires a multi-disciplinary approach and often involves several modes of treatment including: pharmacological, rehabilitative, psychological, and interventional therapies. For this last type of treatment, pain specialists at the Mayo Clinic use fluoroscopic guidance in a full-service OPC with appropriate sedation and nursing care available to appropriately treat patients. The specific procedures include epidural steroid injections, facet joint injections, neurolytic blocks, radiofrequency lesioning, neurostimulation, and neuraxial infusions.

It is clear there are many different pain procedures, however, the durations of most of the procedures are very similar. This relative consistency allows a scheduling system that groups the procedure type into five categories (I-V). Type I includes the shortest and simplest procedures and Type V has the longest and most complex set of procedures, often requiring multiple techniques and advanced imaging.

The original Pain Clinic procedural area was a sub-section of a larger out-patient procedure center which had been designed around procedures which did not necessarily fit the Pain Clinic model. The out-patient procedure center had been designed with a number of pre/post rooms which served as both intake and recovery for the procedures performed on the floor. These rooms had the benefit of not being dedicated to a specific patient during the entire procedure. Patient belongings were stored in movable lockers which would allow pre/post room usage while the patient was in the procedure room, allowing a more flexible arrangement of pre and post procedure functionality.

While this design worked well for most of the procedures performed in the area, short duration procedures (such as pain treatment) did not benefit. There was little benefit in moving a patient's

Figure 1. Basic schematic of original pain clinic

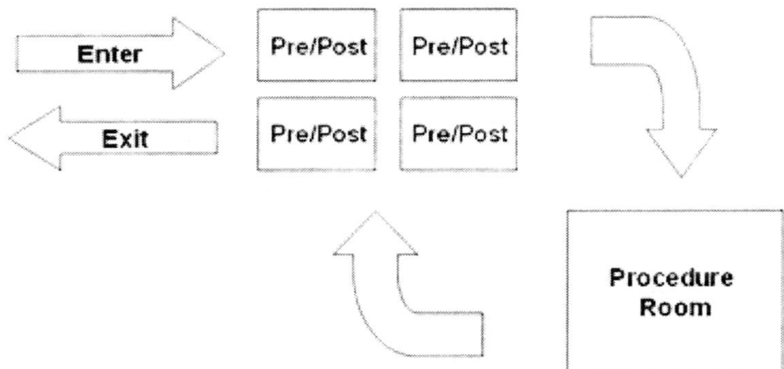

belongings out of a pre/post room during a procedure if the patient was expected to return in a short period of time. As a result the pre/post rooms being used for pain treatment were somewhat under utilized.

Additionally, the demand for pain treatment exceeded the capacity of the single treatment room available. The combination of increasing demand, and inefficient use of pre/post room space resulted in the plan to move the pain clinic to a different OPC with a design for improved patient flow throughout the process. While the primary motivation for the move was to handle increased demand, this redesign also allowed for streamlined patient flow.

Because the Pre/Post room method was not efficient, the plan was to move to dedicated rooms for pre-procedure and recovery. Each individual procedure room would have a dedicated "Vitals Booth" which served the purpose of pre-procedure activities. Patients would go to a bank of four recovery bays after their procedures. The size of the Vitals Booths and the Recovery Rooms would also be much smaller than the existing Pre/Post rooms, yet adequate for their purposes. So even though their number would double, their total space would not increase. The only real increase in floor space would be for the additional three Procedure Rooms.

Although this redesign began prior to the use of simulation modeling, simulation was used to evaluate the design for possible issues which could be addressed before the new unit opened. Because the Vitals Booths were very small and not designed

Figure 2. Basic schematic for proposed pain clinic

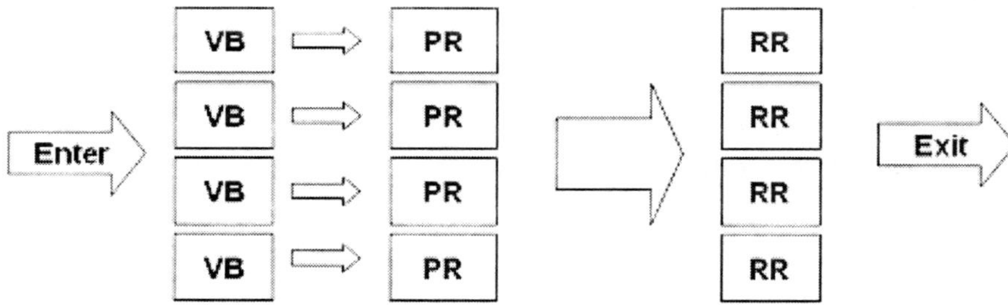

for patient comfort but rather clinical necessity, administrators at the Pain Clinic were particularly focused on minimizing patient waiting time at this stage of the process. Further, there was a concern that delays in patient recovery could create a bottleneck and limit efficient flow of patients through the procedure rooms.

The new design would also involve some staffing changes. The original process had one nurse serving two pre/post rooms, with their primary functions being patient movement to and from the procedure rooms, pre-procedure processing (e.g., checking vitals), and post-procedure recovery observation. The proposed process would still have nurses performing these duties, but it was unclear what staffing levels would be required to address the increase in patient loads, and how some small shifting of work to more dedicated tasks would work. Nurses would be dedicated to either the Vitals Booths or the Recovery Bay, with one nurse in the Recovery Bay and an undetermined number serving the Vitals Booths.

USING SIMULATION TO ASSIST REDESIGN OF THE PAIN CLINIC

The process for building the simulation model generally followed the classical approach discussed in Law and Kelton (2000). After identifying the problems discussed in the previous section, we collected the data required to drive the model. Historical data from the original pain procedural area were available and generally applicable to the new design. Probability distributions were estimated using a year's worth of data. Because the new facility required some process changes, new data was required for some aspects. For example, the pre-procedure activities of the nurses were not directly available from the historical data. Observations of these activities were performed and used to fit a triangular distribution to obtain a reasonable input to the model.

The model was built using Arena 10.0 (Software developed by Rockwell Automation Technologies, Inc., version 10.0, 2005). Specific model building activities will be discussed further in following paragraphs, however, once a base model was built it was verified by walking through each logical step in the computer model and observing the animation of the process. The model was validated to ensure it was a reasonable representation of the new facility by soliciting expert opinion from administrators familiar with the original practice. With a valid model, experiments and appropriate analyses were performed as discussed in the following sections.

Throughout the simulation process, communication with administrators from the Pain Clinic was maintained. Similar to the approach discussed in Lane et al. (2003), we were careful to use the time of the client staff as wisely as possible, but we also ensured we had sufficient information to complete an analysis that would be useful to the Clinic administrators.

The model for this project was based on an existing model that had already been simulated and validated as part of a larger simulation (Huschka 2007) looking at scheduling within an OPC and how the use of "Hedging" patient release could be used to maintain patient throughput while also reducing patient wait times. Hedging is a way of dealing with the natural uncertainty in the treatment process. By adding extra "safety time" to the release of patients into their treatment process over and above the mean procedure time, patients wait less when there is significant variability in the procedure times. This approach is similar to using safety stock in inventory systems (Silver et al., 1998) or safety staff in hospitals (Bekker and deBruin, 2010). For the Pain Clinic, a hedge was added to spread the scheduled arrival of patients.

The original model was modified to fit the proposed design and baseline simulations were performed. One of the first aspects to determine was how to pull patients into the system. The original model's Pre/Post rooms were comfortable

Table 1. Initial simulation model results to determine best time to pull patients into a procedure room

Trigger to Move into Vitals Booth	As soon as available	After Pre-incision	After Procedure
Wait in Vitals Booth	14.6 Minutes	10.3 Minutes	1.6 Minutes
Wait for Recovery	3.4 Minutes	3.4 Minutes	3.3 Minutes
Avg. Patients Per Day	43.6	43.6	43.5

rooms. Patients had the luxury of a large room with a TV and space for a companion to sit while they waited for their procedure and also during recovery. Additionally, since there was excess Pre/Post space this area was not a bottleneck within the process. The new design did not have this luxury. The Vitals Booths would be small, little more than changing rooms, not designed to serve as a long duration hold for patients prior to their procedures. And with a lack of TV, or much else, it was not desirable to have patients spend excess time in the Vitals Booths.

Fortunately, there were several trigger points which could serve as possible points to have patients enter the Vitals Booths. The actual pain treatment procedure consists of three distinct steps, each of which could serve as a trigger point. The steps were pre-incision (getting the patient positioned and ready for the procedure), procedure (actual pain treatment), and post-procedure (closing or bandaging of treatment location). Thus, patients could enter immediately when the booth was available, after the patient currently in the Procedure Room had completed their pre-incision step of the procedure, or after the patient currently in the Procedure Room had completed their procedure. Technically we could also use the time when the Procedure Room was completely empty (end of post-procedure), however that would cause the procedure room to site idle while the incoming patient was in Vitals Booth so it was not evaluated. Since the two major objectives of the new design were to obtain a capacity of 48 patients per day and also to not have patients wait for a recovery room these two metrics were used to evaluate all stages of the simulation. As Table 1 reveals, it was apparent that the initial design of the new Pain Clinic had some problems.

Not only was the configuration not able to treat 48 patients per day, we also observed patients waiting for a recovery room regardless of when we would pull patients into a procedure room. When the floor space was designed the recovery spaces were based on a 1:1 approach. It was known that recovery time for these procedures was, on average, approximately equal to the procedure time and that the most complicated procedures would have their patients recover in a separate area. However, the variation around the time to recovery was large enough to cause flow problems on a regular basis. Additionally, the rareness of the complicated procedures was such that a very low number of patients would be assigned to the alternate recovery area.

Fortunately, there were ready solutions to these problems. The new Pain Clinic area was again to be part of a larger OPC; this time of more closely related activities. These other activities had pre/post rooms similar to the previous Pain Clinic location, one of which had already been designated as an alternative recovery area for the complicated patients. Thus, the easiest solution would simply be to use the alternative recovery area whenever the primary area was full, regardless of the procedure being performed. This provided a valuable option for Pain Clinic patients whenever the regular recovery rooms over flowed and the simulation showed this would not happen too frequently.

Additionally, the initial simulation provided valuable insight as to when to move patients into

Table 2. Late stage simulation results using post procedure start as the trigger

Hedge	10 Minutes	15 Minutes
Wait in Vitals Booth	0.4 Minutes	0.2 Minutes
Wait for Recovery	0.0 Minutes	0.0 Minutes
Procedure Room Utilization	67.2%	61.3%
Avg # Patients per Day	52.8	48.3
Patients Going to Secondary Recovery	1.9	1.1

the procedure room. As discussed earlier, having patients wait in the Vitals Booth was not desirable, and it appeared that having patients move into the Vitals Booth after the current patients completed their procedure, but prior to the end of their post-procedure, would work well.

Also, we gained some insight into the scheduling of patients. The initial simulation used the scheduling routine from the old Pain Clinic, however, research into scheduling (Huschka et al., 2007) examined the benefits of scheduling heuristics, primarily the use of *hedging* patient arrivals in order to optimize patient throughput and minimize patient waiting time within the waiting room. By inserting an appropriate "hedge" time, patient waiting time is reduced without significantly reducing patient throughput.

Using the insight from hedging, the use of an alternate recovery room when the primary is full, and the optimized trigger point for pulling patients we explored several scenarios to determine which would work best. There were several iterations of going back and forth with the operational administrators of the area to ensure that we did not miss anything important from a practical implementation perspective. The final simulation results are shown in Table 2.

As the Table 2 shows, the simple use of a smart trigger, and the use of a secondary recovery along with hedging of patient arrivals predicted that the new Pain Clinic would be able to obtain the desired results. What is most interesting is that the use of the secondary recovery area is quite small under either hedge scenario, yet that small difference makes a significant difference in overall throughput by eliminating blocking of the procedure room while a patient waited for a regular recovery room.

The final aspect of the model to evaluate was proper staffing. The models to this point were based on the assumption of one nurse for each Vitals Booth who would perform duties only associated with the Vitals Booth. Staffing for the other areas was generally predictable based on existing areas, but the Vitals Booth area was an unknown. After some additional simulation scenarios it was determined that a model with one nurse working two Vitals Booths would only slightly reduce the total patient throughput while still maintaining all other important considerations. At that point it was really a financial decision of whether one or two additional patients per day were worth the cost of additional nursing staff in the area.

One Year Later: A Check on Validity

A year later the model was re-evaluated. The Pain Clinic had since moved into the new area, and we were curious as to how the new design was actually working when compared to the simulation model. The two graphs in Figure 3 show that the simulated and the actual patient processing are very similar. Each line represents one patient in the procedure room throughout the day. An actual and simulated day that had 12 patients was chosen for comparison purposes with the time being represented in military time along the horizontal axis. Due to the way patients enter into the area the actual arrival time associated with waiting

Figure 3. Comparison patient times: actual and simulated

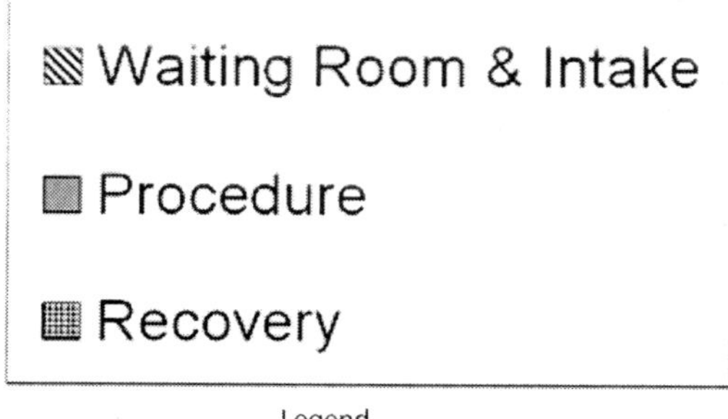

Legend

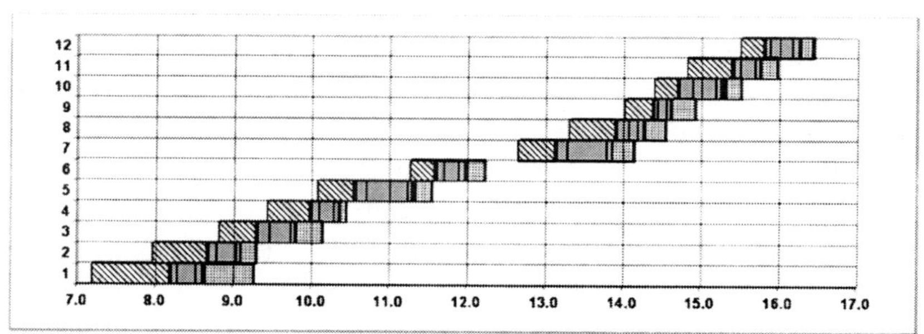

Randomly Sampled Actual Day

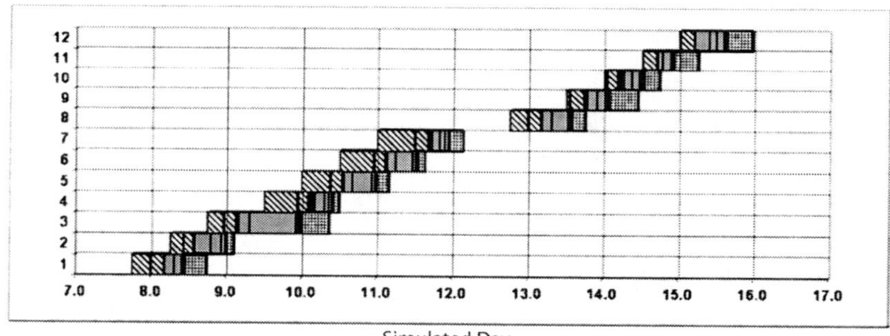

Simulated Day

and entry into the vitals booth is not collected completely, so those times are collapsed in order to have a consistent graph between the simulation and actual data.

At the time this follow-up analysis was performed, the new pain clinic was not at full operation so it was not possible to obtain full floor data for comparison purposes, however, it appeared that the floor was operating very closely to what the simulation model predicted. Area administrators were also pleased with the results from the simulation. This had been our first attempt to simulate an area which did not already exist at Mayo Clinic, so it was very pleasing to see such highly valid results and usefulness to the clinical area.

Another Use for the Model

Another year later we were again asked to examine the Clinic. The new Pain Clinic was still not running at the target patient volumes, but it was sufficiently close to capacity that the area was starting to see some bottleneck problems related

Table 3. Vitals Booth nursing options

Model	Current	No Turnover	No Turnover No Rooming	Current plus one float nurse
5th %	3:49 PM	2:48 PM	2:31 PM	2:40 PM
Med	4:27 PM	3:27 PM	3:07 PM	3:09 PM
95th %	5:15 PM	4:16 PM	3:48 PM	3:52 PM
MEAN	**4:30 PM**	**3:34 PM**	**3:06 PM**	**3:11 PM**
SD	21 minutes	28 minutes	25 minutes	23 minutes

to the nursing staff working the Vitals Booths. This was not immediately troubling to us. The simulation model had shown that having one nurse in charge of two Vitals Booths would be the best approach, but that this approach would make it difficult to reach the full 48 patients per day. As we had determined during the original analysis, the addition of another nurse or two would make only a very small increase in the total number of patients seen. However, the problems they were seeing exceeded what the model had predicted. It was becoming exceeding difficult to have all patients through recovery by 4:00 pm and the procedure rooms were experiencing some waiting for their next patient.

As with all modeling of complex environments, particularly those with human resources, some small tasks are easy to miss or misunderstand. Such was the case with this model. The assumption was that the nurses working the Vitals Booths would only serve that function. In reality they were also cleaning (turnover) the Vitals Booths between patients. They also physically moved the patients into the procedure rooms. The model assumed the procedure room staff would bring them into the room. Although this was a small amount of time, as the floor started to get closer to full capacity it started to become a bottleneck within the system.

The actual data from the Pain Clinic was not really helpful for diagnosing the cause of the problem. They did not have a large sample of data at this time but it was obvious that they were having a hard time maintaining the 4:00 pm departure goal, and the general feeling was one of being rushed on the floor by the Vitals Booth nurses as well as frustration within the procedure rooms when they were waiting for patients. So we re-examined the model and looked more closely at the timings, specifically at the end of a shift, to see if we could get insight in to what was happening.

The "Current" column in Table 3 gave us a sense of what was going on from a time perspective. By having the simulation model include the time required to turnover the Vitals Booths we saw that the end of a full day will run late on average. Although the turnover time was very short (3 to 5 minutes) over a day with 10 or more patients this time really started to add up. Table 3 also shows other options we explored to mitigate the problem. They could shift the turnover task to other staff, they could also shift the procedure room rooming task to other staff, or they could add an additional staff member to float between the four vitals booths while still performing the turnover and rooming tasks.

It would then be up to the administrators in the area to determine whether an additional nurse would be feasible, or if a clinical assistant or some other less expensive staff would be better suited to performing the rooming and turnover.

CONCLUSION

In summary, this chapter discussed a case study of using discrete-event simulation modeling as a tool to assist in the design and implementation of new space and processes for an outpatient procedure center at Mayo Clinic. Specifically, the model suggested several operational changes to meet the objectives of the Pain Clinic. By determining an appropriate time to release patients for their procedures, using a planned "hedge" to delay patient release, and a identifying a limited need for additional recovery resources, our model helped the Clinic meet desired patient volumes while minimizing patient waiting during the process. This approach is in keeping with the desire at the Mayo Clinic to maximize the value of its health care to patients (where value is defined as quality (outcomes, safety, and service) divided by cost).

As an engineering management method discrete-event simulation provides what-if capability to explore options before making expensive changes to existing facilities or asking employees to change processes and then finding out the changes are not effective. The science of a tool like DES helps in gaining acceptance by decision makers and those affected by recommendations. Our study highlights the need for continual engagement between those in charge of designing or administering health care processes and those who are building the model. This active dialog should continue beyond the completion of a particular project. In our study we found an additional use of the model to propose alternative options for work allocation and staffing levels to ensure the smooth flow of patients.

At the time of this writing the Pain Clinic is still moving towards full capacity after which time the model will likely be evaluated again to see how well it matches the current operation and to determine if it could plan another role in clinic improvement. Regardless of any future usage, the model has proved to be extremely valuable in the progression of the Pain Clinic from a simple one procedure room process within an existing OPC to an entirely new four procedure room unit on a different floor.

ACKNOWLEDGMENT

We gratefully thank the many Mayo Clinic staff who assisted with this study. In particular, we wish to recognize the contributions of Dr. Bradley Narr and Adam Thompson. This project was funded in part by grant CMMI-0620573 (Denton) from the National Science Foundation.

REFERENCES

Bailey, N. T. (1952). A study of queues and appointment systems in hospital outpatient departments. *Journal of the Royal Statistical Society. Series A (General)*, *14*(2), 185–199.

Bekker, R., & de Bruin, A. M. (2010). Time-dependent analysis for refused admissions in clinical wards. *Annals of Operations Research*, *178*(1), 45–65. doi:10.1007/s10479-009-0570-z

Blake, J. T., Carter, M. W., & Richardson, S. (1996). An analysis of emergency room wait time issues via computer simulation. *INFOR*, *34*(4), 263–272.

Chand, S., Moskowitz, H., Norris, J. B., Shade, S., & Willis, D. R. (2009). Improving patient flow at an outpatient clinic: Study of sources of variability and improvement factors. *Health Care Management Science*, *12*(3), 325–340. doi:10.1007/s10729-008-9094-3

Clague, J. E., Reed, P. G., Barlow, J., & Rada, R. (1997). Improving outpatient clinic efficiency using computer simulation. *International Journal of Health Care Quality Assurance*, *10*(5), 197–201. doi:10.1108/09526869710174177

Davies, R. (1994). Simulation for planning services for patients with coronary artery disease. *European Journal of Operational Research*, *72*(2), 323–332. doi:10.1016/0377-2217(94)90313-1

Fischman, D. (2010). Applying lean six sigma methodologies to improve efficiency, timeliness of care, and quality of care in an internal medicine residency clinic. *Quality Management in Health Care*, *19*(3), 201–210.

Gupta, D., & Denton, B. (2008). Appointment scheduling in health care: Challenges and opportunities. *IIE Transactions*, *40*(9), 800–819. doi:10.1080/07408170802165880

Hall, R. W. (Ed.). (2006). *Patient flow: Reducing delay in healthcare delivery*. Los Angeles, CA: Springer.

Haraden, C., & Resar, R. (2004). Patient flow in hospitals. *Frontiers of Health Services Management*, *20*(4), 3–15.

Harper, P. R., & Gamlin, H. M. (2003). Reduced outpatient waiting times with improved appointment scheduling: A simulation modelling approach. *OR-Spektrum*, *25*(2), 207–222. doi:10.1007/s00291-003-0122-x

Ho, C., & Lau, H. (1992). Minimizing total cost in scheduling outpatient appointments. *Management Science*, *38*(12), 1750–1764. doi:10.1287/mnsc.38.12.1750

Huschka, T., Denton, B., Gul, S., & Fowler, J. (2007). Bi-criteria evaluation of an outpatient procedure center via simulation. *Proceedings of the 2007 Winter Simulation Conference*, (pp. 1510-1518).

Huschka, T. R., Denton, B. T., Narr, B. J., & Thompson, A. C. (2008). Using simulation in the implementation of an outpatient procedure center. *Proceedings of the 2008 Winter Simulation Conference*, (pp. 1547-1552).

Jun, J. B., Jacobson, S. H., & Swisher, J. R. (1999). Applications of discrete-event simulation in health care clinics: A survey. *The Journal of the Operational Research Society*, *50*(2), 109–123.

Kopach, R., DeLaurentis, P.-C., Lawley, M., Muthuraman, K., Ozsen, L., & Rardin, R. (2007). Effects of clinical characteristics on successful open access scheduling. *Health Care Management Science*, *10*(2), 111–124. doi:10.1007/s10729-007-9008-9

Kros, J., Dellana, S., & West, D. (2009). Overbooking increases patient access at East Carolina University's student health services clinic. *Interfaces*, *39*(3), 271–291. doi:10.1287/inte.1090.0437

LaGanga, L. R., & Lawrence, S. R. (2007). Clinic overbooking to improve patient access and increase provider productivity. *Decision Sciences*, *38*(3), 251–276. doi:10.1111/j.1540-5915.2007.00158.x

Lane, D. C., Monefeldt, C., & Husemann, E. (2003). Client involvement in simulation model building: Hints and insights from a case study in a London hospital. *Health Care Management Science*, *6*(2), 105–116. doi:10.1023/A:1023385019514

Lane, D. C., Monefeldt, C., & Rosenhead, J. V. (2000). Looking in the wrong place for healthcare improvements: A system dynamics study of an accident and emergency department. *The Journal of the Operational Research Society*, *51*, 518–531.

Law, A. M., & Kelton, W. D. (2000). *Simulation modeling & analysis* (3rd ed.). New York, NY: McGraw-Hill, Inc.

Merkle, J. F. (2002). Computer simulation: A methodology to improve the efficiency in the Brooke Army Medical Center Family Care Clinic. *Journal of Healthcare Management*, *47*(1), 58–67.

Noon, C. E., Hankins, C. T., & Cote, M. J. (2003). Understanding the impact of variation in the delivery of healthcare services. *Journal of Healthcare Management*, *48*(2), 82–98.

Silver, E. A., Pyke, D., & Peterson, R. (1998). *Decision systems for inventory management and production planning and control* (3rd ed.). New York, NY: Wiley.

Sinreich, D., & Marmor, Y. (2005). Emergency department operations: The basis for developing a simulation tool. *IIE Transactions*, *37*(3), 233–245. doi:10.1080/07408170590899625

VanBerkel, P. T., & Blake, J. T. (2007). A comprehensive simulation for wait time reduction and capacity planning applied in general surgery. *Health Care Management Science*, *10*(4), 373–385. doi:10.1007/s10729-007-9035-6

ADDITIONAL READING

Denton, B., Viapiano, J., & Vogl, A. (2007). Optimization of surgery sequencing and scheduling decisions under uncertainty. *Health Care Management Science*, *10*(1), 12–24. doi:10.1007/s10729-006-9005-4

Gupta, D., Natarajan, M. K., Gafni, A., Wang, L., Shilton, D., & Holder, D. (2007). Capacity planning for cardiac catheterization: a case study. *Health Policy (Amsterdam)*, *82*, 1–11. doi:10.1016/j.healthpol.2006.07.010

Harper, P. R., & Pitt, M. A. (2004). On the challenge of healthcare modelling and a proposed project life cycle for successful implementation. *The Journal of the Operational Research Society*, *55*, 657–661. doi:10.1057/palgrave.jors.2601719

Ho, C. J., & Lau, H. S. (1999). Evaluating the impact of operating conditions on the performance of appointment scheduling rules in service systems. *European Journal of Operational Research*, *112*, 542–553. doi:10.1016/S0377-2217(97)00393-7

Kumar, A., & Shim, S. J. (2005). Using computer simulation for surgical care process reengineering in hospitals. *INFOR*, *43*(4), 303–319.

McLaughlin, D. B., & Hays, J. M. (2008). *Healthcare Operations Management*. Chicago: Health Administration Press.

Nickel, S., & Schmidt, U.-A. (2009). Process improvement in hospitals: a case study in a radiology department. *Quality Management in Health Care*, *18*(4), 326–338.

Rohleder, T. R., & Klassen, K. J. (2000). Using client-variance information to improve dynamic appointment scheduling performance. *Omega*, *28*, 293–302. doi:10.1016/S0305-0483(99)00040-7

Rohleder, T. R., & Klassen, K. J. (2002). Rolling horizon appointment scheduling: a simulation study. *Health Care Management Science*, *5*, 201–209. doi:10.1023/A:1019748703353

Visser, J., & Beech, R. (2005). *Health operations management: patient flow logistics in health care*. London: Routledge.

Young, T. (2005). An agenda for healthcare and information simulation. *Health Care Management Science*, *8*, 189–196. doi:10.1007/s10729-005-2008-8

Chapter 11
Reducing Consultation Waiting Time and Overtime in Outpatient Clinic:
Challenges and Solutions

Zhu Zhecheng
Health Services & Outcomes Research, Singapore

Heng Bee Hoon
Health Services & Outcomes Research, Singapore

Teow Kiok Liang
Health Services & Outcomes Research, Singapore

ABSTRACT

Outpatient clinics face increasing pressure to handle more appointment requests due to aging and growing population. The increase in workload impacts two critical performance indicators: consultation waiting time and clinic overtime. Consultation waiting time is the physical waiting time a patient spends in the waiting area of the clinic, and clinic overtime is the amount of time the clinic is open beyond its normal opening hours. Long consultation waiting time negatively affects patient safety and satisfaction, while long clinic overtime negatively affects the morale of clinic staff. This chapter analyzes the complexity of an outpatient clinic in a Singapore public hospital, and factors causing long consultation waiting time and clinic overtime. Discrete event simulation and design of experiments are applied to quantify the effects of the factors on consultation waiting time/clinic overtime. Implementation results show significant improvement once those factors are well addressed.

DOI: 10.4018/978-1-60960-872-9.ch011

INTRODUCTION

An outpatient clinic is a private or public healthcare facility which is devoted to diagnosis and treatment of non-emergency patients (Gupta & Denton, 2008). There are many types of outpatient clinics and the functions and settings of outpatient clinics vary from country to country (Chand, et al., 2009; Wijewickrama, 2006; Zhu, Heng, & Teow, 2009). In Singapore, there are three types of outpatient clinics: general practitioner (GP), polyclinic and specialist outpatient clinic (SOC). A GP is a private medical practitioner who provides primary care in the community neighbourhood. Polyclinic is a government clinic covering a wide range of subsidized primary care services. Both GP and polyclinic cater mainly to walk-in patients. Specialist outpatient clinics (SOCs) are clinics belonging to hospitals and medical centres. They offer specialized services for the diagnosis and treatment for more complex medical conditions that usually cannot be treated at the primary care, and include specialties such as Orthopaedics, Surgery, Eye, Ear, Nose and Throat. An SOC mainly accepts patients with appointments.

Patients are referred to SOCs from various sources such as GPs, polyclinics or within the same hospital's emergency and inpatient departments. There are also many cross referrals from other specialty SOCs within the hospital. All the referrals enter the SOC's appointment system. A free time slot is assigned to each request. The assignment practice follows various policies. For instance, a first-come-first-serve policy will give the incoming request an earliest available time slot. However, some time slots may also be reserved for requests that need urgent attention. The capacity of a SOC is usually measured by the number of free time slots. The capacity depends on many factors such as consultant workload, space constraint and target revenue.

Outpatient clinics with appointment system have several advantages over those for walk-in patients. Firstly, demand fluctuation can be absorbed by the appointment system. Over-utilization or under-utilization is less likely to happen than in walk-in based outpatient clinics. Secondly, appointment-based outpatient clinics provide a better patient experience than walk-in-based outpatient clinics. Patients are able to choose their preferred doctors and continue to see the same doctor for their follow-up visits in appointment-based outpatient clinics. The patient waiting time of well planned appointment based clinics are shorter because the uncertainty of patient arrivals is mitigated by the pre-defined time slots. This chapter mainly focuses on appointment-based outpatient clinics. Henceforth, outpatient clinics mentioned in this chapter refer to appointment-based outpatient clinics.

There are a few performance measures for an outpatient clinic. Two commonly used measures are waiting time and overtime. According to Gupta & Denton (2008), there are two types of waiting times in a typical outpatient clinic: indirect waiting time and direct waiting time. Indirect waiting time represents the time between a confirmed request and the assigned time slot. It is also known as appointment lead time. Indirect waiting time is usually determined by the demand/supply relationship. A long indirect waiting time indicates a possible inaccessibility of healthcare facility and may cause higher no-show rate. Direct waiting time represents the physical waiting time a patient spends in the waiting area of the clinic. Long direct waiting time may affect patient satisfaction negatively (Gupta & Denton, 2008). Clinic overtime represents the extended opening hours. Overtime overuses the clinic resources, and can cause negative effects on the morale of both physicians and other clinic staff. Direct waiting time and overtime are usually determined by the appointment schedules and administrative efficiency. The study focuses on the direct waiting time and overtime. Henceforth, waiting time mentioned in this chapter refers to the direct waiting time.

In recent years outpatient clinics face increasing pressure to handle more appointment requests than before due to aging and growing population (www.moh.gov.sg, 2010). In order to mitigate the pressure of the increasing appointment lead time, more time slots are arranged in each working day to maintain a constant lead time. However, the rising workload per working day causes other problems. The overloaded clinic becomes more congested and patients have to wait longer for their consultations. There is also a higher chance of overtime. One approach to reduce the patient waiting time and clinic overtime is to add more resources (consultants, equipment, consultation rooms). As such an approach is expensive; a more cost-effective approach is to fully utilize the current resources to handle the increasing pressure through better outpatient clinic planning.

The clinics are complex systems with various patient flows and sources of uncertainties. Although a "basic" patient flow is a three-step procedure: reception, consultation and departure, the actual patient flow is highly patient-specific. For instance, a patient may undergo medical tests prior to the consultation. The consultant may request laboratory tests during the consultation of a patient. When the patient is on his way to the requested laboratory tests, the consultant may see the next patient. The consultation of the patient then continues after the laboratory test results are out. The amount of variation depends on patient condition, clinic type and consultant pattern.

Outpatient clinic also faces many uncertainties. For instance, the appointment system does not eliminate the randomness in patient arrival. Patients may not show up on the day of their appointments and thus waste the time slots. A common practice to compensate no-show is to double-book: more appointments are booked in the available time slots. Other than no-show, patients may arrive earlier or later than their given appointments. All these factors increase the variation of the patient arrivals. Consultation time is another source of uncertainty as the duration of each patient's consultation varies due to patient's condition and the specific physician. These factors increase the variations of the outpatient clinic and make the outpatient clinic planning a challenging task.

Both the external workload pressure and internal outpatient clinic complexity have negative impact on patient waiting time and clinic overtime. Since the workload pressure is almost inevitable and extra resources are not always available, healthcare service providers are interested in the approaches of reducing waiting time/overtime without reducing the workload or increasing resources. Many have studied various approaches to reduce waiting time/overtime in outpatient clinics. One well studied approach is via better appointment rule (Bailey, 1952; Cayirli & Veral, 2003; Ho & Lau, 1999). An appointment rule defines how the time slots are distributed over the time horizon of the working hours (known as a session) and how different types of appointments are arranged in the time slots. A good appointment schedule helps to reduce waiting time/overtime by better utilizing the session. Another approach is to detect the factors causing long patient waiting time/clinic overtime in outpatient clinics; such as patient no-show/double booking (Chand, et al., 2009; Green & Savin, 2008; Robinson & Chen, 2009), patient and consultant punctuality (Blance & Pike, 1964; Fetter & Thompson, 1966). Certain factors are caused by the uncertainties beyond the control of outpatient clinics, while others are caused by administrative or planning factors which can be detected and removed to improve the efficiency of the clinic.

Discrete event simulation (DES) has been widely applied in healthcare system to test the what-if scenarios in different hospital sections including emergency department (Best & Sage, 1992; Connelly & Bair, 2004; White, Su & Shih, 2003a), inpatient department (Cahill & Render, 1999; Costa at el., 2003; Kim at el., 1999; Ridge at el., 1998), and outpatient clinics (Hutzschenreuter, 2004; Cayirli, Veral and Rosen, 2004, 2006; Su &

Shih, 2003b; Wijewickrama, 2006; Zhu, Heng, & Teow, 2009; Klassen & Rohleder, 1996; Harper & Gamlin, 2003). A properly constructed and calibrated DES model provides a robust test field where the healthcare service providers are able to arbitrarily modify the current clinic settings or test certain process improvement to evaluate the corresponding consequences or effects. The simulation results of the DES model could also be a useful reference during the implementation phase.

The purpose of this chapter is to propose an approach to reduce long patient waiting time and clinic overtime in outpatient clinics without decreasing workload and introducing additional resources. We build models and use data from an outpatient clinic to detect the possible factors causing long patient waiting time/clinic overtime. Improvements are proposed based on the significant factors. A DES model is constructed to simulate the patient flow in a generic outpatient clinic and is used to quantify the effects of different improvement settings. The simulation results then guide the implementation in an actual practice.

Figure 1. Patient flow of a generic outpatient clinic

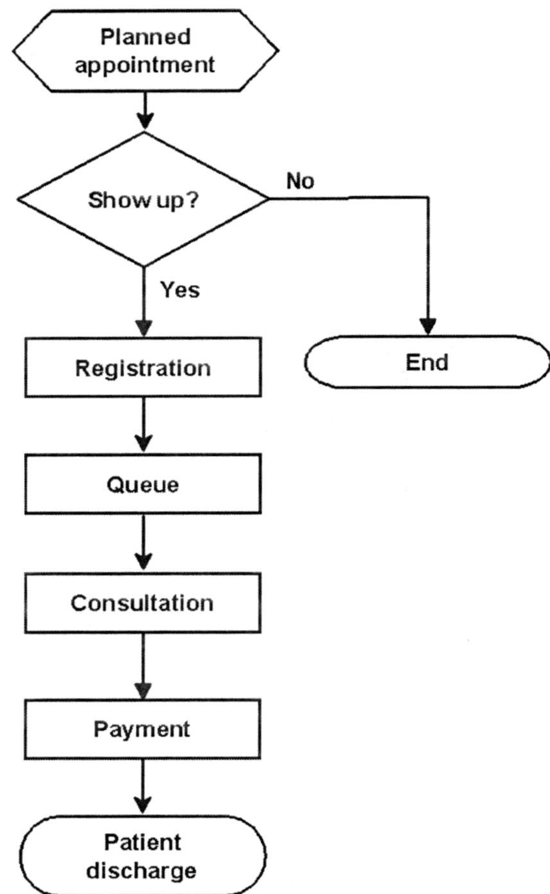

PATIENT FLOW OF A GENERIC OUTPATIENT CLINIC

Figure 1 illustrates the patient flow of a generic outpatient clinic which caters to appointment-patients (no walk-in patient is considered). Patient may skip his/her appointment for various reasons. If he/she turns up, he/she will register at the registration counter and be issued with a queue number. He/she then waits till his/her number is called and proceeds to the consultation with the physician. When the consultation is over, the patient proceeds to the payment counter, makes the payment and ends his/her visit. The whole procedure comprises of three steps: registration, consultation and payment. Among the three steps, consultation is the most time-consuming and variable, and the key factor contributing to patient waiting time/clinic overtime. Registration and payment are less variable and their processing times are shorter, hence they are not considered in the remaining chapter.

Gantt chart (Pinedo, 1995) is widely applied to visually describe the scheduling practice in manufacturing systems. The concept of Gantt chart is adapted in this chapter to describe the patient flow in the outpatient clinic. Figure 2 illustrates the patient flow of a complete session in the outpatient clinic, as explained:

- The vertical black lines represent the session start time (9:00) and close time (12:30). The duration of the session is 210 minutes.

Figure 2. Gantt chart representation of the patient flow: an ideal situation

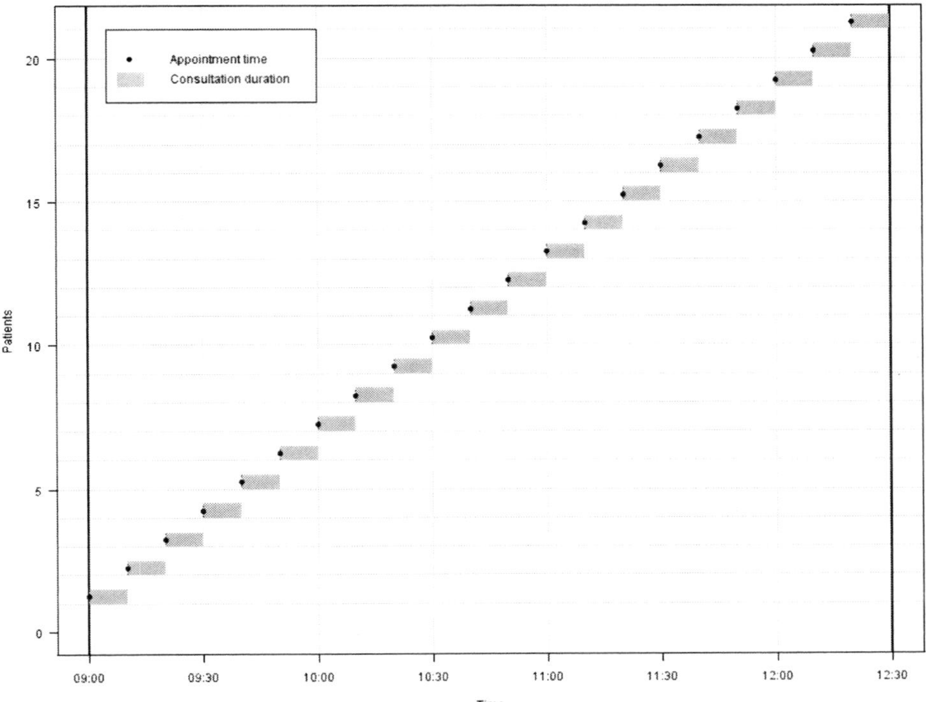

- A black dot represents the appointment time of each patient. There are 21 time slots in the session. As an illustration, the interval between two adjacent time slots is fixed at 10 minutes. Each time slot is occupied by one appointment.
- A grey solid block represents the consultation of each appointment, with the length of the block indicating the duration of the consultation. As an illustration, the consultation duration of all appointments is fixed at 10 minutes.

Figure 2 illustrates an ideal session where no variation or uncertainties exist in the outpatient clinic. All patients are punctual. The interval between two adjacent time slots perfectly matches the consultation durations. The clinic operates like a streamlined production line. The next consultation starts immediately after the completion of the previous consultation. The whole session is fully utilized and there is no waiting time and overtime. However, such an ideal situation does not exist in reality.

Figure 3 illustrates the patient flow with variation in patient arrival and consultation duration. The triangle represents the patient arrival time, the arrow indicates a patient arrives later than his/her appointment time, and the dotted line indicates that the patient arrives earlier than his/her appointment time. The shaded block represents the patient waiting time. The patient waiting time is defined as follows: if the patient arrives later than his/her appointment time, it is the period from arrival time to consultation start time; if the patient arrives earlier than his appointment time, it is the period from appointment time to consultation start time. Overtime is also shown in Figure 3, defined as the period between the session close time and the consultation end time of the last patient.

Figure 3. Patient flow considering the uncertainty of patient arrival and the variation of consultation duration

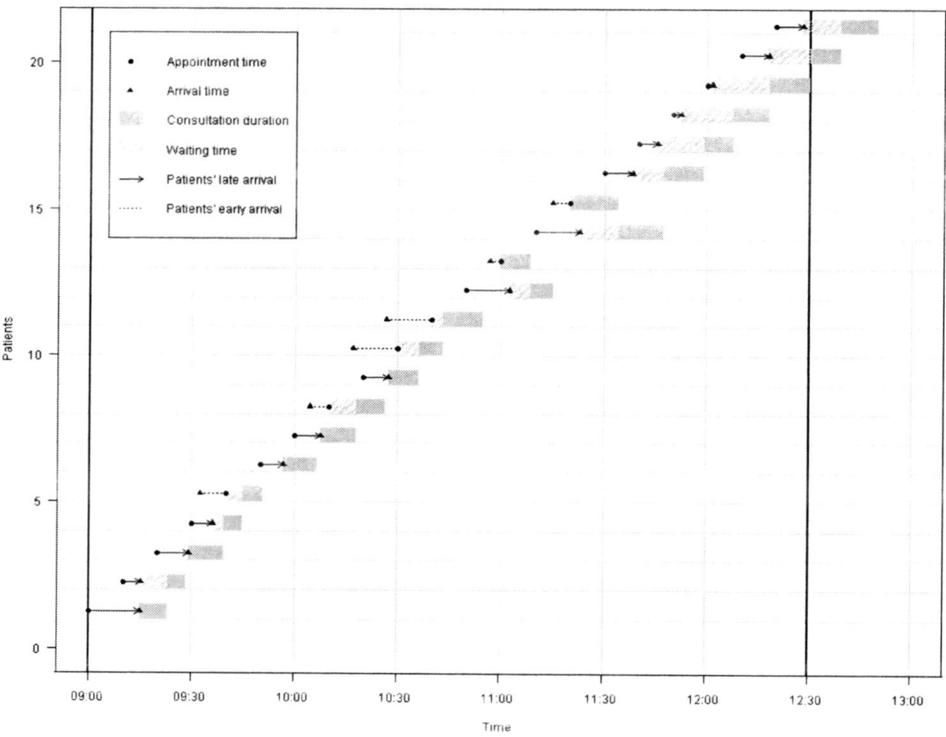

The patient flows illustrated in Figures 2 and 3 show that all time slots are evenly distributed throughout the clinic session. The interval between two time slots is fixed and each time slot is assigned with one and only one appointment. Such appointment rule is helpful when the consultation durations are homogeneous and no-show/double booking does not exist. It takes two steps to generate an appointment schedule: distribute the time slots over the session, and arrange the sequence of different types of appointments in the fixed time slots. Various rules to generate appointment schedules under various conditions have been proposed. In the well known Bailey's rule (Bailey, 1952), two appointments are booked at the beginning of a session, known as initial block. Successive appointments are then booked at the interval of mean consultation time. Similar rules were proposed in Welch & Bailey (1952) and Welch (1964). Other than booking one patient in one time slot, several researchers proposed the idea of booking multiple patients in one time slot. Soriano (1966) proposed to book two patients in each time slot. Liu & Liu (1998) and Vanden Bosch at el. (1999) argued that it was better to book different number of patients in different time slots. All the appointment rules mentioned above have fixed intervals between two adjacent time slots.

There are also rules with flexible intervals, for which there are two approaches. The first approach determines the intervals by patient type. Such an approach is quite popular in real application. It is a common practice for SOC schedulers to assign different intervals for new (first-time) patients and follow-up patients (Lau & Lau, 2000). Ho

Figure 4. Patient flow of an actual session in an outpatient clinic

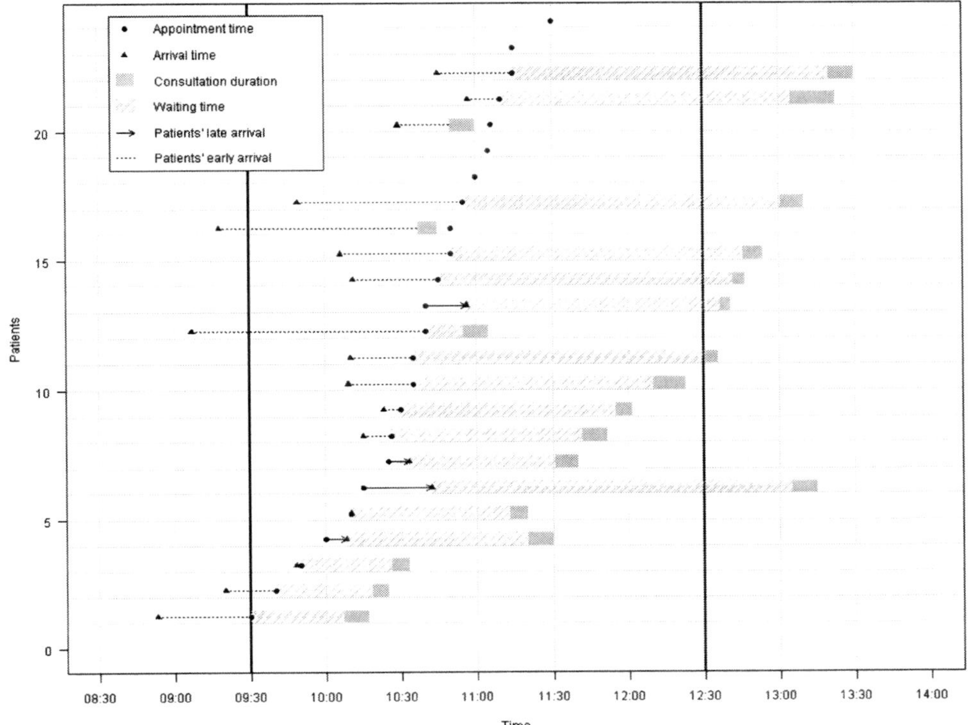

& Lau (1992) and Wang (1993) classified the patients into "high variance patient" and "low variance patient", and then assigned them with different intervals. The second approach adjusts the intervals according to different time of the session. Cayirli, Veral and Rosen (2004) pointed out that it is helpful to arrange a longer interval at the latter part of the session compared to the early part of the session. Ho & Lau (1999) pointed out that the intervals should follow an increasing rather than a decreasing manner. A more comprehensive review of appointment rules can be found in Cayirli & Veral (2003) and Ho & Lau (1999).

CASE STUDY

The patient flows described in Figures 2 and 3 do not reflect fully the actual situation. Figure 2 does not consider any uncertainties and variations, and Figure 3 only considers the variation of patient arrival times and consultation durations. Data was collected from an SOC of a Singapore government hospital over 13 sessions to appreciate the possible extent of variations in an actual situation. We collected information on appointment type, detailed timing and staff remarks. "Appointment type", which is known prior to the visit, tells if patient is new or follow-up which could be useful to explain the variation. Detailed timings of each patient (appointment time, arrival time, consultation start time, consultation end time) were recorded by clinic staff during the session. During the data collection period, the clinic staff also recorded remarks which could be useful to explain the phenomenon in the outpatient clinic. Figure 4 illustrates the Gantt chart of an actual session in the outpatient clinic. Some observations are made:

1. Among the twenty actualized appointments, four patients arrived late. This is undesirable as it can be slot wasted, and if it occurs near the end of the session, it may cause overtime. However, majority of the patients arrived earlier than their appointment time. Nevertheless, too much of early arrival is also undesirable because it then causes congestion in the waiting area. Figure 4 showed that four patients arrived even before the session opening time. Under this type of arrival pattern, it then may be unnecessary to book two appointments at the session beginning, as Bailey's rule suggested.
2. Consultation duration was highly variable due to the complexity of patients' conditions. The distribution of consultation duration is usually right-skewed due to complex and time-consuming cases.
3. The last time slot was planned one hour before session end time. In practice, the clinic is reluctant to arrange an appointment near the end of a session because of the possibility of running into overtime. This large buffer time inevitably compresses the distribution of the time slots and causes congestion.
4. Time slots were unevenly distributed among the whole session. For instance, there were 4 slots from 9:30 to 10:00 and 9 slots from 10:20 to 10:50. These could be due to different appointment types and practice of double-booking.
5. There were 7 no-shows/overbooked appointments in the session. Patient no-show is one major variation in clinic scheduling. According to Chand at el. (2009), longer appointment lead time usually leads to higher no-show rate. High no-show rate wastes allocated time slots. Overbooking is usually then applied to mitigate no-show (Kim & Giachetti, 2006; LaGanga & Lawrence, 2007). In this case, the number of overbooking was estimated to compensate no-shows based on historical data. Overbooked appointments usually take the time slots with some of the original appointments. This practice causes unequal time slot distribution and increases waiting time.
6. The first time slot was 9:30 and the first consultation started at 10:09, which was 39 minutes late. Such type of delay can be due to (a) unavailability of the physician; (b) missing/incomplete patient information; or (c) insufficient preparatory work. This again has a significant impact on both patient waiting time and clinic overtime.
7. Irregular calling sequence existed in the session, where a later appointment slot was called before the patient in an earlier slot (patient 16 and 21 in Figure 4). According to the staff remarks, there were several reasons for the irregular calling sequence. Firstly, some patients left the outpatient clinic temporarily after they registered. When there was no response when the name was called, the next patient was called instead. Secondly, some patients arrived much earlier than their appointment time and waited long. They then complained to the clinic staff so the clinic staff put them ahead. Irregular calling sequence generally increases the variation of waiting time.
8. There were times when there was no patient in the consultation room while there were patients in the waiting area. Figure 4 shows such unused periods from 11:05 to 11:12 and 12:01 to 12:10. However, the "unused" time was probably for report writing, or waiting for result and administrative tasks.

Based on the above observations, Table 1 lists 8 possible factors for the long patient waiting time/clinic overtime in the SOC. These factors can be classified into three categories.

1. Patients' early or late arrival (factor 1) and consultation duration (factor 2), both beyond

Table 1. Factors causing long patient waiting time/clinic overtime

	Factor	Category
1	Patients' early/late arrival	System uncertainty
2	Consultation duration	System uncertainty
3	No-show/double booking policy	Appointment schedule
4	Uneven distribution of time slots	Appointment schedule
5	Compressed session time	Appointment schedule
6	Irregular calling sequence	Administrative issue
7	Clinic delay	Administrative issue
8	Unused session time	Administrative issue

the control of the outpatient clinic, are classified as system uncertainties.

2. No-show/double booking policy, uneven distribution of time slots and compressed session time (factors 3-5) are related to appointment scheduling.
3. Irregular calling sequence, clinic delay and unused session time (factors 6-8) are administrative issues.

Factors 3-8 can be mitigated by better appointment schedule and more efficient administration.

DISCRETE EVENT SIMULATION MODEL AND VALIDATION

A discrete event simulation (DES) model is constructed using Simul8 2008 Profession (Simul 8 Corporation, 2008; simul8.com, 2010) to simulate the patient flow of the outpatient clinic. Model parameters are based on the 13 sessions of actual data collected. Table 2 summarises the type of data collected and the corresponding parameter settings. $\bar{X}$ denotes the mean and S denotes the standard deviation. In the DES model, the parameters settings of session duration, number of time slots, percentage of no-show, percentage of overbooking, percentage of patients arriving late and percentage of clinic delay take the same value as the collected data. Gamma distribution $Gamma(k,\theta)$ is applied to fit the skewed distributions of patients' late arrival, consultation duration, session start time punctuality.

A two-step model validation procedure is applied. Open box validation (Fletcher & Worthington, 2009; Pidd, 1999) was first applied. Patient flow of the model and parameter settings were presented to the clinic staff to make sure that the model patient flow was a valid mapping of the actual patient flow and the parameter settings were reasonable estimates of the actual practice. Black box validation (Pidd, 1999) was next applied. The simulation results were compared to the performance measures derived from the actual data. In this study, three performance measures were considered: 50th percentile patient waiting time, 95th percentile patient waiting time, and clinic overtime. We ran each scenario with 100 simulations. Table 3 lists the results of black box validation. The simulation results are close to the actual data with t-test showing no significant difference between the actual data and the simulation results (p-values > 0.05).

DESIGN OF EXPERIMENTS

As discussed in the previous section, six of the eight factors responsible for the long patient waiting time/clinic overtime are related to appointment scheduling and can be improved through process

Table 2. Summary of data collection and the DES model parameter setting

Denotation	**Data collection**	**DES model parameter**
Number of sessions	13	*NA*
Session duration	180 minutes	180 minutes
Number of time slots per session	25	25
Percentage of no-show	30%	30%
Percentage of overbooking	30%	30%
Percentage of patient arriving late	15%	15%
Percentage of clinic delay	40%	40%
Percentage of unused session time	10%	10%
Percentage of irregular calling sequence	10%	10%
Distribution of patients arriving late	$\bar{X}$ =14.3, S=5.7	*Gamma*(15,1)
Distribution of consultation duration	$\bar{X}$ =6.5, S=2.3	*Gamma*(6,1)
Distribution of clinic delay	$\bar{X}$ =31.2, S=5.8	*Gamma*(30,1)
Distribution of unused session time	$\bar{X}$ =9.4, S=2.9	*Gamma*(9,1)

$\bar{X}$: mean; S: standard deviation

Table 3. Model validation

Performance measure	$\bar{X}$		***p-value*** **(t-test)**
	Actual	**Simulation**	
50th%tile waiting time	45.3	40.0	0.7923
95th%tile waiting time	72.4	70.2	0.7103
Overtime	19.1	17.1	0.7898

$\bar{X}$: mean

improvement. Design of experiments (DOE) is applied to quantify the effects of these six factors on the performance measures. To maintain a controllable experiment scale, uneven distribution of time slots and compressed session time are combined into one factor: time slot distribution. Clinic delay and unused session time are combined into one factor: session utilization. Hence the four factors considered in the DOE include: no-show/overbooking (Factor A), time slot distribution (Factor B), irregular calling sequence (Factor C), and session utilization (Factor D). Each factor has an original setting (0) and an improvement setting (1). Table 4 lists the factors and levels of the DOE. Details of original and improvement settings are as follows:

Table 4. Factors and levels of the DOE

Factor	Level	
	0 (Original)	**1 (Improvement)**
A (No-show/overbooking)	Shared time slot	Individual time slot
B (Time slot distribution)	Variable	Fixed
C (Irregular calling sequence)	Yes	No
D (Session utilization)	Unpunctual session start time and unused session time	Punctual session start time and fully used session time

A. No-show/overbooking: in both the original and improvement settings, the number of overbooked appointments is set equal to the expected number of no-shows. In the original setting, overbooked appointments share the same time slots with some of original appointments. In the improvement setting, each appointment has its own time slot, and the interval between two adjacent appointments is equal and fixed.

B. Time slot distribution: in the original setting, the plan horizon is 120 minutes, and the intervals between two adjacent appointments are variable. In the improvement setting, the plan horizon is extended to 170 minutes by pushing the last time slot to ten minutes before the planned session end time. The intervals between two adjacent appointments are fixed and calculated by 170/(N-1), where N denotes the sum of the original and overbooked appointments.

C. Irregular calling sequence: in the original setting, there is a 10% chance of irregular calling sequence. Such practice is assumed to be eliminated in the improvement setting.

D. Session utilization: in the original setting, there is a 40% chance of a delayed session and a 10% chance of unused session time. In the improvement setting, all sessions are assumed to start on time and there is no unused session time.

The above mentioned DOE has 16 factor combinations. One of the 16 combinations represents the baseline scenario in which all factors are set to 0 (no change made to the current situation), while the other 15 combinations represent the possible improvement scenarios in which one or more factor are set to 1. The outcomes of each factor combination are represented by three performance measures: 50th percentile waiting time, 95th percentile waiting time and overtime. DES model is used to simulate all 16 factor combinations and then measure the outcomes. In this study, 100 simulation runs are conducted for each factor combination and the means of the runs reported.

SIMULATION RESULTS AND DISCUSSION

Table 5 lists the simulation results of the 16 scenarios. Each scenario corresponds to one factor combination. C_{95} denotes the confidence interval at the 95% confidence level. The results show that scenario 16 (all improvement settings applied) significantly outperforms scenario 1 (the baseline scenario) in all three performance measures. This indicates that the improvement factors effectively reduce waiting time and overtime. Another observation is that the four factors have different effectiveness. A factorial analysis was conducted to study the significance of individual factor and interaction between factors.

Table 5. Simulation results of patient waiting time/clinic overtime

Factor combination	A	B	C	D	Performance (minutes)					
					50th percentile waiting time		95th percentile waiting time		Overtime	
					$\bar{X}$	C_{95}	$\bar{X}$	C_{95}	$\bar{X}$	C_{95}
1	0	0	0	0	40.0	(36.4;43.6)	70.2	(65.6;74.8)	17.1	(13.6;20.6)
2	1	0	0	0	38.1	(34.6;41.6)	66.7	(62.4;71.0)	16.0	(13.5;18.5)
3	0	1	0	0	17.4	(14.7;20.1)	31.2	(28.0;34.4)	16.8	(14.3;19.3)
4	0	0	1	0	39.4	(35.9;42.9)	67.8	(63.5;72.1)	15.7	(12.8;18.6)
5	0	0	0	1	33.2	(31.3;35.1)	64.2	(61.1;67.3)	9.9	(7.6;12.2)
6	1	1	0	0	16.2	(13.4;19.0)	28.8	(26.8;30.8)	16.8	(13.5;20.1)
7	1	0	1	0	37.9	(34.5;41.3)	64.3	(60.2;68.4)	15.5	(12.6;18.4)
8	1	0	0	1	30.9	(29.0;32.8)	60.3	(57.6;63.0)	9.6	(7.5;11.7)
9	0	1	1	0	17.2	(14.5;19.9)	28.9	(26.1;31.7)	16.4	(13.3;19.5)
10	0	1	0	1	11.2	(9.8;12.6)	24.2	(22.2;26.2)	9.7	(7.3;12.1)
11	0	0	1	1	33.2	(31.3;35.1)	60.9	(58.2;63.6)	9.5	(7.3;11.7)
12	1	1	1	0	15.9	(13.1;18.7)	26.7	(24.8;28.6)	16.8	(13.5;20.1)
13	1	1	0	1	8.8	(7.7;9.9)	21.4	(19.5;23.3)	9.4	(7.1;11.7)
14	1	0	1	1	30.7	(28.8;32.6)	58.3	(55.7;60.9)	9.2	(7.3;11.1)
15	0	1	1	1	11.2	(9.8;12.6)	22.8	(20.8;24.8)	9.5	(7.3;11.7)
16	1	1	1	1	8.7	(7.5;8.7)	19.8	(17.9;21.7)	9.4	(7.4;11.4)

A, B, C and D: base factors

$\bar{X}$: mean

C_{95}: confidence interval at the 95% confidence level

Table 6 lists the results of the factorial analysis including intercept, base factors (A, B, C and D) and two-way interactions (AB, AC, AD, BC, BD, CD). Three-way and four-way interactions are excluded in the factorial analysis. Several observations are made:

1. Time slot distribution (factor B) is the most significant factor affecting 50th percentile waiting time, followed by session utilization (factor D), then no-show/overbooking (factor A). Irregular calling sequence (factor C) does not significantly affect the 50th percentile waiting time.
2. Time slot distribution (factor B) is the most significant factor affecting 95th percentile waiting time, followed by session utilization (factor D), then no-show/overbooking (factor A) and irregular calling sequence (factor C). All four factors significantly affect the 95th percentile waiting time.
3. Session utilization (factor D) is the only significant factor affecting overtime. All

Table 6. Factorial analysis of the simulation results

Factors	Performance (minutes)					
	50th percentile waiting time		95th percentile waiting time		Overtime	
	c	*p-value*	*c*	*p-value*	*c*	*p-value*
Intercept	24.38	<0.0001	44.78	<0.0001	12.95	<0.0001
A	-0.98	<0.0001	-1.49	<0.0001	-0.11	0.1116
B	-11.11	<0.0001	-19.30	<0.0001	0.14	0.0668
C	-0.10	0.0493	-1.09	<0.0001	-0.20	0.0203
D	-3.39	<0.0001	-3.29	<0.0001	-3.43	<0.0001
AB	0.05	0.2532	0.19	0.1010	0.11	0.1116
AC	0	1.0000	0.08	0.4380	0.09	0.1883
AD	-0.24	0.0017	-0.04	0.6690	-0.01	0.9231
BC	0.02	0.5471	0.16	0.1400	0.13	0.0862
BD	0.04	0.3774	-0.13	0.2310	-0.16	0.0407
CD	0.06	0.1675	0.05	0.5850	0.08	0.2441

A, B, C and D: base factors
AB, AC, AD, BC, BD, CD: two-way interactions
c: regression coefficient of the factorial analysis

other factors do not significantly affect the overtime.

4. None of the two-way interactions significantly affect performance measures.

The above observations reveal that time slot distribution is the most significant factor affecting patient waiting time (both 50th percentile and 95th percentile). One reason is that patient arrivals are compressed into a shorter period in the original scenario. This causes mismatch between demand (patient arrival) and supply (clinic capacity). Moreover, variable time slot intervals aggravate the mismatch. Such mismatch is relieved in the improvement setting by expanding the slot horizon and spacing out the time slots.

No-show/double booking also significantly affects both 50th percentile and 95th percentile waiting time. The practice of sharing one time slot in the original scenario adds extra variation (batching) to the time slot distribution.

Session utilization has significant effects on both patient waiting time and clinic overtime. If one session is delayed, the whole patient flow of that session is shifted (as shown in Figure 4), which causes extra waiting time and overtime. Unused session time has a similar effect.

Irregular calling sequence results in some patients' consultation start times being moved forward and others' being delayed. While such practice does not affect the average waiting time significantly, it causes extra variation among patients' waiting time. Hence 95th percentile waiting time is affected.

Simulation results and factorial analysis conclude that the four factors improve one or more performance measures in the following order: time slot distribution, session utilization, no-show/double booking and irregular calling sequence.

IMPLEMENTATION RESULTS AND DISCUSSION

Motivated by the positive simulation results, recommendations were made to the outpatient

Table 7. Comparison of performance between original, implementation and simulation results

Performance measure (minutes)	Original		Implementation		Simulation*	
	$\overline{X}$	C_{95}	$\overline{X}$	C_{95}	$\overline{X}$	C_{95}
50th%tile waiting time	45.3	(34.0;56.6)	20.8	(14.9;26.7)	8.7	(7.5;9.9)
95th%tile waiting time	72.4	(60.4;84.4)	42.0	(35.9;48.1)	19.8	(17.9;21.7)
Overtime	19.1	(9.2;29.0)	13.4	(7.4;19.4)	9.4	(7.4;11.4)

$\overline{X}$: mean
C_{95}: confidence interval at the 95% confidence level
*: best possible, using all 4 factors combined

clinic to improve their clinic performance. All four improvement settings were suggested and 13 sessions of data were collected to evaluate the effectiveness. Table 7 compares the performance measures among the original, implementation and best possible simulation results. The implementation significantly outperformed the original setting in all three performance measures: the 50th percentile waiting time was reduced by 54%, the 95th percentile waiting time was reduced by 42% and the overtime was reduced by 36%. However, probably as the four improvement settings were not fully executed, implementation results were not as good as the simulation. For instance, the implementation data shows that although the session start times were more punctual than before, some sessions were still later than their planned start time for various reasons. The suggested time slot distribution was not fully implemented either. Equal and fixed interval between two successive appointments was not achieved in some sessions due to last minute booking. Irregular calling sequence and two appointments sharing the same time slot could be found in the implementation results, although less frequently. The gap between the implementation and simulation results indicates that reducing patient waiting time and clinic overtime should be a continuous improvement process. In order to achieve a significant and sustainable improvement, it is critical for the whole outpatient clinic to work together and fully apply the improvement factors.

CONCLUSION AND FUTURE RESEARCH DIRECTION

This chapter focuses on two common problems in outpatient clinics: long patient waiting time and clinic overtime. Data was collected from an outpatient clinic of a Singapore government hospital to feed into subsequent modelling. The data included appointment time slots, patient arrivals, patient waiting time and clinic overtime, etc. Eight factors were identified as possible causes of the long patient waiting time/clinic overtime: patients' early/late arrival, consultation duration, no-show/double booking, uneven distribution of time slots, compressed session time, irregular calling sequence and clinic delay. Among the eight factors, patients' early/late arrival and consultation duration are beyond the control of the outpatient clinic and the remaining six factors can be mitigated by better appointment schedule and more efficient administration. DOE with 16 factor combinations was then applied to test the impact of the factors on three performance measures: 50th percentile waiting time, 95th percentile waiting time and overtime. A DES model was applied to simulate all the factor combinations. Factorial analysis was then carried out on the simulation results. Analysis results show that all four factors except irregular calling sequence significantly affect both 50th percentile and 95th percentile patient waiting time. Time slot distribution is the most significant factor. Session utilization is the only significant factor affecting clinic overtime. Irregular calling sequence significantly affects 95th percentile waiting time. Motivated by the positive simulation results, all four improvement factors were implemented in the outpatient clinic and the implementation results significantly outperformed the original ones in all three performance measures. There are two possible directions of future research: firstly, the current implementation results are not as good as the simulation results. Future study could focus on improving the implementation results. Secondly, the performance measures considered in the study are patient waiting time and clinic overtime. Future study could include more performance measures such as appointment lead time and patient satisfaction.

REFERENCES

Bailey, N. (1952). A study of queues and appointment systems in hospital outpatient departments, with special reference to waiting-times. *Journal of the Royal Statistical Society. Series A (General)*, *14*, 185–189.

Blanco, W. M. J., & Pike, M. C. (1964). Appointment systems in out-patients' clinics and the effect of patients' unpunctuality. *Medical Care*, *2*(3), 133–145. doi:10.1097/00005650-196407000-00002

Cahill, W., & Render, M. (1999). Dynamic simulation modelling of ICU bed availability. *Proceedings of the 1999 Winter Simulation Conference*, *2*, (pp. 1573-1576).

Cayirli, T., & Veral, E. (2003). Outpatient scheduling in health care: A review of literature. *Production and Operations Management Society*, *12*(4), 519–549. doi:10.1111/j.1937-5956.2003.tb00218.x

Cayirli, T., Veral, E., & Rosen, H. (2004). *Assessment of patient classification in appointment systems*, 1st Conference of the POMS College of Service Operations.

Cayirli, T., Veral, E., & Rosen, H. (2006). Designing appointment scheduling systems for ambulatory care services. *Health Care Management Science*, *9*, 47–58. doi:10.1007/s10729-006-6279-5

Chand, S., Moskowitz, H., Norris, J. B., Shade, S., & Willis, D. R. (2009). Improving patient flow at an outpatient clinic: Study of sources of variability and improvement factors. *Health Care Management Science*, *12*, 325–340. doi:10.1007/s10729-008-9094-3

Connelly, L. G., & Bair, A. E. (2004). Discrete event simulation of emergency department activity: A platform for system-level operations research. *Academic Emergency Medicine*, *11*(11), 1177–1185. doi:10.1111/j.1553-2712.2004.tb00702.x

Costa, A. X., Ridely, S. A., Shahani, A. K., Harper, P. R., De Senna, V., & Nielsen, M. S. (2003). Mathematical modeling and simulation for planning critical care capacity. *Anesthesiology*, *58*, 320–327.

Fetter, R., & Thompson, J. (1966). Patients' waiting time and doctors' idle time in the outpatient setting. *Health Services Research*, *1*, 66–90.

Fletcher, A., & Worthington, D. (2009). What is a generic hospital model?—A comparison of generic and specific hospital models of emergency patient flows. *Health Care Management Science*, *12*(4), 374–391. doi:10.1007/s10729-009-9108-9

Green, L. V., & Savin, S. (2008). Reducing delays for medical appointments: A queueing approach. *Operations Research, 56*(6), 1526–1538. doi:10.1287/opre.1080.0575

Gupta, D., & Denton, B. (2008). Appointment scheduling in health care: Challenges and opportunities. *IIE Transactions, 40*, 800–819. doi:10.1080/07408170802165880

Harper, P. R., & Gamlin, H. M. (2003). Reduced outpatient waiting times with improved appointment scheduling: a simulation modelling approach. *OR-Spektrum, 25*(2), 207–222. doi:10.1007/s00291-003-0122-x

Ho, C., & Lau, H. (1992). Minimizing total cost in scheduling outpatient appointments. *Management Science, 38*(12), 1750–1764. doi:10.1287/mnsc.38.12.1750

Ho, C., & Lau, H. (1999). Evaluating the impact of operating conditions on the performance of appointment scheduling rules in service systems. *European Journal of Operational Research, 112*, 542–553. doi:10.1016/S0377-2217(97)00393-7

Hutzschenreuter, A. (2004). *Waiting patiently: An analysis of the performance aspects of outpatient scheduling in health care institutes. BMI Paper*. Amsterdam, The Netherlands: Vrije Universiteit.

Kim, S., & Giachetti, R. E. (2006). A stochastic mathematical appointment overbooking model for healthcare providers to improve profits. *IEEE Transactions on Systems, Man, and Cybernetics – Part A, 36*(6), 1211-1219.

Kim, S. C., Horowitz, I., Young, K. K., & Buckley, T. A. (1999). Analysis of capacity management of the intensive care unit in a hospital. *European Journal of Operational Research, 115*, 36–46. doi:10.1016/S0377-2217(98)00135-0

Klassen, K. J., & Rohleder, T. R. (1996). Scheduling outpatient appointments in a dynamic environment. *Journal of Operations Management, 14*(2), 83–101. doi:10.1016/0272-6963(95)00044-5

LaGanga, L. R., & Lawrence, S. R. (2007). Clinical overbooking to improve patient access and increase provider productivity. *Decision Sciences, 38*(2), 251–276. doi:10.1111/j.1540-5915.2007.00158.x

Lau, H., & Lau, A. H. (2000). A fast procedure for computing the total system cost of an appointment schedule for medical and kindred facilities. *IIE Transactions, 32*(9), 833–839. doi:10.1080/07408170008967442

Liu, L., & Liu, X. (1998). Block appointment systems for outpatient clinics with multiple doctors. *The Journal of the Operational Research Society, 49*(12), 1254–1259.

Pidd, M. (1999). *Tools for thinking: Modelling in management science*. Wiley and Son.

Pinedo, M. (1995). *Scheduling theory, algorithms and systems*. Prentice Hall.

Ridge, J. C., Jones, S. K., Nielson, M. S., & Shahani, A. K. (1998). Capacity planning for intensive care units. *European Journal of Operational Research, 105*, 346–355. doi:10.1016/S0377-2217(97)00240-3

Robinson, L. W., & Chen, R. R. (2009). *The effects of patient no-shows on traditional and open-access appointment scheduling policies*. (UC Davis Graduate School of Management Research No. 16-09 / Johnson School Research Paper Series No. 43-09). Retrieved June 1, 2010, from http://papers.ssrn.com/ sol3/ papers.cfm?abstract_id= 1478736

Simul8 Corporation. (2008). *Simul8 user manual*. Simul8 Corporation.

Soriano, A. (1966). Comparison of two scheduling systems. *Operations Research, 14*, 388–397. doi:10.1287/opre.14.3.388

Su, S., & Shih, C. L. (2003a). Modeling an emergency medical services system using computer simulation. *International Journal of Medical Informatics*, *72*, 57–72. doi:10.1016/j.ijmedinf.2003.08.003

Su, S., & Shih, C. L. (2003b). Managing a mixed-registration-type appointment system in outpatient clinics. *International Journal of Medical Informatics*, *70*(1), 31–40. doi:10.1016/S1386-5056(03)00008-X

Vanden Bosch, P. M., Dietz, C. D., & Sumeoni, J. R. (1999). Scheduling customer arrivals to a stochastic service system. *Naval Research Logistics*, *46*, 549–559. doi:10.1002/(SICI)1520-6750(199908)46:5<549::AID-NAV6>3.0.CO;2-Y

Wang, P. P. (1993). Static and dynamic scheduling of customer arrivals to a single-server system. *Naval Research Logistics*, *40*, 345–360. doi:10.1002/1520-6750(199304)40:3<345::AID-NAV3220400305>3.0.CO;2-N

Welch, J. D. (1964). Appointment systems in hospital outpatient departments. *Operational Research Quarterly*, *15*(3), 224–237. doi:10.1057/jors.1964.43

Welch, J. D., & Bailey, N. (1952). Appointment systems in hospital outpatient departments. *Lancet*, *259*, 1105–1108. doi:10.1016/S0140-6736(52)90763-0

White, C. R., Best, J. B., & Sage, C. K. (1992). Simulation of emergency medical service scheduling. *Hospital Topics*, *70*, 34–37.

Wijewickrama, A. (2006). Simulation analysis for reducing queues in mixed-patients' outpatient department. *International Journal of Simulation Modelling*, *5*(2), 56–68. doi:10.2507/IJSIMM05(2)2.055

Zhu, Z. C., Heng, B. H., & Teow, K. L. (2009). Simulation study of the optimal appointment number for outpatient clinics. *International Journal of Simulation Modelling*, *3*, 156–165. doi:10.2507/IJSIMM08(3)3.132

Chapter 12
Reducing Patient Waiting Time at an Ambulatory Surgical Center

David Ben-Arieh
Kansas State University, USA

Chih-Hang Wu
Kansas State University, USA

ABSTRACT

This chapter describes a methodology to reduce patient waiting time in a for-profit ambulatory surgical center. Patients in this facility are scheduled in advance for the various operations, and yet operations start late, last longer than expected creating undesired delays. Although this facility is limited to ambulatory surgery, it provides a large number of different surgeries, which are scheduled using "block" scheduling approach. The methodology presented generates a more accurate schedule by creating better time estimates for the operations and with lower variability. The effect of sequencing the surgeries, such that the ones with lower variability are performed earlier in the day, is also discussed.

INTRODUCTION

This chapter describes a methodology that reduces patient waiting time in a for-profit ambulatory surgical center. Patients in this facility are scheduled in advance for the various operations, and yet operations start late, or last longer than expected creating undesired delays. The facility is of small size having the potential capacity of 30 hours of surgery scheduled in any given day.

Currently, surgeries are scheduled by a scheduler using the "block" scheduling approach. Although the facility is limited to ambulatory surgery, we counted about 300 different surgery types, with a staff of quite a few surgeons. Using the block scheduling approach each group of doctors who utilizes the surgery center are assigned one or more half-day blocks in which they can schedule any

DOI: 10.4018/978-1-60960-872-9.ch012

procedure at anytime, given that no other doctor is using that time slot. As the doctors call in and request an operation room, the scheduling nurse allots an amount of time for each surgery based on previous experience. However, the combinations of surgeries and physicians are quite large, adding to the variability that is a part of the process, making the nurse's estimates quite inaccurate.

The objective of this chapter is to present a method that will create a more accurate scheduling by increasing the accuracy of the operations' time estimates, reducing the variability in the operations and sequencing the operations in a more effective manner.

Background

When scheduling surgeries one has to deal with three types of surgeries: elective, urgent or emergency. Elective surgeries can be delayed or scheduled with the least priority, while urgent operations need to be done as soon as possible, many times on a short notice. Emergency surgeries have the highest priority and many times introduce a dynamic scheduling approach by changing the planned schedule as the need for emergency operations arises. This chapter deals with the first category of elective surgeries only, which usually simplifies the analysis.

Scheduling operating rooms is a complex problem that has to be solved both at a strategies level and a shorter term tactical level. At the strategic level there are three common planning strategies (Fei, et.al, 2009): Open schedule, Block schedule, and Modified Block schedule. The open schedule allows the surgeon to choose and time slot for a case, while a block schedule assigns blocks of time and an operating room to each surgeon. Within that block the surgeons can schedule their cases as they see fit. The Modified Block schedule allows more flexibility by keeping some operating rooms unassigned to a block.

Most research work defines the operating rooms scheduling problem as the problem of which the overall objective is to allocate the patients to the various blocks and sub-specialties, during the planning period (Testi and Tandani, 2009). This objective usually uses a 2 step process: the first to allocate the blocks to the surgical sub-specialties (MSSP: Master Surgical Schedule Problem) and then to allocate the patients to each block (termed as SCAP: Surgical Case Assignment Problem). This planning problem is solved using a 0-1 Linear Programming with the objective of minimizing the damage caused to the patients by waiting for the operation. Another method using a two step approach for operating rooms scheduling is presented in (Jebali etl al, 2006).

A slightly different approach is presented in the planning of cardiothoracic surgeries (Adan et. Al, 2009). In this case, also, the problem is defined in a two-levels hierarchy: The tactical level that creates a master surgical schedule that operates on a given number of patients and optimizes the utilization of the resources required at the operating theater. The detailed level assigns patients to rooms and time slots. This approach also has been solved using mixed integer programming while the patients length of stay can be assume deterministic (as for example in Vissers et. Al, 2005) or stochastic (Adan et. Al, 2009; Denton et al, 2007).

Some operation scheduling approach the problem as a three stage problem: stage one assigns the operating room time to the various specialties. The second stage allocates time to the various blocks and assigns the specialties to each block. The third stage deals with the detailed schedule assigning individual patients to the available time slots (Santibanez at. Al, 2007). A similar three phase approach is analyzed in (Testi et. al, 2007). A common solution approach uses a mixed integer-programming model (for example Blake et. Al, 2002; Visser, 1998).

Various constraints are considered as the limiting factor on the schedule, usually the limiting factors are the operating rooms themselves as well as the human resources such as specialists, and nurses (e.g. Roland 2010). In some cases the capacity of the downstream resources such as IC and recovery rooms is considered (e.g. Adan et. Al, 2009).

A more comprehensive scheduling approach can be used as a decision support system weighing different options and objectives. Such as system reported in Belien at. Al (2009) considers three main objectives: balanced bed occupancy at the hospital, allocating operating rooms to single specialties as much as possible, and creating a simple and repetitive schedule. This is achieved using mixed-integer programming and the simulated annealing heuristic.

A different approach towards scheduling operating rooms uses simulation to analyze complex and more realistic situations. Such simulation models are used to analyze the performance of operating rooms, allowing the analyst to examine different process flows such as induction of anesthesia to the next patient while an operation is still being performed on the previous patient (Riitta et. al, 2009). Often the simulation is used to assess impact of various policies in complex scenarios that cannot be evaluated analytically (e.g. Santibanez et. al, 2009).

Scheduling ambulatory care has developed its own methodology such as sequencing rules (Cayirli et. Al) (for a comprehensive review of scheduling ambulatory care see Cayirli and Veral, 2003).

There have been various attempts to deal with the inherent uncertainty of the operation times. This uncertainty has inspired a stochastic optimization approach reported by Denton et. al (2007). This approach is solved as a two-stage stochastic programming model generating an optimal schedule considering the tardiness of the schedule, the patients waiting time and the idle time of the rooms.

A critical component in effective scheduling of the operating rooms is an accurate estimate of the surgery durations. It is well understood that the performance of the schedule is highly dependent on the accuracy of the surgery time estimates. The need for accurate estimates for surgery times is demonstrated in Does et. al (2009) where a loss of 40 minutes of surgery times in a 13 operating rooms hospital can be translated to a loss of more than $3 million a year. One approach to increase the accuracy of the estimates is to use real time data on each patient combined with historical data from nursing and anesthesia documentation (Page, 2009).

Attempts to approximate surgical times are reported in Zhou and Dexter (1998), by using log-normal distributions. Similarly attempts to estimate the post-anesthesia durations are assessed by Marcon and Kharraja (2002).

Operating rooms represent a bottleneck in most hospitals (Gordon et al., 1988). Of course in our case the operating rooms consist of the entire clinical operation and their efficiency is of outmost importance. Thus, in this chapter we explore block scheduling in which the blocks are released to surgeons rather than groups of specialists similar to the case described in (Fei et. al, 2010). The objective of this chapter is to suggest a methodology that improves the scheduling of the operating rooms by providing better time estimates of the surgeries.

CURRENT PROCESS

Pre-Op Process

The Surgical Center uses four pre-operational bays, four operating rooms, four PACU I recovery bays and eight PACU II recovery bays (PACU stands for Post Anesthesia Care Unit). On an average day, this combination of rooms is more than adequate for the Center's surgeries. However, on days with many short procedures a fifth bay is required for pre-operation and PACU I procedures. Opening a fifth bay in pre-operation area accommodates the doctors that bounce between two rooms performing the surgery and allows an

Figure 1. The preoperative process: nurse perspectives

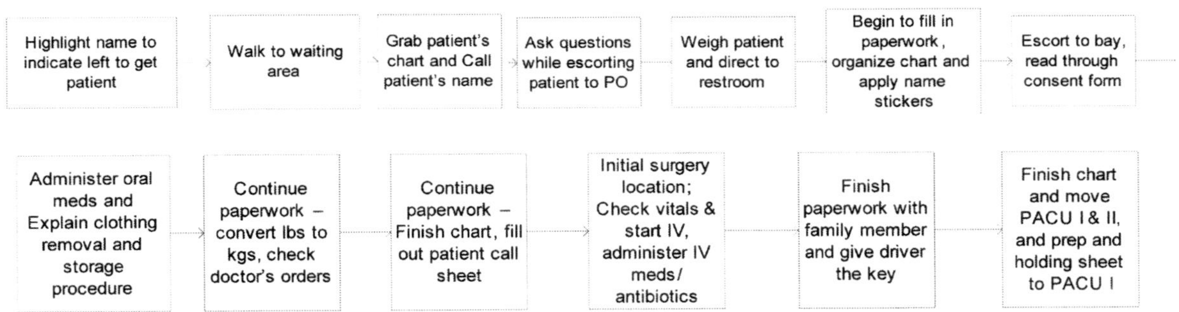

assistant to suture the patient. Of the patients that are served during a given day approximately 10% stay overnight. These overnight patients do not go to either stage of recovery (PACU), but remain in their bed and go directly to the overnight rooms.

Currently, pre-operation nurses contact patients scheduled for a surgery by phone the night prior to the surgery. This call is to confirm the scheduled operation time, give before-surgery instructions, describe what to expect and answer any questions the patient may have. Patients are asked to arrive 60 minutes prior to the scheduled operation time. During this time frame, patients must check in at the front desk as well as complete several pre-operational procedures. Of these 60 minutes, 30 - 45 minutes are required for these procedures. The variance in pre-operational procedures is due to the differences in patients' physiology (i.e. hard to access veins, necessary testing, etc). While it seems sufficient to ask the patients to arrive only 30 minutes before the scheduled operation times, patient arrival time in relation to operation time varies from patient to patient. Nurses and staff have noticed that patients may arrive up to 15 minutes early or late.

Pre-operation nurses use this fifteen minute variance to accommodate multiple patients simultaneously. Within the pre-operational procedures, some tasks require only the patient (i.e. changing garments, completing paperwork) and other tasks require only the nurse. This process is depicted in Figure 1.

As the day progresses and unexpected events occur, delays in the planned schedule occur. Long delays in the schedule extend waiting times by an hour or two. To be courteous to the patients affected by these delays, the patients are advised to remain in the facility as the staff are nearly ready or they are told to go home and expect a phone call as the operation rooms are running behind schedule. If the patient has not yet arrived, the staff in the surgical center makes a phone call home to tell the patients there is no need to come in at the scheduled time. The information the patient receives depends on how far behind the schedule are the operating rooms.

Operations Procedures

The OR is set up for current surgery once the room has been cleaned from the previous surgery. All procedure baskets for the day are placed in the OR the morning before each day starts. Once cleaning of the room is complete, nurses pull the contents from the procedure baskets, open relevant surgical packs, and place any needed equipment At this point the patient is brought into the surgery room. The center always allots 15 minutes for turnover of a room and any setup required for the next surgery.

Once the patient is brought into the operating room, a series of activities that prepare the patient for the actual procedure take place. However, before any of these steps begin, the patient is put under anesthesia. First the patient is moved from the gurney to the operating table. Then they are positioned so as to eliminate any pressure points on the body being aggravated, helping to keep the patient as comfortable as possible once the surgery is completed. The time required to accomplish this can vary depending on the patient.

Next, the patient is hooked up to monitoring equipment and the area of their body that is to be operated on is cleaned. The patient is draped with medical drapes, which isolate the area of the body to be worked on. Once these steps are completed, the first incision is made.

After the surgery is completed, the patient is bandaged, undraped and then moved to a gurney or to an in-patient bed. A patient is not allowed to come out of the OR until he/she has a score of at least five on the checklist for PACU I. Until this happens the patients stays in the OR and a Certified Registered Nurse Anesthesiologist (CRNA) stays with them. Each patient requires a different amount of time to be released to PACU I. Release time depends on how much anesthesia the patient required during surgery and how quickly the patient metabolizes the anesthesia drugs out of their system.

Turnover time for an OR varies depending also on the procedure that was preformed. Some procedures like shoulder or total hip replacement require more time including the cleaning. Others such as inserting ear-tubes require far less time. Independent of the procedure, there are at least two and often three professionals in charge of turning over an OR. They include a nurse, a scrub technician and a charge nurse, who is the nurse in charge of the turnover process. On some occasions, there will be one or two other nurses available who will help with the turnover process as well. In this paper we are interested in the patient waiting time before the surgery, being the critical component of the process.

PROBLEMS WITH THE CURRENT OPERATION

The center currently schedules the surgeries according to a block schedule. In this scheduling approach each group of doctors who utilizes the surgical center are assigned one or more half-day blocks in which they can schedule any procedure at anytime given that no other doctor is using that time slot. As the doctors call in and request an operation room the scheduling nurse allots an amount of time for each surgery based on her previous experience. There is apparently no set timetable for any surgery, so the nurse simply decides on a time that she considers to be adequate for the given procedure. Currently, the estimated surgery time of the scheduler deviates on average by 24 minutes from the actual time, with a large standard deviation as shown in the Figure 2 (presented in absolute value).

In addition to the variation of surgery times, we documented the pre-operation procedures and found that on average they require 30-45 minutes. A prophylactic antibiotics must be administered within 60 minutes of incision, so large deviation in the per-operational or operations' times could cause delays in the surgeries which can become quite costly.

With this current scheduling system, there are surgeries that run anywhere from just a few minutes to several hours longer than expected which translates into patients with procedures later in the day waiting a longer amount of time. In addition, if procedures with greater time variability are scheduled earlier in the day, this effect will be compounded throughout the day, resulting in longer delays as the day progresses.

Figure 2. Deviation between estimated and actual surgery times

Difference Between Actual and Current Process Allocation

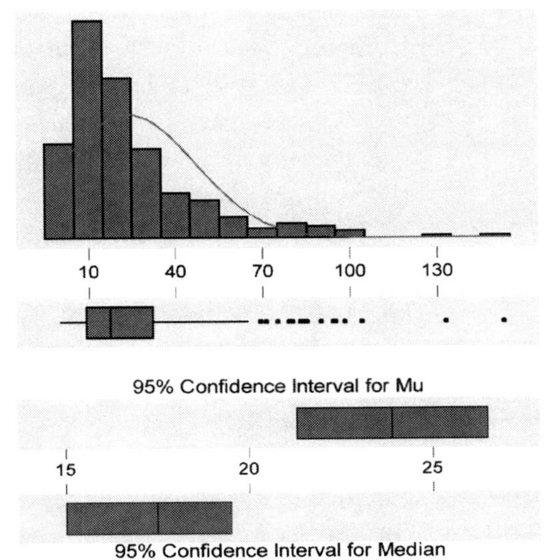

Surgery Time

Anderson-Darling Normality Test

A-Squared:	15.579
P-Value:	0.000
Mean	23.9007
StDev	23.0036
Variance	529.166
Skewness	2.04400
Kurtosis	5.57723
N	302
Minimum	0.000
1st Quartile	9.000
Median	17.500
3rd Quartile	32.000
Maximum	153.000

95% Confidence Interval for Mu

21.296 26.506

95% Confidence Interval for Sigma

21.304 25.001

95% Confidence Interval for Median

15.000 19.502

CLUSTERING SURGERIES TO REDUCE OPERATION TIME VARIANCE

The first step towards a solution is to create clusters of similar operations, using combinations of physicians and surgeries.

The clustering was done using the following assumptions:

1. A decision table was created using the total time the patient was in the operation room. This includes the variable amount of time that is required to prepare the patient for the operation once they are in the OR as well as the fifteen-minute turnover time at the end of the operation.
2. If a procedure runs over, the next procedure will be late by at least the amount of time the previous procedure was over plus any other additional considerations.

In order to simplify the data analysis, a more concise method of identifying the doctors and the procedures performed at the center, is needed. This is achieved by using a "service code" for each procedure. This code is an identifier that is used to denote what procedure or procedures are performed during a given operation. If more than one procedure is performed then there would be more than one service code entered into the data sheets for that particular surgery.

The first step in creating the reference tables is to analyze the complete schedule of an entire "typical" month. This information includes the service code(s) performed in each surgery, the doctor(s) that performed it and the time the patient entered and left the operation room. This allows calculation of the total time each patient was in the OR.

In order to de-personalize the data, the service code identifying each surgery and the doctor performing each surgery were converted into a

Table 1. A partial list of services and codes

Service	Service Code
ARTHPAI	3
ARTHPAI, ACLKNEE	5
BMWT	9
BMWTADE	10
BUNION	14
BUNION, NEUROMA	15
CARPTUNN	19
DIAGLAP	32
DIAGLAP, LSO	33
DIAGLAP, OVARCYST	34
DIAGLAP, OVARCYST, RSO	35
DIAGLAP, TAH, LAPVHYST	36
ESWL	43
ESWL, CYSTROTRO	44
EXCCERND	45
EXCCYST	46
EXCFINMA	47

numerical identifier. A partial list of services and their codes is provided in Table 1.

Each operation type is analyzed for its duration and variability, independent of the doctor as shown in Table 2. This analysis is performed on each of the 300 and more operation types.

Moreover, each surgeon was analyzed for his average surgery time and variability as Figure 3 shows graphically.

This analysis is summarized in a table that lists the surgery time for each operation type and doctor as shown in Table 3.

The last column (N) in Table 3 represents the number of surgeries (observations) of a certain type preformed by a certain doctor. This number of trials is especially important, since it can be assumed that if a large number of trials are present, the mean and standard deviation data will give an accurate estimate of surgery time. If the number of trials is small, then the estimate may not be very reliable.

Table 2. Partial analysis of each operation type (in minutes)

Service Code	Mean	Standard Deviation	N
ARTHPAI	70.45	23.07	31
ARTHPAI, ACLKNEE	180.7	27.7	6
BMWT	17.67	5.55	9
BMWTADE	47.2	6.5	5
(1) BUNION; (2) BUNION, NEUROMA	79.6	43.1	5
CARPTUNN	41.5	15.7	4
(1) DIAGLAP; (2) DIAGLAP, LSO; (3) DIAGLAP, OVARCYST; (4) DIAGLAP, OVARCYST, RSO; (5) DIAGLAP, TAH, LAPVHYST	71.75	25.5	8
(1) ESWL; (2) ESWL, CYSTROTRO	44.15	13.9	20
(1) EXCCERND; (2) EXCCYST; (3) EXCFINMA; (4) EXCGANG; (5) EXCISION; (6) EXCISVAG; (7) EXCLESN; (8) EXCLYMP; (9) EXCMASS; (10) EXCNEVUS; (11) EXCULNST	61.24	18.16	17
GREENLIG	61.4	8.65	5
INGHERNI	64.88	12.51	8
LAPCHOL	66.36	19.98	14
LAPVHYST	101.25	25.23	8

Figure 3. Analysis of doctor time (in minutes)

Descriptive Statistics

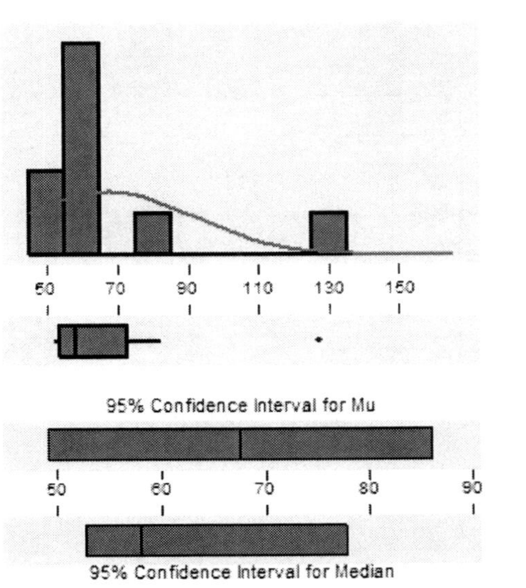

Variable: Time
Doctor: 18

Anderson-Darling Normality Test

A-Squared:	1.250
P-Value:	0.001
Mean	67.5556
StDev	24.1097
Variance	581.278
Skewness	2.30453
Kurtosis	5.49581
N	9
Minimum	52.000
1st Quartile	53.500
Median	58.000
3rd Quartile	72.500
Maximum	127.000

95% Confidence Interval for Mu
49.023 86.088

95% Confidence Interval for Sigma
16.285 46.189

95% Confidence Interval for Median
52.684 77.670

The last step of the analysis is to cluster the operations into a manageable number of groups that include the operation type and the surgeon. A partial list of the clustered operation is shown in Table 4 below (the complete list is too long). These times are referred to as "Standard Operating Procedures" (SOP) and provide the guidance to the scheduling nurse. This table helps the scheduling nurse to decide on how much time to allocate to each combination of surgeon and surgery type.

As a result, by using the table as a decision tool to estimate the duration of each surgery, the difference between the estimated time of the surgery and the actual type is significantly reduced, improving the accuracy of the schedule and reducing the patient waiting time. The average difference is shown in Figure 4.

Figure 4 shows that the new "group" time estimates are much more accurate. Thus, using the SOP table as a decision tool reduces the difference between the allotted surgery time and actual surgery time by nearly 60%. The mean allotted times are different by only nine minutes (with the greatest difference as high as 90 minutes). Furthermore, this Figure shows that half the procedures analyzed ran over their allotted time by only three minutes and 75% of the procedures were less than 12 minutes over. By the end of a day with four surgeries on average running behind schedule, excess waiting time was decreased by 56 minutes. This analysis was conducted on actual schedules using the new time estimates.

MOVING HIGH VARIABILITY SURGERIES TO THE END

Next, given that there is natural variability in the operation time, we measured the effect of starting the day with surgeries of low variability, and assigning the operations with larger variability later in the day. We used simulation to assess the effect of this policy on the lateness of surgeries throughout the day. In this case we found a

Table 3. A partial surgery time table (in minutes)

Service	Doctor	Time (mean)	Std. Dev.	N
ABDPLAST	1	154	*	1
ADEN CH	2	49	*	1
ARTHPAI	3	85	12.06	4
	4	72	*	1
	5	80.14	11.32	7
	6	107.2	41.2	5
	7	82.56	24.11	9
	8	73.67	5.51	3
	9	88	4.24	2
ARTHPAI, ACL/HAM	5 9 10	274	*	1
	5	222	*	1
ARTHPAI, ACLKNEE	3	190	*	1
	5	204.5	43.1	2
	7	203	31.1	2
	9	169	*	1
ARTHROD	8	190	*	1
BICEPTEN	7	140	*	1
BLEPHARO, BROWLIFT	2	130	*	1
BMWT	11	30	2.6	4
	2	34.8	6.72	5
BMWTADE	11	63.67	3.51	3
	2	60	11.31	2
BONEGRFT	8	128	*	1
BREASTBX	12	50	*	1
BREAUGU	1	101.33	8.08	3

Table 4. Clustering Surgeries by physician and surgery type (partial list, in minutes)

Service Code	Doctor Code	Mean	Standard Deviation	N
3	8	70	12.06	4
3	16	65.14	11.32	7
3	18	67.56	24.11	9
3	20	58.67	5.51	3
3	22	73	4.24	2
5	8	175	*	1
5	16	189.5	43.1	2
5	18	188	31.1	2
9	1	15	2.16	4

Figure 4. Measuring similarity between the assessed and actual surgery times (in minutes)

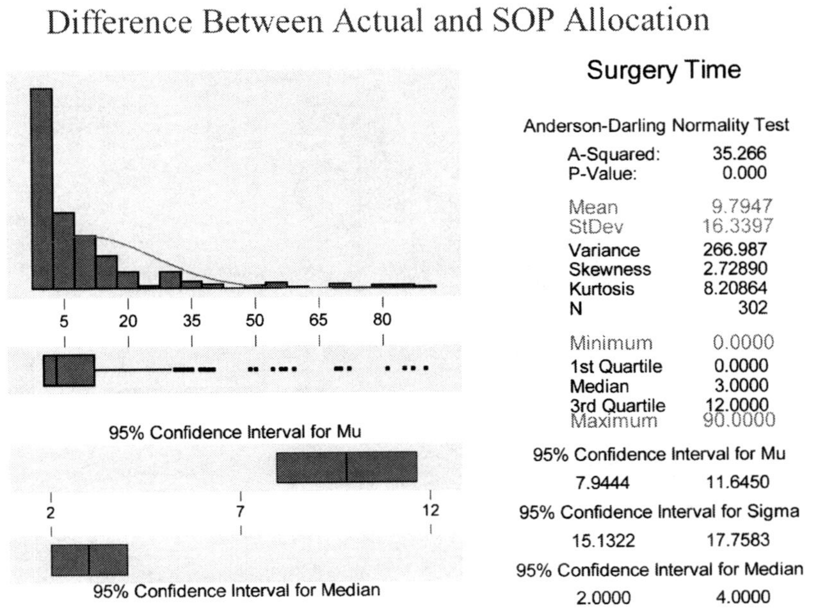

Difference Between Actual and SOP Allocation
Surgery Time
Anderson-Darling Normality Test
A-Squared: 35.266
P-Value: 0.000
Mean 9.7947
StDev 16.3397
Variance 266.987
Skewness 2.72890
Kurtosis 8.20864
N 302
Minimum 0.0000
1st Quartile 0.0000
Median 3.0000
3rd Quartile 12.0000
Maximum 90.0000
95% Confidence Interval for Mu
7.9444 11.6450
95% Confidence Interval for Sigma
15.1322 17.7583
95% Confidence Interval for Median
2.0000 4.0000
5 20 35 50 65 80
95% Confidence Interval for Mu
2 7 12
95% Confidence Interval for Median

Figure 5. Mean and variance of operation time for all surgeons (in minutes)

Descriptive Statistics
Variable: Time
Service: 32
Anderson-Darling Normality Test
A-Squared: 0.916
P-Value: 0.010
Mean 71.7500
StDev 25.5049
Variance 650.5
Skewness 2.18776
Kurtosis 5.35151
N 8
Minimum 51.000
1st Quartile 55.250
Median 63.500
3rd Quartile 76.000
Maximum 131.000
95% Confidence Interval for Mu
50.427 93.073
95% Confidence Interval for Sigma
16.863 51.909
95% Confidence Interval for Median
52.871 80.475
30 75 120 165 210
95% Confidence Interval for Mu
50 60 70 80 90
95% Confidence Interval for Median

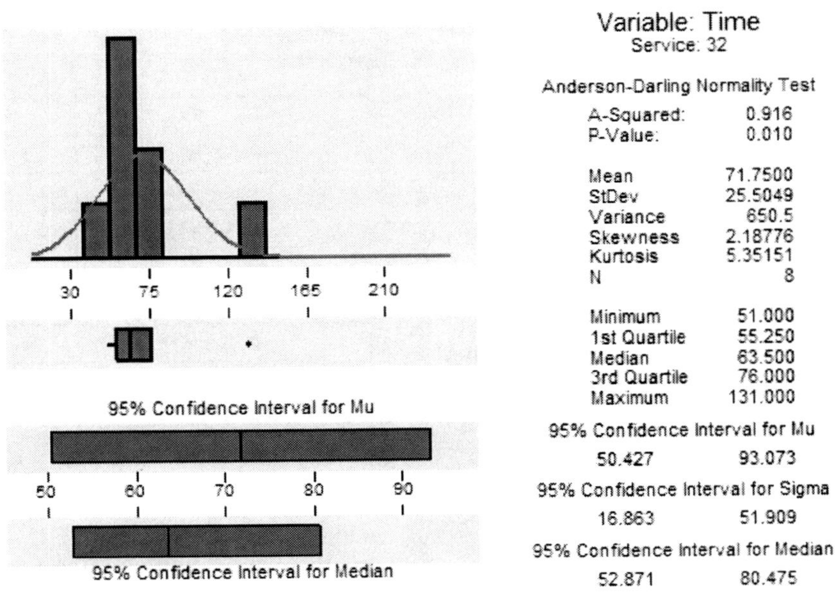

Figure 6. An example of the simulation screen

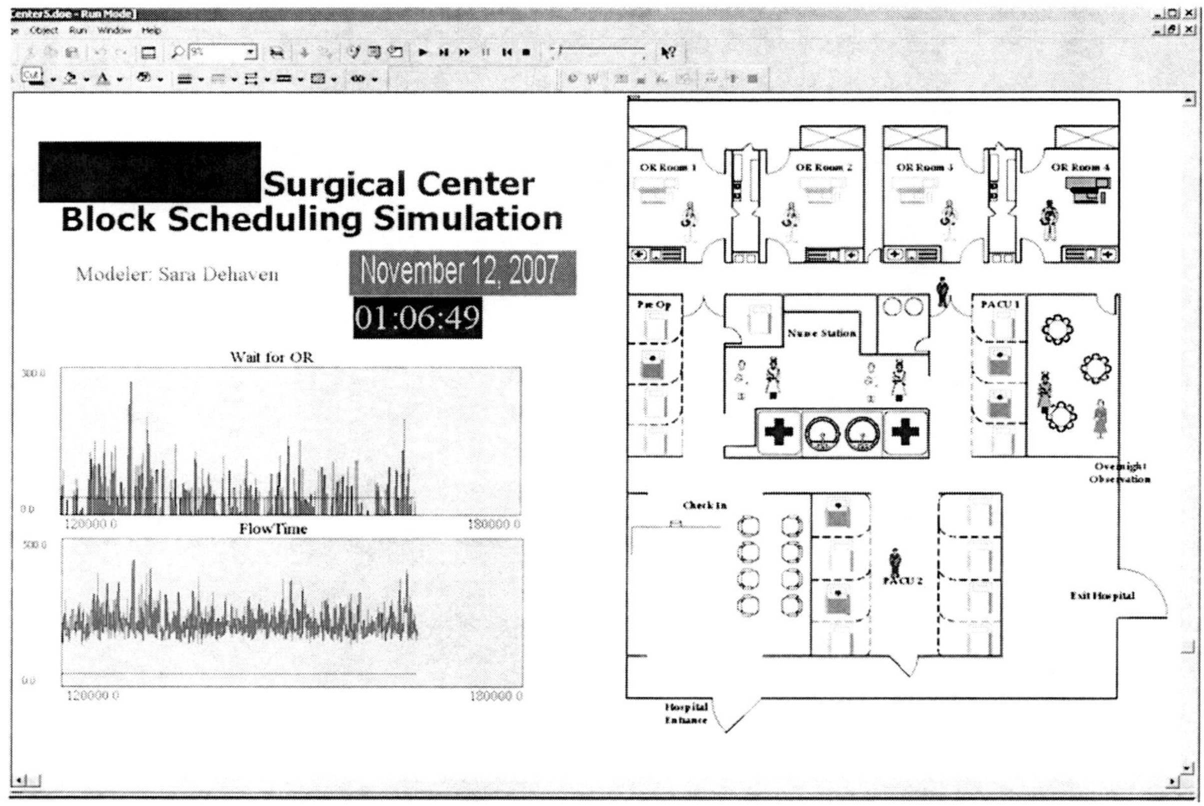

reduction of about 40% in the waiting times (or lateness) for surgeries. This is in addition to the savings achieved using the SOP as the predicted surgery times.

An analysis of each operation type for all doctors shows a fairly considerable variability. An example is shown in Figure 5.

The last part of the method was to simulate the new process in order to check for capacity of the clinical and administrative staff. We found that this process allows the surgical center to conduct 10 more operations per week, without the need to hire any new personnel.

Simulation Analysis

In this section we present four simulation experiments as follows:

Table 5. Base case operations data

Function	Utilization
Nurse_R1	0.48
Nurse_R2	0.29
Nurse_R3	0.45
Nurse_R4	0.61
Nurse_R5	0.21
Nurse_R6	0.06
OR_Room1	0.49
OR_Room2	0.48
OR_Room3	0.49
OR_Room4	0.49

Base case: Surgical times are taken from the actual log book. The sequence of operations is the actual schedule operation sequence. The Opera-

Figure 7. Average time related performance of base case (in minutes)

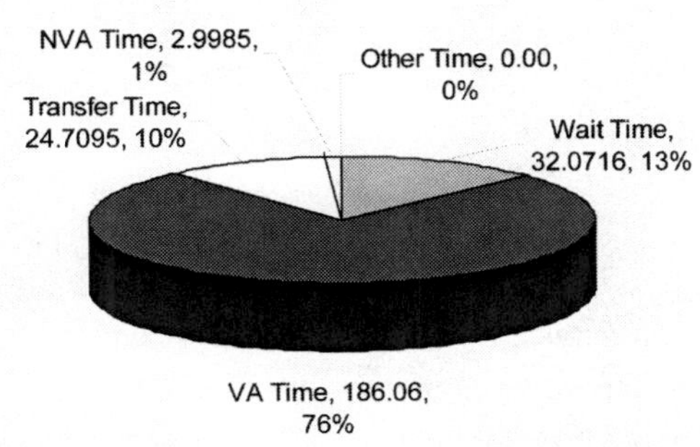

Figure 8. Performance of using random schedule

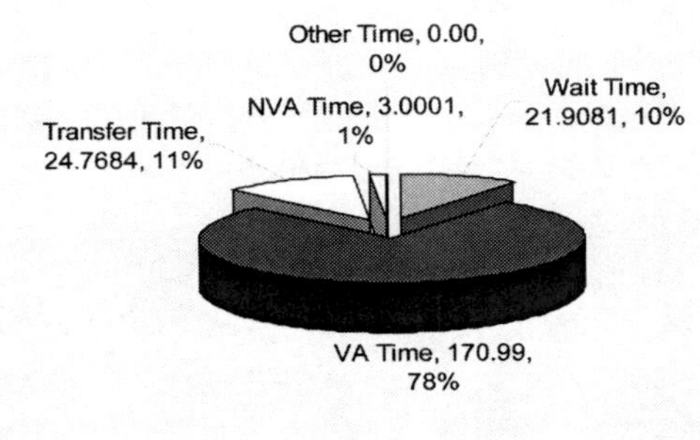

tion Room schedules are taken from the actual log book as well.

Case 2: Surgical times are taken from the same log book – but the sequence of operations is randomly generated from the population of surgeries performed that month (with the same proportions).

Case 3: Surgeries or doctors with large variation are scheduled later in the day.

Case 4: The schedule places operations with high variability earlier in the day, representing a "worst case analysis".

An example of the simulation screen is presented in Figure 6.

Simulation Results

Case I

The results are presented in Table 5.

This Table shows the utilization of the nurses as well as the four operating rooms. Clearly the operating rooms are utilized at about 50% only, and the patients' waiting time as shown in Figure 7 is 32 minutes in average.

Figure 7 shows the total time spent in the system, waiting time, Value Added Time (time of actual surgery excluding preparation time and recovery time), time spent being moved to/from OR and recovery rooms, and total non-value adding time. The total time spent in the system is 245 minutes with average waiting time of 32 minutes representing 13% of the overall time spent at the facility. Overall Value Added time represents 76% which is quite efficient.

Case II: Scheduling the Surgeries in a Random Manner

In this case the total waiting time is 220 minutes with the other properties shown in Figure 8.

In this case the sequence of operations throughout the day is randomly decided without regard to variability. The proportions of operation types is accurately maintained. Surprisingly, this case shows a moderately improved performance! Thus we concluded that the current sequencing of operations is done based on the demands of the surgeons which is worse than a randomly generated sequence. For example, in many cases the physicians prefer to start the day with the hard cases that have higher variability.

Case III: Low Variability First

Here the total time is 215 minutes with waiting time of 19 minutes only. This is the best achievable case, as shown in Table 6.

In this case we schedule the operations such that the ones with large variance are scheduled at a later time in the day. The Table shows that the waiting time is significantly reduced. The average total time patient spent in the facility is also reduced (as well as the value added time) which allows for more surgeries to be performed during the day.

Case IV: High Variability First

In this case, the average total time patient spent in the facilty is 257 minutes with average waiting time of 41 minutes – the poorest performance as expected.

CONCLUSION

This chapter presents a methodology to improve the schedule of a for-profit ambulatory surgical facility. This facility is characterized by a large variety of surgeries, surgery types and doctors who perform them creating high variability in the operations' times. The schedule of these surgeries suffered from inaccurate estimated time used by the scheduling nurse. In addition, the surgeries were scheduled without regard for the inherent variability of the operation.

The approach presented herein creates a decision table based on Standard Operating Procedures that helps the scheduler to make a more accurate time estimate for each surgery. This table is created by clustering the surgeries and doctors into groups with similar properties. This decision table therefore helps to reduce the patients' waiting time. The decision table allows the surgery scheduler to look up the amount of time allotted for an individual doctor performing a specific

Table 6. Performance under low variability first

	Average	Half Width	Minimum	Maximum
Total Time	215.63	1.37005	121.29	592.17
Wait Time	19.4741	1.24534	0.00	386.86
VA Time	168.41	0.297259002	83.2312	283.82
Transfer Time	24.7455	0.043245203	16.9395	38.9327
NVA Time	3.0024	0.003635410	2.1180	3.7084
Other Time	0.00	0.000000000	0.00	0.00

procedure. This table can be updated easily with or without external assistance. Schedulers will require only a short training session to learn how to use a decision table.

This work also examined the issue of variability of surgery times. This variability can be caused by the difference between individual patients, as well as the difference between surgeons. Thus, in this chapter we analyzed the results of shifting low variability operations towards the beginning of the day, and scheduling the high variability ones later on. This means that more complicated patients or surgeons with higher variability will be scheduled later. As a result this will reduce the average waiting times from 32 minutes to 19.5 minutes, a significant reduction.

Combining both approach of using better time estimates for the schedule, and shifting high variability surgeries into the later part of the day will greatly improve the operations.

REFERENCES

Adan, I., Bekkers, J., Dellaert, N., Vissers, J., & Yu, X. (2009). Patient mix optimisation and stochastic resource requirements: A case study in cardiothoracic surgery planning. *Health Care Management Science*, *12*(2), 129. doi:10.1007/s10729-008-9080-9

Belien, J., Demeulemeester, E., & Cardoen, B. (2009). A decision support system for cyclic mater surgery scheduling with multiple objectives. *Journal of Scheduling*, *12*, 147–161. doi:10.1007/s10951-008-0086-4

Blake, J. T., Dexter, F., & Donald, J. (2002). Operating room manager's use of integer programming for assigning block time to surgical groups: A case study. *Anesthesia and Analgesia*, *94*, 143–148.

Cayirli, T., & Veral, E. (2003). Outpatient scheduling in health care: A review of literature. *Production and Operations Management*, *12*(4), 519–549. doi:10.1111/j.1937-5956.2003.tb00218.x

Cayirli, T., Veral, E., & Rosen, H. (2006). Designing appointment scheduling systems for ambulatory care services. *Health Care Management Science*, *9*, 47–58. doi:10.1007/s10729-006-6279-5

Denton, B., Viapiano, J., & Vogl, A. (2007). Optimization of surgery sequencing and scheduling decisions under uncertainty. *Health Care Management Science*, *10*, 13–24. doi:10.1007/s10729-006-9005-4

Does, R., Vermaat, T., Verver, J., Bisgaard, S., & Van Den Heuvel, J. (2009). Reducing start time delays in operating rooms. *Journal of Quality Technology*, *41*(1), 95–109.

Fei, H., Chu, C., & Meskens, N. (2009). Solving a tactical operating room planning problem by a column-generation based heuristic procedure with four criteria. *Annals of Operations Research*, *166*, 91–108. doi:10.1007/s10479-008-0413-3

Fei, H., Meskens, N., & Chu, C. (2010). A planning and scheduling problem for an operating theatre using an open scheduling strategy. *Computers & Industrial Engineering*, *58*(2), 221. doi:10.1016/j.cie.2009.02.012

Gordon, T., Lyles, A. P. S., & Fountain, J. (1988). Surgical unit time review: Resource utilization and management implications. *Journal of Medical Systems*, *12*, 169–179. doi:10.1007/BF00996639

Jebali, A., Hadi Alouane, A. B., & Ladet, P. (2006). Operating rooms scheduling. *International Journal of Production Economics*, *99*, 52–62. doi:10.1016/j.ijpe.2004.12.006

Marcon, E., & Kharraja, S. (2002). *Etude exploratoire sur la strategie de dimensionnement d'une SSPI.* Actes de la 2 Conference Internationale Francophone d'Aitomatique, Nantes, France.

Marjamaa, R. A., Torkki, P. M., Hirvensalo, E. J., & Kirvelä, O. A. (2009). What is the best workflow for an operating room? A simulation study of five scenarios. *Health Care Management Science*, *12*(2), 142–147. doi:10.1007/s10729-008-9073-8

Page, D. (2009). Taking the guesswork out of scheduling surgeries. *Hospitals & Health Networks*, *83*(6), 12.

Roland, B., Di Martinelly, C., Riane, F., & Pochet, Y. (2010). Scheduling an operating theatre under human resource constraints. *Computers & Industrial Engineering*, *58*(2), 212. doi:10.1016/j.cie.2009.01.005

Santibanez, P., Begen, M., & Atkins, D. (2007). Surgical block scheduling in a system of hospitals: An application to resource and wait list management in a British Columbia health authority. *Health Care Management Science*, *10*, 269–282. doi:10.1007/s10729-007-9019-6

Santibáñez, P., Chow, V. S., French, J., Puterman, M. L., & Tyldesley, S. (2009). Reducing patient wait times and improving resource utilization at British Columbia Cancer Agency's ambulatory care unit through simulation. *Health Care Management Science*, *12*(4), 392–407. doi:10.1007/s10729-009-9103-1

Testi, A., & Tànfani, E. (2009). Tactical and operational decisions for operating room planning: Efficiency and welfare implications. *Health Care Management Science*, *12*(4), 363. doi:10.1007/s10729-008-9093-4

Testi, A., Tanfani, E., & Torre, G. (2007). A three-phase approach for operating theatre schedules. *Health Care Management Science*, *10*, 163–172. doi:10.1007/s10729-007-9011-1

Visser, J. M. H. (1998). Patient flow-based allocation of inpatient resources: A case study. *European Journal of Operational Research*, *105*, 356–370. doi:10.1016/S0377-2217(97)00242-7

Vissers, J. M. H., Adan, I. J. B. F., & Bekkers, J. A. (2005). Patinet mix optimization in cardiothoracic surgery planning: A case study. *IMA Journal of Management Math*, *16*, 281–304. doi:10.1093/imaman/dpi023

Zhou, J., & Dexter, F. (1998). Methods to assist in the scheduling of add-on surgical cases: Upper prediction bounds for surgical case durations based on log-normal distribution. *Anesthesiology*, *89*(5). doi:10.1097/00000542-199811000-00024

Chapter 13
Scheduling Healthcare Systems:
Theory and Applications

Arben Asllani
The University of Tennessee - Chattanooga, USA

ABSTRACT

This chapter offers a series of scheduling techniques and their applications in healthcare settings. Healthcare administrators, physicians, and other professionals can use such techniques to achieve their operational goals when resources are limited. Implementing scheduling techniques in healthcare is difficult. Healthcare systems are complex, and the scheduler must be able to connect the scheduling theory with suitable algorithms for implementation. The chapter covers a wide spectrum of scheduling models, from single server and deterministic models to the more difficult ones, those which consider several servers and stochastic variables. A strong emphasis is placed on the practical aspects of scheduling techniques in healthcare.

INTRODUCTION

Scheduling plays a crucial role in healthcare organizations. The pressure to reduce costs has an impact on the quality of service. Healthcare schedulers must find a line between reducing cost and caring for people. Application of scheduling techniques in healthcare can reduce costs and improve the quality of medical treatments.

DOI: 10.4018/978-1-60960-872-9.ch013

Healthcare systems are complex because of their complicated design, multifaceted objective functions, and stochastic nature. Consider an emergency department at a hospital. There are several ambulances, emergency technicians, nurses, and doctors. Patients arrive and wait in several service areas: triage, waiting room, emergency room, beds, X-ray machines, and laboratory stations. All these "server stations" differ with respect to their operational characteristics, such as processing capacity, processing times, and operational goals. The system becomes even more complex when considering that upon arrival, patients may go through several stations which often are determined dynamically as patients move from one station to another. In this complex scheduling system, the primary goal is to provide high quality treatment. This goal, however, must be achieved while costs of patients' care are kept as low as possible.

In addition, there are difficult questions of medical scheduling ethics. For example, should the physician schedule an untested and expensive treatment or a more traditional and less expensive one? Should a doctor see his patients according to the First Come First Served (FCFS) rule or Shortest Case First (SCF) heuristic? The FCFS rule provides an equal waiting time for patients and is a known to be "a fair" scheduling heuristic. On the other side, the SCF heuristic may seem "unfair" to patients but it may significantly increase utilization of doctors, nurses, and other resources of the healthcare clinic.

Another challenge of healthcare scheduling is that healthcare systems have a high degree of patient contact and are difficult to control and rationalize. For example, patients arrive randomly and as such they can always make an input to, or cause a disruption in, the healthcare service. Besides patient arrivals, treatment times are often random in nature. Consider the oncology department in the same hospital. Planning and scheduling radiotherapy treatments seems to be an uncomplicated task for the scheduler. A patient will typically visit the treatment center several times a week for a given number of consecutive weeks as described in his or her treatment plan. The goal of such a patient scheduling system is to ensure the delivery of the right treatment at the right time while maximizing the utilization of equipment and other resources. However, this is not a simple task because treatment time for each patient is random. Under such environment, it is difficult to minimize waiting times for patients, idle times for equipment, or overtime for nurses and technicians.

In general, the implementation of operations research models and scheduling techniques in real life problems is difficult. Such a challenge is related to the scheduler's inability to connect a theoretical model with an appropriate approach for implementation. There are two main objectives of the chapter: (a) describe a series of scheduling models in healthcare organizations, and (b) provide practical solutions and algorithms which can be used by healthcare practitioners to achieve their operational goals.

The next section of the chapter will describe a framework of scheduling models in the healthcare industry. According to this framework every scheduling model in healthcare has two dimensions: number of treatment stations and nature of scheduling problems. A scheduling environment may involve one or many servers (stations) and the nature of the problem may be deterministic or stochastic. If the processing times of treatments and patient arrivals can be ascertained with certainty, then the model represents a deterministic scheduling problem. Those models where the processing and arrival times are considered as random variables represent stochastic scheduling problems.

The chapter continues with detailed investigations of a series of scheduling situations according to the above framework. For each case, scheduling theory is consulted and the most practical possible solution is offered. The suggested algorithm for each case can be extended to similar scheduling situations which belong to the same scheduling category, that is, the same number of stations and the same problem type. The chapter concludes with a summary of assumptions used in the models and with a discussion of implementation issues of the offered heuristics.

BACKGROUND

There is a broad selection of research about the applications of scheduling techniques in healthcare. Several books (Brandeau, Sainfort, & Pierskalla, 2004; Ozcan, 2005; Pinedo, 2009) contain one or more chapters with a special focus on planning and scheduling applications in healthcare. Literature reviews show that operations research techniques have mostly been used in the healthcare industry to solve specific and independent problems (Pinedo, 2009; Ozcan, 2005). A survey of heuristic algorithms for various scheduling problems encountered in healthcare is provided in Beliën (2007).

Among those individual scheduling models, special attention is given to scheduling operating rooms or theatres. Surgeries are considered to be the engine of the hospital: they are the most costly and also the main generators of hospital revenues (Denton, Viapiano, & Vogl, 2007). Many other healthcare units are scheduled around the surgery rooms or theatres. The deterministic case of the single operating room is first discussed in Weiss (1990). Denton, Viapiano, & Vogl (2007) analyze the stochastic case of the single operating room and Fei, Meskens, & Chu (2010) suggest a genetic algorithm to generate a weekly surgery schedule in an operating theatre. A review of recent operational research on operating room planning and scheduling is provided in Cardoen, Demeulemeester, & Beliën (2010).

Radiotherapy treatment scheduling has also been studied extensively in the literature. A recent study by Conforti, Guerriero, & Guido (2008) offers a mathematical formulation of the radiotherapy treatment problem. Systematic analysis of hospital administration has been generally ignored by decision scientists. The main reason for this neglect is that healthcare systems are very complex and attempting to derive optimal solutions for the whole system often becomes unrealistic. This chapter tackles the above challenge by offering a scheduling framework and placing a series of healthcare scheduling problems into this framework. A healthcare practitioner can investigate the algorithm or the heuristic of a particular problem in the framework and can relate that model to other scheduling problems which belong in the same category. Figure 1 indicates an overall schema of scheduling problems.

Figure 1. Overall classification of healthcare scheduling problems

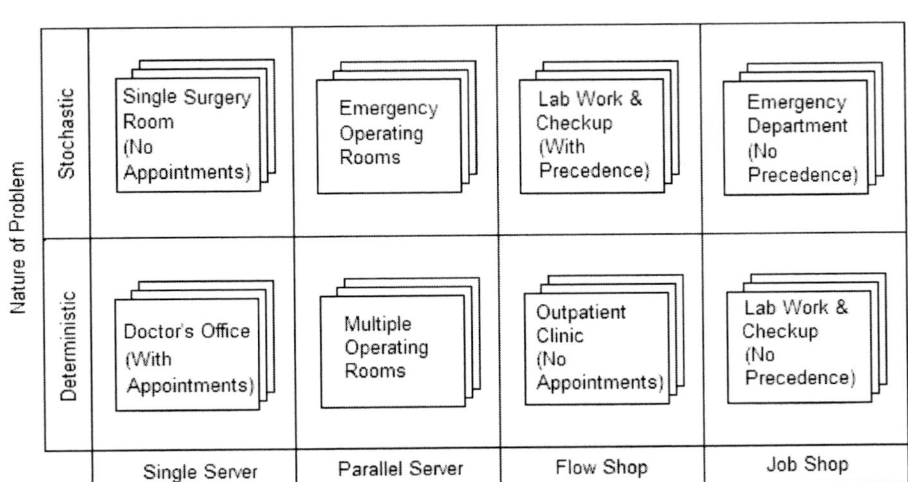

One dimension of the above matrix is based on the number of servers or treatment stations. From now on, the terms "server" and "treatment stations" are used interchangeably and refer to either physical stations such as surgery rooms, hospital beds, the emergency department, or human resources, such a physician, nurse, or technician. From this perspective, healthcare scheduling models are grouped into a single server or many servers. When patients are treated in one station, this scheduling problem is known as a single server case. Examples of single server cases include scheduling an operating unit, a doctor's office, a nursing station, and so on. The goal in the single server case is to find the best sequence in which patients should be processed through the server. Understanding the single server scheduling model is important for two main reasons: it lays the foundations for more complex, multi-server cases (Pinedo, 1995) and it is useful to model and study patient bottleneck problems, which occur frequently on healthcare scheduling situations.

Many-server scheduling problems in healthcare can be further grouped into three configurations: parallel server, flow shop, and job shop. A scheduling model is said to have parallel server configuration when there are a number of one-procedure treatments, which can be processed in any of the stations (Pinedo, 1995). Examples of parallel server models may include outpatient clinics with many doctors, triage areas with many nurses, and so on.

Scheduling theory defines flow shop models as those situations in which servers and workstations are arranged in a serial fashion and each job (in our case, each patient) has to pass through each station (Pinedo, 1995). Patient treatments in this model are multistage in nature. Consider a situation when the scheduler must book several surgeries in a given day. Scheduling the operating room can be modeled as a single server problem. However, when considering other treatments for each patient (anesthesia, surgery, post-surgery recovery), the option would be to use a flow-shop model.

Finally, the most complex of all cases is the job-shop configuration. In this model patients' treatments vary, they are not always in a predetermined order, and patients are equally likely to be assigned to any station for treatment. Scheduling resources in the emergency department is a good representative of healthcare job-shop scheduling configuration.

The remainder of the chapter discusses a series of scheduling problems as shown in Figure 1. The complexity and difficulty of scheduling models is expected to gradually increase as the discussion moves from the single server models to the job shop models. In general, simple scheduling problems can be solved with straightforward and practical heuristics. On the other side, complex scheduling problems require more sophisticated and often impractical algorithms.

Often, a scheduler must decide between complexity and practicality. For example, consider an outpatient clinic with several doctors who process patients as they arrive randomly. If the goal of the scheduler is to minimize doctors' downtime, an integer 0-1 linear programming (LP) model can be used. However, it is often impractical for the scheduler to generate a large LP problem every day with hundreds of constraints and decision variables. Instead, the decision maker can either use pre-designed software templates or can reasonably assume the whole clinic as one single server and then use proven heuristics, such as Shortest Case First, Longest Case First, First Come First Served, or other scheduling heuristics. While those techniques may not provide optimal solutions, they provide good solutions, which are also practical.

SCHEDULING SINGLE SERVER HEALTHCARE SERVICES

There is a wide range of healthcare situations which fit the characteristics of a single server model. A flu vaccination station, a doctor's office, and an operating table are examples of single server scheduling environments. Techniques and results that are obtained from single server models can be used as the basis for more complicated scheduling environments. In fact, scheduling problems in more complex scheduling environments can be reduced into a single server model. For example, consider an emergency center that has many workstations (servers) and resources (nurses, technicians, and doctors). In an emergency situation, when arrivals of patients significantly increase, the operation room of the center becomes a single bottleneck in the operation of the emergency department. In such a situation, eliminating the bottleneck and applying single server techniques in the operating room is the most efficient scheduling effort one may consider. For the single server environment, the deterministic and stochastic cases are discussed.

Single Server Deterministic Model

The first step of any scheduling effort is to identify an appropriate objective function. Probably, the most important scheduling goal in healthcare is the *makespan*. The *makespan* is "equivalent to the completion time of the last job to leave the system" and a "minimum *makespan* implies a high utilization of workstations (Pinedo, 1995, p. 13). In healthcare, minimization of the *makespan* implies the minimum possible time when the last patient completes treatment. However, in most single server cases, the *makespan* does not depend on the sequence of treatments. In such cases, there are two meaningful objective functions: *total weighted completion time* and *early due dates*.

The Total Weighted Completion Time

Total completion time is calculated as the sum of completion times of all treatments and is often referred to as *flow time*. *Total* ***weighted*** *completion time* is referred to as *weighted flow time* and the weight may be regarded as an importance factor. For example, several patients may need to be treated on the same day, which usually is "right away." The triage nurse can indicate how urgent the treatment is, or how severe it would be to postpone treatment at a later time. Such importance or priority of treatment *j* is indicated by w_j.

If there are *n* patients to be treated in a single server environment and if each treatment lasts p_j, then the *total weighted completion time* is calculated as $\Sigma w_j C_j$. In this case $C_j = p(1) + p(2) \ldots + p(j)$ is the time when patient *j* completes the treatment and the station becomes available for the next patient. It is shown that the *Weighted Shortest Case First (WSCF)* rule is optimal in this situation. Please refer to Pinedo (1995, p. 27) and (Smith, 1956) for proof of this rule. According to the *WSCF* rule patients need to be ordered in the decreasing order of w_j/p_j.

Example: Appointment scheduling at the doctor's office is an example of single server scheduling. Patients call in to request an appointment and the doctor's nurse will obtain the information about their medical concerns. We assume that the patients do not require emergency or immediate attention because in such cases they are asked to call 911 or go to the emergency department. However, each patient may be in a different degree of pain, or they need to see the doctor as soon as possible due to other factors, such need for medication, risk of the illness becoming worse, and so on. Considering these factors, the nurse assigns a priority to each patient, indicating how important it is to complete the treatment as soon as possible. This weight is shown by a number from 1 to 10 where 1 means that the patient can be seen late in the day and 10 means that the patient must be seen as soon as possible. Based on previous experience and recorded data, the nurse can also estimate how long it will take for the office to treat a patient. This information is shown in Table 1.

Solution: A step by step approach to this scheduling heuristic is provided below:

Table 1. Priority and treatment times

Patient	1	2	3	4	5	6	7
Priority	1	9	6	4	4	8	6
Treatment Time (in minutes)	70	60	60	50	40	80	90

- **Step 1:** Record patient arrivals (calls), estimate processing times, and assign priorities
- **Step 2:** Calculate the wj/pj ratio for each patient and reorder patients in the decreasing order of this ratio to generate an optimal sequence
- **Step 3:** Calculate completion time and appointment time for each patient in the optimal sequence
- **Step 4:** Call patients and confirm appointments according to those times.

It is suggested that the scheduler allow idle time between patients to compensate for unexpected possible variations of patient arrivals or treatment times. Table 2 shows the implementation of this heuristic. The results are also compared with the results of the FCFS rule, a rule which would normally be implemented in this scheduling environment. Once the w_j/p_j is calculated, the second part of the table shows the same set of patients arranged in the decreasing order of w_j/p_j. The new sequence {2, 3, 5, 6, 4, 7, 1} indicates the optimal schedule. As shown, while the total completion time (450) does not change when patients are

Table 2. Comparison of FCFS and WSCF

Patient Scheduling Using FCFS Rule							
Patient	1	2	3	4	5	6	7
Priority (wj)	1	9	6	4	4	8	6
Treatment Time (in minutes, pj)	70	60	60	50	40	80	90
wj/pj	0.01	0.15	0.10	0.08	0.10	0.10	0.07
Completion Time	70	130	190	240	280	360	450
Weighted Objective Function	70	1,170	1,140	960	1,120	2,880	2,700
Total Weighted Objective Function	70 + 1,170 + 1,140 + 960 + 1,120 + 2,880 + 2,700 = 10,040						
Patient Scheduling Using WSCF Rule							
Patient	2	3	5	6	4	7	1
Priority (wj)	9	6	4	8	4	6	1
Treatment Time (in minutes, pj)	60	60	40	80	50	90	70
wj/pj	0.15	0.10	0.10	0.10	0.08	0.07	0.01
Completion Time	60	120	160	240	290	380	450
Weighted Objective Function	540	720	640	1,920	1,160	2,280	450
Total Weighted Objective Function	540 + 720 + 640 + 1,920+ 1,160 + 2,280 + 450 = 7,710						

rearranged, the weighted total completion time is reduced from 10040 to 7710. The new sequence considers the priority and the importance of seeing patients according to their priority needs.

Due Date Related Scheduling

Patient treatments are often constrained by a certain due date. They either need to be completed as early as possible or they must be completed before a certain date. For example, when a patient has to undergo a surgery, the physician may indicate a due date for the surgery and the goal of the scheduler is to assign the operation schedule before or as close as possible to the due date. In such cases, the objective function of the scheduling model will be to minimize *maximum lateness* (L_{max}). In this case, lateness (L_j) *is* defined as C_j-d_j, where C_j is the completion time of treatment *j* and d_j is the due time of treatment *j*. Accordingly, L_{max}= max $\{L_j\}$ for all $j = 1...n$ where *n* is the number of treatments to be scheduled. A practical heuristic for such a situation is *Earliest Due Date (EDD) First,* that is, treatments must be scheduled in the increasing order of their due dates.

In other situations, due date is so critical that the scheduler must only consider those treatments for which the due date requirement is met. If a patient cannot be scheduled within the due date then the patient may be sent to another facility. The scheduler's goal is to minimize the number of treatments that are sent away, which leads to another important objective function: minimizing *the number of tardy treatments* (ΣU_j). In this situation, the scheduler must create two sets: acceptable treatments (AT) for which the due date can be met and unacceptable treatments (UT) for which the due date is not met and those treatments must be send to another operating unit. The goal here is to minimize the number of treatments in the UT. Pinedo (1995, pp. 38-39) provides an optimal algorithm and the proof for this scheduling heuristic. According to Pinedo (1995), the algorithm is simple:

*Treatments are added to the AT set in increasing order of due dates. If the inclusion of treatment j*results in this treatment being completed late, the scheduled treatment with the largest processing time is moved from AT to UT.*

The following example illustrates both due date related single server cases: *minimizing maximum lateness* and *minimizing the number of tardy treatments*.

Example: Operating room is another good example of single server environments in healthcare. Scheduling surgeries must consider very expensive resources involved in this operation: the cost of rooms, surgeons, and anesthesiologists. Also, operating rooms are considered to be the hospitals' engines (Pinedo, 2009, p. 292) because surgeries drive the demand for Intensive Care Units (ICUs), doctors, nurses, beds, and so on.

Consider a situation in which there are five surgeries to be scheduled in an operating room of the emergency department. While each surgery must be completed as soon as possible, the surgeon has indicated the time when the surgery must be completed, or the patient may have further complications or his life is in danger. For example, the surgery for the first patient must be completed within 190 minutes; the surgery for the second patient must be completed within 170 minutes, and so on. Also, surgery time is estimated based on the nature of the surgery and patient's age as shown in Table 3.

Solution: A solution to this scheduling problem is shown in Table 4. The upper part of this table indicates scheduling results if patients are assigned to the operating room based on their arrival order (FCFS). In this pattern, there will be three late completions of surgeries and the maximum lateness is 200. As shown earlier, there are two approaches to improving the schedule. When the goal is to *minimize maximum lateness*, then the EDD rule is the best. The middle part of Table 4 indicates scheduling according to the EDD

Table 3. Operating and due times for each patient

Patient	1	2	3	4	5
Operating Time (in minutes)	60	90	70	70	40
Due Time (in minutes)	190	170	210	90	180

heuristic. The best sequence is {4, 2, 5, 1, 3} and maximum lateness is reduced to 120 minutes.

However, the EDD rule still allows three surgeries not able to be completed on time. The *AT-UT algorithm* can be applied. Patients 4 and 2 can be positioned first and second in the sequence with both surgeries being completed on time. Putting patient 5 into third position causes problems. The surgery completion time will be 200 minutes whereas its due time is 180 minutes. The *AT-UT algorithm* requires that the patient with the largest surgery time among those three patients

Table 4. Comparison between FCFS, EDD, and EDD & AT-UT

Patient Scheduling Using FCFS Rule					
Patient	1	2	3	4	5
Operating Time(in minutes)	60	90	70	70	40
Due Time (in minutes)	190	170	210	90	180
Completion Time (in minutes)	60	150	220	290	330
Lateness (in minutes)	0	0	10	200	150
Maximum Lateness (in minutes)	200				
Number of Late Surgeries	3				
Patient Scheduling Using EDD Rule					
Patient	4	2	5	1	3
Operating Time(in minutes)	70	90	40	60	70
Due Time (in minutes)	90	170	180	190	210
Completion Time (in minutes)	70	160	200	260	330
Lateness (in minutes)	0	0	20	70	120
Maximum Lateness (in minutes)	120				
Number of Late Surgeries	3				
Patient Scheduling Using AT-UT Algorithm					
Patient	5	1	3	4	2
Operating Time(in minutes)	40	60	70	70	90
Due Time (in minutes)	180	190	210	90	170
Completion Time (in minutes)	40	100	170	240	330
Lateness (in minutes)	0	0	0	150	160
Maximum Lateness (in minutes)	160				
Number of Late Surgeries	2				

be removed from the sequence (AT) and placed into the UT set. As such, patient 2 with operating time of 90 minutes is deleted from the schedule and patients 4 and 5 remain in the first and second positions. If patient 1 is now placed in the third position following patient 5, it is completed on time at 170 minutes. However, if patient 3 follows patient 1 in the fourth spot, it is completed late (240) when the due time for this patient is 210. The algorithm then requires that job 4, with the largest processing time be removed from the scheduled spots. So the optimal schedule is {5, 1, 3, 4, 2}. This schedule has the minimum number of tardy completion (2).

Single Server Stochastic Model

In the previous section, processing times of medical treatments are assumed to be known and deterministic. However, in the healthcare practice, the scheduler must recognize that many treatments are random and the schedule must consider *expected* processing times. The stochastic counterpart of the single server case is more complex. Due to the uncertain processing times, some treatments may be completed earlier than expected, whereas some others may be completed later. When a certain procedure finishes earlier than expected, then the server such as the operating room or the intensive care unit remains idle until the next scheduled appointment which results in resource under-utilization. On the other hand, if a procedure is completed later than expected, the next patient has to wait for the preceding patient and the procedure will start later than the original appointment time. This is the main source of patient waiting times and often causes overtime for other resources, such as surgeons, nurses, and technicians.

To avoid such inefficiencies, the scheduler must a) plan the best possible schedule of medical treatments, and b) dynamically revise the previously defined schedules to make sure that expected times and actual times do not differ significantly. Dynamic revision of appointment scheduling requires simple and practical scheduling heuristics. Fortunately, the algorithms for the stochastic models are similar to those discussed in the deterministic counterparts. Minimization of weighted completion time $\Sigma w_j C_j$, maximum lateness L_{max}, and number of tardy treatments ΣU_j that we discussed in the previous section are still relevant in the stochastic model.

Total Weighted Completion Time

The weighted completion time for the stochastic version of the single server model can be minimized when using the *weighted shortest expected case first (WSECF)* rule. This rule schedules the treatments in decreasing order of the ratio $w_j/E(X_j)$ where w_j is the weight (importance or seriousness) of the treatment and $E(X_j)$ is the expected time of medical treatment for patient *j*.

Example: Consider the set of surgeries to be scheduled in the operating room as shown in Table 5. The processing times for each surgery are random variables.

Solution: As shown in Table 5, there will be different surgeons assigned to each surgery and they will charge different hourly rates. In this situation, the weight or priority is the hourly

Table 5. Physicians' rates and expected surgery times

Surgery	1	2	3	4	5	6
Physician Rate	$100	$900	$600	$400	$400	$800
Expected Operating Times (in hours)	0.5	1	1	0.8	0.7	1.2

surgeon's rate. The goal of the scheduler here is to minimize surgeons' idle time, and assuming that doctors are available at the beginning of their shift (emergency shift), the sooner the surgery is completed the less idle time.

Table 6 compares the *FCFS* rule with *WSECF*. In the upper part, when the FCFS rule is used, the expected value for the total weighted completion time is $9,980. This amount represents the total payments to all surgeons for all surgeries. The lower part of Table 6 indicates the new schedule according to the *WSECF* rule, which leads to the following schedule of surgeries: {2, 4, 5, 3, 6, 1} for a total weighted completion time of $8540 and the emergency room is expected to save $1,440.

Due Date Related Scheduling Model

Consider the single case server where treatment times have arbitrary distributions and deterministic due dates. The EDD rule minimizes expected maximum lateness for the single server stochastic problem, just as in the deterministic counterpart. Also, the AT-UT heuristic minimizes the expected number of late treatments.

Example: It is now 10:00 AM and the scheduler of the emergency room has received several surgeries to be scheduled. The on-call physician has indicated due times when each surgery must be completed and their expected processing times as shown in Table 7. Treatments have arbitrary distributions of processing times but deterministic due dates.

Table 6. Comparison between FCFS and WSECF

Surgery Scheduling Using FCFS Rule						
Surgery	1	2	3	4	5	6
Physician Rate (wj)	$100.00	$900.00	$600.00	$400.00	$400.00	$800.00
Expected Treatment Times (pj)	0.50	1.00	1.00	0.80	0.70	1.20
E(wj/pj)	$200.00	$900.00	$600.00	$500.00	$571.43	$666.67
Expected Completion Time	0.50	1.50	2.50	3.30	4.00	5.20
Expected Physician Fee	$50.00	$ 1,350.00	$ 1,500.00	$ 1,320.00	$ 1,600.00	$ 4,160.00
Expected Total Physician Fee	$50.00 + $ 1,350.00 + $1,500.00 + $1,320.00 + $1,600.00 +$4,160.00 = $9,980.00					
Surgery Scheduling Using WSECF Rule						
Surgery	2	4	5	3	6	1
Physician Rate (wj)	$ 900.00	$800.00	$600.00	$400.00	$400.00	$100.00
Expected Treatment Times (pj)	1.00	1.20	1.00	0.70	0.80	0.50
E(wj/pj)	$ 900.00	$666.67	$600.00	$571.43	$500.00	$200.00
Expected Completion Time	1.00	2.20	3.20	3.90	4.70	5.20
Expected Physician Fee	$ 900.00	$ 1,760.00	$ 1,920.00	$ 1,560.00	$ 1,880.00	$520.00
Expected Total Physician Fee	$900.00 + $1,760.00 + $1,920.00 + $1,560.00 + $1,880.00 + $520.00 = $8,540.00					

Table 7. Operating and due times for each patient

Surgery	1	2	3	4	5
Operating Time (in hours)	0.5	1.0	1.5	3.0	2.0
Due Time	11:00 AM	10:30 AM	4:00 PM	12:00 PM	11:00 AM

Solution: The solution to this problem is shown in Table 8 and is similar to the deterministic counterpart of single server scheduling. This case demonstrates again how different scheduling heuristics provide different optimal solutions for given objective functions. The upper part of Table 8 shows scheduling on a FCFS rule. The maximum lateness for this solution is 7 hours and 3 surgeries are completed after the due time. The EDD rule is very efficient in this situation. Although all 5 surgeries are completed late, there is a significant reduction in the maximum lateness (4 hours).

When applying the AT-UT algorithm, the first surgery to be placed in the first spot according to the EDD rule is surgery 2. However, this surgery

Table 8. Comparison between FCFS, EDD, and EDD & AT-UT

Surgery Scheduling Using FCFS Rule					
Surgery	1	2	3	4	5
Operating Time	0.5	1.0	1.5	3.0	2.0
Due Time	11:00 AM	10:30 AM	4:00 PM	12:00 PM	11:00 AM
Completion Time	10:30 AM	11:30 AM	1:00 PM	4:00 PM	6:00 PM
Lateness	0.00	1.00	0.00	4.00	7.00
Maximum Lateness	7				
Number of Late Surgeries	3				
Surgery Scheduling Using EDD Rule					
Surgery	2	1	5	4	3
Operating Time	1.0	0.5	2.0	3.0	1.5
Due Time	10:30 AM	11:00 AM	11:00 AM	12:00 PM	4:00 PM
Completion Time	11:00 AM	11:30 AM	1:30 PM	4:30 PM	6:00 PM
Lateness	0.5	0.5	2.5	4.5	2
Maximum Lateness	4.5				
Number of Late Surgeries	5				
Surgery Scheduling Using AT-UT Algorithm					
Surgery	1	3	2	5	4
Operating Time	0.5	1.5	1.0	2.0	3.0
Due Time	11:00 AM	4:00 PM	10:30 AM	11:00 AM	12:00 PM
Completion Time	10:30 AM	12:00 PM	1:00 PM	3:00 PM	6:00 PM
Lateness	0.0	0.0	2.5	4.0	6.0
Maximum Lateness	6.0				
Number of Late Surgeries	3				

will be tardy since it is now 10:00 AM, the surgery must be completed before 10:30 AM, and the surgery itself lasts 1 hour. The scheduler sends this patient to another surgery room and places surgery 1 in the first spot. This surgery is due at 11:00 AM and will be completed at 10:30 AM. Next is surgery 5. It will be tardy, and since surgery 5 has the largest expected processing time, it is moved to another surgery room. The same process occurs with surgery 4. Surgery 3 is finally placed in the second spot and it is not tardy.

SCHEDULING PARALLEL SERVER HEALTHCARE SERVICES

The parallel server scheduling model is a generalization of the single server. The occurrence of similar (parallel) workstations with similar operating characteristics is common. Examples of such situations include a series of vaccination stations, an outpatient clinic with many available doctors, hospital beds, and ICUs.

Parallel Server Deterministic Model

In this section, parallel server models with the following two objective functions are considered: the minimization of *makespan* and the *total completion time*. When dealing with servers in parallel, *makespan* becomes a very important indicator of operational efficiency. Minimization of *makespan* ensures that the set of medical treatments are completed as early as possible. Assuming the same arrival time, *total completion time* will, on the other hand, be an indirect indicator of patient waiting times. The second scheduling goal is important because studies show that patient waiting times are directly correlated with patient satisfaction.

Minimizing Makespan

Minimization of *makespan* in a parallel server environment is of special interest for the healthcare practitioner. It not only minimizes the time when the last patient leaves the system but also has the effect of balancing the load over various servers. In the parallel server environment the *Longest Case First (LCF)* rule is recommended (Graham, 1969). According to this rule, if there are m treatment stations the m longest processing treatments are assigned at the start of the scheduling period. After that, once a station is freed, the longest unscheduled treatment is assigned to that station. The *LCF* rule will generally place the shortest treatments toward the end of the scheduling period where they can be used for load balancing. It is important to note that this heuristic does not guarantee the minimum possible *makespan*; however, it can be proved that it guarantees a very good solution (Pinedo, 1995).

Example: Hospitals generally have more than one operating room. The collection of operating rooms in a healthcare center is sometimes called an operating theatre. Scheduling these theatres may be regarded as a parallel server scheduling problem. Daily schedule of four similar operating rooms is considered. There are nine surgeries and the surgery times, which also include setup times, are shown in Table 9.

Solution: When surgeries are assigned according to their arrival time (FCFS), the sequence is shown in Figure 2. The first four surgeries are assigned to the four operating rooms. The first operating room to be freed is OR2 and surgery 5 is assigned to this room. Continuing with this heuristic the *makespan* is 420.

Now, the LCF rule is implemented. The first four surgeries to be assigned in the four operating

Table 9. Surgery times for each patient (in minutes)

Patient	1	2	3	4	5	6	7	8	9
Operating Time	140	80	120	120	100	300	80	120	130

Figure 2. Surgery assignments according to the FCFS rule

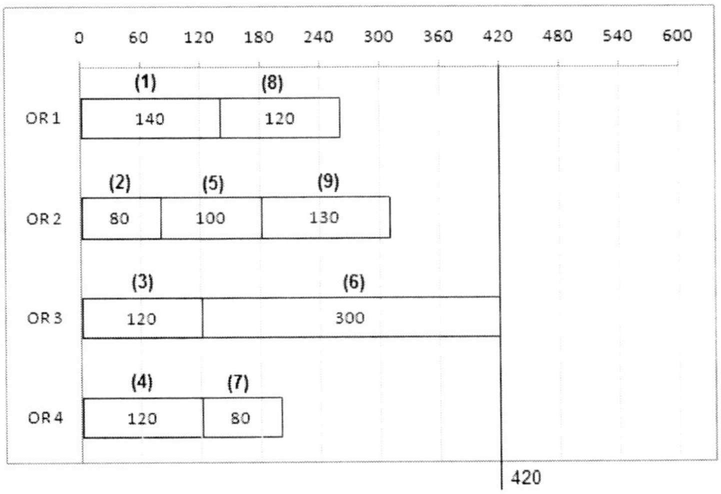

0
60
120
180
240
300
360
420
480
540
600
OR1
(1)
140
(8)
120
OR2
(2)
80
(5)
100
(9)
130
OR3
(3)
120
(6)
300
OR4
(4)
120
(7)
80
420

rooms are surgeries {6, 1, 9, 3}. Operating room OR4 is the first room to become available and the surgery with the next longest operating time, surgery 4, is assigned to this room. Then, at time 130 OR3 becomes available and surgery 8 is assigned there. Once all surgeries are assigned based on the LCF rule, the *makespan* is 320.

As shown in Figure 3, the LCF rule provides a shorter *makespan* for the *many* parallel server environments. In addition, a shorter *makespan* provides better resource utilization. For example, the FCFS rule has an overall idle time of 490. Specifically for each operating room, idle time in minutes is:

OR1: 420 – (140 + 120) = 160
OR2: 420 – (80 + 100 +130) = 110
OR3: 420 – (120 + 300) = 0
OR4: 420 – (120 + 80) = 220

Figure 3. Surgery assignments according to the LCF rule

0
60
120
180
240
300
360
420
480
540
600
OR1
(6)
300
OR2
(1)
140
(5)
100
(7)
80
OR3
(9)
130
(8)
120
OR4
(3)
120
(4)
120
(2)
80
320

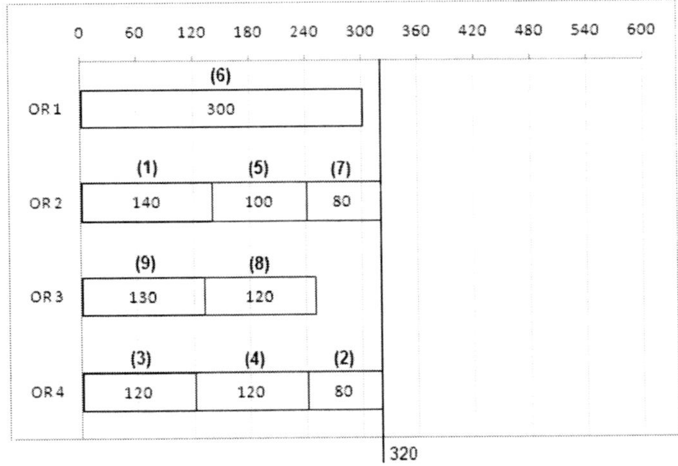

Table 10. Surgery times for emergency patients (in minutes)

Patient	1	2	3	4	5	6	7	8	9	10	11	12
Operating Time	120	80	40	120	100	60	80	60	60	50	120	130

On the other side, the LCF rule has an overall idle time of only 90 minutes and for each operating room the idle time in minutes is:

OR1: 320 – (300) = 20
OR2: 320 – (140 + 100 +80) = 0
OR3: 320 – (130 + 120) = 70
OR4: 320 – (120 + 120+ 80) = 0

Less idle time means better utilization of operating rooms and other resources such as doctors and nurses. The LCF rule provides the best utilization of resources, a shorter *makespan*, and a balanced load between medical stations. However, such a rule is not intended to minimize patient processing times and as a result does not necessarily minimize patients' waiting times. The next section discusses the Shortest Case First rule which tends to minimize patient waiting times.

Minimizing Total Completion Time

As mentioned in the single server case, total completion time is calculated as the sum of completion times and is also known by the practitioners as the *flow time*. If there are n patients to be treated in an m server environment and if each treatment lasts p_j, then the total completion time is calculated as ΣCj, *where* $C_j = p(1) + p(2) \ldots + p(j)$.

It is shown that the *Shortest Case First (SCF)* rule is optimal for this scheduling model (see Pinedo, 1995, pp. 79-80). According to the *SCF* rule patients need to be ordered in the increasing order of treatment times.

Example: Consider an emergency department at a local hospital with 5 surgery rooms. The goal of the scheduler is to minimize total patient treatment time. Processing times for each surgery are estimated and shown in Table 10:

Solution: Figure 4 shows patient assignments according to their arrival time, FCFS. The first five surgeries are assigned to each operating room. The first operating room to be freed is OR3 and surgery for patient 6 is assigned in this room. Then, OR2 becomes available and surgery for patient 7 is assigned there. Continuing in this heuristic (FCFS), the total completion time in minutes for all twelve patients is:

120+170+80+160+40+100+160+120+240+100 +160+290 = 1740

Now, the SCF rule is implemented. As shown in Figure 5, the first five surgeries to be assigned in the five operating rooms are surgeries {3, 10, 6, 8, 9}. Operating room OR1 is the first room to become available and the surgery with the next shortest operating time, surgery 7, is assigned in this room. Then, at time 50 room OR2 becomes available and surgery 2 is assigned there. When all surgeries are assigned based on the SCF rule, the total completion time in minutes for all patients is:

40+120+240+50+130+260+60+160+60+180+6 0+180 = 1540.

Parallel Server Stochastic Model

Consider the stochastic counterpart of the models discussed in the previous section. As processing times become random, the scheduler must use *expected* processing times. In general, as the number of treatment stations increases, the complexity of the scheduling model increases. Although mod-

Figure 4. Surgery assignments according to the FCFS rule

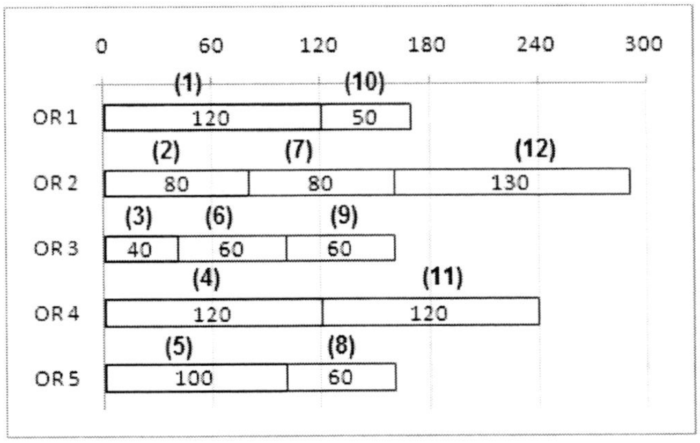

0 60 120 180 240 300
(1) (10)
OR 1 120 50
(2) (7) (12)
OR 2 80 80 130
(3) (6) (9)
OR 3 40 60 60
(4) (11)
OR 4 120 120
(5) (8)
OR 5 100 60

els become more complex, the same principle is suggested: the scheduler must a) plan the best possible schedule of medical treatments, and b) must revise the previously defined schedules continuously. For simplicity, the discussion of the stochastic parallel server scheduling is limited to **two** servers.

Minimizing Expected Makespan

Consider two treatment stations with similar processing characteristics. There are n patients and processing time for each patient is a random variable X_j that is exponentially distributed. Treatments are placed in a list and the first two treatments in the list are assigned to each station at time *0*. Once a station becomes free, the next treatment in the list is assigned to that station. The goal is to identify the order of treatments in the list so the expected value of makespan is minimized. In order to minimize the expected makespan, the *longest expected case first (LECF)* rule is suggested. This heuristic works well for *many* stations and is optimal for two stations when treatment times are assumed to follow exponential distribution.

An illustration of this case is already provided when the deterministic counterpart is discussed earlier in the chapter. The LECF algorithm is the

Figure 5. Surgery assignments according to the SCF rule

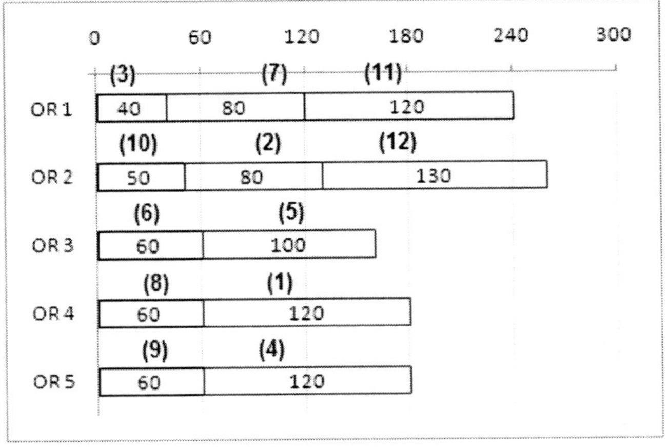

same as the LCF rule with the only difference that data shown in Table 9 are assumed to represent the *expected* processing times for the surgeries.

Minimizing Expected Number of Late Treatments

Assume that n treatments with random processing times (X_j) are to be scheduled in *two* stations. Treatment times have arbitrary distributions and due dates are known and deterministic. The goal is to minimize the expected number of treatments which are completed after the due date. This problem is significantly hard because the actual realization of processing times and due dates are not known a priori. However, a practical heuristic for such situations can be implemented by modifying the *earliest due date (EDD)* algorithm which is suggested for the single server counterpart. As a reminder, in the single server case, if a patient could not be scheduled within the due date then the patient may be sent to another facility. In our case, the next facility is replaced by the next available treatment station. Here are the steps of the algorithm:

- **Step 1:** *Place all incoming treatments in a list of accepted treatments (AT) in increasing order of due dates.*
- **Step 2:** *Continue to update the list of AT as new treatments arrive using the same EDD rule.*
- **Step 3:** *Add treatments to the first station (k=1) according to the order from list AT.*
- **Step 4:** *If the inclusion of a certain treatment results in this treatment being late, the scheduled treatment in station k with the largest processing time is removed from machine k and placed in station k+1. If station k+1 cannot accommodate this treatment, attempt to accommodate treatment in the next station until k=m. If treatment cannot be accommodated in any station, then place treatment into list UT so the patient can be sent to another facility.*
- **Step 5:** *Continue Steps 2 through 4 until no more treatments are waiting in list AT.*

Example: Consider a set of surgeries with arbitrary distribution of treatment times and deterministic due dates. These times are shown in Table 11. There are two surgery rooms available.

Solution: The solution to this problem is shown in Tables 12, 13, and 14. The performance of the FCFS rule (Table 12) is compared to the performance of the EDD heuristic (Table 13), and to the performance of the proposed EDD/AT-UT algorithm (Table 14). According to the FCFS rule, surgeries are scheduled in the following order: {1, 4, 6} for Operating Room 1 (OR1) and {2, 3, 5, 7, 8, 9} for Operating Room 2 (OR2). As shown in Table 12, when sequenced according to the FCFS rule, three surgeries {6, 8, 9} are completed late. When the surgeries are selected according to EDD or the combination of EDD and the AT-UT algorithm, only one surgery {6} is completed late.

SCHEDULING FLOW SHOPS HEALTHCARE SERVICES

In many healthcare facilities a number of treatments have to be performed on every patient.

Table 11. Expected operating times and due times (in hours)

Patient	1	2	3	4	5	6	7	8	9
Operating Time	1.4	0.8	1.2	1.2	1	3	0.8	1.2	1.3
Due Time	6	5	8	5	3	5	6	3	2

Table 12. Solution for FCFS Algorithm

Patient	**1**	**2**	**3**	**4**	**5**	**6**	7	**8**	**9**			
Operating Time	1.4	0.8	1.2	1.2	1	3	0.8	1.2	1.3			
Due Time	6	5	8	5	3	5	6	3	2			
	Surgery Number	Operating Time	Surgery Number	Operating Time	Surgery Number	Operating Time	Surgery Number	Operating Time	Surgery Number	Operating Time	Surgery Number	Operating Time
OR1	**1**	1.4	**4**	1.2	**6**	3						
OR2	**2**	0.8	**3**	1.2	**5**	1	**7**	0.8	**8**	1.2	**9**	1.3
OR1	6	1.4	5	2.6	5	5.6						
OR2	5	0.8	8	2	3	3	6	3.8	3	5	2	6.3
	Due Time	Completion Times	Due Time	Completion Time	Due Time	Completion Times	Due Time	Completion Times	Due Time	Completion Times	Due Time	Completion Times
Late Surgery	Total Number of Late Surgeries =											3
OR1					Late							
OR2									Late		Late	

Table 13. Solution for EDD Algorithm

Patient	**9**	**5**	**8**	**4**	**2**	**6**	7	**1**	**3**			
Operating Time	1.3	1	1.2	1.2	0.8	3	0.8	1.4	1.2			
Due Time	2	3	3	5	5	5	6	6	8			
	Surgery Number	Operating Time	Surgery Number	Operating Time	Surgery Number	Operating Time	Surgery Number	Operating Time	Surgery Number	Operating Time	Surgery Number	Operating Time
OR1	**9**	1.3	**4**	1.2	**6**	3						
OR2	**5**	1	**8**	1.2	**2**	0.8	**7**	0.8	**1**	1.4	**3**	1.2
OR1	2	1.3	5	2.5	5	5.5						
OR2	3	1	3	2.2	5	3	6	3.8	6	5.2	8	6.4
	Due Time	Completion Times	Due Time	Completion Time	Due Time	Completion Times	Due Time	Completion Times	Due Time	Completion Times	Due Time	Completion Times
Late Surgery	Total Number of Late Surgeries =											1
OR1					Late							
OR2												

Table 14. Solution for EDD & AT-UT Algorithm

Patient	9	5	8	4	2	6	7	1	3			
Operating Time	1.3	1	1.2	1.2	0.8	3	0.8	1.4	1.2			
Due Time	2	3	3	5	5	5	6	6	8			
	Surgery Number	Operating Time	Surgery Number	Operating Time	Surgery Number	Operating Time	Surgery Number	Operating Time	Surgery Number	Operating Time	Surgery Number	Operating Time
OR1	9	1.3	4	1.2	7	0.8	3	1.2				
OR2	5	1	8	1.2	2	0.8	1	1.4	6	3		
OR1	2	1.3	5	2.5	6	3.3	8	4.5				
OR2	3	1	3	2.2	5	3	6	4.4	5	7.4		
	Due Time	Completion Times	Due Time	Completion Time	Due Time	Completion Times	Due Time	Completion Times	Due Time	Completion Times		
Late Surgery	Total Number of Late Surgeries =											1
OR1												
OR2									Late			

Often, these treatments must be performed on all patients in the same order, which implies that patients have to follow the same route. Medical stations or servers are assumed to be set up in series and the environment is referred to as a *flow shop*. Optimization of flow shop models in healthcare is primarily concerned with the utilization of workstations. As such, the makespan is a very important objective function in the following flow shop models.

Dual Server Deterministic Model: Johnson's Rule to Minimize Makespan

In the early days of operations research, S.M. Johnson offered the rule that minimizes the makespan for a flow shop model with two stations (Johnson, 1954). A potential environment where Johnson's rule can be applied is as follows: there are n patients to be scheduled in a treatment which consists of two stages. Processing time of patient j in the first stage is p_{1j} and in the second stage is p_{2j}. Johnson's rule is also known as SPT(1)-LPT(2) which in the case of healthcare scheduling is the same as SCF(1)-LCF(2). Here are the steps to implement the SCF(1)-LCF(2) heuristic as provided by Johnson (1954):

- **Step 1:** *List the treatment times for each patient on both stations.*
- **Step 2:** *Select the shortest treatment time.*
- **Step 3:** *If the shortest time is for the first station, assign the patient first; if it is for the second station, assign the patient last. In case of a tie, assign the patient first.*
- **Step 4:** *Repeat Steps 2 and 3 for each remaining patient until the schedule is complete.*

Example: A physician and her nurse are running behind with their schedule in the Saturday clinic. They have been seeing their patients on a FCFS basis. It is 5:00 PM and the clinic is closed for the day. However, there are still five patients in the waiting room. Typically a patient goes through a two-stage routine. First, the patient is seen by the nurse who gathers information about the patient's condition, measures body temperature, records blood pressure, and asks about previous medications or related questions. Second, the patient is seen by the physician who examines the patient further, recommends treatment, or prescribes a medication. Table 15 indicates the expected times for each patient:

Figure 6 indicates a Gantt representation of the solution when patients are scheduled on a FCFS basis. Figure 7 indicates the solution for the same group of patients when they are scheduled according to Johnson's Rules. FCFS scheduling leads to an overall makespan of 155 minutes and the physician is idle for 60 minutes. Patients B and C will have to wait 5 minute between the nurse and the physician. On the other side, Johnson's Rules lead to an overall makespan of 130 minutes, the physician is idle for 35 minutes, and patient C will wait 5 minutes.

Table 15. Expected times for each patient (in minutes)

Patient	Nurse	Physician
A	20	10
B	5	25
C	25	15
D	35	15
E	40	30

According to Johnson's Rules, Patient B has the overall lowest processing time (5), and since this time belongs to the first stage, this patient is placed in the first spot. Patient A has the next shortest treatment time (10) in the second stage, and since this time belongs to the second stage, it is placed as late as possible, in the last spot. The next shortest treatment time (15) belongs to patients C (stage 2) and D (stage 2). Since the first stage of patient C is shorter than the first stage of patient D (25<35), patient D is placed in the latest available position, just ahead of patient A. Then, C is placed ahead of patient D, which leaves patient E in the second position and the optimal sequence is {B, E, C, D, A}. This sequence will ensure that the physician and her nurse complete their day at the clinic as early as possible.

Many Servers Deterministic Model: Critical Path Method

There are no analytical methods that can be used to find an optimal schedule for a *many* server flow shop model. However, it is suggested that the scheduler identify the bottleneck in the flow shop and try to improve the flow of patients using Johnson's Rules. Once a good schedule is generated, the critical path method can be used

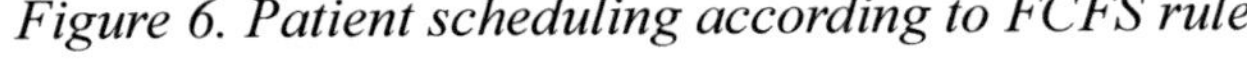
Figure 6. Patient scheduling according to FCFS rule

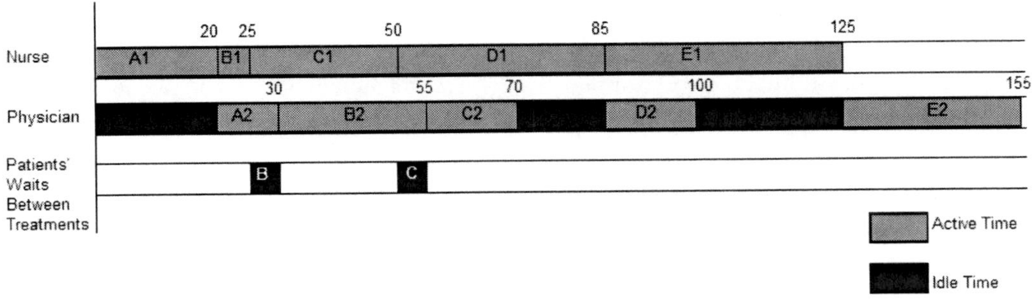

Figure 7. Patient scheduling according to Johnson's rules

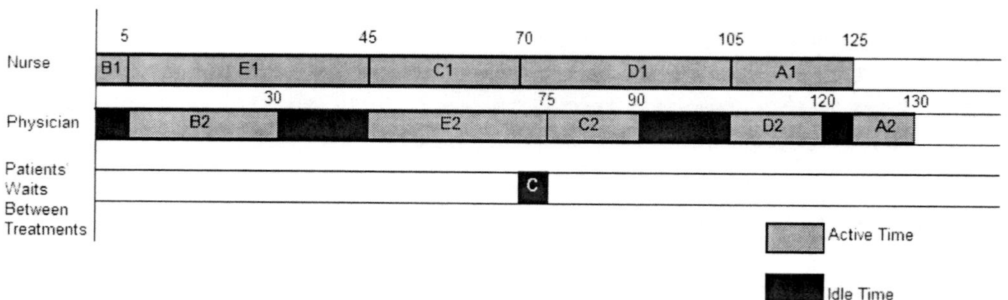

to identify critical treatments. The critical path of treatments in a healthcare flow shop with m stations is the sequence of treatments which forms the longest chain of treatments with no room for slack. Placing more resources in those critical activities can reduce the overall *makespan*.

The following presents a list of steps to follow when using the critical path method for scheduling n patients in **two** stations in a flow shop environment.

- **Step 1:** *Divide the workstations into two groups and apply Johnson's Rules to derive a sequence of patients.*
- **Step 2:** *Construct a network reflecting the precedence relationships.*
- **Step 3:** *Determine critical path and the makespan.*
- **Step 4:** *Create a Gantt chart to investigate those critical treatments and allocate additional resources to reduce makespan.*

Example: As indicated in the previous example, the physician and her nurse are able to schedule patients using Johnson's Rules and can minimize the makespan. However, the earliest possible time to complete seeing patients is 130 minutes. Since the nurse has no idle time, there may be a need to request additional nurses. Figure 8 shows the solution with two nurses and one physician. The overall *makespan* is now only 110 minutes and idle time for the physician is only 15 minutes. This solution will likely increase patients' wait times between two processes, from when they have seen the nurse until they see a physician. In the example above, patients C, A, and D wait for a total waiting time of 95 minutes.

Flow Shop Stochastic Models with Two Stations

Consider n patients to be treated for two procedures in workstation 1 and 2. The processing time of patient j in the first treatment is X_{1j}, exponentially distributed with rate λ_j. The processing time of patient j in the second treatment is X_{2j}, exponentially distributed with rate μ_j. Just like the deterministic counterpart, this model has a very simple solution when the objective function is the minimization of makespan. Pinedo (1995, p. 232) indicates that the optimal sequence can be achieved when patients are ordered in the decreasing order of $\lambda_j - \mu_j$.

Example: There are six patients for their annual physician checkup. Assume that the overall process has two major processes: (1) laboratory testing and waiting for the lab results, and (2) physician checkup and consultation. Also, assume that the checkup and consultation always follows the laboratory testing its results. Based on previously recorded data, it is anticipated that these two processes will follow exponential distributions.

Figure 8. Using critical path method to improve patient scheduling

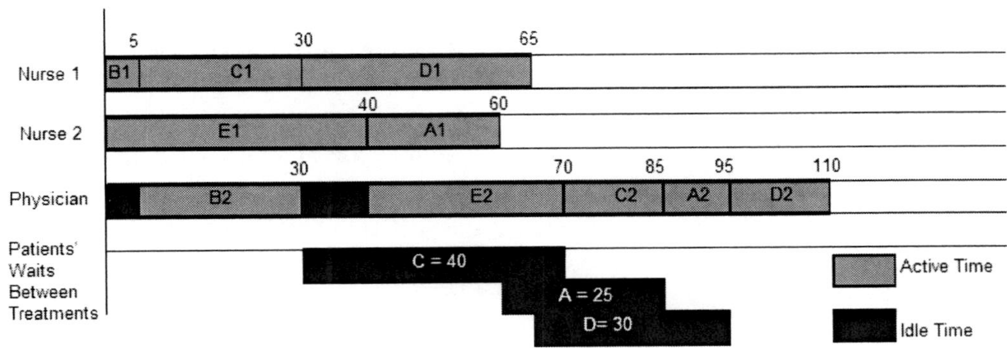

Specifically, the expected rate for each patient for each process is shown in Table 16.

As indicated in Table 17, applying the decreasing order of $\lambda_j - \mu_j$ leads to the following sequence {4, 1, 3, 5, 6, 2}. This sequence is expected to reduce the makespan when both sets of treatment times are exponential distributions. For practical reasons, the decreasing order of means can be used even when the sets of treatment times are not exponential.

SCHEDULING OPEN AND JOB SHOPS HEALTHCARE SERVICES

This section deals with multi-treatment models, which are different from the flow shop models discussed in the previous section. In the flow shop model, all patients follow the same route. However, in practice patients are often given different combinations of treatments as decided by their physician. This situation is referred to as *open shop* models, and when the treatments are fixed but not the same for each patient, the model is referred as *job shop*.

Minimizing Makespan in Two Stations: Deterministic

Consider a situation when n patients require two treatments. A patient can receive treatment 1 or 2 in any order; the scheduler may determine the route. For example, patients arrive at the laboratory clinic to perform two types of tests. Processing times for each patient for each test may vary. The order in which tests are taken is not important. In such situations, an optimal scheduling heuristic exists and it is known as the *longest alternate*

Table 16. $\lambda - \mu$ for each patient

Patient	Stage 1 (λ)	Stage 2 (μ)	λ−μ
1	20	10	10
2	5	25	-20
3	25	15	10
4	35	15	20
5	40	30	10
6	65	65	0

Table 17. Solution using λ-μ

Patient	Stage 1 (λ)	Stage 2 (μ)	λ−μ
4	35	15	20
1	20	10	10
3	25	15	10
5	40	30	10
6	65	65	0
2	5	25	-20

case first (LACF) rule (Pinedo, 1995). According to this rule, whenever a workstation is freed, the scheduler must select the patient waiting for treatment with the longest treatment time in the other workstation (Pinedo, 1995, pp. 120-121).

More often, patients have to be treated in a predetermined route. Some patients have to go first through workstation 1 and then go through workstation 2, while some other patients have to follow the opposite route. In this situation, referred to as *job shop*, and similar to the LACF rule, patients must be processed as follows: patients who have been treated in workstation 1 have the lowest priority in workstation 2, and vice versa; patients who have been treated in workstation 2 are given lowest priority in station 1. The remaining question is: how should a starting sequence be selected before applying the LACF rule? In this situation, the SCF(1)-LCF(2) rule is suggested.

Example: Consider the same set of patients as in the previous in the example of the Flow Shop Stochastic Models with Two Stations when six patients needed to be scheduled for the annual physician checkup and laboratory testing (Table 16). There are two changes in the assumptions of the previous example: treatment times are deterministic and there are no precedence constraints. The second assumption implies that patients can see the physician or perform the laboratory test in any order as determined by the nurse. Once the SCF(1)-LCF(2) rule is applied the sequence of patients is {2, 6, 5, 3, 4, 1}. Following this sequence, patient 2 is assigned in first for treatment 1 and patient 6 is assigned first for treatment 2. Automatically, patient 2 will be the last one to be assigned for treatment 2 and patient 6 will be the last one to be assigned for treatment 1. The application of the LACF rule suggests the {2, 5, 3, 1, 4, 6} sequence of patients for the laboratory test (treatment 1) and {6, 4, 1, 3, 5, 2} for the physician checkup (treatment 2). This solution will reduce the makespan from 255 minutes (according to FCFS) to 190. This solution is shown in Figure 9.

Minimizing Makespan in Two Stations: Stochastic

The algorithms suggested for the stochastic open shop models are different from the deterministic model. Instead of the LACF rule, the literature suggests that in order to minimize makespan, priority must be given to those patients that have not yet undergone treatment on either machine. This rule is known as the *longest expected remaining case first (LERCF)* rule.

The algorithm for the stochastic job shop is an extension of the heuristic suggested for the stochastic flow shop model. Recall that in the flow shop case, the rules suggest selection of the job with the longest difference of processing expected times in each workstation ($\lambda_j - \mu_j$). Using the same principle, the scheduler of a job shop in a

Figure 9. Patient scheduling according to the LACF rule

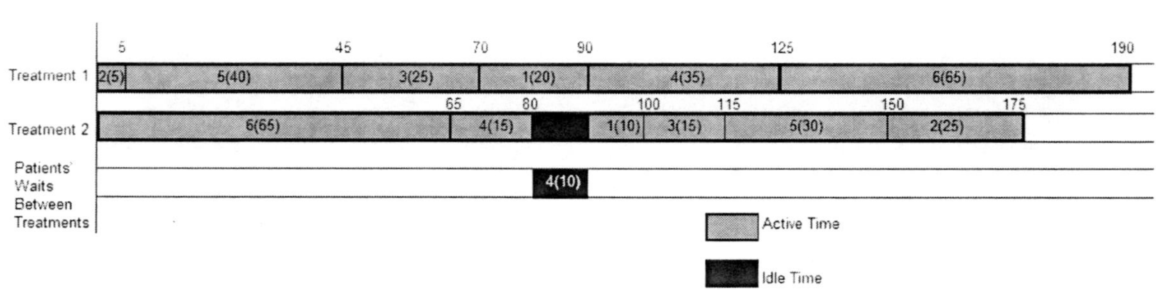

stochastic environment must follow the algorithm described below:

Create two sets of patients: J12 is the set of patients have to first undergo treatment 1, and J21 is the set of patients have to first undergo treatment 2. When workstation 1 is freed, the scheduler must select from J12 the patient with the highest $\lambda_j - \mu_j$. *If all patients from J12 are treated in workstation 1, then the scheduler may assign any patient from J21. When workstation 2 is freed, the scheduler must select from J21 the patient with the highest* $\lambda_j - \mu_j$. *If all patients from J21 are treated in workstation 2, then the scheduler may assign any patient from J12.*

Example: An emergency department situation can be used to illustrate the above algorithm. Arriving patients can see the doctor or perform laboratory work in any order as determined by the triage station. Some patients do not need to perform laboratory work. Also, it is still assumed that treatment times of these two processes follow exponential distributions and the expected rates for each patient for each process are shown in Table 18.

First, two sets J12 = {1, 2, 4, 5, 7, 10} and J21 = {1, 2, 3, 4, 5, 6, 7, 8, 9, 10} are created. Patient 4 with the highest $\lambda_j - \mu_j = 40$ is assigned first for laboratory work. Following the highest priority of $\lambda_j - \mu_j$, patients are assigned for laboratory work in the following order {4, 7, 1, 5, 2, 10}. Similarly, patients are selected for checkup according to the highest $\lambda_j - \mu_j$ which leads to the following sequence {4, 7, 1, 5, 2, 10, 3, 6, 8, 9}.

CONCLUSION AND IMPLEMENTATION CONCERNS

A summary of scheduling rules discussed in this chapter is provided in Table 19. This table lists healthcare scheduling environments, the objective functions, and appropriate scheduling heuristics for a series of scheduling problems, from single server models to many server models, from deterministic problems to stochastic ones. It is hoped that the decision maker will investigate these scheduling problems and implement the suggested heuristics in similar scheduling problems encountered in the everyday operations of healthcare systems.

The techniques described in this chapter are based on mathematical models. An attempt is made to offer practical solutions to complicated healthcare scheduling environments. The scheduler must be aware that some assumptions may not be completely accurate in real world healthcare situations. This chapter favors the *practicality* of the algorithm over the *accuracy* of optimal solutions. In this context, a few assumptions are discussed and practical recommendations of how to deal with them are provided:

Patient Arrivals

- **Assumption:** Suggested algorithms assume that there are *n* patients to be scheduled and those patients are present at the beginning of the scheduling period. In real situations new patients are added continuously. Appointment scheduling has to be

Table 18. Expected Times for Each Patient in the ER (in minutes)

Patient	Lab Work	Checkup	λ-μ
1	20	10	10
2	5	25	-20
3		15	
4	55	15	40
5	40	30	10
6		65	
7	45	25	20
8		40	
9		45	
10	25	80	-55

Table 19. Summary of healthcare scheduling environments and suggested heuristics

Scheduling Environment	Scheduling Goal(s)	Suggested Algorithm
Single Server: Deterministic	Minimization of Total Weighted Completion Times	Weighted Shortest Case First (WSCF)
	Minimization of Maximum Lateness	Earliest Due Date (EDD)
	Minimization of the Number of Late Treatments	Acceptable Treatments -Unacceptable Treatments (AT-UT)
Single Server: Stochastic	Minimization of Total Weighted Completion Times	Weighted Shortest Expected Case First (WSECF)
	Minimization of Maximum Lateness	Earliest Due Date (EDD)
	Minimization of the Number of Late Treatments	Acceptable Treatments -Unacceptable Treatments (AT-UT)
Parallel Server: Deterministic	Minimization of Makespan	Longest Case First (LCF)
	Minimization of Total Completion Time	Shortest Case First (SCF)
Parallel Server: Stochastic	Minimization of Expected Makespan	Longest Expected Case First (LECF)
	Minimization of Expected Number of Late Treatments	Combination of EDD and AT-UT
Flow Shop: Deterministic	Minimization of Makespan	Johnson's Rules (Dual Server Case)
		Combination of Johnson's Rules and Critical Path (Many Server Case)
Flow Shop: Stochastic	Minimization of Expected Makespan	Longest λ_j- μ_j First
Job Shop: Deterministic	Minimization of Makespan	Longest Alternate Case First (LACF)
Job Shop: Stochastic	Minimization of Expected Makespan	Longest Expected Remaining Case First (LERCF)

done with no complete information of the near future.

- **Recommendation:** Schedulers may need to plan for unexpected patient arrivals by allowing slack times in the appointment slots.

System Disruptions

- **Assumption:** Suggested models assume no changes in the system while patients are processed during the scheduling period. In practice, unexpected events occur and they require modifications in the existing schedule.
- **Recommendation:** There is a trade-off to be considered in this situation: continue with the existing schedule and achieve a less than expected good solution OR place additional time and effort to reschedule the system and achieve better solutions.

System Constraints

- **Assumptions:** Healthcare models in the real world are more complicated than those considered in this chapter. Treatment restrictions and medical constraints may be involved.
- **Recommendation:** The primary goal of scheduling techniques in healthcare is to increase utilization of medical equipment and human resources, such as doctors and nurses. However, if necessary, medical considerations must always supersede cost and efficiency concerns.

First Come First Served Approach

- **Assumptions:** The FCFS is the most popular scheduling heuristic, the one which equalizes patients' waiting times. This heuristic is also known as the "fair" scheduling rule and patients expect to be treated according to this rule. However, as the chapter indicates, FCFS is not necessarily as efficient as other heuristics offered by the literature and explained in the chapter.
- **Recommendation:** While FCFS is not an efficient rule, it does not contradict other scheduling rules. In general, if the medical stations are better utilized then they can process more patients and as such patient waiting times will be reduced. Many medical facilities operate under the following heuristics:
    - **Emergency cases first:** Emergency patients are always served first. In general, waiting patients will accept that an emergency patient is processed before them.
    - **FCFS:** While patients stay in the waiting area, it is recommended that patients are called in according to their arrival time.
    - **Suitable Scheduling Heuristic:** Once a nurse screens them, patients are seen by the doctor or called for treatment according to the most efficient scheduling heuristic as discussed in the models in this chapter.

While healthcare practitioners need to recognize the complexity of healthcare scheduling systems, they may use the provided framework as a practical tool for better scheduling techniques. In order to practically implement the various scheduling scenarios discussed in this chapter, the hospital or clinic scheduling staff could prepare templates using MS Excel. This will allow for easier implementation and faster scheduling calculations.

REFERENCES

Beliën, J. (2007). Exact and heuristic methodologies for scheduling in hospitals: Problems, formulations and algorithms. *4OR: A Quarterly Journal of Operations Research, 5*(2), 157-160.

Brandeau, M. L., Sainfort, F., & Pierskalla, W. P. (2004). *Operations reserach and health care-A handbook of methods and applications*. Springer.

Cardoen, B., Demeulemeester, E., & Beliën, J. (2010). Operating room planning and scheduling: A literature review. *European Journal of Operational Research, 201*(3), 921–932. doi:10.1016/j.ejor.2009.04.011

Conforti, D., Guerriero, F., & Guido, R. (2008). Optimization models for radiotherapy patient scheduling. *4OR: A Quarterly Journal of Operations Research, 6*(3), 263-278.

Denton, B., Viapiano, J., & Vogl, A. (2007). Optimization of surgery sequencing and scheduling decisions under uncertainty. *Health Care Management Science, 10*(1), 1–12. doi:10.1007/s10729-006-9005-4

Fei, H., Meskens, N., & Chu, C. (2010). A planning and scheduling problem for an operating theatre using an open scheduling strategy. *Computers & Industrial Engineering, 58*(2), 221–230. doi:10.1016/j.cie.2009.02.012

Graham, R. L. (1969). Bounds on multiprocessing timing anomalies. *SIAM Journal on Applied Mathematics, 17*, 263–269. doi:10.1137/0117039

Johnson, S. M. (1954). Optimal two- and three-stage production schedules with setup times included. *Naval Research Logistics Quarterly, 1*(1), 61–68. doi:10.1002/nav.3800010110

Ozcan, Y. A. (2005). *Quantitative methods in health care management*. San Francisco, CA: John Wiley & Sons.

Pinedo, M. (1995). *Scheduling: Theory, algorithms, and systems*. New Jersey: Prentice Hall, Inc.

Pinedo, M. L. (2009). *Planning and scheduling in manufacturing and services*. New York, NY: Springer. doi:10.1007/978-1-4419-0910-7

Smith, W. E. (1956). Various optimizers for single-stage production. *Naval Reserach Logistic Quarterly*, *3*(1-2), 59–66. doi:10.1002/nav.3800030106

Weiss, E. N. (1990). Models for determining estimated start times and case orderings in hospital operating rooms. *IIE Transactions*, *22*(2), 143–150. doi:10.1080/07408179008964166

Chapter 14
Appointment Order Outpatient Scheduling System with Consideration of Ancillary Services and Overbooking Policy to Improve Outpatient Experience

Yu-Li Huang
New Mexico State University, USA

ABSTRACT

Patient wait time and access to care have long been a recognized problem in modern outpatient healthcare delivery systems. In spite of all the efforts to develop appointment rules and policies, the problem of long patient waits persists. Despite the reasons, the fact remains that there are few implemented models for effective scheduling that consider patient wait times, physician idle time, overtime, ancillary service time, as well as individual no-show rate, and are generalized sufficiently to accommodate a variety of outpatient clinic settings. The goal of this chapter is to improve the quality and efficiency of healthcare delivery by developing a physician schedule that meets the clinical policies without overbooking using an innovative wait ratio concept, a patient arrival schedule from the physician schedule accounting for ancillary services, an evidence-based predictive model of no-show probability for individual patient, and a model-supported dynamic overbooking policy to reduce the negative impact of no-shows.

DOI: 10.4018/978-1-60960-872-9.ch014

INTRODUCTION

Patient wait time and access to care have long been a recognized problem in modern outpatient healthcare delivery systems which impact patient and medical staff productivity and stress, the quality and efficiency of the medical care, the cost of healthcare. Despite all the efforts to develop appointment rules and policies, the problem of long patient and appointment availability during a clinic day persists. Regardless of the reasons for this problem, there are few implemented models for effective scheduling that consider patient wait time, physician idle time, overtime, ancillary service time, as well as individual no-show rate and that are generalized sufficiently to accommodate a variety of outpatient health care settings.

The goals of this chapter are to improve healthcare delivery by reducing patient wait time and increasing access to care; and to allow physicians to see the desired number of patients, while providing quality care across various outpatient clinic settings and specialties. To accomplish this goal, the four specific aims of developing a scheduling system are:

1. To develop a physician treatment schedule by using a 'wait ratio' concept instead of the traditional cost ratio that best accommodates the variation in visit types, treatment time, and clinic constraints, without overbooking.
2. To develop patient arrival schedule, based on the physician treatment schedule, accounting for ancillary services required before physician's visits (such as x-rays) minimizing patient wait time and eliminating unnecessary first consultations by the physician.
3. To develop evidence-based overbooking policies by understanding the cause of patient no-show, using a predictive statistical model that can estimate the probability of no-show rate for any individual patient that incorporates the patient's characteristics, environmental concerns, and preference.
4. To incorporate a model-supported, dynamic overbooking policy into the scheduling system that minimizes the costs of patient wait, physician idle, and clinic overtime.

This chapter provides a step-by-step method for improving patient scheduling including data collection, determination of the best scheduled time interval for each visit type, creation of a physician schedule, a corresponding patient arrival schedule appropriate for required pre-activities such as x-ray and lab tests, and development of the evidence-based dynamic overbooking policies. The successful implementation of this approach will provide evidence to build a patient-centric outpatient environment, improving outpatient experience in terms of waiting and access to care.

By achieving the specific aims of this research, systemic wait times are expected to be reduced for both physician and patient and improve patient access to care by determining the most adequate treatment time interval for treating each patient type equally in terms of the 'wait ratio' under clinic constraints, taking into account any ancillary services required prior to physician's visit, and incorporating an overbooking policy that considers individual patient's characteristics and preferences. Access to care and efficiency of healthcare delivery will be improved, as well as the overall quality of healthcare. Since reduced patient wait times have the potential to reduce clinic and practitioner stress levels, turnover is expected to be reduced in the clinic, which will lead to improved overall quality of care. In short, the success of implementing the approach will improve the outpatient experience for both patients and medical staff and create outpatient clinics as healthier, more cost-efficient, and more approachable environments to ultimately improve the quality of care.

BACKGROUND

Patient wait time in outpatient health care delivery systems has been a long-recognized issue of reduced quality of care. Huang (1994) indicated patient satisfaction on waiting in an outpatient clinic is a crucial part of improving health service quality and efficiency. As competition has increased for limited health care dollars, efforts have been made to increase efficiency and reduce costs, yet only limited gains have been made in terms of reducing patient wait time. Ironically, one of the main strategies to decrease overall healthcare cost has been to shift traditionally inpatient services to an outpatient setting, effectively increasing the burden on outpatient facilities to efficiently manage health care delivery. Being able to reduce patient wait time and improve patient access to care in an outpatient facility by introducing a more effective scheduling scheme has become an important topic of quality of care.

The problem of limited access to healthcare due to patient no-show has also been recognized. Many studies report the no-show rate based on the location and clinic types as low as 10% (Warden, 1995; Casey et al., 2007; Corfield, Schizas, Noorani and Williams (2008). Deyo and Inui (1980) noted that broken appointment (no-show) rates generally range from 15-30% in general adult and pediatric clinics (primary care setting). Rust, Callups, Clark, Jones and Wilcox (1995) reported an even wider range of no-show rates, 3-80%, from public pediatric clinics. Hixon, Chapman and Nuovo (1999) reported no-show rates above 20% in a teaching clinic, which both reduces the educational opportunity in the residency program and the productivity of the clinic. The common impacts are reduced clinic efficiency, provider productivity, wasted medical resources, increased health care cost, and limited patient access to care. Patient no-shows create unexpected idle time for medical staff. These unanticipated idle times for a physician and support staff are virtually unrecoverable. Hence, developing a policy in a scheduling system to proactively identify and reduce the negative impact of no-shows becomes an important task to improve health-care delivery systems.

The evolution of the outpatient scheduling methods started in the 1950's. Bailey (1952) and Welch (1964) first proposed the individual appointment scheduling rules with fixed interval on the average service time. Then the block appointment rules (multiple-block systems) with fixed interval, two or more patients scheduled at the same time, were developed and studied (Blanco White and Pike, 1964; Soriano, 1966). Later on, Variable-block systems (different block sizes) were developed (Villegas, 1967; Rising, Baron, and Averill, 1973; Fries and Marathe, 1981). Ho and Lau (1992) proposed a more complicated individual block with variable interval. Since 1990, a number of studies have been developed and evaluated for appointment rules or policies for efficient scheduling and modeling the probability of no-shows (Ho and Lau, 1992; Ho, Lau and Li, 1995; Klassen and Rohleder, 1996; Yang, Lau and Quek, 1998; Vanden Bosch and Dietz, 2000; Harper and Gamlin, 2003; Cayirli, Veral and Rosen, 2006; Wijewickrama, 2006; Kaandorp and Koole, 2007). Despite the insights generated by research, the developed appointment rules (policies) do not seem to be broadly adopted by outpatient clinics because they are complex, difficult to follow, and include no clear explanation as to which rules are most appropriate in which type of outpatient environments. These researchers present the impact of no-shows on waiting but do not focus on how to reduce the negative impact of no-shows, per se. Also, actual case studies with implementation results are not available to support the feasibility of the theoretical appointment rules. This leaves a significant gap between the theoretical constructs and the realities of practical applications. Furthermore, regardless of how sophisticated the proposed appointment rules are or how significantly they have impacted the current scheduling systems, the variability in patient treatment time has not been addressed under clinical conditions. In essence, this simply means that patients are scheduled to accommodate the physician's schedule. The basic model of patient scheduling, employed by most of the approaches and models presented in the literature focuses on minimizing total cost using the cost ratio approach while still trying to accommodate variation in patient treatment time. However, by doing so, this inherently favors the reduction of physician idle time and often results in the inappropriate treatment time intervals. Moreover, to the best of our knowledge, virtually none of the research ever addresses clinic policy or constraints on a schedule, such as the time at which the last patient should be seen in a session or when the session should end.

Some approaches presented in the literature are case specific, which precludes generalization. One group used simulation approaches to design patient process for a specific clinic (Swisher, Jacobson, Jun and Balici, 2001; Guo, Wagner and West, 2003; Wijesickrama and Takakuwa, 2005). Those simulation studies, regardless of their focus, arrived at similar conclusions regarding the influence of patient flow and admission policies. Other studies have relied on trial and error to select the best schedule for a particular clinic from a range of possible solutions such as Meza (1998), Harper and Gamlin (2003), Klassen and Rohleder (2004). Other research resulted in the proposed Open Access approach using the philosophy of "doing today's work today" (Murray and Tantau, 1999; O'Hare and Corlett, 2004; Bundy, 2005; Giachetti, Centerno and Sundaram, 2005; O'Connor et al., 2006; Robinson and Chen, 2009; Liu et al., 2009; Phan and Brown, 2009). This approach seems to improve patient access and no-show rate, but practically burden patients in attempting to get appointments, which may drive away patients and leads to profit losses. Due to the nature of this approach, overtime is allowed to occur when the demands are high. This, in turn, increases the cost for clinics and burdens clinics' management. Mehrotra, Keehl-Markowitz and Ayanian (2008) studied the implementation of open access and find it is difficult to achieve the same-day access. Liu et al. (2009) concluded open access worked better when the patient load is relatively low. Open access fundamentally did not focus on reducing patient wait time, especially the wait time before seeing a physician, but exclusively attempted to fill up the clinic day so that the resources could be fully utilized. Similarly, some researchers suggest that overbooking would reduce physician idle time and increase profitability for healthcare providers (Kim and Giachetti, 2006; LaGanga and Lawrence, 2007; Kros et al, 2009). They focus on minimizing the total cost including physician idle time, overtime and patient wait time. They did not capture the likelihood of individual patient characteristics and conditions, thus their models inherently favor the reduction of physician idle time and overtime. Muthuraman and Lawley (2008) developed a sequential scheduling algorithm with considering no-show probability into patient groups. This approach basically limits patients' options to choose time slots. Those approaches tend to increase patient wait time significantly, which contributes to further no-shows, and may not be manageable easily by clinics.

Cayirli and Veral (2003) conducted a comprehensive review of the literature on the topic of outpatient scheduling appointments, which highlights the problems related to the definitions and formulations of outpatient appointments, the performance measurements and evaluations, and historically used analysis methods. They concluded more than one major limitations in the past literature: 1. most studies are case specific and, therefore, difficult to generalize; 2. the patient flow modeling are based on unrealistic assumptions, which does not reflect reality; 3. the studies focus on developing appointment rules to accommodate more possible clinical scenarios as opposed to exploring the variation and uncertainty in patient flow; 4. the appointment rules has not been widely adapted, presumably due to a lack of understanding of how rules are prioritized and implemented in practice.

While many researchers worked on developing appointment rules to minimize cost, patient wait time and physician idle time, they believed that wait times were mainly due to the uncertainty of physician service time. Some research has modeled the multiple-server system, including ancillary services in the clinical environment (Cox, Birchall and Wong, 1985; Rising et al., 1973). They proposed additional rules beyond appointment rules to prioritize the second consultation of patients returning from ancillary service. However, none of the research proposed to account for the variation in time required for ancillary services in the scheduling system. Most clinic scheduled appointment intervals represent visit time with the physician, and offer no guidance for patient arrival time. In order to proactively capture patients' requirement for ancillary services during appointment scheduling, the patient arrival time should be distinguished from physician visit time. None of the studies addressed the importance of a two-schedule appointment system.

DESIGN OF APPOINTMENT SCHEDULING

Issue, Controversies, Problems

Past research has placed little importance on the role of data collection in the clinic setting. In fact, the majority of the outpatient clinics do not base their scheduling policies on historical treatment time data. Huang (2009) demonstrate through simulation how much even small errors in time estimation, such as one minute, can affect patient wait time, physician idle time, and finish time in the course of a single day. They believe that long wait times in current outpatient scheduling systems occur primarily due to inaccurate estimates of treatment time and concluded that patient wait time increases dramatically, especially when both the scheduled time and the actual average treatment time are greater than or equal. Under these conditions patient wait time starts to accumulate. As wait time starts to accumulate, the physician idle on average begins to drop. Another major concern pointed out by Huang (2009) is whether physicians can see all scheduled patients without using their lunch hours, breaks, delaying finish time, or rescheduling patients. Their findings indicate that if the average treatment time is equal to or greater than the scheduled time interval, a physician will encounter overtime to see all patients. This is compounded by the normal variation in treatment times that can occur over a given session. Needless to say, a physician may actually finish earlier than scheduled if the average treatment time is less than the scheduled time. Their major conclusion is that failure to determine the treatment time interval based on actual treatment time can significantly impact patient wait time, physician idle time and overtime.

The basic existing scheduling models by the past researchers emphasize on preventing physicians from idling. These models, such as Single-block, Individual-block/Fixed-interval with or without an initial block, Multiple-block/Fixed-interval with or without an initial block, Variable-block/Fixed-interval, and Individual-block/Variable-interval, present physician-centric solutions. These models either overbook (scheduling multiple patients at the same time) or determine the scheduled interval based on minimizing total cost using the cost ratio approach. The cost relative to physician idle time tends to be much higher than to patient wait time due to the perception of higher physician compensation and cost of medical facility (Keller and Laughhunn, 1973; Yang et al., 1998). Hence, these basic models inherently favor the reduction of physician idle time. Huang (2009) propose an objective way to determine the time interval using the concept of wait ratio with the available clinic constraints such as clinic session finish time, time of last appointment, number of patients to be seen, and average patient wait time.

Wait ratio is an innovative and useful measure of the relative comparison of patient wait time and physician idle time. Considering these two variables together provides an advantage over the traditional cost ratio to prevent the 'physician centric' solution. Using the wait ratio also offers benefits for patients being treated equally regardless their visit types and conditions and for clinics fully utilizing their resource capacity.

In addition, the distinction between patient arrival time and the actual appointment time, which is defined as service start time, is often blurred in practice. Therefore, it is not uncommon for a patient to arrive on time for the scheduled appointment, but be delayed at the front desk completing necessary paperwork or other ancillary services required before seeing the physician. Even though the patient may not perceive this as wait time, physicians often regard this unplanned delay as idle time. It is also not uncommon for physicians to fill this idle time with activities which, in turn, may often extend beyond the initial delay causing a cascade that compounds patient wait time throughout a given session. Hence, to eliminate the discrepancy between what patients understand as arrival time and clinic staff regard as service start time, a distinction between arrival time and appointment time has to be made in the scheduling models. Furthermore, how much earlier a patient should arrive if ancillary services such as an x-ray are required before their encounter time with the physician is also an important issue. In theory, patient wait time increases when ancillary service time is overestimated due to early completion from ancillary service and also when ancillary service time is underestimated because of the patients' delay for being seen by the physician. Ideally, ancillary service time should be considered to the point where the physicians can maintain their schedules without contributing significantly to patient wait time.

As for overbooking to prevent no-shows, clinic no-shows are when a patient does not arrive to a previously scheduled clinic appointment. This is problematic for multiple reasons. For example, patients in need of an urgent clinic appointment cannot be seen when the schedule if full even if a last minute opening occurs due to a no-show. It also deprives the clinic of needed revenue since an empty visit slot results in non-billable "down time". One way to help avoid this problem is to overbook appointments where more than one patient is scheduled at the same time. This is similar to how airlines operate with flight reservations. This can also create significant problems because if all patients do arrive for their appointments the wait times can be very long, which may lead to clinic overtime, and will result in significant patient and family dissatisfaction. Currently clinics often try to deal with overbooking by making a flat overbooking percentage (perhaps 5% of visits) or based on the no-show rate to achieve the expected number of patients to be seen such as Shonick and Klein (1977), Vissers (1979) without regard to the probability that each patient may actually arrive or no-show. A better system would be to provide a prediction for the best time to overbook a patient based on the highest probability for when a currently scheduled patient is likely to no-show. This provides a dynamic way to overbook patients considering individual probability of no-show so that the expected total costs of patient wait time, physician idle time, and overtime can be minimized.

Solutions and Recommendations

A step by step approach from data collection, model development, to implementation with expected outcomes is explained. The following diagram, Figure 1, provides an overview of the relationship between project components and the anticipated outcomes:

Data Collection Design and Scheme

The data collected includes the actual treatment time with patients from the physician, residents (if

Figure 1. Overview of project activities and anticipated outcomes

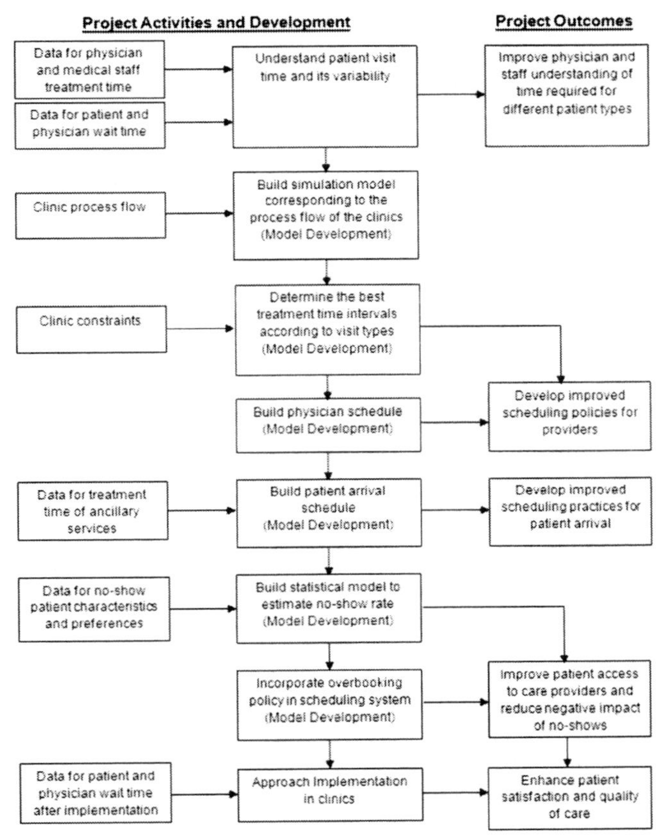

applied), technicians (x-ray, lab test), registered nurses and medical assistants along with patient visit type. Digital time clock can be equipped and attached on the door of each exam room for medical providers to write the time of entering and exiting. The primary reason for collecting treatment time data is to understand the actual treatment time and its variation for each visit type for different medical providers and for any ancillary services. One of the important arguments of this research is that designing a scheduling time interval for any visit without consideration of its actual duration and variation has proven to be inefficient and insensitive to patient wait time and physician idle time (Huang, 2009). The collected data is used to develop the research approach. In addition, these data will be very valuable to help physicians to understand the length of time they spend on particular types of patients.

Another data is collected for building predictive statistical model to estimate the probability of no-show of individual patient or patient group. Many researchers have studied contributing factors to no-shows, in particular clinic environments. Such documented factors include gender, age, the length of waiting time for the appointment, and deprivation (Sharp, 2001). Bean and Talaga (1995) identified no-show factors such as service quality and direct patient costs, distance to the clinic, and a lack of a personal relationship with their physicians, especially in pediatric clinic settings. They also found that appointment no-shows can be predicted by the number of days to the scheduled appointment, the doctor's specialty, and the patient's age and gender. Turner, Weiner, Yang and TenHave (2004) found adherence to physician visits significantly increases attendance for the first appointment. Kruse and Rohland (2002) studied follow-up patients' characteristics impacting their attendance. McCarthy, McGee and O'Boyle (2000) stated the perception of long waiting times in a clinic increases no-show rates. Gallucci, Swartz and Hackerman (2005) found the delay in scheduling appointments negatively impacts the rate of kept appointments. Grunebaum, Luber, Callahan and Leon (1996) found the longer lead time from referral date to the appointment date significantly increases no-show rates in a primary care clinic. Many causes were documented to try to understand the reasons for no-shows. Many researchers have also used the existing data to predict the probability of no-shows, but with limited factors (Dervin, Stone and Beck, 1978; Goldman, Freidin, Cook, Eigner and Grich, 1982; Gruzd, Shear and Rodney, 1986; Glowacka, Henry and May, 2009). Hence, there is not a well-defined model that consists of all these potential factors for predicting patients' no-show rates. Most clinics should have enough existing data plus some external data that can be used to predict patient no-shows. Therefore, historical data needs to be collected. The data should include at least: 1. patient characteristics such as gender, location, age, insurance status and mobility. 2. patient conditions, such as the reason(s) for the visit. 3. environmental factors such as weather and traffic information. This predictive model is the most critical component when defining the overbooking policy. The more accurate the model is, the better the no-show variation can be captured. Thus, the validation of the model accuracy is important.

Model Development

After collecting data and observing clinic process flow, simulation models will be built according to individual practices of each physician. The primary goals of the simulation models are to determine the best scheduled time interval for each visit type under clinic policies and constraints, the time needed for any required ancillary services, and the overbooking scheme. The basic model of patient flow in a clinic has been widely done by many researchers such as Ho and Lau (1992). The interrelationship among the parameters such as appointment time and length, the length of service time, the service starting time and finish time has been well established. These successful models allow researchers to calculate the important performance measurements such as physician idle time, patient wait time, and overtime. This chapter adopts these existing basic models to develop a more patient-centric solution that helps to alleviate patient congestion in a clinic day and improve patient access to care.

Determination of the Best Scheduled Time Interval Using Wait Ratio

A successful appointment system should minimize patient delays while fully utilizing medical resources. However, there is a tradeoff in that reducing patient wait time may increase physician idle time and vice versa. Hence, this research balances patient wait time and physician idle time by determining the Wait Ratio between them. This in turn allows us to determine the treatment or service time interval for each type of visit for a given Wait Ratio. Determining the treatment time intervals across different visit types by the same Wait Ratio is to ensure every patient is treated equally in terms of waiting. The best scheduled time interval is defined as the maximum scheduled time interval for each visit type that satisfies medical and clinic constraints. This best scheduled time interval ensures a good patient flow in a clinic session, which is the foundation of accounting for ancillary services and overbooking scheme, assuming all scheduled patients show up on time for their appointments. The simulation optimization model to determine the best scheduled time interval using wait ratio concept is developed by Huang (2009). Parameters required in this model include: 1. T_i is the physician's service time to treat patient *i where* i=1,2,3,...,n. T_i follows a probability distribution with mean μ and standard deviation σ. Treatment or service time is defined as the time from which a physician enters the exam room to the time at which the physician finally exits the exam room and includes any additional physician service for that patient such as reading charts or dictating. This is the result from treatment time data collection. 2. n is the number of patients scheduled per session (a day, a morning or an afternoon). With these two clinic input information, X (the scheduled time interval for a patient in minutes) can be determined, $X=\mu+d\sigma$, d is the decision variable (the number of standard deviation away from the mean μ), given a wait ratio, R, which is the degree to which average patient wait time $\left(\overline{W}\right)$ exceeds R physician idle time $\left(\overline{P}\right)$, $where\ \ R = 1,2,3,\cdots,l\ and\ l \in R^+$ or $\overline{W}/\overline{P} = R$. Then a number of simulation runs are needed to conclude average schedule time interval, $\overline{X}$, for each visit type. The common visit types are: NP (new patient), RV (return visit), FU (follow-up), HP (pre-operation), and POP (post-operation). To assure that the model does reflect actual clinic operation, certain clinic policy or constraints such as clinic or session finish time, time of last appointment, number of patients to be seen (or number of desired appointment slots) in a given session, average patient wait time, maximum patient wait time, average physician idle time, maximum physician idle time and the sequence of the various visit types, are critical in finalizing the best wait ratio and generating the best treatment time interval $\overline{X}^*$ for each visit type. Some studies concluded that the scheduling sequence of the various visit types in a clinic session has significant impact on patient waiting (Klassen and Rohleder, 1996; Harper and Gamlin, 2003). However, each clinic management team should decide its own sequence for an individual physician to meet patients' needs without any restriction. In addition, Huang (2009) pointed out from three case studies most clinics designed their time intervals much shorter than actual treatment time, which resulting in the insufficient length for a visit. Therefore, one critical constraint to ensure the adequate length of time interval of $\overline{X}^*$ is $\Pr\left(T_i \le \overline{X}^*\right) \ge 0.5$; that is the probability of a wait less than or equal to 50%.

In short, this model does not attempt to force the clinic setting to fit the solution, but rather aims at fully utilizing the available resources and capacity to achieve the best solution. Although clinic policy and constraints above are not addressed in the literature, they are used here to determine a wait ratio to replace conventional cost ratios. The concept of 'wait ratio' is novel. Its advantage over the traditional cost ratio is due to physicians' tendency to over-estimate the cost of their time as opposed to patient time, most likely due to their lack of criteria for accurately evaluating time cost for the patient. This proposed method effectively eliminates introduced bias by assuming the cost of patient time in favor of clinic defined policy and constraints.

An example is presented to demonstrate how to find the best treatment time interval. Assuming a clinic with two scheduling visit types, NP (new patient) and RV (return visit), would like to have a scheduling template of 32 patients including 8 NPs and 24 RVs and distribute the patient types evenly throughout a clinic day. The only constraint is to finish a clinic day in 7 hours (8:00 am to 3:00 pm). Assuming the treatment time distributions of NP follows Gamma with mean of 15.7 minutes and standard deviation of 9.2 minutes and of RV also follows Gamma with mean of 11.1 minutes and standard deviation of 6.1 minutes. To be noted, Gamma distribution was one of service distributions used by many researchers such as Yang et

Figure 2. The summary results for the example

Wait Ratio (R)	Average time interval $(\bar{X})$		Average Patient wait time	Average Physician idle time	Finish time
	NP	RV			
1	20.2	14.1	6.2	3.3	491.2
2	18.9	13.1	8.7	2.4	159.6
3	18.2	12.6	10.6	2.0	444.2
4	17.8	12.3	11.9	1.7	434.8
5	17.5	12.1	12.9	1.5	428.0
6	17.2	11.9	13.8	1.4	422.9
7	17.0	11.8	14.5	1.3	418.9
8	16.8	11.7	15.1	1.2	415.6
9	16.7	11.6	15.7	1.1	412.8
10	16.6	11.5	16.3	1.1	410.5
11	16.5	11.4	16.8	1.0	408.4
12	16.4	11.3	17.3	1.0	406.5
13	16.3	11.3	17.7	0.9	404.8
14	16.2	11.2	18.1	0.9	403.3
15	16.1	11.1	18.5	0.9	401.9
16	16.0	11.1	18.9	0.8	400.6
17	16.0	11.1	19.3	0.8	399.4
18	15.9	11.0	19.6	0.8	398.3
19	15.8	11.0	19.9	0.7	397.3
20	15.8	10.9	20.3	0.7	396.3

al. (1998). Therefore it is chosen to demonstrate the approach throughout the entire chapter. Using the proposed model, the results from different wait ratios are in Figure 2. Base on the constraint of 7 hours (420 minutes), the optimal wait ratio is 7 at finish time of 418.9 minutes, which corresponding to the best treatment time interval should be 17 minutes for NP and 11.8 minutes for RV. The choice ensures the minimal patient wait time while uses the maximum clinic capacity. The corresponding probabilities of not waiting are 63% and 62%, respectively. If the clinic adds additional constraint of average patient wait time less than 20 minutes, this indicates the wait ratio of 19. In this case, the optimal wait ratio is still 7, since it satisfies both constraints.

Provider Schedule

Based on the best scheduled time interval for each visit type, the provider schedule is constructed so that appointment slots are consecutive, without overbooking or double-booking. For the physician, this schedule represents the actual time at which each patient encounter should begin. This schedule can also provide a timeline for physicians to best utilize their 'idle' time in between patients. Continuing the example, assuming starts at 8 am, the provider schedule should be constructed as shown in Figure 3. NP is scheduled at 17 minutes and RV is scheduled at 11.8 minutes. The scheduled sequence for the first four patients is RV, NP, RV, and RV. The scheduled provider time is 8:00, 8:12 (8:00 + 11.8 minutes), 8:29 (8:12 + 17 minutes), and 8:41 (8:29 + 11.8 minutes), respectively.

Patient Arrival Schedule

Once a physician schedule is established, then the corresponding patient arrival schedule must be determined. The main concept behind the arrival schedule is to provide sufficient time between the patient arrival at the clinic and the actual examination time for the patient to complete activities and required ancillary services such as signing in, filling out paperwork, having vitals taken, having an x-ray taken, providing a specimen, and moving between lab or x-ray room and exam room. The time assigned to pre-visit activities will differ from clinic to clinic and between specialties. However, if the time needed for these activities is not well defined, wait time will be compounded

Figure 3. The scheduling scheme for the example

Patient Type	Scheduled Time	Required Lab Tests	Arrival Time	Actual Arrival Time
RV	8:00	Y	7:29	7:30
NP	8:12	N	8:12	8:12
RV	8:29	Y	7:58	8:00
RV	8:41	Y	8:10	8:10
RV	8:52	Y	8:21	8:20
NP	9:04	N	9:04	9:05
RV	9:21	Y	8:50	8:50
RV	9:33	Y	9:02	9:00
RV	9:45	N	9:45	9:45
NP	9:56	N	9:56	9:55
RV	10:13	N	10:13	10:15
RV	10:25	N	10:25	10:25
RV	10:37	Y	10:06	10:05
NP	10:49	Y	10:18	10:20
RV	11:06	Y	10:35	10:35
RV	11:18	N	11:18	11:20
RV	11:29	N	11:29	11:30
NP	11:41	Y	11:10	11:10
RV	11:58	Y	11:27	11:25
RV	12:10	Y	11:39	11:40
RV	12:22	N	12:22	12:20
NP	12:33	N	12:33	12:35
RV	12:51	Y	12:20	12:20
RV	1:02	N	1:02	1:00
RV	1:14	N	1:14	1:15
NP	1:26	N	1:26	1:25
RV	1:43	Y	1:12	1:10
RV	1:55	N	1:55	1:55
RV	2:06	Y	1:35	1:35
NP	2:18	Y	1:47	1:45
RV	2:35	Y	2:04	2:05
RV	2:47	N	2:47	2:45

for either physician or patient. Ideally, the physicians should be able to maintain their schedules without contributing significantly to patient wait time. Ancillary services such as x-ray, lab test, diagnosis vascular studies, and electrocardiogram (EKG) are important to assist the physician in making an accurate assessment and are most likely required prior to a physician visit in many outpatient clinics. The focus here is for clinics which prefer both ancillary and physician services to be done in one visit.

Ancillary services impact patient wait time, as demonstrated in our previous studies. Ironically, patient wait time increases by both underestimating and overestimating the length of time required for ancillary services. When ancillary service time is overestimated, increased wait times result from early completion before the physician is ready for the patient. When ancillary service time is underestimated patients experience delays in being seen by the physician. The time assigned to pre-visit activities will differ from physician to physician. Hence, the best scheduled ancillary service time to be considered in scheduling should be determined according to individual physician's schedule and needs. The approach to scheduling patient arrival requires schedulers to 'triage' patients, asking questions that help the scheduler to determine: first, if a patient actually needs an ancillary service, and secondly, how much must be done prior to the physician visit. A simulation model is needed to determine the most appropriate time so that the patient waiting can be minimized. Three additional parameters are needed: ancillary service time, A_i, follows a probability distribution with mean of μ_A and standard deviation of σ_A, the probability of patients who need ancillary services, and number of available ancillary service resources. Average patient wait time $\left(\overline{W}\right)$ includes both from ancillary service and physician. Let Y be the scheduled time interval of ancillary service for a patient in minutes where $Y = \mu_A + k\sigma_A$. k is the number of standard deviation away from the mean. The objective is to minimize $\overline{W}$ by changing k in order to find the optimal k^*. Therefore, the optimal scheduled time interval (Y^*) for each patient should be $Y^* = \mu_A + k^*\sigma_A$ *where* $0 \leq \Pr\left(A \leq Y^*\right) \leq 1$, $\Pr\left(A \leq Y^*\right)$ is the probability of ancillary service time of distribution $D\left(\mu_A, \sigma_A^{\ 2}\right)$.

Continuing with the example, the clinic required some patients to have lab tests prior to physician visit. The clinic has only one test machine, about 50% of patients required lab tests, and the test time distribution follows Gamma distribution with mean of 29.3 minutes and standard deviation of 12.9 minutes. After running simulations on this model, the result of the probability of ancillary service time, $\Pr(A \leq Y^*)$, that minimizes the average patient waiting is 0.6; see Figure 4, which translates the optimal scheduled time interval (Y^*) to be 30.7 minutes. This means patients who need lab tests are required to arrive 30.7 minutes earlier on average. With this information, the patient arrival schedule can be constructed; see Figure 3. The first RV patient is scheduled to see physician at 8:00 am and is required to have lab tests done. Hence, he/she needs to arrive 31 minutes earlier, which is 7:29 am. Normally, clinics should communicate the arrival time with patients in a 5-minute interval. Therefore, 7:29 am will be rounded to the nearest 5-minute interval, which is 7:30 am.

Overbooking Policy

The majority of clinics have overbooked slots (at least two patients to be scheduled at the same starting time) in their scheduling systems regardless the probability of no-shows at any given slot. This chapter proposes to redefine overbooking policies based on the probability of no-shows of a scheduled patient to determine if an overbooking is appropriate so that the total costs (patient wait time, physician idle time and overtime) can be minimized. There are two major components here. First, a statistical prediction model will determine the probability of no-shows given patient characteristics and considered with other environmental factors. Then, a simulation optimization model will find the optimal threshold of no-show rate obtained from the prediction model to minimize the total costs. The most critical parameter for this model to work is the predicted probability of no-show for patient j at time slot i, $p_{i,j}$. Let p be the threshold of no-show rate for each time slot. At any time slot, overbooking can be

Figure 4. Average patient wait time with various probability of lab test distribution indicates 30.7 minutes is optimal at 60% of ancillary service time of distribution

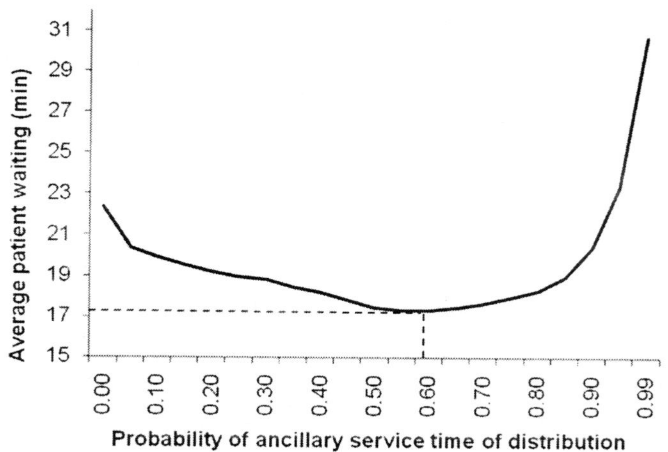

performed as long as the joint probability at a slot is still greater than the threshold, $\prod_j p_{i,j} \geq p$. Let W be the total patient wait time, P be the total physician idle time, and O be the overtime for a clinic day. Given c_w is the cost of patient wait time per minute, c_p is the cost of physician idle time per minute, c_o is the cost of overtime per minute, and c_T is the total cost of patient wait time, physician idle time and overtime. Therefore, $c_T = c_w W + c_p P + c_o O$. The objective is to find the optimal value for the threshold of no-show rate (p^*) that minimizes c_T.

Continuing the example, assuming $c_w = 0.25, c_p = 5, c_o = 7.5$, and $p_{i,j}$ follows Gamma distribution with mean of 0.3 and standard deviation of 0.1, the result shown in Figure 5 indicates that c_T is minimized at no-show threshold (p^*) equal to 0.26. The number of patients overbooked is 18. Hence, the total number of scheduled patients in this case is 50. The overbooking scheme for the example is presented in Figure 6. This means that clinics will overbook a patient where the predicted probability of no-show scheduled in a time slot is greater or equal to 0.26. This approach provides a dynamic way to overbook patients based on the prediction of no-shows for each patient.

Summary of Research Design

This approach uses an interesting concept of 'wait ratio' instead of traditional cost ratio of the patient wait time and the physician idle time. As many researchers have used traditional cost ratios, the issue of the long patient waits in a physician's office still exists. Based on results from previous studies (Huang, 2009), significant reduction in patient wait time, as much as 56%, can be achieved. In addition, this research demonstrates a step-by-step, easily implemented approach for patient scheduling developed to reduce patient wait time, enhance patient flow, and improve patient access to care, without significantly increasing physician idle time. The approach allows clinic management to quickly determine the best scheduled time interval for different visit types and then integrate clinical policies or constraints to produce two scheduling templates, one for the physician encounter and one for patient arrival. Separating the two schedules will make it possible to create a template for patient arrival that

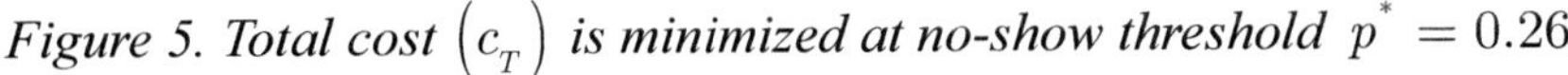

Figure 5. Total cost (c_T) *is minimized at no-show threshold* $p^* = 0.26$

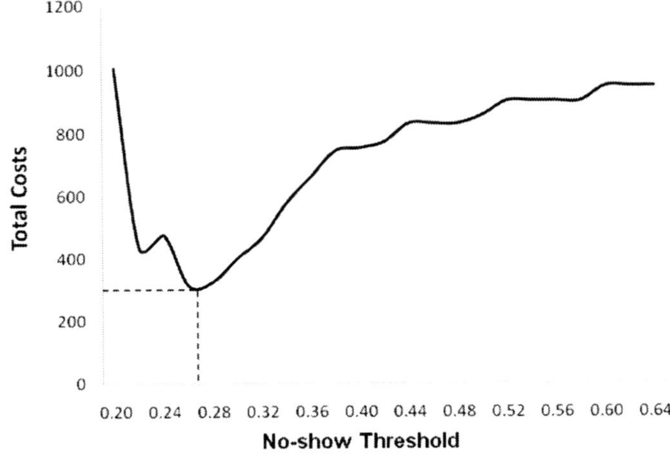

Figure 6. The overbooking scheme for the example

i	Schedule Time Slots	Patient Type	1st patient booked	1st patient no-show rate ($p_{i,1}$)	2nd patient overbooked if $p_{i,1} \geq p^*$	2nd patient no-show rate ($p_{i,2}$)	Joint no-show rate $p_{i,1} \times p_{i,2}$	3rd patient overbooked if $p_{i,1} \times p_{i,2} \geq p^*$	Overbooked	Total Booked
1	8:00	RV	1	0.14	0				0	1
2	8:12	NP	1	0.37	1	0.38	0.14	0	1	2
3	8:29	RV	1	0.21	0				0	1
4	8:41	RV	1	0.51	1	0.42	0.21	0	1	2
5	8:52	RV	1	0.22	0				0	1
6	9:04	NP	1	0.37	1	0.16	0.06	0	1	2
7	9:21	RV	1	0.59	1	0.38	0.22	0	1	2
8	9:33	RV	1	0.21	0				0	1
9	9:45	RV	1	0.24	0				0	1
10	9:56	NP	1	0.36	1	0.32	0.12	0	1	2
11	10:13	RV	1	0.21	0				0	1
12	10:25	RV	1	0.25	0				0	1
13	10:37	RV	1	0.24	0				0	1
14	10:49	NP	1	0.23	0				0	1
15	11:06	RV	1	0.10	0				0	1
16	11:18	RV	1	0.32	1	0.18	0.06	0	1	2
17	11:29	RV	1	0.34	1	0.33	0.11	0	1	2
18	11:41	NP	1	0.32	1	0.34	0.11	0	1	2
19	11:58	RV	1	0.34	1	0.41	0.14	0	1	2
20	12:10	RV	1	0.27	1				1	2
21	12:22	RV	1	0.28	1	0.39	0.11	0	1	2
22	12:33	NP	1	0.27	1				1	2
23	12:51	RV	1	0.28	1	0.38	0.11	0	1	2
24	1:02	RV	1	0.28	1	0.35	0.10	0	1	2
25	1:14	RV	1	0.29	1	0.33	0.10	0	1	2
26	1:26	NP	1	0.25	0				0	1
27	1:43	RV	1	0.49	1	0.27	0.13	0	1	2
28	1:55	RV	1	0.14	0				0	1
29	2:06	RV	1	0.22	0				0	1
30	2:18	NP	1	0.42	1	0.15	0.06	0	1	2
31	2:35	RV	1	0.41	1	0.26	0.11	0	1	2
32	2:47	RV	1	0.18	0				0	1
								Total	**18**	**50**

accommodates any patient processing tasks or ancillary services that need to be conducted in conjunction with a given physician service. This will reduce the unnecessary first consultation and improve the timely delivery and patient access. Moreover, the common issue of no-shows is considered into the scheduling system and the approach provides a cost-efficient dynamic way of overbooking patients without burdening clinic flow. The conceptual and theoretical framework of this chapter allows the changes of input parameters such as provider treatment time, ancillary service time(s), number of patients seen and no-show rates among physicians in a variety of clinic settings. This approach allows clinic management to input its own parameters such as physician treatment time, scheduling sequence of visit types, types and times of ancillary services, and no-show rates to accommodate the difference of each clinic or physician's practice.

Implementation and Outcomes

After each model development, implementation needs to be in place to provide quantitative feedback to validate the effectiveness of this approach. As mentioned in the section of Summary of Research Design, the work was implemented in part by Huang (2009). The results were very promising. The continuous implementation is needed especially in consideration of ancillary services and overbooking. Each implementation includes system redesign (accommodation) and adjustments. Two important outcome measurements of the demonstration from this proposed approach are: patient wait time and patient access to care. The ultimate goal is to improve outpatient experience for both patients and medical providers. There are intermediate goals for each activity and development. Initial data analysis provides medical providers understanding of time required for different patient types. For each developed model, it should be evaluated through a data collection for patient wait time. At the end of a project, a final data collection will be done to provide evidence of reduced patient wait time as well as the reduction of the unnecessary first consultation and the negative impact of patient no-shows, which will lead to the increase of access to care. The evaluation on the improvement of access to care is measured by number of patients actually seen per clinic day, which is fairly easy to obtain. As a result, patients will be more satisfied in terms of waiting during their visit and obtaining an appointment, which will change the perception of long waits in a physician's office and improve the outpatient experience for both patients and medical providers.

FUTURE RESEARCH DIRECTIONS

Many scheduling approaches have been proposed since the 1950's, especially in the direction of appointment order scheduling systems. Unfortunately, not many of them have been implemented in current scheduling systems. The long patient waits in being able to see a physician and to get an appointment is still demanding. The proposed approach in this chapter is unique and has been demonstrated to be effective in reducing patient wait time (Huang, 2009). The challenge remaining is to implement the approach in different clinic scheduling systems. Hence, an important goal for future research is to further extend this scheduling approach to accommodate a larger range of specialties and clinic management systems. This will allow us to understand systematic difficulties in order to further generalize the approach for adaptability. Furthermore, a perfect scheduling scheme will not be the only solution to improve outpatient experience. Other aspects such as reminder, cancellation and walk-in policies are also an important part of outpatient experience. To the best of the author's knowledge, there are not many studies addressing these issues in terms of the best practices. A telephone survey was conducted over 40 outpatient clinics nationwide regarding the policies of reminder, cancellation and walk-in. The preliminary results indicate that 25% of surveyed clinics do not use any reminder system at all and 10% of the clinics which have reminder system use at least two methods multiple times. The majority of clinics use reminder calls a few days before patients' scheduled appointment. The current reminder practices do not seem to be efficient and may have increased clinic workload. As for cancellation policy, the survey results indicate that more than 50% of surveyed clinics do not have any policy at all. For those that do have a policy, a 24-hour notice is the common practice. However, this 24-hour policy has no logic or mathematical basis to support its effectiveness. A better policy should consider the fill rate for appointments and the patient no-show rate together so that the overall costs of the clinic can be minimized. In terms of walk-in policy, the survey said that about 50% of clinics do not allow walk-in patients at all and for those allowing walk-in patients, 90% of them allow walk-ins at any time. Generally, walk-in patients would have to wait for an opening in between appointments. This random walk-in policy will certainly burden clinic workflow and patient flow. These problems have clear negative impacts to patient satisfaction and quality care. A well-defined policy that can achieve efficiency and cost effectiveness for reminder, cancellation and walk-in is desired for improving outpatient experience.

CONCLUSION

Wait ratio is a novel concept of the relationship between patient wait time and physician idle time. This concept provides an advantage over the traditional cost ratio to prevent from the 'physician centric' solution to ensure patients being treated equally regardless their visit types and conditions, as well as full utilization of clinic resource capacity. The main reason that cost ratio favors physician wait time is due to the definition of cost values assigned to both patient wait time and physician idle time. Keller and Laughhunn (1973) used the hourly pay for the cost of physician idle time and minimum wage to reflect the cost of patient wait time. Realistically, the cost of physician idle time is much higher than that of patient wait time. Hence, the high cost ratio between physician and patient wait time becomes the most dominant factors when deciding patient scheduling time intervals. Since then, the cost ratio has not been defined otherwise. Therefore, it is much more objective to consider wait time itself instead of placing a cost value to wait time, which is basically impossible. By adopting wait ratio allows a clinic to actually take into account clinic constraints or policies, such as time to finish a clinic day, for determining appointment schedule to generate a better patient flow.

Secondly, the novel concept of two scheduling systems, physician and patient arrival schedules, has not been discussed when scheduling appointments. According to the findings from interviewing clinic management regarding what the patient scheduled time means, the general answer has been the scheduled time is the time for a patient to see the physician. This indicates that the pre-activities such as sign-in are completely neglected, which tends to compound the impact of waiting from the beginning of a clinic session. Separating two schedules makes it possible to schedule any ancillary services before seeing the physician in order to customize patients' needs and conditions. In addition, most clinics assume the same amount of time to complete the required ancillary services, for example, 10 minutes for any patients who needs x-rays. This assumption does not account for the variation of ancillary service time at all, which generates waiting for both patients and physicians. Therefore, considering individual requirement of ancillary services is a critical piece for a better scheduling system.

Third, even though overbooking approaches have been widely used in most scheduling systems, traditionally, most of the overbooking slots are designed into the scheduling systems before actually scheduling patients. This traditional approach does not consider the probability of no-show for the individual patient, without understanding patients' characteristics and preferences. This means the majority of time when two patients actually show up at the same time, one of them is bounded to wait for service. This chapter provides an overbooking policy that dynamically accounts for the individual patient's probability of no-show based on patient characteristics (age, gender, location, mobility) and preferences including environmental factors (weather and traffic conditions). In addition, this proposed overbooking policy should be easily adopted into any scheduling systems. This innovative policy will provide a cost-effective way to overbook patients without overloading clinic resources.

In conclusion, one of the major concerns from literature is the gap between theoretical concepts and feasibility in reality. This chapter provides a step-by-step solution for execution the proposed approach conceptually and theoretically from initial data collection and model development to implementation of the approach. This project will not only close the gap between theory and practices but also provide evidence of applicability for any physicians in any specialties. In short, we believe the successful demonstration of this proposed approach will shift the perception of long waits in a physician's office, transform outpatient environment to be much more pleasant, and ultimately improve the outpatient experience.

REFERENCES

Bailey, N. (1952). A study of queues and appointment systems in hospital outpatient departments, with special reference to waiting-times. *Journal of the Royal Statistical Society. Series A (General)*, *14*(2), 185–199.

Bean, A. G., & Talaga, J. (1995). Predicting appointment breaking. *Journal of Health Care Marketing*, *15*(1), 29–34.

Bundy, D. G. (2005). Open access in primary care: results of a North Carolina pilot project. *Pediatrics*, *116*(1), 82–87. doi:10.1542/peds.2004-2573

Casey, R. G., Quinlan, M. R., Flynn, R., Grainger, R., McDermott, T. E., & Thornhill, J. A. (2007). Urology out-patient non-attenders: Are we wasting our time? *Irish Journal of Medical Science*, *176*(4), 305–308. doi:10.1007/s11845-007-0028-8

Cayirli, T., & Veral, E. (2003). Outpatient scheduling in health care: A review of literature. *Production and Operations Management*, *12*(4), 519–549. doi:10.1111/j.1937-5956.2003.tb00218.x

Cayirli, T., Veral, E., & Rosen, H. (2006). Designing appointment scheduling systems for ambulatory care services. *Health Care Management Science*, *9*(1), 47–58. doi:10.1007/s10729-006-6279-5

Corfield, L., Schizas, A., Noorani, A., & Williams, A. (2008). Non-attendance at the colorectal clinic: A prospective audit. *Annals of the Royal College of Surgeons of England*, *90*(5), 377–380. doi:10.1308/003588408X301172

Cox, T. F., Birchall, J. F., & Wong, H. (1985). Optimizing the queuing system for an ear, nose and throat outpatient clinic. *Journal of Applied Statistics*, *12*(2), 113–126. doi:10.1080/02664768500000017

Dervin, J. V., Stone, D. L., & Beck, C. H. (1978). The no-show patient in the model family practice unit. *The Journal of Family Practice*, *7*(6), 1177–1180.

Deyo, R. A., & Inui, T. S. (1980). Dropouts and broken appointments: A literature review and agenda for future research. *Medical Care*, *18*(11), 1146–1157. doi:10.1097/00005650-198011000-00006

Fries, B., & Marathe, V. (1981). Determination of optimal variable-sized multiple-block appointment systems. *Operations Research*, *29*(2), 324–345. doi:10.1287/opre.29.2.324

Gallucci, G., Swartz, W., & Hackerman, F. (2005). Brief reports: Impact of the wait for an initial appointment on the rate of kept appointments at a mental health center. *Psychiatric Services (Washington, D.C.)*, *56*(3), 344–346. doi:10.1176/appi.ps.56.3.344

Giachetti, R. E., Centeno, E. A., Centeno, M. A., & Sundaram, R. (2005). Assessing the viability of an open access policy in an outpatient clinic: A discrete-event and continuous simulation modeling approach. *Proceedings of the 2005 Winter Simulation Conference*.

Glowacka, K., Henry, R., & May, J. (2009). A hybird data mining/simulation approach for modelling outpatient no-shows in clinic scheduling. *The Journal of the Operational Research Society*, *60*(8), 1056–1068. doi:10.1057/jors.2008.177

Goldman, L., Freidin, R., Cook, E. F., Eigner, J., & Grich, P. (1982). A multivariate approach to the prediction of no-show behavior in a primary care center. *Archives of Internal Medicine*, *142*(3), 563–567. doi:10.1001/archinte.142.3.563

Grunebaum, M., Luber, P., Callahan, M., & Leon, A. C. (1996). Predictors of missed appointments for psychiatric consultations in a primary care clinic. *Psychiatric Services (Washington, D.C.)*, *47*(8), 848–852.

Gruzd, D. C., Shear, C. L., & Rodney, M. (1986). Determinants of no-show appointment behavior: The utility of multivariate analysis. *Family Medicine*, *18*(4), 217–220.

Guo, M., Wagner, M., & West, C. (2003). Outpatient clinic scheduling – A simulation approach. *Proceedings of the 2004 Winter Simulation Conference*.

Harper, P. R., & Gamlin, H. M. (2003). Reduced outpatient waiting times with improved appointment scheduling: A simulation modeling approach. *OR-Spektrum*, *25*(2), 207–222. doi:10.1007/s00291-003-0122-x

Hixon, A. L., Chapman, R. W., & Nuovo, J. (1999). Failure to keep clinic appointments: Implications for residency education and productivity. *Family Medicine*, *31*(9), 627–630.

Ho, C., & Lau, H. (1992). Minimizing total cost in scheduling outpatient appointments. *Management Science*, *38*(12), 1750–1764. doi:10.1287/mnsc.38.12.1750

Ho, C., Lau, H., & Li, J. (1995). Introducing variable-interval appointment scheduling rules in service systems. *International Journal of Operations & Production Management*, *15*(6), 59–68. doi:10.1108/01443579510090345

Huang, X. (1994). Patient attitude towards waiting in an outpatient clinic and its applications. *Health Services Management Research*, *7*(1), 2–8.

Huang, Y. L. (2009). *An alternative outpatient scheduling system*. Germany: VDM Publishing House Ltd.

Kaandorp, G., & Koole, G. (2007). Optimal outpatient appointment scheduling. *Health Care Management Science*, *10*(3), 217–229. doi:10.1007/s10729-007-9015-x

Keller, T. F., & Laughhunn, D. J. (1973). An application of queuing theory to a congestion problem in an outpatient clinic. *Decision Sciences*, *4*(3), 379–394. doi:10.1111/j.1540-5915.1973.tb00563.x

Kim, S., & Giachetti, R. E. (2006). A stochastic mathematical appointment overbooking model for healthcare providers to improve profits. *IEEE Transactions on Systems, Man, and Cybernetics*, *36*(6), 1211–1219. doi:10.1109/TSMCA.2006.878970

Klassen, K. J., & Rohleder, T. R. (1996). Scheduling outpatient appointments in a dynamic environment. *Operations Management*, *14*(2), 83–101. doi:10.1016/0272-6963(95)00044-5

Klassen, K. J., & Rohleder, T. R. (2004). Outpatient appointment scheduling with urgent clients in a dynamic, multi-period environment. *International Journal of Service Industry Management*, *15*(2), 167–186. doi:10.1108/09564230410532493

Kros, J., Dellana, S., & West, D. (2009). Overbooking increases patient access at East Carolina University's student health services clinic. *Interfaces*, *39*(3), 271–287. doi:10.1287/inte.1090.0437

Kruse, G. R. (2002). Factors associated with attendance at a first appointment after discharge from a psychiatric hospital. *Psychiatric Services (Washington, D.C.)*, *53*(4), 473–476. doi:10.1176/appi.ps.53.4.473

LaGanga, L. R., & Lawrence, S. R. (2007). Clinic overbooking to improve patient access and increase provider productivity. *Decision Sciences*, *38*(2), 251–276. doi:10.1111/j.1540-5915.2007.00158.x

Liu, N., Ziya, S., & Kulkarni, V. G. (2009). Dynamic scheduling of outpatient appointments under patient no-shows and cancellations. *Manufacturing & Service Operations Management*, Articles in Advance. DOI: 10.1287/msom.1090.0272

McCarthy, K., McGee, H. M., & O'Boyle, C. A. (2000). Outpatient clinic waiting times and non-attendance as indicators of quality. *Psychology Health and Medicine*, *5*(3), 287–293. doi:10.1080/713690194

Mehrotra, A., Keehl-Markowitz, L., & Ayanian, J. Z. (2008). Implementing open-access scheduling of visits in primary care practices: A cautionary tale. *Annals of Internal Medicine, 148*(12), 915–922.

Meza, J. (1998). Patient waiting times in a physician's office. *The American Journal of Managed Care, 4*(5), 703–712.

Murray, M., & Tantau, C. (1999). Redefining open access to primary care. *Managed Care Quarterly, 7*(3), 45–55.

Muthuraman, K., & Lawley, M. (2008). A stochastic overbooking model for outpatient clinical scheduling with no-shows. *IIE Transactions, 40*(9), 820–837. doi:10.1080/07408170802165823

O'Connor, M. E., Matthews, B. S., & Gao, D. (2006). Effect of open access scheduling on missed appointments, immunizations, and continuity of care for infant well-child care visits. *Archives of Pediatrics & Adolescent Medicine, 160*(9), 889–893. doi:10.1001/archpedi.160.9.889

O'Hare, C. D., & Corlett, J. (2004). The outcomes of open access scheduling. *Family Practice Medicine, 11*(2), 35–38.

Phan, K., & Brown, S. (2009). Decreased continuity in a residency clinic: A consequence of open access scheduling. *Family Medicine Journal, 41*(1), 46–50.

Rising, E. J., Baron, R., & Averill, B. (1973). A system analysis of a university health service outpatient clinic. *Operations Research, 21*(5), 1030–1047. doi:10.1287/opre.21.5.1030

Robinson, L., & Chen, R. (2009). A comparison of traditional and open-access policies for appointment scheduling. *Manufacturing & Service Operations Management*, Articles in Advance. DOI: 10.1287/msom.1090.0270

Rust, C. T., Callups, N. H., Clark, W. S., Jones, D. S., & Wilcox, W. E. (1995). Patient appointment failures in pediatric resident continuity clinics. *Archives of Pediatrics & Adolescent Medicine, 149*(6), 693–695.

Sharp, D. J. (2001). Non-attendance at general practices and outpatient clinics: Local systems are needed to address local problems. *British Medical Journal, 323*(7321), 1081–1082. doi:10.1136/bmj.323.7321.1081

Shonick, W., & Klein, B. W. (1977). An approach to reducing the adverse effects of broken appointments in primary care systems: Developing a decision rule based on estimated conditional probabilities. *Medical Care, 15*(5), 419–429. doi:10.1097/00005650-197705000-00008

Soriano, A. (1966). Comparison of two scheduling systems. *Operations Research, 14*(3), 388–397. doi:10.1287/opre.14.3.388

Swisher, J. R., Jacobson, S. H., Jun, J. B., & Balci, O. (2001). Modeling and analyzing a physician clinic environment using discrete-event (visual) simulation. *Computers & Operations Research, 28*(2), 105–125. doi:10.1016/S0305-0548(99)00093-3

Turner, B. J., Weiner, M., Yang, C., & TenHave, T. (2004). Predicting adherence to colonoscopy or flexible sigmoidoscopy on the basis of physician appointment–keeping behavior. *Annals of Internal Medicine, 140*(7), 528–532.

Vanden Bosch, P. M., & Dietz, D. C. (2000). Minimizing expected waiting in a medical appointment system. *IIE Transactions, 32*(9), 841–848. doi:10.1080/07408170008967443

Villegas, E. L. (1967). Outpatient appointment system saves time for patients and doctors. *Hospitals, 41*(8), 52–57.

Vissers, J. (1979). Selecting a suitable appointment system in an outpatient setting. *Medical Care, 17*(12), 1207–1220. doi:10.1097/00005650-197912000-00004

Warden, J. (1995). 4.5-million outpatients miss appointments. *British Medical Journal, 310*(6988), 1158–1158.

Welch, J. D. (1964). Appointment systems in hospital outpatient departments. *Operational Research Quarterly, 15*(3), 224–232. doi:10.1057/jors.1964.43

White, M. J. B., & Pike, M. C. (1964). Appointment systems in outpatients' clinics and the effect on patients' unpunctuality. *Medical Care, 2*(3), 133–145. doi:10.1097/00005650-196407000-00002

Wijewickrama, A., & Takakuwa, S. (2005). Simulation analysis of appointment scheduling in an outpatient department of internal medicine. *Proceedings of the 2005 Winter Simulation Conference*.

Wijewickrama, A. K. A. (2006). Simulation analysis for reducing queues in mixed-patients' outpatient department. *International Journal Simulation Model, 5*(2), 56–68. doi:10.2507/IJSIMM05(2)2.055

Yang, K. K., Lau, M. L., & Quek, S. A. (1998). A new appointment rule for a single-server, multiple-customer service system. *Naval Research Logistics, 45*(3), 313–326. doi:10.1002/(SICI)1520-6750(199804)45:3<313::AID-NAV5>3.0.CO;2-A

ADDITIONAL READING

Bailey, N. (1952). A Study of Queues and Appointment Systems in Hospital Outpatient Departments, with Special Reference to Waiting-Times. *Journal of the Royal Statistical Society. Series A (General), 14*(2), 185–199.

Cayirli, T., & Veral, E. (2003). Outpatient Scheduling in Health Care: A Review of Literature. *Production and Operations Management, 12*(4), 519–549. doi:10.1111/j.1937-5956.2003.tb00218.x

Glowacka, K., Henry, R., & May, J. (2009). A hybird data mining/simulation approach for modelling outpatient no-shows in clinic scheduling. *J Opl Res Soc, 60*(8), 1056–1068. doi:10.1057/jors.2008.177

Harper, P. R., & Gamlin, H. M. (2003). Reduced outpatient waiting times with improved appointment scheduling: a simulation modeling approach. *OR-Spektrum, 25*(2), 207–222. doi:10.1007/s00291-003-0122-x

Ho, C., & Lau, H. (1992). Minimizing Total Cost in Scheduling Outpatient Appointments. *Management Science, 38*(12), 1750–1764. doi:10.1287/mnsc.38.12.1750

Ho, C., Lau, H., & Li, J. (1995). Introducing variable-interval appointment scheduling rules in service systems. *International Journal of Operations & Production Management, 15*(6), 59–68. doi:10.1108/01443579510090345

Huang, Y. L. (2009). *An Alternative Outpatient Scheduling System*. Germany: VDM Publishing House Ltd.

Kim, S., & Giachetti, R. E. (2006). A Stochastic Mathematical Appointment Overbooking Model for Healthcare Providers to Improve Profits. *IEEE Transactions on Systems, Man, and Cybernetics, 36*(6), 1211–1219. doi:10.1109/TSMCA.2006.878970

Klassen, K. J., & Rohleder, T. R. (1996). Scheduling Outpatient Appointments in a Dynamic Environment. *Operations Management, 14*(2), 83–101. doi:10.1016/0272-6963(95)00044-5

Kros, J., Dellana, S., & West, D. (2009). Overbooking Increases Patient Access at East Carolina University's Student Health Services Clinic. *Interfaces*, *39*(3), 271–287. doi:10.1287/inte.1090.0437

LaGanga, L. R., & Lawrence, S. R. (2007). Clinic Overbooking to Improve Patient Access and Increase Provider Productivity. *Decision Sciences*, *38*(2), 251–276. doi:10.1111/j.1540-5915.2007.00158.x

Liu, N., Ziya, S., & Kulkarni, V. G. (2009). Dynamic Scheduling of Outpatient Appointments under Patient No-Shows and Cancellations. *Manufacturing & Service Operations Management*, Published online in Articles in Advance, October 2, 2009. DOI: 10.1287/ msom.1090.0272

Muthuraman, K., & Lawley, M. (2008). A stochastic overbooking model for outpatient clinical scheduling with no-shows. *IIE Transactions*, *40*(9), 820–837. doi:10.1080/07408170802165823

Robinson, L., & Chen, R. (2009). A Comparison of Traditional and Open-Access Policies for Appointment Scheduling. *Manufacturing & Service Operations Management*, Published online in Articles in Advance, October 2, 2009. DOI: 10.1287/ msom.1090.0270

Vanden Bosch, P. M., & Dietz, D. C. (2000). Minimizing Expected Waiting in a Medical Appointment System. *IIE Transactions*, *32*(9), 841–848. doi:10.1080/07408170008967443

Vissers, J. (1979). Selecting a Suitable Appointment System in an Outpatient Setting. *Medical Care*, *17*(12), 1207–1220. doi:10.1097/00005650-197912000-00004

Welch, J. D. (1964). Appointment Systems in Gospital Outpatient Departments. *Operational Research Quarterly*, *15*(3), 224–232. doi:10.1057/jors.1964.43

Yang, K. K., Lau, M. L., & Quek, S. A. (1998). A New Appointment Rule for a Single-Server, Multiple-Customer Service System. *Naval Research Logistics*, *45*(3), 313–326. doi:10.1002/(SICI)1520-6750(199804)45:3<313::AID-NAV5>3.0.CO;2-A

KEY TERMS AND DEFINITIONS

Cost Ratio: The ratio between the cost of patient wait time and the cost of physician idle time.

Individual-Block: Only a patient is scheduled in each block, time slot.

Multiple-Block: At least two patients are scheduled in each block, time slot.

No-Show Rate: The probability of patients missed their appointments.

Overbooking: At least two patients are scheduled at the same time.

Scheduled Time Interval: The length of time scheduled between two consecutive patients.

Wait Ratio: The ratio between patient wait time and physician idle time.

Section 3
Electronic Health Records

Chapter 15
Electronic Health Record:
Adoption, Considerations and Future Direction

Janine R. A. Kamath
Mayo Clinic, USA

Amerett L. Donahoe-Anshus
Mayo Clinic, USA

ABSTRACT

Over the last two decades there has been considerable deliberation, experience, and research in the arena of Health Information Technology (HIT), Electronic Medical Records (EMR), Electronic Health Records (EHR), and more recently, Electronic Personal Health Records (PHR). Despite the challenges involved in adopting these systems and technologies, there is consensus that they bring significant value to the delivery of trusted and affordable healthcare. The investment involved and the impact on customers, clinical and non-clinical staff, and processes are significant and far reaching. This chapter attempts to synthesize the vast amount of information, experience, and implementation perspectives related to Electronic Health Records with the intent of assisting healthcare institutions and key stakeholders make informed choices as they embark on designing, developing, and implementing an EHR. EHR considerations, challenges, opportunities, and future directions are also addressed. The chapter highlights the power of management engineering to facilitate planning, implementation, and sustainability of the EHR, a critical asset for a healthcare organization and the overall healthcare industry.

DOI: 10.4018/978-1-60960-872-9.ch015

INTRODUCTION

Providing high-quality, safe, integrated, affordable, efficient and sustainable care should be the hallmark of healthcare organizations. This is a promise we have to make and keep to our patients, their families and other key stakeholders in the healthcare delivery process. A critical component in facilitating this kind of care and an overall excellent patient experience is an EHR. An EHR is defined as an electronic record of health-related information on an individual that conforms to nationally recognized interoperability standards and that can be created, managed, and consulted by authorized clinicians and staff across more than one healthcare organization. An electronic medical record (EMR) is different in that the record is used by authorized clinicians within one healthcare organization. "The principal difference between an EHR and an EMR is the ability to exchange information interoperably," National Alliance for Health Information Technology (NAHIT) says in its April 28, 2008 report, *Defining Key Health Information Technology Terms.*

The benefits of an EHR have been published and contested (Ludwick et al., 2009). Paperwork has been reported to take up to a third of a physician's workday and a national survey of residents shows that they spend as much as six hours per day documenting (Chen, 2010). The ability to access information, leverage best practice, support individualized medicine, minimize inappropriate variation in health care and enable timely interventions are all perceived advantages of an EHR. The availability of patient data together with the expert knowledge of qualified clinicians helps to assure the best care for every patient, every day. The hope is that the EHR provides an infrastructure to support the best patient care and experience. Like most health care systems though, electronic health records are complex. The ability to collect and store data (e.g. textual, imaging, administrative) has led to a data explosion which if not properly managed can lead to difficulty finding and synthesizing pertinent information. To meet the needs of multispecialty and multidisciplinary healthcare providers, EHRs must balance application data granularity and the interoperability needed to integrate data and communicate across systems. Implementation of an EHR must be carefully planned and executed to leverage the benefits and avoid the risks introduced by immature, misaligned and poorly implemented technology.

In addition to effectively and efficiently supporting the clinical practice, the EHR must also facilitate research, education, and operational aspects of healthcare delivery. The EHR is critical for analyzing large amounts of patient information more efficiently, and for providing decision support and best practice guidance at the appropriate points in the care process. The EHR supports applying new research findings to continually enhance patient care, wellness and prevention, comply with ever increasing regulations, assist with revenue recognition opportunities and minimize the administrative healthcare overhead.

The EHR is very important in enabling patients and families to actively participate in the healthcare process, access and enter information online (e.g. review lab results and dismissal instructions, monitor vital signs, schedule appointments) in a patient friendly and safe manner and communicate with their care providers. In an increasingly knowledge and information centric service like healthcare, the intellectual assets and expertise embodied in people and contained in the EHR are central to global competitiveness, population health and economic growth.

The objectives of this chapter are to:

1. Discuss the value of an EHR and the role of management engineering.
2. Highlight key enablers and considerations for successful EHR adoption.
3. Recognize the potential of knowledge management and decision support.
4. Share EHR challenges and implications.

5. Suggest future opportunities to leverage management engineering and advances in technology.

BACKGROUND

Despite the significant value of an EHR, over the last decade only about 15-20% of healthcare institutions have implemented one. As mentioned above, the clinical, operational and administrative benefits have been well documented in the literature. However, cost, complexity of the clinical process, clinician buy–in, privacy and confidentiality, and maturity of EHR systems are a few of the concerns that have deterred institutions from embarking on the EHR journey. Recognizing the importance of an EHR in delivering high value healthcare, the *American Recovery and Reinvestment Act of 2009 (ARRA) was signed into law on February 17th* (Boyd et al., 2010).

This law provides major incentives for health care providers and hospitals to improve caregivers' decisions and patients' outcomes through the use of certified HIT. The Health Information Technology for Economic and Clinical Health Act (HITECH) allows $27 billion in incentive payments through Medicare and Medicaid to caregivers and hospitals when EHRs are used to achieve improved patient care. It is hoped that increased use of EHRs will eventually lead to the creation of a nationwide system of EHRs which will improve healthcare quality and efficiency and the health of populations (Blumenthal, 2009).

HITECH specifically supports the "meaningful use" of EHRs, i.e. EHR use to achieve improvements in patient care processes and outcomes. The Department of Health and Human Services (DHHS) published the final 2011-2012 criteria for EHR "meaningful use" on July 13, 2010. The criteria include core objectives, the basic functions that enable EHRs to support improved care and additional tasks to move toward full EHR implementation and meaningful use. The HITECH act also requires electronic reporting of three core quality measures for 2011-2012: blood pressure, tobacco status and adult weight screening and follow-up. Three other measures can be selected from a list. Finally, HITECH requires the certification of EHRs using the DHHS standards published on June 18, 2010 (Blumenthal, 2009). If however, physicians and hospitals do not adopt this new technology, they will face reduced Medicare payments beginning in 2015 (Health Care Advisory Board (HCAB), 2010).

Health Information Exchange (HIE) is another requirement to prove meaningful use of an EHR and to qualify for the incentives offered by the HITECH Act. The vision of HIE is the seamless exchange of discrete encoded data elements, which can be processed and are human readable in formats that facilitate patient care in a variety of practice settings.

These recent national policies and incentives add an important new dimension for healthcare organizations to consider as they implement new EHR systems or upgrade existing ones. The implications also impact vendors, regulatory and compliance bodies, insurance companies and other key stakeholders in the healthcare industry. We predict that significant changes and new developments will emerge as all the impacted stakeholders move rapidly to leverage the new incentives. Healthcare organizations will benefit by closely monitoring the EHR landscape over the next few years.

MANAGEMENT ENGINEERING SUPPORT FOR EHRs

Experience has shown that developing and implementing an EHR that supports delivering trusted and affordable healthcare is a monumental effort. From a management engineering perspective, one key reason for EHR implementation being so difficult is that healthcare is not like other traditional systems. Healthcare behaves more like a complex adaptive system (CAS) with different implications for system design and management when compared to a traditional system. Some of the characteristics of a CAS are that it is non-linear and dynamic, composed of independent agents with goals and behaviors that might conflict, self-organizing and often with no single point of control (Rouse, 2007). Understanding these important behavioral differences of a healthcare system will help to model, design, develop and implement for a CAS.

Being innovative and proactive in leveraging proven management and systems engineering approaches is another key to success in this difficult journey. Institutions like Mayo Clinic, Kaiser Permanente, and Cleveland Clinic are examples of healthcare organizations that have demonstrated the value of successfully applying engineering principles, methods and tools in implementing an EHR while still being sensitive to the human impacts of an EHR, primarily on patients and staff. Examples include current and future state process mapping, detailed requirements gathering, simulation, process and usability laboratory studies, staffing and workload modeling, and impact evaluations. Engineering emphasizes the importance of designing right from the start, for instance, an EHR that supports the needs of primary care, specialty care, internal medicine and a procedural/surgical practice. The clinical and operational needs of these practices can be quite different. The EHR should balance and optimize the needs of these various practices while maintaining a patient-centric focus. An engineering approach would proactively consider related EHR factors such as technical hardware, facility design, space needs, ergonomics and compliance requirements. Another example is modeling how an EHR can be integrated into decision making processes, much like how evidence-based knowledge can be integrated into daily clinical practice. Mayo Clinic formally established its internal business consulting and management engineering expertise in 1947. This expertise was invaluable to develop and sustain an integrated paper medical record that was transported through a network of carefully engineered chutes and a pneumatic tube system. The integrated record and transport system ensured that clinical information was available at the right time, in the right place and to the right care providers. Subsequently, the management engineering team partnered closely with IT and the clinical practice to transition the paper record and associated workflow processes to an EHR.

In the recent report prepared by the Agency for Healthcare Research and Quality (AHRQ) and the National Science Foundation (NSF) the importance of technology systems being information and patient optimized was highlighted (Sheth Valdez et al., 2010). The report mentions that clinical and process learning should routinely be fed back into the EHR for continuous improvement from existing and newly created knowledge. Using a management engineering approach will help to systematically and proactively analyze, design and implement an EHR that supports the complexity and subtle nuances prevalent in a CAS-like healthcare.

CONSIDERATIONS FOR EHR ADOPTION

The current adoption rate for EHR implementation has been estimated to be about 50% (Jarvis, 2009). A case study identified some of the reasons for slower adoption as inadequate training, lack of time to learn and practice, lack of ongoing support, technical issues with logon time, systems that are not intuitive, and attitudes and expectations (Rahimi et al., 2008).

To assist with successful EHR implementation, setting up a governance and oversight structure approved by senior leadership early in the journey is essential. Also, involving clinical staff in development and implementation is vital. Various planning tools exist to facilitate and guide implementation planning including a comprehensive project or work plan which documents tasks, assigns responsibilities to vendor and organizational resources, and establishes timelines for an effective implementation (Rutherford, 2007) (Mustain et al., 2008). Specific tasks within the project plan may include establishing a strategy, documenting functional and system requirements, usability and system load testing, pre- and post- implementation metrics, risk management, contingency planning, change management, and implementation plans for communication, training/education and go-live support. A few of these key tasks are detailed in the following sections.

EHR Governance

Effective governance and senior leadership involvement is imperative for the successful and timely implementation of an EHR. Mayo Clinic developed an EHR governance and oversight structure which was physician-led and included representatives from the clinical practice, IT and the management engineering division. In addition to a governance group, there were three major oversight groups for orders and medications, documentation tools and user experience and interfaces. This structure effectively supported the initial transition to an EHR and continues to support the ongoing maintenance and evolving requirements for the EHR. The EHR vision, strategy and goals must be shared by senior leadership with customers and staff so they understand the rationale behind this major change. Senior leadership needs to explain how the EHR investment will align with the organizational strategy and improve quality, costs, revenue, efficiencies, error rates, etc. They need to build the "case for change". The EHR governance and decision making authority must be communicated widely. Ongoing clinical involvement is needed at a governance level to ensure improved clinical care, outcomes and workflow. The clinicians involved will help to champion the EHR and get clinician buy-in. To assure alignment with the clinical practice at Mayo Clinic, the physician leader of the EHR is a member of the Clinical Practice Committee. Accountability for measuring and delivering tangible results along with the identification of which institutional processes will benefit from the EHR is the responsibility of the governance structure. Sustainable business plans and financial considerations must be developed and championed for the initial capital expense and as importantly, for ongoing operating expenses (Yoon-Flannery et al., 2008). In our experience one of the critical success factors for EHR adoption has been a deliberate and clearly outlined governance structure with visible senior leadership support during and after the EHR implementation.

Implementation Strategy

Implementation of an EHR may occur through a phased rollout of functionality, by a phased rollout to practice settings, or by big-bang implementations (Karnas et al., 2007) (Ludwick et al., 2009). Whichever method is chosen, clear strategies, objectives and plans for implementation must be established to minimize the impact and disruption to the organization, customers and staff while ensuring a successful EHR roll out. One strategy suggested by the Gartner Group in 2008 provides a five generation phasing for the EHR from initially focusing on collecting clinical information, secondly documenting the information, next helping clinicians, then serving as a colleague, and finally being a mentor. See Figure 1 (Handler, 2008), though we recognize Gartner's current views may have evolved from those in 2008.

The EHR strategy must tie to the organization's strategy and areas needing improvement (Glaser, 2009). Mayo Clinic has a "knowledge-to-delivery" strategic requirement to perpetuate its legacy of generating new knowledge, vetting that which is learned by others, managing information, and then bringing it immediately and seamlessly into the practice. Following a nearly 100-year, comprehensive and trusted historical paper medical

Figure 1. Gartner's Five Generations of EMRs. (© 2008, Handler. Used with permission)

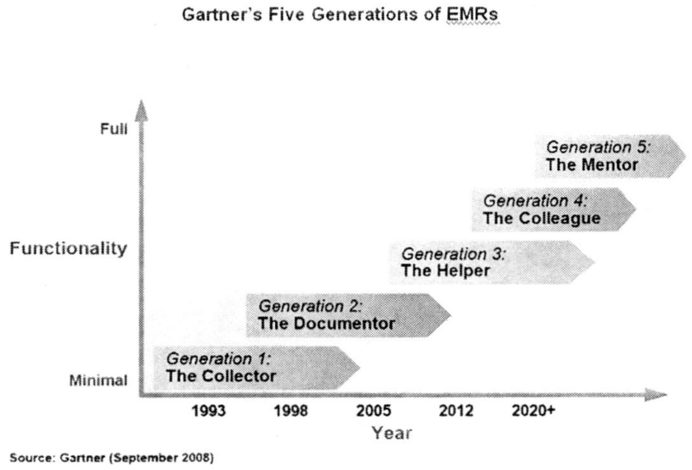

Gartner's Five Generations of EMRs

Full

Functionality

Minimal

Generation 5: **The Mentor**

Generation 4: **The Colleague**

Generation 3: **The Helper**

Generation 2: **The Documentor**

Generation 1: **The Collector**

1993 1998 2005 2012 2020+

Year

Source: Gartner (September 2008)

record, the strategy adopted for implementation of an EHR at Mayo Clinic was a phased approach with three key milestones (see Figure 2): I. Outpatient Provider Chartless, II. New Patient Chartless, and III. Support Staff Chartless.

The first step was to create an infrastructure to enable Mayo Clinic to go chartless and minimize the use of paper. The intent to convert paper to electronic forms and provide backup and business continuity was made clear. As much as possible, standardized processes for clinical and non-clinical staff were created. There was a commitment to provide training and support to facilitate use of the electronic systems. Our experience

Figure 2. Mayo Clinic chartless strategy

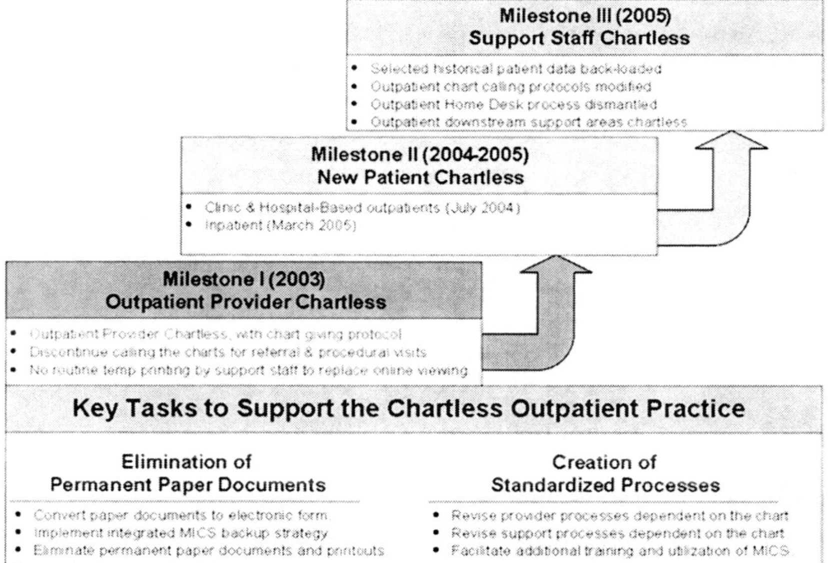

Milestone III (2005)
Support Staff Chartless
Selected historical patient data back-loaded
Outpatient chart calling protocols modified
Outpatient Home Desk process dismantled
Outpatient downstream support areas chartless
Milestone II (2004-2005)
New Patient Chartless
Clinic & Hospital-Based outpatients (July 2004)
Inpatient (March 2005)
Milestone I (2003)
Outpatient Provider Chartless
Outpatient Provider Chartless, with chart giving protocol
Discontinue calling the charts for referral & procedural visits
No routine temp printing by support staff to replace online viewing
Key Tasks to Support the Chartless Outpatient Practice
Elimination of Permanent Paper Documents
Convert paper documents to electronic form
Implement integrated MICS backup strategy
Eliminate permanent paper documents and printouts
Creation of Standardized Processes
Revise provider processes dependent on the chart
Revise support processes dependent on the chart
Facilitate additional training and utilization of MICS

shows that developing the appropriate infrastructure is a critical building block for transitioning to an electronic environment.

In Milestone I, all outpatient paper forms and reports were converted to an electronic solution, appropriate clinical and non-clinical staff could view data online and the routine calling of paper histories was discontinued (though available on an as-needed basis). Milestone II was focused on completing electronic solutions for all paper forms to reduce the dual environment of paper and electronic records. A new summary view was created to support efficient viewing of electronic patient data. Milestone III addressed remaining process issues associated with outpatient visits and inpatient care (e.g. infrastructure and oversight for ongoing support and enhancement of the EHR was established).

Smaller healthcare organizations which might not have the volume, complexity and financial implications of a large academic healthcare organization might benefit from a big-bang strategy. This is definitely more risky and it would be wise to develop an appropriate business continuity plan as well as an IT back-up plan in the event of major EHR system issues. In summary, the implementation strategy adopted needs to consider all the related current and future variables before a decision is made. Major strategy decisions should be endorsed and supported by the governance team and senior leadership.

External Vendor, Internal Development or Hybrid Model

Determining what EHR system will be used requires many considerations. An evaluation of the systems is needed to assure the selected system(s) will meet the customer, staff and business needs. The following list includes examples of such considerations:

- competitive advantage
- functionality
- usability
- customer satisfaction
- reliability
- performance measures
- scalability for size of the organization
- internal IT capability
- financial obligations
- alignment with organization mission and vision
- interoperability
- standards
- customization capability
- timeliness of maintenance, upgrades and enhancements
- vendor financial viability

System selection should also be guided by gathering user requirements and the desired outcome (McGowan et al., 2008). Documenting functional requirements, developing a robust request for information and request for proposal, identifying objective system evaluation criteria and site visits are a few critical factors for selecting the right software. If a vendor cannot meet the organizational and user needs, the system will not be successfully implemented and sustained. Part of the system selection and evaluation must include an objective evaluation of the internal IT capabilities and future vision of the IT department. A number of organizations have elected to develop their own internal EHR and not implement a vended product. This approach offers the customization, contextual understanding and timely response that usually are not offered by vendors.

The hybrid model is another option. This model utilizes mature vendor software for some aspects of the EHR (e.g. laboratory results, monitoring, ordering medications and tests, documentation) while using internal IT staff to develop more customized software or missing functionality (e.g. department or specialty needs, integrated viewers, requirements of cutting edge/ experimental services). The hybrid model attempts to optimize and blend vended and internal IT software to develop a more comprehensive EHR.

Another key consideration in the system selection process is the system architecture. A comparative analysis of system architectures is important. *A client-server based EHR or a web-based EHR?* Recently, this question is often being asked. Server-based EHRs are stored on site, are often thought to be faster, and do not have a dependence on internet connections. They do require local IT expertise and support, including the ability to install software on computers and to back up the server. Web-based EHRs are accessed via a standard internet web browser, making them available anywhere there is internet connection. The vendor pays for the server (data is not stored on site) and for the IT support for the system. Web-based EHRs are dependent on internet connections and the EHR vendor. The appropriate architecture will have to be decided based on factors that include patient volume, cost, complexity of clinical processes, future organizational needs, ongoing maintenance, speed, reliability and HIT skill sets.

Mayo Clinic adopted a hybrid approach with the EHR being primarily a vended product. Some of the specialty practice and complex core process needs are met with other vended or internally-developed software. Key to integrating the multiple software applications from a clinical practice perspective is an internally developed viewing and workflow support application with system interfaces to facilitate navigation, workflow, and an integrated view of the patient record.

Whether vendor purchased, internally developed, server- or web-based or a hybrid, the software must meet the needs of all stakeholders for patients across the continuum of care. Once the EHR is selected, there must be ongoing, clear communication among the vendor, healthcare organization and staff to stay abreast of dynamic requirements and expectations.

System Requirements

Functional requirements are the backbone of a successful EHR implementation. McGowan et al. (2008) suggest that, "Rarely is EHR implementation failure due solely to issues with the technology." They suggest that an EHR that is selected on the basis of organizational needs, goals of key stakeholders and consideration of financial implications should not fail. There is also recognition of the need for user involvement in system selection, requirements gathering and identification of risks and challenges such as system stability and maintenance. Unless these risks and challenges are addressed at the point of selection, large investments may be made without adequate means to address consequences (Sloane et al., 2007).

Thorough identification of system requirements will help to assure that the system goals and objectives are met. The specific deliverables associated with the system requirements should be defined and documented in relation to the clinical workflow (Rutherford, 2007). Clinical workflows for all the disciplines and practices accessing the record for documentation or viewing should be defined. These workflows are multiple and complex. There are also core processes which must be considered (e.g. medication management, ordering and billing,) though they are often difficult to isolate in the complex environment of health care. Not to be forgotten are patient-centered workflows (e.g. check-in, appointment making, scheduling, and follow up on tests and results) which occur across multi-disciplinary teams and care settings. In addition, the processes that involve clinicians' multi-tasking and experiencing regular interruptions must be considered (Wakefield, 2007). Management engineering provides valuable tools (e.g. process mapping, failure mode effect analysis, root cause analysis, control charts, simulation and usability) for evaluating and documenting various processes and dependencies which can then be translated into functional requirements of the EHR system.

Data Standardization and Integration

While unstructured, free-text documentation may be useful for sharing individual patient communications, it is not suitable for sharing data across applications or practices, or for understanding trends and developing reports. The use of standardized, elementized data across care settings and organizations will help the exchange of useful clinical information. It will also minimize duplication of information and rework. While there are some clinical data standards available, they are not widely implemented.

Our experience has shown that to assure data standardization, a data governance structure and process needs to be created by senior leadership and communicated widely. Data governance should provide the policies, resources and tools to help define data, identify what standards exist, document what needs are met with the data and understand what data linkages exist between systems. Without careful data governance, poor data quality may result in incomplete, inconsistent, or duplicate data. Additional issues with data may include:

- dissimilar data definitions or formats
- non-standard terminology
- lack of customer-defined business rules
- inability to accept source data downstream
- lack of data integration
- different context between input and output for the same data element
- human error perpetuated through multiple systems

Data governance also provides metadata which is data about data. In other words, it is a description of a specific data element. The metadata will help assure that if data is changed, moved, deleted, etc., the impact on other systems will be understood. Metadata also provides knowledge about data such as which reports display it, who are the main contacts or experts, what regulations impact it, what is the source, etc.

Medical specialty societies create and publish papers suggesting best practices. If these clinical domain experts also document the single data elements and their attributes, the EHR could enable optimal data use and value. Ideal data structures would support information design that will improve clinicians' ability to quickly review and extract the most pertinent data. Medical informaticists are valuable resources for the design of EMR data structures (Miller, 2008).

The Certification Commission for Healthcare Information Technology (CCHIT) is moving the industry toward data standardization (Hagland, 2009). When EHR databases can share data and become networked to do so electronically, the ability to improve health care will increase exponentially.

System Design: Scope, Testing, and Human Factors

EHRs offer the potential to capture, store, retrieve and synthesize patient data. To be useful, the data must be presented to the right people at the right time and in the right sequence. Carefully designed user interfaces and application flow are important for successful EHR adoption and use. Properly designed, an EHR can be integrated into the health care system, including time-associated dependencies, complexities of clinical tasks and workflows, and care settings and processes which surround the technology.

While the benefits of an EHR may be anticipated, they are not typically realized at the time of implementation. Rather, they are realized after significant user adoption and full functionality of the software is implemented (Doebbeling et al., 2008). The use of engineering studies such as sequential pattern analysis (recurring patterns of use) and first-order Markov chain model (overall sequential order of feature access) can also help to assure ideal design of the EHR. How users access clinical data is reflective of patient care processes and clinical workflow which can be validated with further research such as context inquiry (in what part of the process do they need which data) and ethnographically based observations (within clinical care settings, what is needed to gather pertinent information). Users of the EHR know best what they are looking for and when. Involvement of users in the system design process is critical for user acceptance upon implementation (Rahimi et al., 2008) (Zheng et al., 2009). Human Factors is the science that studies human capabilities as they pertain to the design of systems and products for safe and effective use. Conducting human factors studies to understand user preferences and the impact an EHR has on the practice will provide knowledge and insights to help assure a system design which will best meet user needs. Formal usability testing provides the opportunity to observe users interacting with the EHR and to understand *what they are looking for, what is intuitive, and what are their likes and dislikes.* Conducting usability tests early in the development process will allow time to make design changes. To be most successful, technology needs to be flexible and designed for diverse environments and users. At Mayo Clinic, users were actively involved throughout the design and development process. The formal usability and process flow testing, whether in the specialized Usability/Process Lab or contextually in the clinical practice, proved to be extremely valuable to validate that key functional requirements were met and that the software was intuitive, responsive and usable within various workflows and clinical scenarios.

Education, Communication and Change Management

Even with user-defined functional requirements and input on system design, user adoption upon EHR implementation requires much support. The complexity of computer systems implementation in health care may be found in the interrelationships between technology, information, people and organizational issues (Ludwick et al., 2009). To deal with this complexity, a contextual implementation model was developed at three levels: the organizational level, clinical or departmental level and the individual level. Key dimensions for this socio-technical model are provided at each level. For example, at the organizational level, consideration should be given for the culture, previous implementation experiences, level of management support, and resources available. At the clinical or departmental level, consideration should be given to unique needs, work practices and cultural diversity of each environment. At the individual level, consideration should be given to the differences between care providers in how they use computers in the care process. By using these dimensions pre-, during and post-implementation, difficulties with adoption can be alleviated (Callen et al., 2008).

Comprehensive implementation planning includes consideration of change management principles (Mustain et al., 2008). Using an established change management model, such as Prosci's Awareness-Desire-Knowledge-Ability-Reinforcement (ADKAR) can help guide planning to ease the transition to an EHR. The model reflects stages for an individual's readiness for change and helps guide the education, communication and implementation support required for adoption (Hiatt, 2006). Emphasis is placed on communicating early and often to raise users' awareness of plans for implementation. Including the staff and patient benefits expected from the use of an EHR will also help adoption as users will understand the benefits the EHR will provide them. For example, Kaiser Permanente documented and shared potential operational efficiencies created by their EHR (Chen et al., 2009). However, caution must be used to avoid the creation of unrealistic expectations about the benefits of an EHR.

In addition to recognizing the benefits of an EHR, staff needs to understand the capabilities of the EHR and be competent in using them. It is by use of all EHR functionality that the benefits will eventually be realized. Providing EHR educational offerings such as hands-on classroom computer training, reference materials (electronic and hard copy), time to practice and user support (onsite application team, onsite super user and/or Help Desk support) contributes to the ability to adopt and become proficient with the EHR. Proficiency may also be achieved by allowing time following classroom training to practice, conducting pilots, and/or having parallel systems (current and future) for a period of time. Often, allowing time to practice can enable users to share their own discoveries and best practices among colleagues. Peer education is powerful because of the credibility inherent among colleagues. A comprehensive implementation plan with multiple approaches for training was used by Mayo Clinic, including online courses, quick reference guides, classroom training and short tips/tricks sessions. The plan also included multiple communication approaches, including internal publications, user testimonials, presentations, email, posters and electronic bulletin board notices. Finally, the plan included multiple levels of user support, including onsite support by the project team, local super users, electronic support assistants with advanced training, and remote support by the help desk and command center.

Once implemented, reinforcement of the desired use of an EHR can occur at multiple levels. Senior leadership can share data regarding practice outcomes and adoption rates, operational managers can share efficiencies gained and celebrate achievement of pre-established milestones, and users can provide testimonials on the EHR benefits, such as access to patient information and the ability to get data out of an electronic system (Rahimi et al., 2008).

Carefully planned strategies to increase training, improve ease of use, incentives and mandates (internal or external) may all encourage greater use of EHR features which will ultimately result in improved organizational performance (Poon et al., 2010).

Impact Analysis and Ongoing Evaluation

As mentioned above, there are many projected benefits of an EHR. To understand projected benefits and validate that they have been achieved, baseline measurements must be conducted prior to implementation for comparison post-implementation. An impact analysis provides understanding of the influence an EHR has on the organization and includes both quantitative and qualitative measures. See example measures in Table 1.

The impact analysis should include an evaluation to assess workflows and patient outcomes pre- and post-implementation. This will help to determine if the EHR has improved or worsened outcomes. A study by Wakefield et al. (2007) used a survey, "Information Systems Expectations and Experience", to evaluate staff expectations and the actual experience for nursing practices in four sites. The results highlighted the value of early identification of staff perceptions and concerns which will allow planning for targeted interventions to address issues. As EHRs are dynamic, post-implementation assessments help to point out the need for additional system adjustments and fine tuning. The results of the post-implementation assessment at Mayo Clinic emphasized the importance of iterative adjustments and fine tuning. In addition, it validated that customer satisfaction and cost savings were both realized. For example, customer satisfaction was realized in the availability and legibility of the medical record. Cost savings due to reduced movement of paper records resulted in the reassignment of staff to other areas of the clinical practice or reduction of staff via natural attrition.

The impact analysis should also evaluate risks such as confidentiality and patient data privacy

Table 1. Example measures

Quantitative Measures	Qualitative Measures
• Clinical outcome measures, e.g. EHR-related adverse events or potential hazards, reportable error rates, preventive service screening • Clinical process measures, e.g. % of electronic prescriptions, documentation of allergies and immunizations • Workflow impact measures, e.g. documentation timing study • Financial impact measures, e.g. office visits per member per month • Application reliability, e.g. EHR downtime	• Satisfaction, e.g. provider and patient/family satisfaction • Provider competency and adoption • Improved access to patient records • Enhanced efficiency in workflow, e.g. ease of finding information • Quality of provider-patient communications • Completeness of documentation • Legibility of the EHR

(Yoon-Flannery et al., 2008). A safe, effective EHR should include evaluation of safety issues. EHR certification (for safety, working as designed and fixing defects) and self-assessment of EHR use (competency in EHR use, downtime procedures) are being strongly encouraged. There continue to be suggestions that the Office of the National Coordinator for Health information technology (ONC) create a National EHR Adverse Event Investigation Board to monitor unplanned consequence from EHR use (Sittig et al., 2010).

HEALTH CARE KNOWLEDGE AND DELIVERY

Best care practices are continually being researched, improved upon using rapid cycles, and defined by quality initiatives, professional associations and special interest groups. However, our experience indicates that these best practices are not shared and implemented consistently. There are significant gaps in the management and dissemination of knowledge at the appropriate points in the care delivery process. EHR's do not seem to be mature and sophisticated enough to support knowledge management. Past studies have not shown consistent improvement in quality measures by the use of EHRs. A study regarding the use of specific EHR features (not simply presence of an EHR) in primary care practices did correlate with higher performance on some Healthcare Effectiveness Data and Information Set (HEDIS) quality measures (Poon et al., 2010). It has been recognized that EHRs can improve the health care system by reducing inappropriate variation (Hannan, 1999). Some of the opportunities for influencing variation are discussed below, in the decision support section. Management Engineering methodologies and tools (such as process mapping and LEAN methodology) are effective in reducing variation. Guiding best care practice, however, is dependent on successful adoption of EHR functionality.

Knowledge Management

There is an exponential volume of electronic data now available from various sources, (e.g. medical devices, documentation tools, compliance reports, external patient data). The difficulty for the clinical practice is bringing all the data, knowledge and best practice together in a way that allows the clinician to synthesize information accurately and quickly. For information coming from multiple systems, the challenge of data interoperability is that "… flaws, delays, and failures can be life-critical" (Sloane et al., 2007). EHRs have the potential to support providers in the care of their patients and in conformance to practice standards.

Knowledge management is a discipline that ensures that the intellectual capabilities of an organization are shared, maintained and institutionalized. It offers a process of capturing, organizing, and storing the expertise and experiences of staff and groups within an organization and making it available to others in a manner which enables adoption of insights and experiences.

Knowledge management systems in healthcare store clinical knowledge and allow easy access to knowledge from the EHR at the time it is needed to support the clinical practice. Mayo Clinic recognizes knowledge management as one of its strategic objectives. Part of this objective includes the active management of internal or external healthcare knowledge and information and providing it to the practice. Mayo has developed a centralized knowledge system called "Ask Mayo Expert (AME)" to store expert knowledge, references and subject matter experts. Electronic alerts in the EHR prompt care providers that AME information is available and provide a link to the information.

Tools which healthcare organizations have used to enable knowledge management include expert learning systems (best information for patients' conditions), information systems that interface research and education with the practice, data warehouses, and real time clinical decision support systems.

DECISION SUPPORT

Computer-based Clinical Decision Support (CDS) is a complex, highly integrated clinical system functionality that has been identified as an important tool for improving quality, preventing medical errors and reducing costs in healthcare

(Lin et al., 2008) (Zheng et al., 2009) (Bates, 2010). Like other large healthcare organizations, Mayo Clinic is leveraging CDS to assist providers in delivering best practice care by getting the right information to the right person at the right time. This is achieved by a blend of electronically triggered rules which can generate alerts, send a message to providers and/or provide a link to internal knowledge management systems. It is well recognized that the use of decision support requires iterative learning and continual refinement.

Point of Care Knowledge Delivery

The following stages in the patient care process have been identified as critical for Clinical Decision Support: proactive/preventive care, real time and monitoring of care, and retrospective review.

Proactive/Preventive Care: Finding pertinent information for preventive services and chronic disease management in the EHR can be labor intensive and the information can be difficult to synthesize. This is due to the multiple locations and volume of documentation in the EHR. Decision support mechanisms need to provide timely, pertinent information and care recommendations based on best practices. This level of decision support could improve the quality of patient care and decrease costs by creating a list of patients due for preventive screening or chronic disease surveillance, prompting the scheduling of appropriate appointments for preventive screening, therapeutic interventions and/or closer monitoring and follow-up management of patients with chronic disease (Bates, 2010). A challenge for the EHR continues to be to support coordination of this kind of care.

Real Time and Monitoring of Care: Relying on humans to remember to check for lab or test results, recognize declining symptoms, place all the appropriate orders for all conditions, and recognize medication allergies or intolerances in a fast-paced, complex healthcare environment is no longer sustainable. Technology is able to help flag values outside of normal ranges, to recognize patterns of changing vital signs, to alert providers to published best practices and to prompt interventions for specific disease states. Real-time notification with ongoing monitoring and feedback will effectively facilitate compliance with clinical utilization and documentation requirements. The technologies need to be easily accessible within the clinician's work flow at the time that they need to take action to address patient needs. As an example, the monitoring and timely diagnosis of patients developing sepsis can positively impact patient recovery.

Retrospective Review: Comparing individual and organizational performance with published best practices provides pertinent feedback for changing behavior. Likewise, understanding the overall health of populations and variations in outcomes are important drivers of excellence in patient care. An example is the Minnesota Community Measurement which compares diagnosis-specific population data (e.g. asthma, diabetes, high blood pressure).

Tools for Decision Support

The specific tools available for clinical decision support are numerous, including passive and active mechanisms. The effectiveness and efficacy of decision support tools are critical to assure the best tool is used for each need. Caution must be used to avoid over-alerting or under-alerting which can diminish the effectiveness of rules designed to guide clinical practice.

The following list illustrates a sample of clinical decision support tools which are actively used at Mayo Clinic and other major healthcare institutions.

- **Expert Rules:** active or passive notifications to facilitate workflow
- **Secure Messaging:** secured electronic communications/reminders to providers and services
- **Centralized Problem List:** historical and current diagnoses to prompt interventions
- **Order Sets and Protocols:** standardized and approved best-practice interventions for identified problems
- **Panel Query:** a providers' list of patients who may meet certain criteria

While there are clear benefits of leveraging the EHR to provide clinical decision support, there are challenges yet to be addressed. Some of these include the multiple databases in which pertinent data resides, resource constraints to support a dynamic clinical practice and external reporting needs, care provider alert fatigue, and an over-dependency on or complacency about decision support.

EHR CHALLENGES AND CONCERNS

Adoption of HIT and an EHR is often envisioned as facilitating the development of an ideal health care delivery system. However, as with any significant and invasive change, the EHR has its set of challenges and setbacks. It is important for healthcare institutions to recognize these challenges and prepare to work through them in a proactive and deliberate manner.

Financial Implications

Many healthcare executives still believe the financial return from investing in EHRs is a myth. On July 3, 2008, the *New England Journal of Medicine* published eye-opening research regarding the rate of electronic health record (EHR) adoption in the United States (Jarvis, 2009). Based on anecdotal evidence, the study reveals that the two most significant barriers to EHR utilization are "fear" and "funding." Many physician practices fear that the conversion will be too difficult and disruptive. At the same time, they are concerned about how they will be able to fund the investment, and the impact the transition will have on their bottom line. The study also revealed that often workflow processes are not reengineered and hence even the best manual system will fail within an automated environment. The reengineered processes need to be patient-centered and optimized for the entire continuum of care (e.g. pre-visit, visit and post-visit) or core process (e.g. medication management, ordering, scheduling and orders cycle), and not just for local practice groups or areas.

Another challenge is to define the real cost involved in implementing an EHR. Often, only the installation price of the software, which is the "tip of the iceberg" and may represent 50% or less of the entire project cost, is included (Jarvis, 2009). However, it is critical to factor in expenses related to hardware purchases, infrastructure upgrades, paper record scanning or abstraction, staff training time, and a temporary decrease in productivity. It is also important to consider which software features will increase efficiency and improve outcomes, and consider how the technology will support the institution and providers over the long term. While the task of obtaining funding can be ominous, healthcare institutions should continually be on the lookout for new funding opportunities. Patient advocacy groups are playing an ever-increasing role, particularly in the development of PHRs. Likewise, malpractice carriers view EHRs as a viable strategy to reduce exposure to risk. One Ohio practice, for example, used its EHR to negotiate a 50% reduction in annual premiums – from $400,000 to $200,000 (Jarvis, 2009). However, the focus needs to be on value and not just on cost. Overall, the EHR is an investment and the qualitative as well as quantitative aspects need to be considered.

Impact of Government and Regulatory Policies

The current national policies pushing the rapid implementation of meaningful use are a challenge that could result in undesirable and unintended consequences (Boyd et al., 2010). For example, pressure for rapid adoption of an EHR may inhibit or prohibit the involvement of key stakeholders. Also, it may inhibit or prohibit the use of appropriate design and implementation strategies, resulting in suboptimal technologies and poor integration into practice. Meaningful use varies with context, institution, clinician, patient, secondary use of the data and third-party payers. The questions that need to be seriously considered are: *Meaningful to whom?, Meaningful for what purpose(s)?, and Meaningful under what circumstances?* (Boyd et al., 2010). Furthermore, the current high cost of EHRs and the push at a national level for implementation is likely to prevent institutions from continually investing in new/upgraded systems, potentially resulting in stagnation of EHR improvement and innovation.

Meaningful use brings another concern related to HIEs. Despite considerable promise, few examples of well-functioning and sustainable HIEs exist to serve as models. A 2007 survey revealed that of more than 100 regional health information organizations, 25% were defunct and only 15 were of at least modest size and exchanging data across a range of populations (Rudin et al., 2009). Integrating HIEs into clinical workflows is expected to be challenging even when performance levels are high. The experiences of the 3 collaborative pilot communities provide a revealing characterization of the perspectives of key HIE stakeholders. Critical success factors for HIEs, from the stakeholders' perspectives, included community-wide trust, strategic interests of individual health care providers and the medical community as a whole, and benefits derived from measuring quality of care. It remains to be seen whether this effort or any other HIE in the United States can provide direct benefits from quality measurements or other activities. Without such benefits, the sustainability of HIEs and the accompanying increases in clinical data available for public health practice and research may remain precarious. There is a lot more learning that needs to take place in the HIE arena. The HIE vision mentioned above will have to be achieved in a phased manner with iterative learning (Rudin et al., 2009).

Management Engineering Support

When it comes to leveraging management engineering for implementing and sustaining an EHR there is still limited understanding of what tools, techniques, and methods are most appropriate to use and under what circumstances they are most effective. As mentioned before, healthcare institutions like Mayo Clinic, Kaiser Permanente and Cleveland Clinic, who continue to leverage and learn from the use of engineering models and methods for EHR implementations, would be valuable resources to institutions who will be involved in EHR implementation. Particularly important and relatively new are the unexpected problems being raised based on evidence, related to EHRs. Some of these problems include EHRs adversely affecting clinical care by generating more work or new work for clinicians, causing workflow problems, creating a sense of complacency because of embedded decision support and alerting mechanisms, or even by generating new kinds of errors (Brokel, 2009). It will be important for experts in the fields of management and systems engineering to explore, develop, and test tools that can be used to support large, multisystem and multidisciplinary EHR implementations as well as to solve current and new issues related to EHRs.

EHR Vendor Incentives

A significant challenge is vendor incentives that are currently short-term oriented and misaligned. The struggle to develop and implement "best of breed" versus "integrated systems" continues in the vendor community as well as in healthcare institutions. As a result, there is no desire for mid-to-long term analyses or support to optimize large complex adaptive systems such as healthcare. Complex adaptive systems have a strong tendency to learn, adapt, self-organize and manage to maximize value (Rouse, 2007). Hence, there clearly is a need to design and develop an EHR for managing complexity and change in various forms: balancing between the needs of primary care, specialty care, internal medicine and procedural/surgical practices from a patient-centric perspective, focusing on the benefits of organizational outcomes and not only on inputs like revenue, supporting a global healthcare system, enabling chronic disease management and longitudinal care, and assisting with monitoring of the entire healthcare system or a subsystem effectively and efficiently.

Privacy, Security and Confidentiality

Ensuring the privacy and security of patient information, and associated public relations issues is still a challenge. Medical identity theft seems to be a disturbing and growing trend. Many positive strides have been made through legislation, consumer advocacy and media attention to improve this arena. For example, fines under the Health Insurance Portability and Accountability Act (HIPAA) for unlawfully disclosing patient data can be as high as $250,000 and, if convicted, a person could face up to 10 years in prison (Civelek, 2009). HIT and EHR security vendors continue to explore better ways to handle this issue by building security in layers with the goal to make access difficult enough to deter thieves and hackers, but not so difficult that users take shortcuts around security safeguards. However, the concern continues to be significant and real. A vast majority of health executives surveyed in 2009 (over 80 percent) cited privacy, legal implications, and public relations ramifications as significant concerns (Civelek, 2009).

Patient and Family Role

Increasing patient and family motivation, and changing long-term habits to better leverage an EHR will need attention in the years ahead. To date, the involvement of patients and/or families in using the EHR and virtual opportunities like portals, have been limited. Some of the factors that have adversely impacted the growth in patient and family involvement include:

- comfort with using technology
- cost factors
- reliability
- reach of technology infrastructure like networks to rural areas
- privacy

The hope is that these challenges will be more deliberately addressed in the near future. It will be important for EHR vendors and internal IT groups to develop patient-friendly and intuitive EHR software to enhance and speed up active engagement. Patients and families need help to understand the value to them, of using the EHR especially if they perceive the patient–physician interaction to be adversely impacted by the use of technology. Voice of the Customer initiatives at Mayo Clinic are helping to assure the patient and family needs are understood as refinements continue to be made to the EHR and other systems.

Dependence on Paper

The dependence on paper even in institutions which have long adopted EHRs continues to be a problem. At Mayo Clinic, the clinical practice and operational teams systematically work with clinical and non-clinical staff to minimize the dependence on paper. The Mayo Clinic Chartless Initiative implemented in 2005 (previously mentioned), is one example of a deliberate and creative approach to move the practice to a more electronic environment. Even though the dependence on paper was minimized by this initiative, as new reports, regulations and new service lines emerged the temptation was to resort to paper. The time delay in EHR upgrades further complicates the paper issue. It is important to recognize that dependence on paper will continue to be a tough challenge to overcome. The lack of reliable and functional point-of-care electronic appliances (e.g. hand-held, portable computers) further compounds this issue. Previous research identified three additional key factors that may lead clinicians to generate paper-based workarounds while using an EHR: (1) poor EHR interface design, (2) poor integration of the EHR into clinical workflow, (3) and an incompatibility between EHR designers' and clinicians' mental models for information access and workflow (Saleem, 2009).

Exponential Growth of Data and Reporting Needs

As more and more health-related information becomes electronic, issues of data capture, redundancy, storage, retrieval, navigation and presentation grow. The impact on clinical workflow, effort and time is significant. Medication management, which is a complex, multifaceted operation involving multiple people, large amounts of data and numerous steps is a good example. The compliance and reporting requirements with medication management are numerous. The impact of diagnostic reports and imaging related data is another key example of an explosion in the volume of electronic data that needs to be managed. Physician documentation in EHRs will be a lynchpin in achieving meaningful use in hospitals and the outpatient setting, but most agree that capturing and reviewing information in the electronic record is still a challenge for clinicians. While structured documentation and templates can reduce the burden of physician typing and data capture, there are still the issues of unstructured notes, redundancy of information and copying and pasting from an existing note to address. Data automatically captured in the EHR through device (e.g. monitors, medical equipment) integration also brings a new set of data challenges and questions like: *how much data?, for how long?, what to store? and, how to display the data?*

The demands of real-time and retrospective reporting (e.g. quality, cost, outcomes, and overall performance) have imposed a substantial burden on healthcare institutions. Although the potential rewards of extracting EHR clinical data for reporting purposes are enormous, the accompanying challenges should not be underestimated. Access to EHR clinical data does not equate to valid and efficient reporting without considerable effort. The complexity of health care and medical decision making demands that careful attention be paid to the process of accessing the correct data and interpreting those data accurately with regard to both content and timing. Even data elements that are anticipated to be reasonably accessible, like medication data, can pose significant data collection and interpretation problems (Roth et al., 2009).

FUTURE EHR RESEARCH AND DIRECTION

As highlighted throughout this chapter, the successful and timely implementation of an EHR is critical to the future survival of healthcare institutions. Patients, staff, regulatory groups, and other key stakeholders will demand its existence. The research, experience and lessons learned by many institutions in implementing EHRs, clearly demonstrate the importance of leveraging management engineering to implement a high-quality, safe, comprehensive and cost-effective solution. In the future, management engineering will also be critical to sustain an EHR in a dynamic and demanding healthcare environment. Based on a literature review, the future direction of government, regulatory bodies and EHR vendors, the experiences of many US and global healthcare institutions, and consumer demands, the following future trends and considerations will be crucial for truly meaningful EHR adoption and use:

EHR Functionality and Maturity

Future EHRs will have to support new healthcare directions in individualized medicine, wellness and prevention, genomics and e-health (e.g. home health, telemedicine, cybermedicine, and patient and family education). In addition, EHR design will need to integrate qualitative and contextual knowledge (e.g., culture, language, ethics, special or relevant personal circumstances) into clinical care so that the healthcare delivery process and staff appropriately consider and respond to these factors. The fast pace of globalization and the obligation of providing appropriate health care to all will demand this enhancement.

The rapid convergence of the World Wide Web with mobile telecommunication devices makes it easier to embed resources in EHRs that could support exchanges of information by customers with health care professionals in a wide range of modalities (e.g. simple text messaging through asynchronous telehealth consultations to live videoconferences). Therefore, healthcare organizations will need to be available and responsive to customers anywhere and at any time. This is a major change and requires thinking through and adapting policies, roles, work processes, and system structures. The healthcare organization could also benefit from tools that enable one-to-many, many-to-one, or many-to-many interactions. The proliferation of generic resources and social media, such as Wikipedia, Facebook, and Twitter, as well as health-specific tools targeting health professionals and customers, is creating new, cost-effective ways to embed powerful tools in the health system. Integrating these tools with the EHR would make them easier to access, while enabling targeted and personalized communication (Shachak et al., 2010).

The healthcare industry is also reaching a point of convergence. After years of growth in their own space, healthcare organizations need to exchange data across healthcare settings (e.g. ambulatory, in-patient), across specialties (e.g. primary care to radiology to the emergency room), and across different healthcare systems. Interoperability of systems will enhance patient safety and accelerate care delivery to patients in need by reducing paperwork and time required for clinical data discovery. It will also contribute to reducing the incidence of redundant or unnecessary procedures thus keeping healthcare costs under better control (Hufnagel, 2009). Key trends that will continue to evolve in the interoperability space include the development, adoption and maintenance of standards, protocols, vocabularies, ontologies and various advanced technologies (e.g. distributed and service-oriented architecture, natural language processing, open source EHRs, portals, mobile computing, and device integration).

As mentioned earlier, the EHR plays a key role in the research realm. In the future, the system will need to better facilitate iterative knowledge development and distribution (e.g. best practices, new treatments and protocols), timely and relevant dissemination of knowledge at the point of care, and seamless knowledge transfer between research and the clinical practice to significantly shorten the "bench to bedside" cycle time. This cycle time involves the time to translate research discoveries and developments from the laboratory to the delivery of enhanced patient care.

Stronger Management and Systems Engineering Role

For true meaningful use the EHR will have to be closely integrated into all aspects of the healthcare delivery process: clinical, research, education and administrative. A stronger role for engineering will be invaluable at all levels and stages. The first key step is to broaden the awareness of engineering and the value engineers provide to successful EHR implementation and adoption. True partnerships between various clinical disciplines and engineers will be crucial. Engaging clinical staff with formal engineering education in technical decision making provides a dual perspective - clinical and engineering. Freeing clinicians from clinical duties could be a challenge, but they still need to be engaged.

The future process will need to leverage management and systems engineering approaches and tools (e.g. computer simulation, workflow modeling, data standards and protocols like HL7 and DICOM, and advanced impact evaluation methods) to design and implement an EHR that supports patient-centric and system-wide optimization, not just sub-system optimization. Also, mandatory or forcing functions will be needed to capture elemental data for system-wide quality and compliance reporting. The value of an engineering and integrated approach is highlighted in the following situations cited in the July-August 2009 AARP bulletin (Yackanicz et al., 2010). A medical computer network linking 6 million patients noted a surge in cases of an intestinal bug causing nausea and vomiting. Within 24 hours, it was traced to an Indianapolis grocery selling tainted custard-filled doughnuts. The second situation relates to Dr. John T. Finnell, a research scientist at Regenstrief and Associate Professor of Emergency Medicine at the Indiana University School of Medicine, who cited an example of a patient admitted to the emergency department with a heart attack. The physician wanted to use heparin but changed his treatment when he read that the person had experienced head trauma two weeks earlier. Dr. Finnell suggested that even a small subset of addictions-related data would make a difference in the life of an emergency room patient by assisting physicians in providing the right care (Yackanicz et al., 2010).

Engineering methods and models will enable the translation of numerical, textual, and computational EHR data into understandable and actionable information for multiple stakeholders (e.g., patients, nurses, primary care and specialty care physicians, or pharmacists) and in different situations (e.g., disease outbreaks like H1N1, error prevention, outcomes studies, and drug recalls). Our experience has been that utilization of enhanced data visualization techniques and graphical user interfaces will be vital with the exponential growth of data and the shrinking time available to clinicians to provide the best care possible.

Leveraging EHR Data

As EHR implementations grow and mature there will be tremendous clinical, research, administrative and financial value latent in this growing health data. This is often referred to as the secondary use of EHR data. The additional value and opportunity that these data offer could include quality measurement, public health surveillance, support for biomedical informatics and clinical and translational research (Hersh, 2007). In 2009, for example, the Centers for Disease Control and Prevention (CDC) selected GE Healthcare to provide extensive surveillance data for H1N1 and seasonal influenza activity throughout the United States every 24 hours. GE Healthcare reports secured and de-identified information from its proprietary Medical Quality Improvement Consortium (MQIC) database, containing more than 14 million patient records. The reports helped the CDC monitor the spread of the H1N1 virus in near real-time (Business wire: GE Healthcare news release, Oct. 28, 2009). Another excellent example is one of Geisinger Ventures' portfolio companies, MedMining, which supports applying Geisinger's health data for a secondary commercial purpose. MedMining provides customized, de-identified data extracts to promote health economics and other biopharmaceutical research (Garrett, 2010).

Continuous Knowledge Sharing

The power and value of global benchmarking, partnerships and sharing of knowledge, as well as lessons learned in the EHR journey have been grossly underestimated. The key stakeholders in the healthcare delivery process would significantly benefit by continuously reviewing the literature to understand if new and more advanced strategies, systems, approaches and learning are available. Building vertical (e.g. EHR vendors, patients, employers, individual healthcare institutions) and horizontal (e.g. collections of healthcare institutions) partnerships to benefit and optimize the whole rather than parts of the process will be critical in the future. A greater commitment to publishing and presenting will facilitate continuous knowledge sharing and learning. Mayo Clinic continues to partner with other organizations and healthcare institutions to share and learn from their experiences. It is through such partnership that the health of the nation and the world will be improved.

CONCLUSION

In conclusion, the EHR is an investment in total practice transformation. It alters the workflow of virtually every care process and significantly impacts most consumers of heath care and those who deliver this vital service. To obtain its full potential, the adoption and implementation of an EHR should be treated as a means of facilitating redesign of outdated, inefficient, and error-prone care processes, and a vehicle for organizational change rather than just another information technology innovation (Brokel et al., 2009). The EHR is not a one-time investment but a journey that will require significant ongoing resources, time and institutional commitment. Hence, the importance of using management and systems engineering approaches and tools to design, develop and implement a robust and dynamic EHR that supports a complex adaptive system like healthcare.

Today and into the near future, government and regulatory incentives will facilitate the adoption and growth of EHRs but with incentives will come compliance, administrative and quality requirements. A proactive, strategic and collaborative approach within and between healthcare organizations will be essential. The vision, goals and principles for an EHR need to be defined upfront and validated along the EHR journey. The future research and direction for EHR adoption holds promise as detailed earlier in this chapter. The promise seems relevant to most healthcare organizations (e.g. smaller physician offices, medium-size hospitals and large academic medical centers) as well as customers.

For now, it is best that healthcare organizations not wait but move ahead quickly and deliberately to implement an EHR. In this endeavor, it would serve organizations well to leverage the vast experience and lessons learned, be realistic about the challenges, continually engage key stakeholders, forge strategic partnerships and proactively plan for the various phases in the EHR journey, keeping in mind exciting future developments.

ACKNOWLEDGMENT

The authors wish to thank the following individuals for their support of and thoughtful feedback on this chapter: Jennifer Ferguson, MS; Karen Larsen, MA, MBA; Thomas Lucas, MA; and Katie Sinning.

REFERENCES

Bates, D. W. (2010). Getting in step: Electronic health records and their role in care coordination. *Journal of General Internal Medicine*, *25*(3), 174–176. doi:10.1007/s11606-010-1252-x

Blumenthal, D. (2009). Stimulating the adoption of health information technology. *The New England Journal of Medicine*, *360*(15), 1477–1479. doi:10.1056/NEJMp0901592

Blumenthal, D., & Tavernner, M. (2010). The meaningful use regulation for electronic health records. *The New England Journal of Medicine*, *363*(6). Retrieved on July 13, 2010, from http://www.nejm.org/doi/full/ 10.1056/NEJMp1006114

Boyd, A. D., Funk, E. A., Schwartz, S. M., Kaplan, B., & Keenan, G. M. (2010). Top EHR challenges in light of the stimulus. Enabling effective interdisciplinary, intradisciplinary and cross-setting communication. *Journal of Healthcare Information Management*, *24*(1), 18–24.

Brokel, J. M. (2009). Redesigning care processes using an electronic health record: A system's experience. *Joint Commission Journal on Quality and Patient Safety*, *35*(2), 82–92.

Callen, J. L., Braithwaite, J., & Westbrook, J. I. (2008). Contextual implementation model: A framework for assisting clinical information system implementations. *Journal of the American Medical Informatics Association*, *15*(2), 255–262. doi:10.1197/jamia.M2468

Chen, C., Garrido, T., Chock, D., Okawa, G., & Liang, L. (2009). The Kaiser Permanente electronic health record: Transforming and streamlining modalities of care. *Health Affairs*, *28*(2), 323–333. doi:10.1377/hlthaff.28.2.323

Chen, P. (2010). Doctors and patients, lost in paperwork. *New York Times,* pp. 1-3.

Civelek, A. C. (2009). Patient safety and privacy in the electronic health information era: Medical and beyond. *Clinical Biochemistry*, *42*(4-5), 298–299. doi:10.1016/j.clinbiochem.2008.09.018

Clancy, T. R., Delaney, C. W., Segre, A., Carley, K., Kuziak, A., & Yu, H. (2007). Predicting the impact of an electronic health record on practice patterns using computational modeling and simulation. *AMIA Annual Symposium Proceedings*, (pp. 145-9).

Corbin, A. (2007). The 360-degree approach. EHRs are only a first step in what should be an effort to integrate clinical and financial applications. *Healthcare Informatics*, *24*(5), 42.

Cross, H. M. (2009). The EHR in our emerging future. *Behavioral Healthcare*, *29*(8), 40.

D'Avolio, L. W. (2009). Electronic medical records at a crossroads: Impetus for change or missed opportunity? *Journal of the American Medical Association*, *302*(10), 1109–1111. doi:10.1001/jama.2009.1319

Dean, B. B., Lam, J., Natoli, J. L., Butler, Q., Aguilar, D., & Nordyke, R. J. (2008). Toward a model of successful electronic health record adoption. *Healthcare Quarterly (Toronto, Ont.)*, *11*(3), 84–91.

DesRoches, C. M., Campbell, E. G., & Rao, S. R. (2008). Electronic health records in ambulatory care: A national survey for physicians. *The New England Journal of Medicine*, *359*, 50–60. doi:10.1056/NEJMsa0802005

Doebbeling, B. N., & Pekny, J. (2008). The role of systems factors in implementing health information technology. *Journal of General Internal Medicine*, *23*(4), 500–501. doi:10.1007/s11606-008-0559-3

Garrett, D. (2010). Tapping into the value of health data through secondary use. *Healthcare Financial Management*, *64*(2), 76–83.

Glaser, J. (2009). Implementing electronic health records: 10 factors for success. *Healthcare Financial Management*, *63*(1), 50–52, 54.

Hagland, M. (2009). A glass slipper? For cash-strapped organizations with EMR dreams, open-source software may be a perfect fit. *Healthcare Informatics*, *26*(8), 32–36.

Handler, T. (2008). Gartner 2008 North American enterprise CPR generation evaluation: Nearly half the products evaluated have finally reached generation 3. *Gartner*, 1-9.

Hannan, T. (1999). Variation in health care – The roles of the electronic medical record. *International Journal of Medical Informatics*, *54*, 127–136. doi:10.1016/S1386-5056(98)00175-0

Health Care Advisory Board. (n.d.). *HHS release meaningful use rule, shaping HER adoption*. Retrieved on July 14, 2010, from http://www.advisory.com/login/ login.aspx?URL=/members/ new_layout/default.asp?contentid=92039&program=1&collect

Hersh, W. (2007). Adding value to the electronic health record through secondary use of data for quality assurance, research, and surveillance. *The American Journal of Managed Care*, *13*(6 Part 1), 277–278.

Hiatt, J. (2006). *Awareness desire knowledge ability reinforcement: How to implement successful change in our personal lives and professional careers*. Loveland, CO: Prosci.

Hufnagel, S. P. (2009). Interoperability. *Military Medicine*, *174*(5), 43–50.

Jarvis, C. W. (2009). Investigate funding alternatives to support successful EHR implementation. *The Journal of Medical Practice Management*, *24*(6), 335–338.

Karnas, J., & Robles, J. (2007). Implementing the electronic medical record: Big Bang or phased rollout? *Creative Nursing*, *13*(2), 13–14.

Knaup, P., Garde, S., & Haux, R. (2007). Systematic planning of patient records for cooperative care and multicenter research. *International Journal of Medical Informatics*, *76*(2-3), 109–117. doi:10.1016/j.ijmedinf.2006.08.002

Leonard, T. (2007). Paving the way for the second wave of EHR adoption. *Health Management Technology*, *28*(2), 24, 26, 28.

Lin, C. P., Payne, T. H., Nichol, W. P., Hoey, P. J., Anderson, C. L., & Gennari, J. H. (2008). Evaluating clinical decision support systems: Monitoring CPOE order check override rates in the Department of Veterans Affairs' Computerized Patient Record System. *Journal of the American Medical Informatics Association*, *15*(5), 620–626. doi:10.1197/jamia.M2453

Ludwick, D. A., & Doucette, J. (2009). Adopting electronic medical records in primary care: Lessons learned from health information systems implementation experience in seven countries. *International Journal of Medical Informatics*, *78*(1), 22–31. doi:10.1016/j.ijmedinf.2008.06.005

McGowan, J. J., Cusack, C. M., & Poon, E. G. (2008). Formative evaluation: A critical component in EHR implementation. *Journal of the American Medical Informatics Association, 15*(3), 297–301. doi:10.1197/jamia.M2584

Miller, D. W., Jr. (2008). The transition from paper to digital: Lessons for medical specialty societies. *AMIA Annual Symposium Proceedings,* (pp. 475-9).

Murer, C. G. (2007). EHRs: Issues preventing widespread adoption. *Rehab Management, 20*(5), 38–39.

Mustain, J. M., Lowry, L. W., & Wilhoit, K. W. (2008). Change readiness assessment for conversion to electronic medical records. *The Journal of Nursing Administration, 38*(9), 379–385. doi:10.1097/01.NNA.0000323956.06673.bf

Nagle, L. M., & Catford, P. (2008). Toward a model of successful electronic health record adoption. *Healthcare Quarterly (Toronto, Ont.), 11*(3), 84–91.

Poon, E. G., Wright, A., Simon, S. R., Jenter, C. A., Kaushal, R., & Volk, L. A. (2010). Relationship between use of electronic health record features and health care quality: Results of a statewide survey. *Medical Care, 48*(3), 203–209. doi:10.1097/MLR.0b013e3181c16203

Rahimi, B., Moberg, A., Timpka, T., & Vimarlund, V. (2008). Implementing an integrated computerized patient record system: Towards an evidence-based information system implementation practice in healthcare. *AMIA Annual Symposium Proceedings,*(pp. 616-20).

Ross, J. (2009). Electronic medical records: The promises and challenges. *Journal of Perianesthesia Nursing, 24*(5), 327–329. doi:10.1016/j.jopan.2009.08.002

Roth, C. P., Lim, Y. W., Pevnick, J. M., Asch, S. M., & McGlynn, E. A. (2009). The challenge of measuring quality of care from the electronic health record. *American Journal of Medical Quality, 24*(5), 385–394. doi:10.1177/1062860609336627

Rouse, W. (2007). Health care as a complex adaptive system: Implications for design and management.

Rudin, R. S., Simon, S. R., Volk, L. A., Tripathi, M., & Bates, D. (2009). Understanding the decisions and values of stakeholders in health information exchanges: Experiences from Massachusetts. *American Journal of Public Health, 99*(5), 950–955. doi:10.2105/AJPH.2008.144873

Rutherford, R. (2007). TimeLine: Visualizing integrated patient records. *IEEE Transactions on Information Technology in Biomedicine, 11*(4), 462–473. doi:10.1109/TITB.2006.884365

Saleem, J. J., Russ, A. L., Justice, C. F., Hagg, H., Ebright, P. R., Woodbridge, P. A., & Doebbeling, B. N. (2009). Exploring the persistence of paper with the electronic health record. *International Journal of Medical Informatics, 78*(9), 618–628. doi:10.1016/j.ijmedinf.2009.04.001

Shachak, A., & Jadad, A. R. (2010). Electronic health records in the age of social networks and global telecommunications. *Journal of the American Medical Association, 303*(5), 452–453. doi:10.1001/jama.2010.63

Sheth, R. S., Ramly, E., & Brennan, P. F. (2010). *Industrial and systems engineering and health care: Critical areas of research.*

Sittig, D. F., & Classen, D. C. (2010). Safe electronic health record use requires a comprehensive monitoring and evaluation framework. *Journal of the American Medical Association, 303*(5), 450–451. doi:10.1001/jama.2010.61

Sloane, E. B., & Carey, C. C. (2007). Using standards to automate electronic health records (EHRs) and to create integrated healthcare enterprises. *Proceedings of the Annual International Conference of the IEEE Engineering in Medicine & Biology Society, 2007*, 6178–6179.

Smalley, H. (1982). Hospital management engineering: A guide to the improvement of hospital management systems.

Wakefield, D. S., Halbesleben, J. R., Ward, M. M., Qiu, Q., Brokel, J., & Crandall, D. (2007). Development of a measure of clinical information systems expectations and experiences. *Medical Care*, *45*(9), 884–890. doi:10.1097/MLR.0b013e3180653625

Yackanicz, L., Kerr, R., & Levick, D. (2010). Physician buy-in for EMRs. *Journal of Healthcare Information Management*, *24*(2), 41–44.

Yellowlees, P. M., Marks, S. L., Hogarth, M., & Turner, S. (2008). Standards-based, open-source electronic health record systems: A desirable future for the U.S. health industry. *Telemedicine Journal and e-Health*, *14*(3), 284–288. doi:10.1089/tmj.2007.0052

Yoon-Flannery, K., Zandieh, S. O., Kuperman, G. J., Langsam, D. J., Hyman, D., & Kaushal, R. (2008). A qualitative analysis of an electronic health record (EHR) implementation in an academic ambulatory setting. *Informatics in Primary Care*, *16*(4), 277–284.

Zheng, K., Padman, R., Johnson, M. P., & Diamond, H. S. (2009). An interface-driven analysis of user interactions with an electronic health records system. *Journal of the American Medical Informatics Association*, *16*(2), 228–237. doi:10.1197/jamia.M2852

Chapter 16
Electronic Medical Records (EMR):
Issues and Implementation Perspectives

Dean E. Johnson
Wellspan Health, USA

ABSTRACT

For many years the electronic medical record has been the holy grail of hospital system integration. Hundreds of millions of dollars have been spent in attempts to develop effective electronic medical records (EMR) to provide clinical care for patients. The advantages of an EMR are listed as reducing error, streamlining care, and allowing multiple people to provide simultaneous care. Unfortunately, most current EMR implementations are developed without completely understanding the processes that are being automated. In some implementations, there is an effort to first outline the process, and then try to create software that will facilitate the existing process, but this effort is not typically done systematically or with the discipline of an engineer. We will discuss the areas that management systems engineers can facilitate the design and implementation of the EMR, reducing the errors in the current processes and preparing the healthcare system for further improvements.

INTRODUCTION

An electronic medical record is the data repository for clinical information regarding the diagnoses, treatment and outcomes for patients in a healthcare system. They range in complexity from a series of scanned images indexed to a patient's name to huge data tables with thousands of pieces of encounter information, each indexed and cross-referenced. The primary purposes of an EMR are to store data in an easily retrievable form, provide clinical data about a patient from other parts of the healthcare system, such as the lab or radiol-

DOI: 10.4018/978-1-60960-872-9.ch016

ogy, and to assist with the management of their treatment. Additionally, a well-designed EMR can serve as a conduit for research and data extraction to measure outcomes.

As an EMR is developed, the usual method is to try to follow the path of a patient during treatment, understand what the interactions with the patient need to be, and provide a system that automates as much of the current care process as possible. This method will work well for some inflexible and narrowly focused clinical areas. This style of EMR implementation may speed up the process of care, but rarely positively affects the improvement of the care, since the old processes remain essentially in place. In other implementations, there is the recognition that current processes will no longer be required, or even desired, in the world of electronic medical records. Both of these development choices are partially correct, but have shortcomings. Although many of these implemented systems offer small areas of improvement, on the whole they end up creating problems that are not anticipated.

If one were to consider the entire healthcare delivery system in a hospital or medical system as an integrated unit, however, the crucial role of the electronic medical record can easily be understood. Correctly identifying a patient, ensuring the proper tracking of information from previous hospital visits and synchronizing records, integration of current clinical data with past clinical data, viewing of radiologic studies, reviewing results and tracking of trends are all possible with an electronic medical record that is designed correctly. In a few years, intelligent systems will be able to assist in the diagnosis and treatment of our patients, although that is still an area in its infancy.

Despite the shortcomings of the current systems for electronic medical records, this area of hospital system integration remains an extremely promising one. The entire healthcare system requires the transfer of vast amounts of information from one caregiver to the next. A simple exam for a patient may have over 100 data points, and the need to document the exams, results and clinical decision-making for patients to be paid for the work that the clinicians and hospital systems are providing becomes more important as the health care dollar becomes the target of ever-increasing scrutiny. Administrative costs for billing are huge, and can be greatly assisted by the systematic application of management engineering design principles in integrating the clinical and administrative electronic records.

I suggest that the implementation of electronic medical records, usually described as a cooperative effort between information technology (IT) departments, administrative personnel and clinicians, would benefit from the management systems engineering approach. Principles of management systems engineering are applicable to any description of the processes that occur within hospital systems and outpatient systems, with examples including project management, measurement of processes, process mapping, descriptions of variation, descriptions of handoffs, information transfer, and process control and financial modeling to support redesigns. Lean systems thinking, error reduction techniques, and andons are all tools that are ignored in EMR design and implementation. The standard work for clinical staff, a term easily understood by the management engineer is not understood by the IT staff, resulting in even more confusion as the IT department tries to fit their systems into the clinical environment. Process mapping, basic to the average management systems engineer, is inconsistently used in the design of software for clinical and healthcare applications. Even the layout of computer equipment is done without flow mapping or an understanding of the labor involved in making the system function in the clinical environment. This inability to understand the role of IT in the system of care in the hospital results in error and waste, but is largely unquantified. Only recently have researchers started to look at the additional complexity generated by electronic medical records, and the errors resulting from the EMR.

This chapter will provide the background needed to understand how an electronic medical record system is currently developed, what its strengths and weaknesses are, and how the skills of a management systems engineer can enhance the installation of an EMR. Later, we will discuss areas that clearly need development, and finally will delve into possible areas for research. The main objectives of this chapter are as follows:

- Describe an electronic medical record.
- Illustrate details in current systems that are controversial or do not work well.
- Provide a framework to understand how these flaws could be improved.
- Provide concrete examples for solutions in current EMR systems.

History and Background

It is important to first understand the purpose and origin of the electronic medical record. Electronic medical records, or EMR, or have also been called clinical data systems, the electronic health record, and hospital or healthcare information management systems. An EMR serves as an interface between the data that is collected for patient care and the administrative tasks and clinical tasks associated with it. So much information is currently gathered during a clinical visit that it becomes very difficult to keep track of it. Before the arrival of the electronic medical record, all of this data was hand written, placed in folders, had a variety of codes and stickers attached to it, and filed in the medical records department of a hospital. Patient care required retrieving the file from storage, transporting the file to the physician caring for the patient and locating the pertinent information within the file. Getting the record to a clinician is the first major challenge. In one study, medical records were unavailable in 30% of patient visits. (Tufo and Speidel, 1971) If the correct record was located, extracting pertinent information was also challenging. It has been demonstrated that at least 10% of the time, physicians could not find the information needed to treat the patient when they have the chart. (Fries, 1974) This has resulted in duplication of testing, misadministration of medication, allergies not being noted in the medical records, and generated frustration for both patients and clinicians. EMRs developed because of the vast amount of information processed and the inability of clinicians to locate the information they needed to treat the patient. The initial electronic medical records were systems developed in the 1970s and 1980s, coinciding with the arrival of more powerful and compact computer systems, and then eventually crafted to fit the clinical environment. The primary functions of early electronic medical records were for administrative purposes, because of the need for tracking information regarding billing and services provided outweighed the utility of the electronic medical record in the hospital. That functional bias still persists in current EMR development with the payer system in the U.S. thought to be one of the principle reasons that the EMR has not developed further, leaving a gap between the clinical needs to treat our patients and the information technology available to assist that treatment. (National Academy of Engineering, 2005)

Initially electronic medical records simply were a representation of the data that was stored on a piece of paper or form, often as simply a scanned image. This initial approach has evolved so that today many systems use a template format to capture discrete data that can be used for quality improvement, research, and measurement. Future systems are being developed with more capability to search natural language text for discrete data to better parse the vast amount of information that can be entered into the EMR.

ISSUES AND CURRENT PROBLEMS

An electronic medical record is a repository for the data that follows the patient through the health care system. This data must be easily accessible, accurate, and protected from individuals who should not be accessing it. The presentation of the data for each patient must be in a format that the provider can use, represent the most current information available, and be updated regularly while notifying the provider of important changes. Although this seems like a relatively straightforward task, the complexity of the clinical care process, the number of conditions that are being treated simultaneously, the number of people involved in the care of any individual patient, and the number of physical spaces that the patient must travel through increases the difficulties of the deployment of electronic medical record exponentially.

Issues surrounding an EMR involve the initial development decisions about proper identification of patients within legacy databases, merging old and new data, securing access for the clinical record, retrieving clinical records in a useful format, and fitting all of these changes into clinical workflow. Also, since one of the most frequently stated reasons for implementing an EMR is improving "quality of care", an EMR must have the potential for measuring clinical outcomes, providing interactive support to the clinical processes, and potentially altering the patient trajectory through the healthcare system.

The above requirements create a huge number of issues surrounding both the development of and implementation of electronic medical records. Starting with the most basic challenges, each record must be properly identified and associated only with the patient that pertains to. In some large healthcare systems, a single patient may have multiple records in different locations with slightly different identifiers on each one. Once properly identified, the goal is to place only accurate information into the chart. Studies done on paper records that indicated that as many as 40% of them can contain incomplete or inaccurate information, even lacking diagnoses, and obviously this data should not be imported into the electronic record (Dawes, 1972) This precludes the simple scanning of all paper within a patients medical chart.

For systems that are transitioning from paper records to electronic records, ensuring that only data pertinent to that particular patient is placed in their electronic medical record is a daunting task. To take these paper records and place them into electronic medical record system, some form of extracting the data is necessary. Typically this is done by typing in the pertinent facts, such as working diagnoses, medications, allergies into a new record associated with a patient that will include patient identifiers such as a medical record number, date of birth, the full name, and address. Handwritten records from electronic charts are then scanned in and saved as image formats to have the information available to clinicians for the first several years of the transition to electronic medical records. From personal experience, clinicians in several systems where there have been new implementations of EMRs have found that a timeframe of 3 years provides a useful history of pertinent clinical information to provide ongoing care. This clinical need can then determine which records will be scanned into the EMR.

Once the initial data is deposited in the electronic medical records for this system, the EMR must be designed to extract that information easily during different care processes for the patient. This extraction process creates design issues such as:

- Who will have access to patient care record?
- What level of access do they require and how much detail should they be allowed to look at?
- What time frame is necessary to understand the record? For example, should the default period include a two week period immediately before the clinical encounter?

- How is the data presented to the care provider?
- Where does the care provider need to access the data?
- What physical methods do care providers have interact with the data?

These issues are the major ones involving the design of the electronic medical record and the implementation of the system. Unfortunately, each issue is often tackled in isolation. An example might be in the development of the display screen for clinical laboratory data. Often the designer, who is not a clinical user of the system, will program the EMR so that data is displayed in a format that will put as much information as possible on the video screen. Clinically important outliers in the data may be represented by display number that is highlighted with additional letter such as H. or L. for high or low respectively, or in a color indicating severity such as yellow for laboratory values that are slightly outside of normal range and red for values that are critically outside of the normal range. How the information is presented on the screen can determine whether physicians are able to pick out the pieces of information needed to care for the patient and correct physiologic parameters that are out of the normal limits. For example, a normal value for a patient's hemoglobin is about 11, and seeing a number on a table that is 10.5 may not trigger any concern. A graphical representation illustrating that the patient's hemoglobin has drifted from 14.2 to this value of 10.5 over one week period, however, may trigger a decision to seek a source of blood loss. It has also recently been demonstrated that for some data seeing a graphical representation and mentally processing that information is faster than seeing the same information in a table form. (Bauer et al, 2010)

The security of electronic medical records is also very important. If, for example a patient has a diagnosis of HIV, they do not wish access to their medical record for people who may potentially reveal to their employer their HIV-positive status. Additionally, many medical conditions come from socially awkward situations that patients do not wish to have widely known. In the United States, The Health Insurance Portability and Accountability Act of 1996 (HIPAA) determines who can have access to patient records; and, other countries, such as those in the European Union, have similar laws. All electronic medical record vendors must ensure that their systems enforce this level of security and perform the data logging that is required to record who accesses the records.

Proper identification of patients, integrity of the system, and representation of the data are all very important issues in the design of the electronic medical record. From the design perspective of using this as part of a healthcare delivery system, a management systems engineer can incorporate these requirements, physical plant requirements, and workflow and assist in integrating all of these components into a complete delivery system. Time-motion studies, for example, of a physician's day might provide information on how long it takes to access the electronic medical record, and what portion of the day is wasted while the variety of data systems exchange information. If, for example simply logging in to access the data record takes 20 seconds but must be done 10 times daily, an engineering analysis of the log-in process and associated delays can save tens of thousands of dollars a year in underutilized labor. This analysis might include looking at alternative login methods, such as using proximity badges or biometric logins, or simply changing the location of terminals so that terminals are not available to people who should not access records.

If the EMR is designed to provide secure, confidential access, is integrated to the workflow of the providers and the clinical pathways of the patient and is providing appropriate clinical alerts, the EMR is functioning relatively well. Unfortunately, putting this information into the EMR does not guarantee that the system can be used to improve the clinical care of the patient. For example, a system currently in place in many hospitals across the world has a specialized report writing language required to extract information from the database. It is very difficult for the clinical staff to create a query like: for all the patients treated in this hospital as inpatients last year, which antibiotic was associated with the shortest time to successful discharge? Which treatments given to these patients seemed to be the most effective at reducing their oxygen needs? Rather than relying on a proprietary method for database extraction, a common data extraction method would make it much easier for physicians to ask these clinical questions, and the EMR would then establish the best practices for treating the patients.

Another current issue in the electronic medical records industry is that each system is vendor-specific. This provides many opportunities for the vendor to sell additional software, but really makes it difficult to integrate separate systems. This issue has been overcome by some people who have created a third software system to interface to others. For example, at Washington Hospital Center in 1996, several enterprising physicians and graduate medical students developed a system that drew information from over 300 different systems. (Microsoft 2009) Some have also tried to use Internet protocols to create larger electronic medical records that span across regions, forming RHIO or Regional Health Information Organizations. The difficulty with this approach is that each health system requires a separate interface, and then the composite database information also must be secured.

One of the most troublesome issues that has arisen as electronic medical records systems become more widely deployed is the increase in time needed to care for an individual patient. There are some studies to indicate that physicians are spending more time on documentation and this time is taken away from direct patient contact.(Asaro et al, 2008) This shift in the utilization of the physician's time is not perceived as being valuable in the eyes of the patient or the physician. In some emergency departments, the throughput decrease after installing an electronic medical record has led to the hiring of an additional person, a scribe, who merely follows around a physician, acting as a personal secretary, to put data into and retrieve data from the electronic medical record. A small clinical practice cannot afford an additional person to enter data into their information system. Also, nurses are now spending more time in front of computers and less time at the bedside in systems that have placed an electronic medical record into their clinical environment. This removes nurses from direct patient care and I have overheard patients stating that "it appears that all of the nurses are sitting in front of computers." Whether this personal observation is borne out in a true study, it does reflect the patient's perception of how an electronic medical record can change their care.

Finally, another issue that is extremely important in healthcare industry is the cost of the electronic medical record system. A large vendor system, such as one from Cerner, AllScripts, or Epic, may require the investment of tens of millions of dollars in the software purchase, installation, design, implementation, hardware support, and ongoing IT support. Even with the newly available funding in the U.S. budget, the $19 billion dollars recently allocated for the national EMR efforts, the 3000 hospitals in the U.S. that answered the survey about EMR use would receive about $6 million dollars apiece. This would be enough for some systems but not enough for most. (Kluger, 2009) This start-up cost for an EMR is thought to be one of the principle reasons preventing their widespread use, and currently the majority of the US does not use an electronic medical record. According to a recent US survey, only 13% of hospitals and 4% of physicians' offices use an electronic medical record. (AHRQ 2010) Since there is no universal standard for information that the electronic medical record must contain, despite the efforts of many organizations, vendors choose to store data in a proprietary format. Additionally, vendors may offer classes to allow a health care system to train employees to customize their deployments, but will often retain portions of their data structures so that there is not an easy interface to another system. This provides them with the business line of developing those interfaces and keeping their programmers employed. The costs of development and implementation keep the small individual practitioner from creating or purchasing their own electronic medical record. When a small practice can afford to purchase an EMR, their individual EMR will often not interface with the hospital to which they send the majority of their patients. Only the larger integrated healthcare systems, which have often purchased the practices of individual physicians, are able to put in an EMR system that supports both the outpatient visit and the inpatient hospitalization. For a rural practitioner, storing the data in electronic form for retrieval and transmission to a hospital tens of miles or hundreds of miles away is simply not a current option.

Current Problems in Existing EMR Systems

Current problems in electronic medical record systems can be divided into two general categories. The first category is the set of unintended consequences of the implementation of an electronic medical record system, including information overload, loss of information through display methods, and the creation of huge supporting infrastructures exclusively for the EMR. The second group of problems centers on the amount of waste that is generated simply by installing an electronic medical record system. This second category appears intuitively backwards, however when careful observations are made, it is possible to see where the systems that were previously optimized for patient and provider interactions now have the electronic medical record system inserted into the interaction. This additional layer of interaction creates waste that is rarely quantified. Both of these categories of problems will be outlined below.

A surprising unintended consequence of an electronic medical record includes providing too much information in a data format that is not easily understandable to the clinical staff caring for the patient. For example, a complete blood count (CBC) may include 24 separate lines of information as shown in Figure 1. Most of that information is extraneous for initial decision-making, and as a physician, I use only 4 of the 24 lines for the majority of my patients. Selected values from this CBC data table may by used by a sub-specialist physician, but are not useful to most physicians taking care of the patient. A better idea is to have a variable display of the information specifically for the specialty of the physician taking care of the patient.

Additionally, many current data tables are cryptic. Looking at the figure, you will notice that not only are all the data values written the same, but each data value has a corresponding acronym (i.e. WBC = White Blood Cell Count, in thousands/

Figure 1. Example of complete blood count table

Hematology	
WBC	6.7
RBC	4.57
HGB	13.6
HCT	40.2
MCV	88
MCH	29.8
MCHC	33.8
Platelet Ct	206
MPV	10.2
RDW-SD	41.3
RDW-CV	12.9
Abs Neut Ct	4.21
Abs Immature Gran Ct	0.01
Abs Lymph Ct	2.04
Abs Mono Ct	0.38
Abs Eos Ct	0.04
Abs Baso Ct	0.01
Mature Neutrophils	63
Immature Gran	0.1
Lymphocytes - Normal	31
Monocytes	6
Eosinophils	1
Basophils	0
RBC Morphology	* Normal

microliter) and no measuring unit designation. This screen has 3 units of measure (thousands/microliter, percentage of a whole and volume in femtoliters) and a comment without a distinction between measuring units. While a data table seems like a reasonable display method, the noise generated by extraneous information can contribute to errors taking care of a patient, and I have encountered this problem daily. Different data should to be displayed in a format to promote understanding of the data, not simply the number. For example, a value such as hematocrit, which is illustrated in the table above with the initials HCT, is better displayed as a label along a trend line giving the numerical value. Rapid changes in hematocrit signal important clinical changes in the patient that may require intervention. This contextual data display should be on a single screen, since it has been shown that processing the information across multiple screens can cause loss of context of the information for the care provider.

Another area with unintended consequences is loss of "information" upon retrieval of data from the electronic medical record, where small data changes may not be noticeable in a sea of a tabular array of values. Not noticing a change in a blood lanoxin value from 1.5 to 2.3 may result in the administration of another dose of the lanoxin, when that second medication dose is not required. Microbiology lab reports are also displayed electronically, and a change in the report may not be fed back to the clinician who originally ordered the test. This can be clinically significant when, for example, a Gram stain on the spinal fluid initially reported by the lab as having a gram-negative value is later changed to become a gram-positive value. This gram stain result can change the selection of antibiotics given to the patient and can affect the decision to notify infectious disease personnel. In current EMR systems, a change such as this will rarely be flagged in order to bring it to the attention of the clinicians. In a paper system, the generation of another piece of paper on the fax machine signals the physician to review the test results. The physician then has that faxed paper in hand as they talk to the patient, without the need to login to a computer screen.

The ease of accessibility of an EMR also works against maintaining patient confidentiality. One of the most widely accepted tenets in medicine is that the information that you provide to your physician is held in high confidentiality. When that information is stored electronically, anyone who can access the database can also access your personal information. There are cases where medical records have been viewed by unauthorized personnel, resulting in a breech of privacy. (Hennessy-Fiske, 2010) Also, records have been stolen or inadvertently lost because they were placed on a laptop or hard drive. (Sturdevant 2009) These incidents generate huge concerns regarding patient confidentiality. When data is physically stored in charts, the only people who can access it must have a physical copy of the chart. Since access to patient data is now an area that is tightly controlled by government regulation, most systems have done a very good job of maintaining several levels of security and ensure that only the proper people are looking at the records. This security requirement creates, however, the need for a security officer and a group of people who ensure the compliance of the system and review the access logs. This additional labor must be factored into the ongoing maintenance costs of electronic medical record.

Along with the problems with information display, results retrieval and security infrastructure that an EMR will create, another unintended consequence of the implementation of an EMR is the creation of large, nonclinical investments in the information technology infrastructure required to run an electronic medical record system. A department that had non-clinical staff who assisted with paper processing finds that it will require an individuals to support the new clinical information system, and the former administrative personnel often remain in place because the computer system generates mounds of paper. This has led to the creation of additional staffing positions in health systems solely to support the EMR. These positions include support for the individual computer system at the desktop, additional people to support the 24-hour nature of health systems delivery in the user help section, additional staffing to run the database backbone, people to maintain the computer equipment and additional security personnel to follow the logging system.

Finally, when implemented, an EMR does not usually replace the medical records section of the hospital because so few hospitals are completely electronic. Until all areas of a health system are electronic, there is a need for a medical records department so that physicians can process signatures for missed orders, retrieve paper records that are generated outside of the electronic system and have a system that can be used when the electronic medical record system fails.

The second major category of problems that an EMR can produce is unintended waste in resource utilization. These resources are the intellectual abilities of clinical personnel, the time for processing patients and the financial resources of the organization. Each of these wastes is discussed below.

In a healthcare system with an EMR, highly skilled and paid physicians and nurses spend more time for documentation and data entry than with traditional paper charting. This results in "overqualified" personnel performing data entry tasks and is usually perceived as an "intellectual waste" that can occur with an EMR implementation. Since it is known that information is lost when a physician leaves a patient's room and tries to recall data, many EMRs have the physicians performing data entry by typing at the bedside, which few physicians are proficient at. (Chisolm, 2008) This data entry is expensive, so in an effort to speed up data entry, physicians have been asked to learn typing, a skill in addition to the technical skills that they have already had to master to be physicians. As an alternative to typing, some systems are starting to use voice recognition; but, in an EMR with voice recognition, talking into a computer while interviewing a patient may appear to be rude or unconcerned. Also, voice recognition software is not the norm, nor is it always tuned to the clinical needs of the physician. Usually, if a physician or nurse is sitting in front of a computer, they are not at a patient's bedside providing direct care, and this difference in focus is often observed by patients.

As if entering the data the first time is not painful enough, many pieces of information are double-entered into the EMR. Reentering data improves the coding level - the method that insurers use to pay for healthcare in the U.S., and is therefore business-value added. As an example, the smoking history of a patient entering an emergency department may be entered in the triage note (of no value there) by a nurse at one skilled salary level and in the physicians' documentation at a salary level four times that of the nurse. This relatively small amount of business-value add however is outweighed by the inefficiency of having the data entered twice.

Sometimes data is entered that few people care about: a skilled nurse is paid to document 4+ pulses in four extremities, which is information stored in a data table but rarely used. The waste is that no physician requires that pulse information unless they are treating a vascular patient. In other words, of 100 patients entering the hospital, perhaps 10 will require the knowledge of all pulses in their extremities. The intellectual wastes of inappropriate task assignation and data entry duplication could be eliminated by proper design.

Besides the intellectual waste generated by the installation of an EMR, time to provide direct patient care is also wasted. A simple example is the time wasted by screen flips and clicks and logins. The most expensive direct labor in the U.S. health system is that of the physicians. If physicians, each making \$2/minute, have 10 logins daily at 20 seconds each, (200 seconds or 3 1/3 minutes daily for 100 physicians) lost labor costs are \$243,000 per year! Unfortunately, many

EMR systems will also freeze up the computers that they run on, since the computer hardware purchased is often not the highest performing equipment available but is bought by looking for the "least expensive solution". This financial shortsightedness can result in a local machine reboot to use the system. Rebooting a computer is often a five minute process before the physician can resume their task, and some systems are requiring a reboot every shift (15 minutes daily, done by the same physicians as above). This can amount to over $1 million in lost labor costs for those 100 physicians yearly. Stated another way, current systems can waste over $2,400 per physician, per year, in just login time. A screen flip that requires one-fourth of a second does not seem like much waste, until the process is noted to occur 1,000,000 times per year. Using the same labor costs as above, these screen flips are responsible for $8,300 in lost wages. This loss of productive time is also frustrating to the physicians who are trying to take care of patients.

Time wasting also occurs when different information systems are not well-integrated. For example, in a current EMR, the cardiology system has the ECG as a document stored in a proprietary format, which then is turned into an image for display. On one computer system, the electrocardiogram for a single patient is stored in a folder labeled "electrocardiogram" and "EKG", with different ECGs stored in two different formats depending upon whether they were input in a recent system or an older system. The clinical staff must open two folders for comparison and opening one file folder automatically closes the other file folder. The radiology image system is similar, and eventually feeds the reports in, but the user must click through several screens to look at an image. A simple viewing solution would be a rollover pop-up window with the image at optimized viewing size. Obtaining the radiology report result requires looking in another area, and if you were to try to include those results in the physician documentation for the patient encounter, you must "cut and paste" between different computer screens, requiring an additional 15-30 seconds per result per patient.

Financial wastes do not only include direct labor costs and lost opportunities for service, but also include material costs. For example, many EMRs require reprinting paper because the printer malfunctions or the software is not easily understood. A common example is the discharge instruction from the emergency department. These are often not read by the patient, not illustrated to enhance understanding, or not at a sixth grade level, and printed several times before a patient leaves. When the visit appears finished, the patient often needs a note stating when the patient can return to work, and it is painful to reopen the chart and to write the note by computer, and is much simpler to hand write it. Family members are not patients and therefore not entered into the EMR but may require school or work excuses as well.

Inefficient work habits also are perpetuated in the current electronic medical record systems. Currently, prescriptions are printed and then handed to the patient. Often these electronic systems will also require a physical physician signature, done by hand and not electronically, resulting in more handling of the same piece of paper. If prescriptions were sent electronically to the pharmacy of the patients choosing, and then there was a feedback loop to the physician indicating that the patient had received the prescription, it would be possible to avoid errors or re-hospitalizations for conditions by following up with patients in a timely fashion. While this is an area that is currently changing, the vast majority of EMR systems print out a piece of paper in a format acceptable to pharmacies according to local regulations.

Finally, even in an EMR, data silos abound. Inpatient episodic care must be followed by long-term outpatient care. Unfortunately, the problems addressed in the hospitalization are not well communicated to the follow-up physicians. Attempts have been made to rectify this information transfer deficiency with varying degrees of success. There are instances where the electronic medical record summary was created automatically, sent to the treating physician, and was unusable because of the format. (Ash, 2004) Realistically, however, most systems do not have standardized medical discharges, or the records from one part of the EMR do not make it back to the outpatient physician, and follow-up care can be inadequate. (Patient Safety Advisory 2008)

MANAGEMENT SYSTEMS ENGINEERING AS A SOLUTION

The unintended consequences and wastes discussed above create a huge opportunity for improvement with the skills of management systems engineers. Management Systems Engineering specializes in understanding the processes, handoffs and interfaces necessary for a system to function smoothly. In contrast, software engineering, which is the major engineering discipline in current EMR development, addresses only those information fragments that are passed back and forth, and does not address the work issues necessary to generate or record the data. If a management systems engineer examined the process of care for a patient as the patient entered the healthcare system, they could produce a process map that could roughly describe the trajectory of the patient. If that process is then converted into a swim lane, and one lane is used for data, it is possible to generate a process map that includes data interchange for clinical care. An example of a swim lane diagram follows in Figure 2, with data, different personnel roles and the patient listed as separate lanes. This can be done with any process to clarify the roles of each resource (person, software or machine).

Mapping the Care Processes

A common task in other industries is the description of a standard work process. Unfortunately, one of the most difficult things in medicine is to define

Figure 2. Swim lane example including the process and data stream. Used with permission from Sueanne McKniff, RN, BSN.

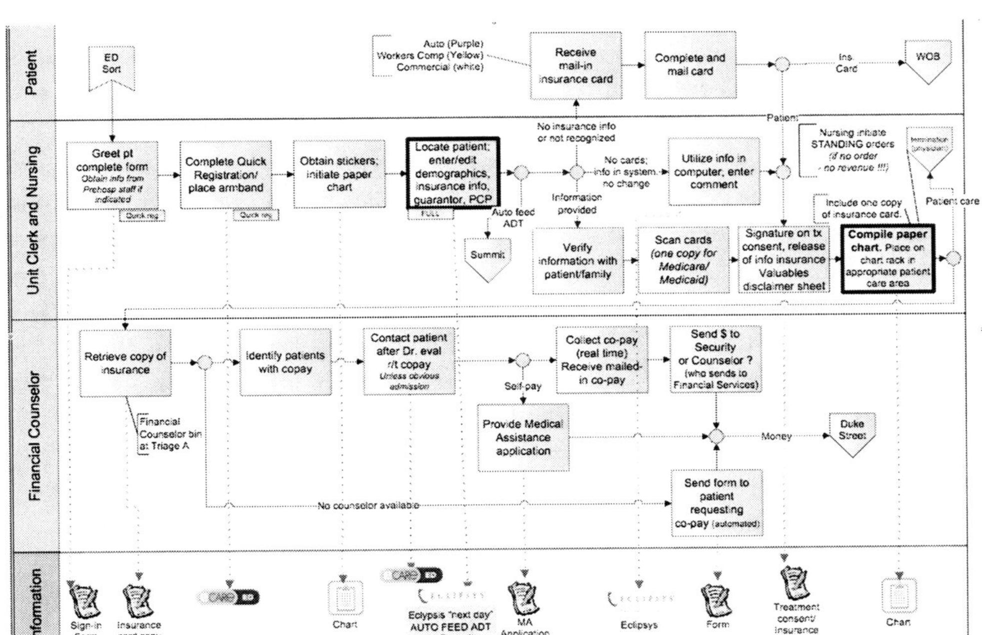

the "standard work" for a clinical job. This task could be easily accomplished by a management systems engineer and is important to understand if you are installing or designing an EMR. For example, in the emergency department, the technician who first meets with a patient may be obtain their temperature, pulse rate and respiration rate (known as "vital signs") while a nurse asks historical questions. Both of these staff positions require the ability to put the data into the EMR, and the ability to easily confirm previous data, but not understanding their individual clinical role makes it impossible to define what data they should access in what order. If you map the care process, and define each positions' role precisely, you also define the software requirements to display and access the underlying data. In most EMR systems, this patient care role definition is done in a vague manner, and extensive and expensive software customization is the norm, rather than the exception.

Illustrating Hand-Offs

One of the strengths of a management systems engineer is their ability to think in terms of a "whole" system, and they understand the importance of hand-offs. In medicine, hand-offs are one of the largest sources of errors (ScienceDaily Feb 2010), and using a management systems engineer to see the hand-offs as software is developed and specified can greatly assist the design and implementation of the EMR. Examples of hand-offs in medicine are easy to find:

A patient is discharged from the hospital, where their stay was tracked in the hospital EMR. They are to follow-up with a primary care physician in a set timeframe to insure that they do not have to be readmitted because in systems that have standardized follow-up, readmissions for certain conditions have been cut dramatically (Jack, 2009). Designing the EMR software so that the encapsulated patient information is sent to the primary care physician, containing a clear summary of the hospital stay, changes to medications, recommendations from inpatient consultants to assist in future care, testing results and specific questions to address, such as did a congestive heart failure patient gain weight since hospital discharge, can improve the efficiency of the outpatient visit, improve the patient's impression of their care, and save the patient and healthcare system money.

A patient has an x-ray done at an outpatient facility. The facility uses PACS, so that the radiologist can read the film remotely, but the reading is then dictated into another system. The ordering outpatient physician must look for the dictation to arrive by mail or fax, or know to look in the EMR at a given time to see the result. If the result is a positive film, a series of phone calls and messages is usually generated. A management systems engineer can observe and illustrate this common process, and define the pieces of information needed to be transferred between the various parties, and then use this information to assist the software engineer in defining the EMR to support this process. Currently, this common scenario may require an additional software purchase as an add-on.

A patient arrives in the ED, having been sent in by his primary care physician, who does not use an EMR (the majority of the cases in the U.S. system at this time). If the primary care physician has called ahead, the note that contains their concerns about the patient and the recommendations from the physician familiar with them is seldom available to treat the patient in the ED. In an EMR that has had this common process looked at by someone familiar with handoffs, this can be a seamless process.

Each of these instances can be easily visualized and illustrated using the tools familiar to management systems engineers.

Illustrating the Future State of the System

With the system engineer's knowledge of the standard work of the clinical staff, the knowledge of the handoffs obtained by studying the system, and basic tools for illustrating and problem-solving common to their background, the management systems engineer can define the future state that the software should help create. This serves a guide for the entire EMR development process. If done, it facilitates software testing, user training and troubleshooting. An illustration of a future state for a triage process is shown in Figure 3, with "UCC" meaning an Urgent Care center for minor ailments and "ED" referring to the main Emergency Department, for more serious medical problems.

Creating the Physical Space Layout

Management systems engineers can also facilitate the design of the work area required when using an electronic medical record. Figure 4 will show this point nicely. The charting area in an emergency department was remodeled to accommodate terminals to input data into the electronic medical record. The physician staff sits on one side of a physical barrier, with five input terminals. They type and selectively dictate into the emergency department electronic medical record. The printer that they must use for patient discharge instructions is located on the other side of a 1.3 meter partition. When a clinician wishes to discharge a patient,

Figure 3. Process map of the revised initial patient stream for an emergency department

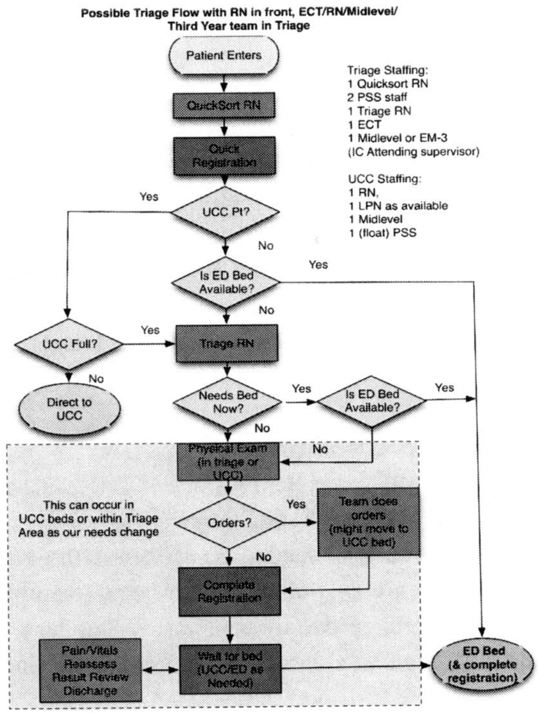

Figure 4. Emergency Department Clinical workstation and printer

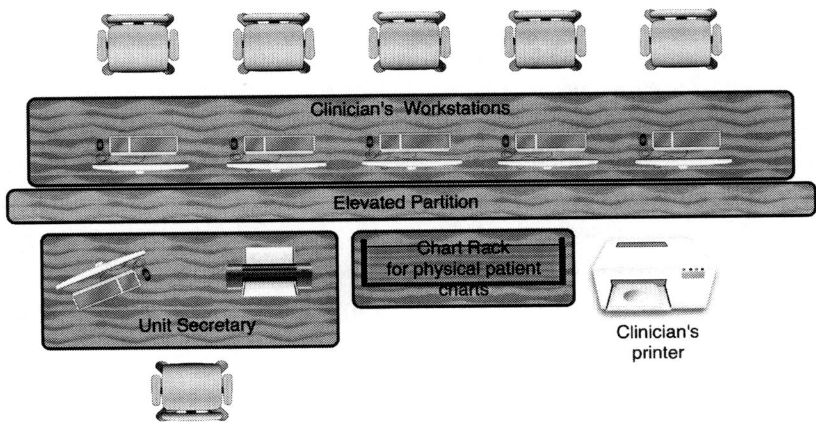

they print discharge instructions, walk from their terminal around the partition to the printer, pickup the discharge instructions, and place these in the chart rack so that nurses can pick them up, and return to their workstation. This printing function has a 5% - 10% failure rate, requiring a reprint. The physicians are the most expensive labor in the department, and they perform this function 50,000 times per year in this facility alone. The nurses then notice a flag set in the EMR to discharge the patient, go to the chart rack to retrieve the discharge papers, take these papers to the patient's rooms, disconnect monitors and intravenous medication lines, review the discharge instructions with the patient, and return to their charting workstations, similar in design to the physicians' workstations. Obviously, this is also done 50,000 times per year in this facility. The dollar value of this waste scales with the department census and direct labor rates of the staff positions.

Work-Cell Creation

Work cell creation is the physical grouping of people and material needed to perform all the steps for taking care of one of person. For example, many emergency departments are set up so that one physician may work with several nurses, and the nurses in turn may have several technicians that work with them. In some hospitals a physician, several nurses, and one or two technicians is grouped together to cover a geographic zone. This is an instance of a small work cell. All the materials, medical supplies, and equipment needed to take care of four or five patients are located in several rooms. The nurses and technicians and physician can all concentrate their efforts on people within that small area, from the time the person arrives in emergency department, is diagnosed, is treated, and is discharged or admitted to the hospital.

Unfortunately, the physical layout of many emergency departments interferes with geographic zone creation, and the electronic medical record is added to a physical space as an afterthought. If one considers the design of electronic medical record, the physical location of the displays and equipment needed for inputs and outputs for each person's various tasks, the integration of data from patients in real-time subject to verification by the staff taking care of the patient, and creates an electronic medical record so that all of these items will work together, it is possible be able to have a significant increase in throughput. This set of principles can be applied to any healthcare facility integrating an EMR.

Ergonomic Design Considerations

Several ergonomic factors also influence the usability of the electronic medical record. These factors include the type of display used (flat-screen, CRT, glossy or matte), the resolution of the display and whether the display has a touchscreen capability, whether color or monochrome, and the location of the displays for the people who are performing the work. For tasks requiring movement to the patient's bedside the portability of data input terminals and ease of use of each terminal are considerations. For more stationary tasks, the physical layout of keyboards, graphical input devices such as tablets, mice, and trackballs can be selected to optimize the interactions with the patient and the EMR. Portable data capture devices will require charging stations, and the management systems engineer can help locate the best locations for these devices to suit the workflow for the department. On computer displays, font choices, colors and display resolutions can also be adjusted to promote the rapid understanding of the information or performance of the next task.

In a private office environment or clinic, the location of the displays, printers, the comfort of the workstations, the ease of changeover of tasks for each person should be considered while designing how the software and workflow work together. An example might be locating the display for the receptionist in a private office such that that individual can both see the person coming into the office to register and the display while looking in the same direction by locating the display below an entrance window. Spaghetti mapping the daily work patterns of the clinic or office can help locate equipment to minimize wasted time walking around.

Designing the System for Future Improvement

One area that management systems engineer can be extremely helpful in is in designing the electronic medical record system to provide the data needed for future enhancements to improve the delivery of healthcare. By understanding measurement principles, and looking at workflow issues while the initial electronic medical record system is being designed, the engineer can prompt the software designers to create data entry points for the information that can later be used to improve the delivery of the service. For example, if an electronic medical record system is being installed into a physician's office with a time-stamp that records when patients arrive and when a patient is placed in a room automatically this data might be useful for optimizing the delivery of care and increasing the throughput of that office. In most healthcare settings this data is never collected. Turnaround times for the most commonly ordered labs and data collection for hospital initiatives can be tracked if designed into the EMR. Also, a management systems engineer can easily design systems that provide alerts to the clinical staff when there are delays in handoffs, improving the efficiency of the care process.

Implementing the Systems

Unfortunately, redesigning the physical plant of a hospital or clinic to accommodate an EMR is not usually possible, so emphasis must be placed on balancing the needs for data functions of an EMR, the people providing care for the patients and the physical plant design. In a large clinic or hospital a physician, who normally goes to the bedside to examine the patient and may move throughout the hospital, requires a mobile, secure, energy efficient device. Most physicians are not content with a heavy laptop that has a two or three hour battery life, but this is often the device purchased for their use. There is also a need to consider where the physician places their input device when they are at the patient's bedside. Nurses who work in a single nursing station may require a fixed workstation for some tasks, and a computer on wheels for other tasks. Certain tasks, such as medication administration, can be handled with a portable data terminal that could scan a barcode, confirm patient information, allow limited input by nursing staff, and then transmit data to the EMR. A patient care technician, whose primary job is performing tasks at the bedside throughout the unit, some of which require immediate recording in the EMR, might be equipped best with a handheld unit, such as a customized smartphone, that is extremely portable and can be dropped into a pocket out of the way when the patient is being cared for at the bedside.

Each of these individuals will have definite roles and interact with only parts of the information system. Each individual may also have a different input device that is required. By providing a system-wide view of the data that each person requires, and integrating that view along with the tasks that the individual must perform, the management systems engineer can add can greatly enhance the design and the workflow of the healthcare system, allowing the efficient use of the EMR.

Management systems engineers also can help in several other key areas. As an EMR is developed, a management systems engineer can insure that the software matches the workflow, and illustrate the staff workarounds that are generated as an EMR is put into place. There are many examples of staff recording vital signs on a piece of tape on their scrubs and then taking this data elsewhere to enter it into the EMR. This inefficiency points out the difficulty with entering data into the EMR.

A management systems engineer could suggest an alternative data capture method, such as having the nurse confirm the machine readings on a touch screen and having this data auto-loaded into the EMR from the vital sign monitors. They would also be capable of calculating the return-on-investment for the hardware and software needed to make this function happen. Besides determining the workflow forced by the implementation of an EMR, the management systems engineer could help find the errors generated by the new workflow, such as the need to register a critically ill patient before retrieving medication from a computer controlled drug dispenser, and help alter the EMR to more accurately reflect the desired workflow.

Once an EMR is implemented, the tasks for the management systems engineer are not complete. Healthcare, like many other industries, changes at an astounding rate. The management systems engineer can describe the current system with the new EMR in place, and look for waste and inefficiencies prompted by new regulatory or business practices. The development of discrete simulations, the application of queuing theory and Little's law and identifying new bottlenecks can improve the delivery of healthcare dramatically. All of these applications are well within the system engineer's abilities.

Future Directions for Research and Care

The biggest change in EMR development would be to just use the simplest tools that an management systems engineer uses. Gantt charts, critical pathways, process diagrams, and spaghetti diagrams are not widespread in healthcare. In an EMR implementation, the usual development method is for a vendor to study an existing process, model their software on that single process, and create modules to fit that process. The vendor may not concern themselves with interfaces and hand-offs of clinical information until their basic user interface is completed and these are often added in at the software implementation stage. Since healthcare is information exchange, methods to facilitate this exchange between clinical staff would be a boon. For example, I know that I need to ask a hand surgeon to repair a flexor tendon in a dominant hand after a table saw injury, but I need to see who's on for hand surgery, page them, wait for them to call back, describe the injury, and then document that they came in and saw the patient. Using an advanced EMR we could, for example, automatically page the correct consultant physician, share a photo of the injury while we discuss it, and press a soft-key to alert the OR staff. At the bedside an RFID tag in the consultant's name tag and the RFID tag on the patient could confirm the exam date, time and duration and automatically enter that into the medical record.

An EMR, if properly designed, could start to capture data on a patient as they arrive, and start to create a list of differential diagnoses, although this is currently beyond our usual software. Vital signs readily identify those who are potentially volume depleted, and have fevers, and this information could be used to start the differential diagnosis. Febrile illness of 104 degrees F (40 C) in a 5-year-old is unlikely to be a simple cold, but may be influenza, meningitis, or roseola. Having this information organized and presented well to the clinician would be a huge improvement over the current system of clinical staff seeking relevant information as they go to see a patient. Old ICU charts were organized so that the clinical staff could see fevers and inputs and outputs easily - since the paper showed the results graphically, but often EMR software does not. Certain trends, such as creatinine and hematocrit are very important clinically, and therefore the default display should be a trend line with an associated value - emphasized for a change greater than 10% or requiring lifesaving intervention. Usually both of these are simply numbers on a table, having the same font size and color as all the other numbers on the table. In an emergency department previous data could be automatically retrieved, and displayed in a usable format. Since it is known that previous laboratory tests including CBC and basic metabolic panel are among the most commonly requested pieces of old data, the values for the CBC and basic metabolic panel could be graphed with their historical and current values to indicate whether or not there is an acute development of an anemia or renal insufficiency (Hripcsak, 2007).

Additionally, it would be helpful if the electronic medical record system had the ability to anticipate what the next part of the treatment plan would be. For a primary care physician seeing a patient with hypertension, it would be helpful to have a list of current medications and doses, have the computer review the interactions between them, and relate them to the recorded blood pressures displayed along a timeline. In a patient that has a urinary tract infection, diagnosed by a bacterial count in a urine sample, the automatic display of any previous urine culture results and their antibiotic susceptibilities could assist in the treatment of this common illness. As lab results became available in an acute care setting, the disposition of the patient could be anticipated (transfer from the ICU, send to the OR, discharge home) by algorithms that assess the number and type of abnormalities and initiate treatment protocols. In the case of a patient that is being referred to a consultant, the ability to automatically collect the type of information that the consultant will require and place it in a format that they can understand intuitively could save time and effort for the referring physician, the patient and the consulting physician. Again this is an example where an intelligent design for a system handoff can be anticipated and handled by people with system engineering skills.

Recognizing that it would be important for the electronic medical record for each patient to track the longitudinal health of the patient, there is a need to develop regional networks of individual medical records that can be transparently accessed from multiple healthcare locations. While some limited networks are growing in the US, others have been developed in other countries throughout the world. At this time the multiple vendors and the multiple methods of displaying the same information make it difficult to navigate through information to provide optimal care of the patient. This results in unnecessary duplication of tests, and additional time attempting to discern what is important. An example of this would be a patient smartcard, a technology that has been developed before but has not yet been perfected, containing the most basic information including medical conditions, medications, allergies, baseline labs, electrocardiogram, imaging studies, and demographics. This would provide a portable data repository that can be carried by the patient. This could be supplemented by a regional database to fill in some of the information when the smart card is not available or the patient is injured and the information is needed urgently. For example, a hypoglycemic diabetic patient involved in a motor vehicle accident with multiple casualties could be quickly identified and treated and their underlying medical condition diagnosed even if they were unconscious.

Finally, research could be performed in real time with the EMR. By having an intelligent data mining agent working in the background, it would be possible to have information to change clinical practice - essentially ongoing clinical trials - on medications and therapies. This goal has been visualized for years, but even a decade after the Institute of Medicine's report 'Crossing the Quality Chasm', the electronic medical record is insufficiently useful to create comparisons between treatments.

CONCLUSION

An EMR is a huge investment in time and money, and when well-implemented, can save patients from adverse drug effects, duplication of testing, and serious harm during their care by insuring that each of the clinical staff caring for a patient has access to needed information. Current EMRs are sporadically implemented, are customized for implementation into a specific healthcare system, and are not interoperable. Management engineers have the abilities to see medical care as a continuum of processes, understand the problems with handoffs and have valuable insights in EMR design, development and implementation. It is only when these needed contributions are more widely accepted that the current design of EMRs, often derided by end-users of these systems, can improve and contribute more significantly to improving healthcare.

REFERENCES

AHRQ. (2010). Electronic medical record systems. Retrieved July 12, 2010, from http://wci-pubcontent/publish/communities/k_o/knowledge_library/key_topics/health_briefing_01232006114616/electronic_medical_record_systems.html

Asaro, P. V., & Boxerman, S. B. (2008). Effects of computerized provider order entry and nursing documentation on Workflow. *Academic Emergency Medicine*, *15*, 908–915. doi:10.1111/j.1553-2712.2008.00235.x

Ash, J. S., Berg, M., & Coiera, E. (2004). Some unintended consequences of Information Technology in healthcare: The nature of patient care Information System-related errors. *Journal of the American Medical Informatics Association*, *11*, 104–112. doi:10.1197/jamia.M1471

Bauer, D. T., Guerlain, S., & Brown, P. J. (2010). The design and evaluation of a graphical display for laboratory data. *Journal of the American Medical Informatics Association*, *17*, 416–424. doi:10.1136/jamia.2009.000505

Chisolm, C. D. (2008). A comparison of observed versus documented physician assessment and treatment of pain: The physician record does not reflect the reality. *Annals of Emergency Medicine*, *52*(4), 383–389. doi:10.1016/j.annemergmed.2008.01.004

Dawes, K. S. (1972). Survey of general practice records. *British Medical Journal*, *3*, 219–223. doi:10.1136/bmj.3.5820.219

Fries, J. F. (1974). Alternatives in medical record formats. *Medical Care*, *12*, 871–881. doi:10.1097/00005650-197410000-00006

Hennessy-Fiske, M. (2010). UCLA is fined $95,000 for violating patient privacy. Retrieved June 30, 2010 from http://latimesblogs.latimes.com /lanow/2010/06/ucla-fined --for-violating-patient-privacy.html

Hripcsak, G., Senqupta, S., Wilcox, A., & Green, R. A. (2007). Emergency department access to a longitudinal medical record. *Journal of the American Medical Informatics Association*, *14*(2), 235–238. doi:10.1197/jamia.M2206

Indiana University School of Medicine. (2010, February 26). The most frequent error in medicine. ScienceDaily. Retrieved July 12, 2010, from http://www.sciencedaily.com /releases/2010/02/100226101330.htm

Jack, B., Greenwald, J., Forsythe, S., O'Donnell, J., Johnson, A., & Schipelliti, L. … Chetty, V. K. (2009). Developing the tools to administer a comprehensive hospital dischargep: The reengineered discharge (RED) program. Retrieved from http://innovations.ahrq.gov/ content.aspx?id=1777

Kluger, J. (2009, March 25). Electronic health records: What's taking so long? Time Online.

National Academy of Engineering. (2005). Building a better delivery system: A new engineering/health care partnership, (p. 64).

Pennsylvania Patient Safety Authority. (2008). Care at discharge—A critical juncture for transition to posthospital care. Pennsylvania Patient Safety Authority, 5(2), 39-43. Retrieved June 20, 2010, from http://patientsafetyauthority.org /ADVISORIES/AdvisoryLibrary /2008/ Jun5%282%29/Pages/39.aspx

Sturdevant, M. (2009, November 19). 1.5 million medical files at risk in health net data breach. The Hartford Courant. Retrieved June 20, 2010, from http://articles.courant.com/ 2009-11-19/ news/ hc-healthbreach1119.artnov 19_1_health-net-data-breach-theft-or-health-united-bank-customer-information

Tufo, H. M., & Speidel, J. J. (1971). Problems with medical records. *Medical Care*, *9*(6), 509–517. doi:10.1097/00005650-197111000-00007

Washington Hospital Center. (n.d.). Electronic medical records help physicians and boost revenues while saving millions. Retrieved June 20, 2010, from http://download.microsoft.com / documents/australia/healthcare /washington.doc

ADDITIONAL READING

Abdelhak, M. (2001). *Health Information: Management of a Strategic Resource*. Philadelphia, PA: W.B.Saunders.

Ball, M. J. (Ed.). (1995). *Healthcare Information Management Systems: A Practical Guide*. New York: Springer-Verlag.

Ball, M. J. (1999). *Performance Improvement Through Information Management: Health Care's Bridge to Success*. New York: Springer-Verlag.

Building a Better Delivery System: A New Engineering/Health Care Partnership. (2005) National Academy of Engineering, Dick, RS & Steen, EB & Detmer, DE (Eds.) (1997) The Computer-Based Patient Record: An Essential Technology for Health Care. Washington, D.C.:National Academy Press.

Drazen, E. L. (Eds.). (1995). *Patient Care Information Systems: Successful Design and Implementation New York*. Springer-Verlag.

Kiel, J. M. (Ed.). (2001). *Information Technology for the Practicing Physician*. New York: Springer-Verlag.

Ozcan, Y. (2005). *Quantitative Methods in Health Care Management: Techniques and Applications*. San Francisco, CA: Jossey-Bass.

Ruffin, M. J. (1999) Digital Doctors. Tampa, Fl: Hillsboro Printing Company

Shortliffe, E. H. (Eds.). (2001). *Medical Informatics: Computer Applications in Health Care and Biomedicine*. New York: Springer-Verlag.

U.S. Congress. (1995). Office of Technology Assessment Bringing Healthcare Online: The Role of Information Technologies. Washington, D.C.: U.S. Government Printing Office.

Chapter 17
Health Information Exchange for Improving the Efficiency and Quality of Healthcare Delivery

Jing Shi
North Dakota State University, USA

Sudhindra Upadhyaya
North Dakota State University, USA

Ergin Erdem
North Dakota State University, USA

ABSTRACT

In healthcare industry, providers, patients, and all other stakeholders must have the right information at the right time for achieving efficient and cost effective services. Exchange of information between the heterogeneous system entities plays a critical role. Health information exchange (HIE) is not only a process of transmitting data, but also a platform for streamlining operations to improve healthcare delivery in a secure manner. In this chapter, we present a comprehensive view of electronic health record (EHR) systems and HIE by presenting their architecture, benefits, challenges, and other related issues. While providing information on the current state of EHR/HIE applications, we also discuss advanced issues and secondary uses of HIE implementations, and shed some light on the future research in this area by highlighting the challenges and potentials.

INTRODUCTION TO EHR AND HIE

Development of EMR/EHR

The adoption of information technology in healthcare has progressed through a series of phases since the 1960s. Initially, health information systems were used in financial industry in the 1960s. These systems aided the organizations' billing, payroll, accounting, and reporting services. During this phase, the use of health information systems was limited to the elimination of clerical work. Primary care clinics took a major initiative during the 1970s in a similar direction and joined

DOI: 10.4018/978-1-60960-872-9.ch017

the bandwagon for implementation of health information systems. In the 1960s, 1970s, and 1980s, the scope of this technology was mostly limited to small areas within the hospitals, such as laboratory, radiology, or administration units (Haux, 2006). After four decades of use, the trend is now to implement an enterprise wide decision support system, including clinical data repositories and fully computerized electronic medical records (EMR) of patients. Meinert (2005) cited a Gartner report which states that EMRs are gradually evolving through five generations with each subsequent generation possessing increasingly sophisticated and integrated functionality.

There are no clear boundaries that outline what constitutes EMR, EHR, computerized patient record (CPR), or other healthcare decision support systems. The US Department of Health and Human Services (HHS) on its website defines EMR as an electronic patient health record that can help care providers in decision making with regards to patients' medical condition. EMR and EHR eliminate manual archiving of medical records and automate access to information, and thus streamline the clinician's workflow. They can also support secondary uses such as claims processing, quality management, outcome reporting, and public health disease surveillance and reporting. The subtle difference between EMR and EHR is that EHR systems usually should have some features related with interoperability to transmit data electronically.

Lærum et al. (2004) stated that using EMR/EHR systems are a prerequisite to improve productivity in healthcare industry. Medical secretaries work as transcriptionists, receptionists and coordinators of patient logistics and the nurses have their own documentation and administrative procedures. The elimination of the paper-based medical records is a radical change in the routines of not just secretaries and nurses but the entire hospital organization. The widespread use of information will lead to reduced medical errors, higher-quality care, and improved efficiency in the healthcare industry (Giannangelo & Fenton, 2008). Central theme to this technology is the automation of patient-specific clinical information. In this process, it is very vital to identify the requirements of both internal and external actors because technology is ubiquitous (Mettler & Vimarlund, 2009). Internal actors represent the personnel involved in the day-to-day functioning of the healthcare organization as well as the patients. External actors correspond to those stakeholders who have a strong influence on the healthcare organization (e.g., insurance companies, suppliers, governmental authorities, other healthcare organizations). EHR helps both the internal and external stakeholders in many different ways such as:

- EHR helps insurance companies make predictions on the future health condition of their clients based on their physical characteristics, family medical history, and lifestyle.
- Public insurance organizations use EHR data to detect frauds and abuses. The data can also be used for improving the social security system to reduce health related expenses.
- Pharmaceutical industry benefits from EHR by analyzing patient-related information and patient preferences for healthcare products.
- Researchers and epidemiologists often base their work on aggregated medical data, including identifiable personal data. EHR systems provide reliable data for such research purposes.
- Law enforcement authorities may be able to limit the number of suspects by using pertinent information on disease and genetic characteristics based on information obtained from EHR (Kokolakis et al., 1999).

Figure 1. Data flow diagram of outpatient triage using EMR (McDonald, 1999)

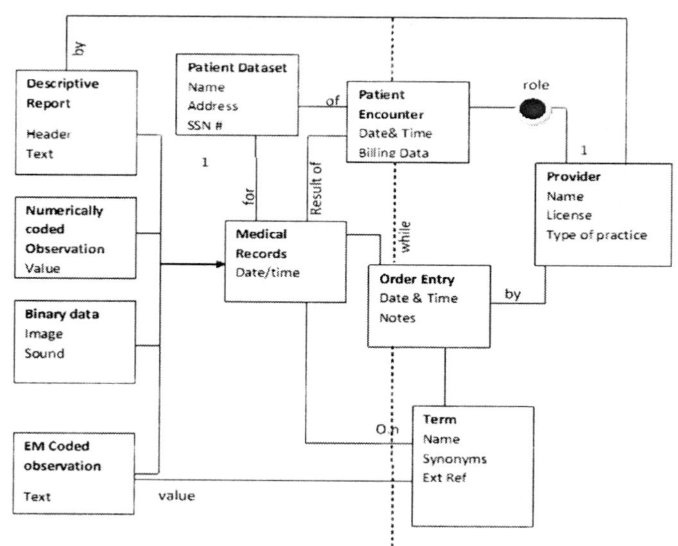

Existing EMR Systems

For a system to be considered as an EMR, it should be able to assist the healthcare institution in different functions such as registering patients, scheduling appointments, providing reminders for patients, nurses and doctors, enabling documentation of patient encounters, and assisting in the billing process and patient education. Figure1 shows the features of basic EMR which uses relational databases with relatively very few files used to store the data. The basic features of EMR as shown in Figure 1 include documenting both structured observations and narrative text reports. EMR also allows archiving and retrieval of radiology reports, thumb nail images, compressed voice, and others. The EMR system also stores term dictionary which defines all the coded elements within the EMR, patient status indicators such as diagnoses, clinical findings, glucose, diastolic blood pressure, Glasgow coma score, etc. These records are indexed based on patient unique identifier, in reverse time order so that response time is less and processing is faster. After identifying patient data, related virtual medical records are displayed.

To date, EMR systems have been regarded as highly decentralized and fragmented systems. Different vendors may offer unique solutions to the same problem for healthcare institutions. KLAS, a company that partners with healthcare professionals, provides a snapshot of EMR segments that are rated based on their importance.

As shown in Figure 2, patient scheduling is the top priority, followed by voice recognition and medical record management for the features of EMR systems. The market for EMR is estimated to reach 53.8 billion USD by 2014, and projections indicate that the market has the potential for further growth because of the demand for general applications which includes EMR, EHR, computerized physician order entry system, and non clinical systems. The current top vendors in this area are Epic Systems Corp, GE Healthcare, McKesson Provider Technologies, and LSS Data Systems (Raths, 2009).

Figure 2. Various features of EMR and their importance (healthcare-informatics.com)

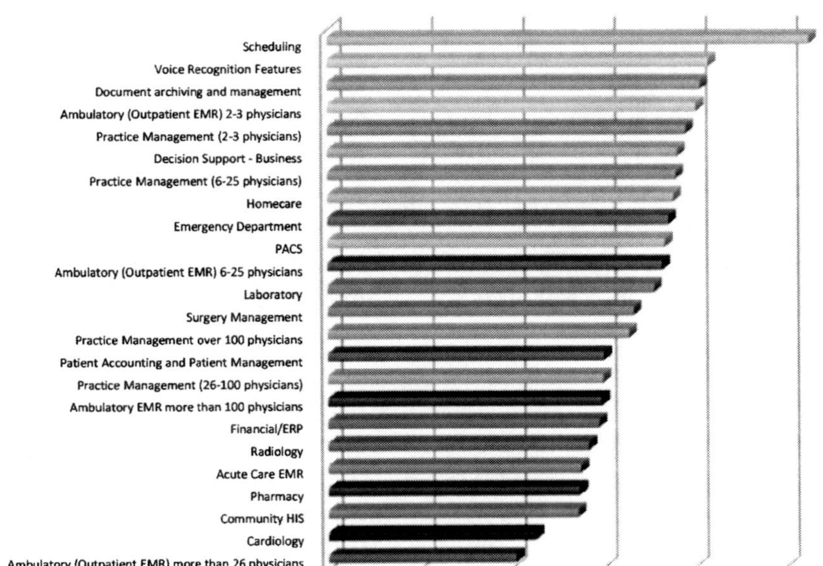

Interoperability Between EMR/EHR Systems

Healthcare process is a collaborative initiative involving doctors, hospitals, pharmacists, staff, patients, payers, regional health information organizations (RHIOs), and many other entities as shown in Figure 3. Interoperability is the ability of these disparate entities interacting with each other during the course of healthcare delivery (Moon et al., 2008). The interoperability among most EHR systems today is unsatisfactory because most of

Figure 3. HIE landscape (Zafar, 2009)

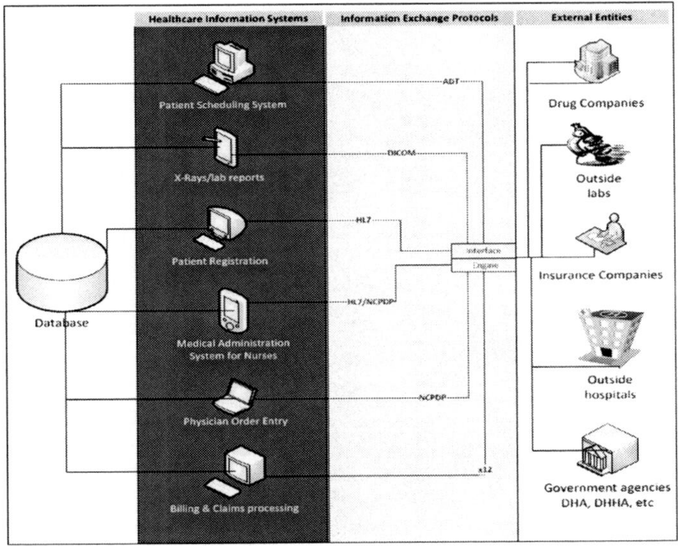

the systems used during the process address just one or a few areas within the healthcare process; they operate in a limited domain and do not support the required functions for a broader perspective. There are many vendors in the market, each arguing about the uniqueness of their solutions and the advantages of their systems over other vendors' solutions. Due to this non-standardized approach and intellectual property issues, the EMR/EHR systems in general fail to provide scalability to promote interoperability.

There are many types of interoperability referred in literature. The most important ones among those are; organizational, operational, systems, semantics, process, and technical interoperability. In this chapter, the scope of discussion is limited to latter three types of interoperability with respect to information exchange within the healthcare industry. As shown in Figure 4, all the three types of interoperability have to be addressed simultaneously in order to achieve better integration among EMR/EHR systems.

Process flows are considered unique to individual healthcare organizations. In 1996, Northern and Yorkshire Regional Health Authority began to explore the capacity of Library and Information Services to support providers and decisions in treating patients (Booth & Falzon, 2001). The initial proposal was to install an identical healthcare system in six healthcare institution libraries. Soon it became clear that it would be more effective for each site to tailor their own package to satisfy and address the needs and expectations of the recipients of healthcare service at local level. In the end, although an approach was made to implement similar systems within the same organization, each location ended up adopting a more customized solution. This example indicates that the inherent process disparity of healthcare organizations is an important factor to be considered for interoperability.

Architectural difference is a persistent problem during the course of implementation of HIE because in many cases, two or more products from the same vendor differ to an extent that the interoperability between those products might be significantly limited. Therefore, it is important to understand the internal architecture and ensure technical interoperability while planning and designing HIE.

Semantic differences exist because of the nature and complexity of healthcare operations. To

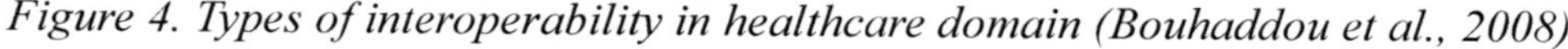

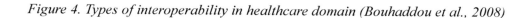

Figure 4. Types of interoperability in healthcare domain (Bouhaddou et al., 2008)

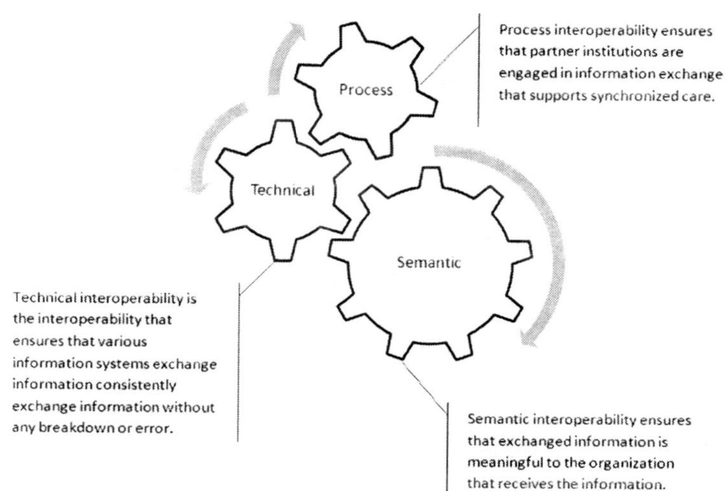

cite an instance, from a pharmaceutical standpoint, two medicines might have the same ingredients but might be different in brand names, or they might be presented in different salt forms. This might cause the clinicians at different hospitals to decide on different pick lists of medications for treating the same ailment (Bouhaddou et al., 2008).

In addition to these differences, there has been lack of national standards in the documenting, archiving, processing, communicating, and presenting healthcare data in the U.S. Sparrow (2008) reported the weakness of The Centers for Medicare and Medicaid Service's (CMS) inability to perform HIE with various stakeholders due to the lack of interoperability. Lack of HIE renders the process incapable of detecting fraudulent schemes such as kickbacks, and false claims for services not provided in CMS. The payment auditing process does not involve any face-to-face contact with providers, and medical records mailed by providers are assumed to be truthful. The information discontinuity creates loopholes in the system for these miscreants to take advantage of the Medicare payment system. An investigation conducted by the Office of Inspector General (OIG) for the Department of Health and Human Services (HHS) discovered that fraud perpetrators such as drug smugglers, terrorists, computer hackers, and thieves submitted fraudulent and fabricated claims on behalf of people who were dead, retired, deported, or incarcerated. Those fraudulent schemes caused CMS to make an overpayment of 23.2 billion USD in 1996.

According to Stiell et al. (2003), the emergency physicians at an emergency department (ED) felt that there was significant information gap in patient services - real time information was not available. The information gaps were more common among the patients referred by a community physician or a nursing home. Lorenzi et al. (2009) conducted a national survey of 2,758 physicians. The survey results showed that only 4 percent of the physicians reported having an extensive electronic records system that was fully functional. The study further stated that the clinicians spent 70 percent of their time on accessing patient data by using medical or nursing notes, computers, telephone and/or internal mail. Adler-Milstein et al. (2009) conducted a survey on RHIOs implementing HIE solutions, and discovered that a significant number of organizations never implemented HIE or ceased to develop HIE solutions. This study raises additional concerns over the current status on proliferation of HIE solutions in healthcare industry.

HIE AND HEALTHCARE DELIVERY

What is HIE?

The Office of the National Coordinator for Health Information Technology (ONC), a unit within the HHS (2008), defines HIE as, "the electronic movement of health-related data and information among organizations according to agreed standards, protocols, and other criteria". A patient in his/her lifetime could visit many medical institutions and each institution may keep only a part of the treatment information for a restricted period of time. Without the access to patients' complete medical history, providers face challenges in deciding appropriate choice of care (Chang et al., 2007). Solution to this problem is an integrated EMR/EHR which can communicate with other stakeholders in the healthcare system based on standard HIE protocol. Hersh (2009) indicated that although healthcare organizations have exemplary EHR systems, they often have difficulty exchanging patient information with other entities in the system. Meanwhile, an increasingly mobile population necessitates the "data following the patients" approach. HIE is the technology that makes this possible.

To promote HIE between medical institutions, American Recovery and Reinvestment Act of 2009 (ARRA) approved approximately 19 billion USD for healthcare institutions investing in health deci-

Figure 5. Healthcare information exchange via HIE protocol

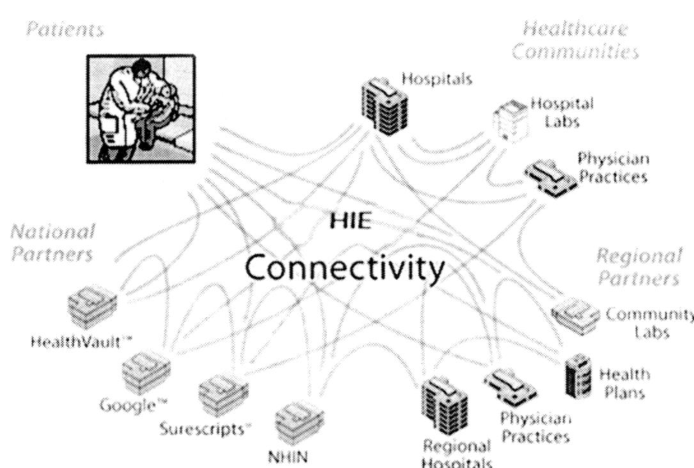

sion support system (HDSS) incentives over five years. This act officially promotes and encourages healthcare institutions nationwide to configure their EMR/EHR systems to support the goal of nationwide interoperable health IT infrastructure. In the U.S., overall 39 statewide HIE initiatives have been reported to date. There are at least 6 county wide HIE initiatives, and some city level HIE initiatives are also undertaken along with the inception of ARRA.

Benefits to Healthcare Delivery

Nationwide interoperable EMR/EHR systems based on a commonly accepted HIE standard carry huge potential. A survey conducted by the Medical Record Institute in 2004 revealed that 80% of the survey respondents believed that sharing patients' records is very important (Chang et al., 2007). This eliminates wastage of resources due to repeated examinations that take place most of the time whenever a patient visits a different medical center. In some cases, the patients are co-treated by more than one physician. In such situations, the lack of HIE incapacitates the provider to access a patient's medical history in a timely manner, and thus negatively affects clinical care. The Levin Group Inc. (2005) reported a study conducted by the Center for Information Technology Leadership to assess the benefits of participating in HIE. It is estimated that, after a 10-year implementation period, the widespread adoption of fully interoperable EMR/EHR based on HIE standards would save the nation approximately 77.8 billion USD annually, or roughly 5% of total healthcare spending. Benefits during the 10-year implementation period amount to 337 billion USD.

HIE contains both extrinsic and intrinsic rewards. According to Hook et al. (2006), interoperability facilitates reduction, eliminates redundant tests, and reduces delays and costs associated with paper-based ordering and reporting. It is estimated that HIE would save the state of New York 2.50 billion USD in laboratory and 1.51 billion USD in radiology annually after full implementation. In addition, some other key benefits due to HIE are:

- Interoperability between outpatient providers and pharmacies would reduce the administrative overhead for transmitting and clarifying prescriptions, saving 221 million USD annually.

- Provider-provider connectivity would save time associated with handling chart requests and referrals, saving 1.01 billion USD annually.
- Payer-provider connectivity would reduce delays and costs associated with paper-based billing, saving an estimated 1.04 billion USD statewide per year. Provider connectivity to the public health system would make reporting of vital statistics and cases of reportable diseases more efficient and complete, saving the state an estimated 15.3 million USD per year.

A fully integrated EMR/EHR transmitting information based on standard HIE protocol can act as a repository for all the scenarios considered, and facilitate consolidation of information by promoting asynchronous interaction among participants (Liu et al., 2007). Such systems can also ease the burden of data collection on care providers, and improve the timeliness, accuracy and value of such information by removing the current inefficient practice of collecting the same data repeatedly for the same patients. Besides, Khoumbati and Themistocleous (2006) classified and generalized the benefits of integration technologies adopted in healthcare organizations, as shown in Table 1.

Existing HIE Rules and Protocols

Regarding the various ways in which information is documented, there are a variety of rules. Medical dictionaries such as Stedman's contain 80,000 or more entries. Systematized nomenclature of human and veterinary medicine (SNOMED) and read codes contain hundreds of thousands of concepts that define how data should be gathered and documented. In addition, ICD10-PCS is a set of tables being developed for healthcare financing administration which contains more than a million procedural codes (McDonald et al., 1998).

The second issue is related with the relay of humongous amount of data. Health Level Seven (HL7) is a widely used format that enables transmitting these codes and information. American Society for Testing Materials (ASTM) 1238, Comite´ Europe´en de Normalisation (CEN) ENV 1613 messages, Digital Imaging and Communications in Medicine (DICOM) messages, and electrocardiography tracings via a CEN standard are also used to transmit radiology and many kinds of clinical observations as well as X-ray reports and images. Similarly, the delivery of admission discharge transfer (ADT) registration information has been mastered via HL7 and CEN ENV 12538, the transmission of community pharmacy information messages via HL7 and National Council for Prescription Drug Programs (NCPDP) messages,

Table 1. Benefits of HIE (Khoumbati & Themistocleous, 2006)

Factors	Benefits of HIE
Productivity & Operations	• Reduced medical errors • Improved patient satisfaction scores. • Reduced paperwork
Cost & Governance	• Higher return on investment for the hospitals. • Reduced the cost of service offered to the patients • Improved accountability due to audit trail capability
Security & Communication	• Electronic transmission of data provides better document control and hence improved patient privacy. • Better compliance with state and federal safety regulations • Improved communication patterns, decision-making, and conflict management.
Technical Infrastructure	• New emerging tools such as Open Source. • Trend in adopting more web based approach for better omnipresence

as well as the transmission of simple claims via Accredited Standards Committee (ASC) X12 messages are few other protocols used to transmit information captured during encounter between patient and the provider. 90% of the healthcare industry in the U.S. has adopted the NCPDP code, and three major companies now provide healthcare institutions with updated NCPDP databases frequently that contain the latest information related to all the approved drugs in the U.S. (McDonald et al., 1998).

Challenges of HIE Implementation

On the average, every year each patient has four outpatient visits with about 50% of the visits to primary care providers, 40% to specialists, and 10% to emergency departments (Kaelber & Bates, 2007). The biggest barrier encountered during patient triage is that healthcare institutions lack timely access to patients' medication and problem lists and are unable to communicate with partner institutions (Harlan et al., 2009). Also, there are huge variations in the communication methods of providers – their preferences for phone, fax, and e-mails are different. In some instances, providers ask residents and students for assistance during patient care. Absence of a universal HIE system makes it difficult to identify the names and contact information of those people aiding the providers during the care delivery process.

Currently, health information technologies (HIT) and EMR/EHR are more focused locally than regionally or nationally and this is an apparent contradiction to the fact that patients may not be solely treated in a single medical facility. During their lifetime, they may be seen by more than one provider separated by distance and time (Dimitropoulos & Rizk, 2009). On the other hand, healthcare institutions must navigate a complex array of federal, state, privacy, and security laws. On the basis of internal requirements, regulations and applicable laws, organizations can take different approaches to develop integrated electronic healthcare system. This creates a challenging environment resulting in wide spread variations during exchanging healthcare related information.

In order to analyze the extent of gap that exists today between the current medical facilities and the nationwide HIE vision, ONC launched a project to assess variation in organization-level business practices, policies, and state laws to help policymakers identify common practices and reduce variation. It was found that health information is protected by a patchwork of practices, policies, and state laws that has evolved over time, without a comprehensive plan or approach. This has resulted in state privacy and security laws that are scattered throughout many chapters of code which might conflict with each other. Most of these laws were made with paper-based systems in mind, and many failed to anticipate a full-scale nationwide HIE (Dimitropoulos & Rizk, 2009).

Although HL7 is very well defined in terms of specifications, many problems in this area arise from blatant vendor deviation because of the lack of technical knowledge on expressing related healthcare information using HL7 (McDonald et al., 1998). For example, for reporting negative test results, one provider might document the incident as "no growth yet" and yet another provider might document the same incident as "no pathogenic throat bacteria recovered". Accordingly, Khoumbati and Themistocleous (2006) stated that healthcare institutions can expect many challenges during the implementation of HIE, and these challenges are listed in the Table 2.

IMPLEMENTATION OF HIE

Generic HIE Procedure

The physical assets are becoming less important in determining the success of a healthcare organization, while the intellectual capital, value of information, and knowledge assets are gaining prominence. Data alone does not add significant

Table 2. Challenges of HIE (Khoumbati & Themistocleous, 2006)

Factors	Challenges
Productivity & Operations	• Lack of management support and training • Loss of productivity during transition phase
Cost & Governance	• High initial capital • Ongoing Integration cost • Cost of data security
Security & Communication	• Inconsistent application of standards makes the system vulnerable for outside attack. • Lack of plug and play type of solutions.
Technical Infrastructure	• Evolving standards. • Inefficiency during merging schema. • Standards for HIE not yet defined by HHS. • Database limitation on space and archiving records.

value. Over the past few decades, healthcare institutions have been gathering data to make informed decisions via EMR/EHR and other decision making systems that are readily available off the shelf or developed in house. These EMR/EHR systems store patient and transaction data, as well as other types of information such as lab and prescription data, provider information, patient electronic medical records, appointment schedules, and imaging results. If defective data is entered into the system at any stage during this process, they spread throughout the system via HIE. This will be an expensive mistake to correct because sound medical decisions can only be made based on reliable medical data. Alshawi et al. (2003) indicated that bad data can cost organizations as much as 10 to 20 percent of the total organization budget, and as much as 40 to 50 percent of IT department budget, and most of the budget is spent in the process of correcting these errors. According to the same study, the framework of archiving interoperable EMRs based on HIE protocol can be addressed using four stages as follows;

Stage 1: Identifying the Root Source of Patient Data

As mentioned earlier, there are many EMRs within the healthcare organizations that archive medical records. In order to ensure high data quality, appropriate measures must be taken. The typical measure is designing appropriate level of checks and validations to prevent bad data being entered into the system. Card et al. (1986) conducted a study to assess the efficiency of human operators while performing manual operations on computers. The study revealed that under normal conditions, a data entry process is 60 percent mental and 40 percent manual, and the error rate of human operators during the process of inputting and processing the data is at least 4 percent. Thus, it is important that EMR/EHR systems have the capabilities for identifying bad data entries.

Stage 2: Assessing the Quality of Data, Data Matching, and Data Mapping by Comparison

The second step is matching or comparing the data elements. Since different EMR/EHR systems are used, it is important to match the data sent from the source before importing it into the target system. For instance, one EMR for scheduling appointments may use "0" to represent male, while another EMR might use "M". Without a thorough process of validation, promoting interoperability based on HIE standards within an organization is meaningless. There are many ways of performing this step. One method involves extracting the data schema from each database that stores EMR data. Data schema is a metadata (i.e., data about the data). Schema matching is a basic problem in many database application domains, and now prevalent during the HIE process for the healthcare industry. This process is the heart of HIE implementation because success or failure in this process largely influences the overall outcome of achieving interoperability. Schema matching can be performed manually, but it has significant limitations. On the other hand, many procedures have been proposed to achieve a partial automation of the matching operation. Figure 6 shows the taxonomy that covers many of these matching approaches (Rahm & Bernstein, 2001). Cannataro et al. (2008) developed a framework of information sharing based on peer-to-peer environment by mapping patient record into an XML-based meta electronic patient record so that users can query the meta record schema for comparison and provide match between source and target data elements. Titus Labs Inc. (2009) designed an enterprise labeling methodology for the same process. Atzeni et al. (2007) developed ModelGen operator that supports model-generic translations of schemas. There are many other models that aim to achieve complete the automated schema translation while implementing HIE, but the major drawback in all these approaches is the difficulty of validating the correctness of complex transformations.

Stage 3: Data Integration or Linking

Once the data elements are identified and mapped between the source and target databases, the next step in this process is the integration of these data elements using XML or other similar formats that can enable connectivity between different systems. This is also the process of consolidating various data elements for seamless data transfer between the source and target databases. Initially a pilot run is performed on these integrated databases and the new data populated from the source EMR system is evaluated. If this appears to match the requirements for interoperability between these two systems, HIE at this stage is considered successful.

Stage 4: Final Checks, Evaluation, Archival and Distribution

Once the data mapping and integration of the source and target systems are performed, the last step in the process is to test the overall integra-

Figure 6. Overview of various database schema matching strategies (Rahm & Bernstein, 2001)

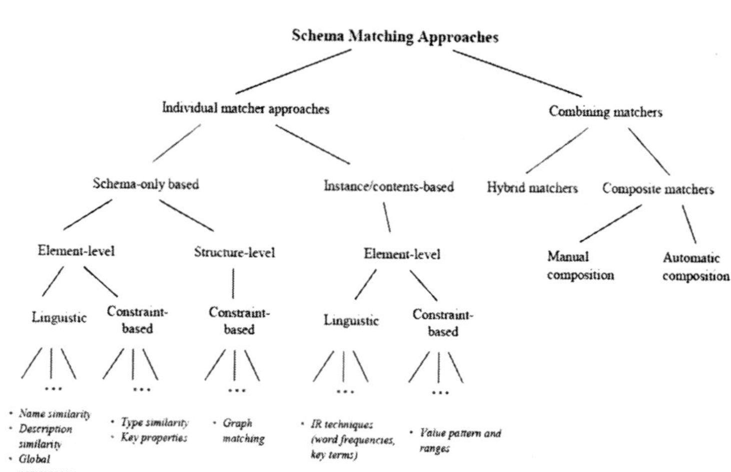

tion and archive the data to prevent misuse of this newly designed interoperable EMR system.

Based on the heterogeneity of the EMR systems from various vendors and the technology used in developing these systems, it is important to choose communication technologies that are capable of achieving interoperability among different systems without data loss or the need for manual intervention in terms of validation. It is almost impossible to achieve a very high accuracy rate during schema translation based on the prevailing market conditions. For this reason, the World Health Organization emphasizes the development based on open source concept. The open source technology enables the access to the source code in an easier manner. EMR/EHR systems based on open source components can support nearly 100% inter-operability based on the nature of scalability, and robustness of this technology as a whole. Nonetheless, the use of open source technology is not possible in all situations. This requires ad-hoc nonstandard solutions to integrate proprietary software from the manufacturer.

Examples of EHR/HIE

Healthcare institutions have made some significant advances in implementing fully functional HIE, but overall development has been sluggish. Few large organizations, notably Department of Veterans Affairs (VA) has implemented a fully integrated electronic records system, other organizations have automated major portions of clinical information systems such as laboratory data, order entry, etc., others are in the process of becoming paperless in the next few years.

Case 1

One of the oldest HIE systems in use is the Regenstrief Medical Record System. It serves more than 1.5 million patients and is used extensively at three hospitals on the Indiana University Medical Center Campus and more than 30 outreach clinics. The basic goals are (1) eliminating the logistic problems of the paper record by providing access for the authorized users to the clinical data stored in electronic format, (2) reducing the clinical book keeping for managing the patients, (3) making the data accessible to the clinical, epidemiologic, outcomes, and the management research. The Regenstrief Medical Record System is a huge system that contains more than 200 million separate coded observations, 3.25 million narrative reports, 15 million prescriptions, and 212,000 electrocardiographic tracings. It has a user group of 1300 medical center nurses, 1000 physicians, and 220 medical students. One distinguishing facet is that this system has been in use for more than 35 years and serving the entire health system of the city of Indianapolis. There are different modules that have been extensively used to facilitate the information flow within this system. For instance, the person identifier module links with data from many hospitals about the patient through the global registry consisting of the separate registration records. These registration records are assigned by each hospital by identifying factors such as the name, gender, birth date, and race. These identifiers would help identify the patient even in situations where patients arrive at the hospital in an unconscious or confused state and are unable to identify themselves. The system has the capability to communicate with the other information systems for various purposes such as acquiring and validating death certificates. A rule based clinical decision support system is implemented with the HIE framework to assist the clinicians. For example, the system might raise a flag against an order of platelet transfusion if the patient's recent count is over certain limit. While the system warns about the ramifications of the order, the physicians are not blocked for completing that order.

Case 2

Both VA and Department of Defense (DOD) have healthcare delivery facilities scattered geographically at various locations nationally. They both share a large patient population. According to Bouhaddou, et al. (2008), the EHR used by VA is VistA, while DoD uses AHLTA. AHLTA stores electronic medical record for more than 8.6 million care recipients scattered throughout the country and VistA stores EMR for 7.5 million veterans throughout the country. DoD and VA set out to implement a comprehensive longitudinal electronic health record system. The objective was to develop an interface between DoD's national clinical data store known as Clinical Data Repository (CDR) and VA's national data store known as Health Data Repository (HDR) to regulate real time bi-directional exchange data for patients, or those patients who receive treatment at both VA and DoD treatment facilities.

The main focus was not an attempt to change the existing standards or repositories between DoD and VA. Both VA and DoD have successfully standardized their terminologies. The patient data collected from the different points of care in both VA and DoD were assembled into one enterprise health data repository for each agency. VA uses HL7 format, while DoD uses HL7 V3 RIM-based model. Enterprise-specific terminology to support mediation is translated from an agency's translation services to the national standard terminologies. This exchange model incorporates a hybrid push and pull model, allowing patient data to be sent automatically upon creation (i.e., push) or upon query (i.e., pull). The two platforms exchange information using a common syntax and common semantics, in compliance with broad HL7 terminology principles. 80% of the effort is spent in standardization of data elements which led to a success rate of more than 90% for bi-directional information exchange. The new HIE architecture performs data exchange and synchronization of database in the range of 12-120 seconds, while previously this operation used to take around 4-5 weeks. In the domain of allergy, there is a 32 percent chance of increase in mediation success from DoD to VA and a 22 percent chance of gain from VA to DoD. Failure rate during their HIE implementation is mostly due to non-standard data. For extreme cases, non-standard data which accounts to 3 to 11 percent of the total volume of the pharmacy data, contributes to around 70 percent of failure in the HIE process.

ADVANCED ISSUES OF HIE TECHNOLOGIES

Experience dealing with large HIE systems leads to the questions about the process and model used to address patient privacy, security, cost, and risks. Failure to assess factors such as patient privacy and security while implementing HIE would definitely contribute to the failure of an HIE system. According to Halamaka et al. (2005), a major challenge in implementing a very broad and inclusive interoperable healthcare system is the secure exchange medium to protect patients' medical information. Many healthcare institutions have invested in internal projects to develop customized, off the shelf solutions to encounter many of the challenges related to standardization, patient data privacy and security.

Security

Undoubtedly, patient information exchange is based on trust. It is assumed that the end users will handle sensitive information in a predictable manner. As such, this transfer of information to partner RHIOs is based on "chain of trust". In 2006, McGraw et al. (2009) conducted a national survey to assess the patients' confidence and they reported that 80 percent of patients surveyed were very concerned about identity theft or fraud, 77 percent were very concerned about use of their medical information for marketing purposes, 56 percent worried that employers would access their health information, and 55 percent were concerned about insurers' seeing their medical history. HHS spent almost six years to provide standards for fair information practice guidelines by dissecting, understanding the myriad of issues, conducting hearings, proposing rules, and analyzing and responding to comments. This effort materialized into a 1,500 pages report that categorically defines the process of keeping the patient data private (McDonald, 2009). Some of the health information exchange principles are only weakly expressed, and others are missing entirely (McGraw et al., 2009). Dimitropoulos and Rizk (2009) stated that in a network where healthcare related information is exchanged between partner institutions, some institutions voiced their concern related to legal responsibility when one institution in the network claimed that its own security program was more secure than the downstream institution's counterpart program. The variation in how organizations secure patient private information has created a sense of mistrust between organizations and raised a concern that the Health Insurance Portability and Accountability Act (HIPAA) measures on information security are also not well understood.

Privacy

HIPAA's protections do not extend to non-identified healthcare information. This allows healthcare institutions to provide non-identified data to third parties for research and business intelligence use and thus circumvents HIPAA guidelines. In turn, these entities may use the related data based on their interest without any restrictions, subject only to the terms of any applicable contractual provisions or state laws that might apply. If a third party who receives this data, re-identifies it using tools and knowledge in its possession, such a case might constitute a violation of HIPAA regulations and might present itself as a potential loophole (McGraw et al., 2009). HIPAA's privacy rules also make it difficult to follow research patients over time, creating problems in bookkeeping for drop-outs and deceased research participants. This also creates problems in designing post-marketing studies. According to McGraw et al. (2009), the definition of marketing in the HIPAA privacy rule often permits the use and dissemination of protected health information without patient's authorization and allows companies to send that patient marketing materials regarding certain healthcare products or services.

All these observations and findings necessitates responding to these privacy and security risks, not just to build trust and avoid individual embarrassment or discrimination, but also to receive accurate and reliable information for maintaining good health status. Without privacy and security assurances, patients might likely withhold information from their providers because of the concern that their personal health information might be used as a source of profit (McGraw et al., 2009). A study indicates that 92 percent of consumers are eager to share their personal health related information with other health professionals involved in their care who are not their primary care provider so that their chances of survival might be improved (Frohlich et al., 2007). It is obvious that if the patients believe that sharing data improves the quality of their life, they are eager to support exchange of information. Yet, at the same time, patients are fearful of others for using their personal medical information that might lead to harmful outcomes (Halamaka et al., 2005). A balanced approach is important in designing/implementing an interoperable EMR/EHR for HIE purposes. Here we refer to the balance between the need to protect privacy and the need for policies, for procedures to be workable; for flawless data exchanges and to improve the quality, safety, efficiency, and affordability of care. In that regard, the guidelines published by HHS as stated by Banning (2008) are noteworthy.

Adaptive and Scalable Mapping Between EHRs

Any attempt to solve patient privacy while implementing an interoperable healthcare system must be premised on a model of patient authorization and control. The system must provide patients sufficient time and space to decide whether or not to participate in sharing personally identifiable information; exercise their rights under HIPAA; and securely share all or portions of their records among institutions. Once patient's consent has been granted for access to a certain type of information, respective entities with relevant rights should be able to access it freely (Halamaka et al., 2005). Meanwhile, Mandl et al. (2007) indicated that the HIE system must address the requirements of federal, state and local statutes, institutions, providers' clinical judgment, and mainly the needs of individuals. RHIOs should start with institution policies as the baseline and incorporate the constantly changing federal and state regulations without any downtime. The success of those measures is strongly dependent on the scalability of the system.

McGraw et al. (2009) stated that, in some instances, hospitals and medical centers partner with third party agencies to manage their patient medical records. In such situations, it is very important that the respective healthcare institutions enforce HIPAA and patient data safety requirements via contractual agreements on other partners in their network. Patient privacy policies in this domain are fragmented and inconsistent, providing neither developers nor consumers the assurances they deserve, especially for services of nationwide reach.

Semantics and Data Mining

Data mining can be defined as the process for analyzing the data and discovering patterns and the correlations using the statistical analytical techniques, computer technologies, and related software to convert the data sets into the meaningful information (Tan et al., 2006). Considering huge amount of data that is used for the EMR and EHR systems, and the need for making the best use of the data in a timely manner, the data mining techniques might serve as an indispensable tool for enhancing the functions of the HIE. Within the context of HIE, data mining techniques address various issues such as handling the complex set of data being utilized by EMR and EHR systems and would help to build a common platform for facilitating the exchange of this information. The data mining might also help to increase the efficiency of the distributed systems where medical information is kept at different sources. In addition, data mining might serve as a valuable tool for supporting the clinical expert systems. Coupled with the effective HIE solutions, the data mining approach might unearth the patterns hidden in the medical data and might be valuable for increasing the overall efficiency of the healthcare delivery systems by assisting the physicians for giving the medical decisions and might possibly reduce the amount of expensive laboratory work that needs to be conducted for diagnosis and subsequent treatment. The HIE promotes and enhances the data mining approach by providing a medium for exchange of the related medical information to be facilitated for the various clinical expert systems.

On the other hand, semantic data mining is a concept for enhancing the data mining process by utilizing the formal procedures, methods and techniques for the integration of the data semantics. The semantics within context of data mining can be considered as a key for deciphering the complex data by integration of the background knowledge and reasoning inferred based on this knowledge (Atzmuller et al., 2009). Incorporating the semantics component in the data mining approach would help identify the relationship between data stored in different repositories and would help promote HIE by bringing forward a common platform for making the best use of the data by introducing the formal guidelines for constructing the relationship between different data types. In a sense, it is an abstraction process that provides the link between the real word and the stored information distributed through the healthcare network. The semantics data mining has been finding more applications especially in the field of the medicine (Cespipova et al., 2004; Kuo et al., 2007). Capturing domain knowledge and incorporating the relation between the components of this domain (i.e., the ontology) through the semantics approach is of help for building common grounds for data mining processes, and improving the quality of the information exchanged between various players in healthcare industry. Without building constructs for exploring the domain knowledge initiated by the semantics approach, it would be highly difficult if not impossible for the system developers who are not well versed in clinical applications to build HIE solutions for promoting the interoperability.

Quantitative Assessment of HIE Impacts

HIE research has been focused on the qualitative analysis and discussion on the benefits and impact of HIE. However, there has been lack of quantitative modeling effort to assess the values of HIE and how HIE affects the decision making in healthcare units. In this regard, the tools from decision sciences, operations research, industrial engineering, and management science are valuable. For instance, the value of information is a well-studied topic in the realm of decision sciences. The modeling approaches might be brought forward for the justification of the HIE and a cost-benefit model can be formed using this approach. However, the quantitative modeling efforts specific to HIE is scarce in literature. Among the most notable one is the approach taken by Walker et al. (2005). A hybrid approach was taken to consider the qualitative and quantitative parts regarding the assessment of the healthcare information exchange and the interoperability. The authors developed an analytical framework and employed decision modeling software accompanied with an influence diagram. Using some underlying assumptions on the price of information, they estimated the potential benefits of implementing HIE.

Quantitative approaches and concepts borrowed from microeconomics theory might be valuable tools for linking HIE with various clinical performance measures. This type of evaluation is important in that HIE is primarily a tool for connecting various EHR systems by enabling the interoperability. Roberts (2007) employed a multivariate approach and discussed about the effect of HIT on various performance measures related with the quality of the healthcare delivery systems such as mortality, financial performance, and patient safety. The author employed the partial least squares approach for analyzing the relation between various components of the HIS, and identified a direct relationship between the complexity of the information technology and the patient safety. Although this study is not related with HIE in a strict sense, it might serve as a guideline for deciding on the level and nature of the information exchange between various HIS for promoting interoperability. In a similar vein, Menon et al. (2000) borrowed some ideas from microeconomics concepts and employed a generic production function for prioritizing the capital investment decisions on non-clinical and clinical components of the information technology. This study might also present some guidelines for managing the deployment of HIE modules to provide the connectivity between various HIT functions.

There is a great deal of research regarding developing mathematical models for investigating the case of information sharing especially for the supply chain applications. Among them, the models that incorporate game theoretical approaches deserve special attention. Healthcare is a complex and competitive industry consisting of many stakeholders. Most of the time, there might be conflicting interests among those stakeholders.

Game theory brings an analytical perspective for capturing the behavior of those stakeholders in a competitive environment where the outcome of the decisions made by one party is dependent on the decisions made by other parties. The game theoretical approach, when applied in information sharing context, might serve as a very valuable tool for analyzing the behavior of the stakeholders in the healthcare industry. We cite a few instances as follows. Galbreth and Shor (2010) employed game theory for analyzing the motives of the malicious market players to attack the information assets for promoting their inferior products. It was concluded that such approaches might be preferable by those malicious players to increase their profits. This study might be adopted in the realm of HIE for the importance of safe-guarding the sensitive patient specific information and emphasize the importance of the medium of trust among the players using HIE applications. Similarly, Zhao and Johnson (2009) developed a game-theoretical approach for the governance of the information. They studied various policies based on the incentives, penalties, and escalation policies and compared the effect of those approaches for governance of the information. This kind of approach might suit well in the context of HIE for developing the escalation policies for providing the flexibility where employees belonging to different organizations might have varying levels of access to the patient-specific information. Yao et al. (2006) developed a slightly more complex approach to model the supply chain consisting of the two retailers and one supplier, and under certain assumptions, they developed the equilibrium conditions which might improve the profitability of the entire supply chain, thus leading to the win-win situations. Although, no horizontal information sharing case was analyzed, the paper provides the valuable insight on how much information to share on the treatment costs of the patient which constitutes the basis of the contractual agreement between the insurers and healthcare institutions for the healthcare delivery systems. Nagarajan and Sosic (2008) presented a game-theoretical approach on the bargaining strategies from the profit allocation and the stability perspective. They investigated the effect of collective bargaining strategies on the allocation of the profit, and the stability concept from the view point of coalition forming was addressed. Stability might be loosely defined as the affinity of the players sticking to the current strategies. The findings of the paper might constitute a good basis for designing the pay-off schemes between the insurer and the healthcare organization and forming the RHIO for facilitating the information flow between the partners in the healthcare network. In addition, through the stability concept, the stated model might serve as a proxy for analyzing the sustainability of the current contracts and information sharing policies in the short run.

SECONDARY USE OF EHR AND HIE

There is no doubt that caregivers are increasingly looking at the role of decision support system and how it can be utilized to help improve the quality of care provided to the patients. Vendors, on the other hand, support this initiative by moving beyond the traditional EMR/EHR used to document patient information and are offering solutions that improve the efficiency of clinical data management systems, site administration, adverse events reporting, and patient diaries. Brown (2004) provided a general summary on the possible secondary uses of EHR and HIE, as shown in the Table 3. On the other hand, the discussion is narrowed down to two aspects of the secondary use.

Disease Management

Obesity is becoming the most common chronic condition. It has been recognized as a leading cause for chronic and serious diseases, such as cardiovascular disease, diabetes mellitus type 2,

Table 3. Secondary use of EHR and HIE (Brown, 2004)

Uses	Notes
Electronic data capture (EDC)	EDC applications such as automatic signature capture
Clinical data management systems (CMDS)	Data repository for clinical trial data as per FDA requirements.
Drug safety monitoring	Document, track, and report adverse medical events during trails.
Trial management	Track the progress of clinical trials
Site management	Monitor the activities of investigators at a large site such as academic medical center.
Vocabulary	Standard vocabulary defined during the trials.
eSubmission	Features that assist submission of clinical data as a part of regulatory process.
Electronic patient dairy	Patient report on quality of life and other information during clinical trial.
IVR or Call IVR	Automated call handling system
Investigator management	Build and manage pool of past and potential investigators to accelerate recruitment.

hypertension, stroke, heart failure, uric acid, and sleep apnea (Polikandrioti & Stefanou, 2009). Recent data suggested that 3 out of every 10 children aged between 2-19 are overweight or obese, and this is higher among African American and Hispanic population and those from lower socioeconomic group. It is recommended that the obese or overweight kids follow up with their primary care physicians once every month regarding the treatment for their chronic condition. However, most obese children are referred to specialists for treatment. This is undesirable because (1) the inadequate number of specialists may lead to long waiting time; (2) it is expensive to consult a specialist while the medical case can be handled by a primary care physician; (3) continuity of care is lost because these children are forced to seek services outside the system. This also makes it difficult for the families to meet different providers at various times. To improve the quality of care, an EHR system was used improve care quality and data reporting. Past data can be compared to current data and provides a quality patient health monitoring system. Such an electronic data management system also allows providers to collaborate with other clinics via teleconference and face to face meetings to share best practices and solve common problems (Anand et al., 2010).

Another example might be provided on tobacco use. Tobacco use is a major cause of morbidity in the U.S., and a brief smoking cessation intervention by clinicians is effective in helping smokers to quit. The U.S. Public Health Service (USPHS) provides guidelines for providers to routinely counsel patients using a five-step algorithm. Accurate measures of providers' adherence to this guideline and to assess the impact of interventions are required. Existing methods for monitoring provider practice patterns include providers' own reports of their behavior, patients' reports of providers' actions, review of medical records, and direct observation of the physician-patient encounter. Each method has limitations. Providers generally overestimate how they counsel patients about smoking. Patients' may underestimate or overestimate the quality of counseling services. The rapid pace of adoption of EMR/EHR has made it easier to study this problem compared to the previous paper records. Also, EMR/EHRs have built-in templates that can easily record standard information, and features that might improve providers' documentation of tobacco counseling activities. Conroy et al. (2005) measured how often primary care physicians and nurse practitioners delivered the USPHS guidelines on smoking intervention at eight primary care clinics that use EMR in Boston area. The authors surveyed the providers, patients, and analyzed the EMR records. The EMR review revealed a low rate of documentation by providers, while patients reported that their physicians conducted the guidelines at a much higher rate. This suggests that physicians failed to document part of their actions. The study shows that EMR is a practical tool of measuring providers' delivery of tobacco treatment services in practice.

Integration of Care

The integration of care is a process that takes place within relationships between individuals. Clinical integration and functional integration describe the phenomena that take place with respect to the analysis in question. Normative integration helps expressing the relationships between various levels. Lastly, systemic integration aims to ensure consistency between the analysis in question and the environment. The integration also involves coordinating clinical practices around the specific health problems of each patient in a sustainable manner. Its goal is to guarantee consistent, comprehensive care; in other words, to ensure that services provided by various professionals, in various locations or organizations, meet the specific needs of each patient, given the knowledge and technology available (Contrandripoulos et al., 2003).

Along with this line, Almborg et al. (2008) surveyed 152 consecutively enrolled relatives (mean age = 60.8 years) of acute stroke patients admitted to a stroke unit about their satisfaction with discharge planning. Discharge planning is a dynamic process that involves the patient, the family, and the caregivers in a dynamic, interactive communication and collaboration regarding a range of specific skills. Survey showed that relatives were often unsatisfied with their perceived involvement in discharge planning and the quality of information they were provided. The families lacked information and felt there was a communication breakdown in connection with discharge process. Families also wanted to participate more in discharge planning. The findings suggest that there is a very strong need to integrate disparate information silos in healthcare industry for effective planning of various services for serving the needs of patients and caregivers.

Vimarlund et al. (2008) expressed the multidimensionality of information in care by highlighting the importance of information and communication technology (ICT) to support integrated healthcare services in elderly homecare. In particular, ICT can enable information exchange, knowledge sharing, and documentation at the point-of-care (POC). In contemporary elderly care organizations, the one-on-one basis healthcare personnel–patient relationship is replaced by a complex relation type where the patient is managed by a team of healthcare professionals, with each professional specialized in different aspects of healthcare and gerontology. Team members do not necessarily belong to the same organizational unit, and they may even provide care outside hospitals or elderly care centers. The efficacy of such shared care depends partly on the interest from the individuals in self-managing their health and on individuals' preference for ageing at home rather than in an institution. This also depends on care providers' ability to easily share information and on the use of appropriate technology to transmit and communicate accurate information between involved actors.

CONCLUSION

Effective decision making based on information technology is the key for the success of healthcare delivery. In addition to the inherent complexity, a striking difference between the healthcare delivery and other systems is that the healthcare systems are less error tolerant. The medical errors not only incur significant costs on the systems, but it might have significant ramifications on the health status of the patients using the system. Due to the lack of the solid standards and the large number of vendors providing customized solutions tailored to the needs of a specific healthcare delivery system, interoperability of EHR/EMR systems has become a major issue. Along with those lines, there is a need for a broad and yet concise discussion of EHR and HIE. To satisfy this need, in this chapter, the functions and benefits of HIE, along with the challenges for implementation are discussed in great detail. Case studies are provided as well. Moreover, the current problems related to handling patient specific data in the context of HIPAA, as well as other state and federal legislations are discussed. In addition, the secondary uses of EHR and HIE systems are discussed.

In conclusion, this chapter serves as a comprehensive reference for EMR/EHR and HIE. HIE offers a great deal of opportunity for improving the healthcare delivery and facilitates system-wide cost savings by integrating data exchange procedures and streamlining the patient flow. However, there are challenges regarding HIE and these should be addressed accordingly. In order to reap the benefits of a fully integrated HIE process, an integrated and comprehensive approach is required during the design and implementation stages. Ultimately, the approaches to implementing EMR/EHR should be aimed at improving efficiency for healthcare delivery and quality of life for the patients.

REFERENCES

Adler-Milstein, D., Bates, D. W., & Jha, K. J. (2009). U.S. regional health information organizations: Progress and challenges. *Health Affairs*, *28*(2), 483–492. doi:10.1377/hlthaff.28.2.483

Almborg, A. H., Ulander, K., Thulin, A., & Berg, S. (2008). Patients` perceptions of their participation in discharge planning after acute stroke. *Journal of Clinical Nursing*, *18*, 199–209. doi:10.1111/j.1365-2702.2008.02321.x

Alshawi, S., Missi, F., & Eldabi, T. (2003). Healthcare information management: The integration of patient's data. *Logistics Information Management*, *16*(3/4), 286–295. doi:10.1108/09576050310483772

Anand, S. G., Adams, W. G., & Zuckerman, B. S. (2010). Specialized care of overweight children in community health centers. *Health Affairs*, *29*(4), 712–717. doi:10.1377/hlthaff.2009.1113

Atzeni, P., Cappellari, P., & Gianforme, G. (2007). MIDST: Model independent schema and data translation. In *Proc. ACM SIGMOD '07*, (pp. 1134-1136).

Banning, P. (2009). Economic-recovery plan to include health info. *MLO: Medical Laboratory Observer*, *41*(2), 48.

Bennett, R. E., Tuttle, M., May, K., Harvell, J., & Coleman, E. A. (2007). *Health information exchange in post-acute and long-term care case study findings: Final report*. submitted to the U.S. Department of Health and Human Services Assistant Secretary for Planning and Evaluation Office of Disability, Aging and Long-Term Care Policy.

Booth, A., & Falzon, L. (2001). Evaluating information service innovations in the health service: If I was planning on going there I wouldn't start from here. *Health Informatics Journal*, *7*(1), 13–19. doi:10.1177/146045820100700104

Bouhaddou, O., Warnekar, P., Parrish, F., Do, N., Mandel, J., Kilbourne, J., & Lincoln, M. J. (2008). Exchange of computable patient data between the Department of Veterans Affairs (VA) and the Department of Defense (DoD): Terminology mediation strategy. *Journal of the American Medical Informatics Association*, *15*(2), 174–183. doi:10.1197/jamia.M2498

Brown, G. E. (2004). *Clinical trials' EDC endgame. Forrester helping business thrive on technology change*. Retrieved from http://www.oracle.com/corporate /analystportal/insider/forrester_clinical_trials_edc_endgame.pdf

Card, S., Moran, T., & Newell, A. (1983). *The psychology of human-computer interaction*. Hillsdale, NJ: Lawrence Erlbaum Associates.

Chang, I. C., Hwang, H. G., Hung, M. C., Lin, M. H., & Yen, D. C. (2007). Factors affecting the adoption of electronic signature: Executives' perspective of hospital information department. *Decision Support Systems*, *44*, 350–359. doi:10.1016/j.dss.2007.04.006

Chu, W. H. J., & Lee, C. C. (2006). Strategic information sharing in a supply chain. *European Journal of Operational Research*, *174*(3), 1567–1579. doi:10.1016/j.ejor.2005.02.053

Conroy, M., Majchrzak, N., Silverman, C., Chang, Y., Regan, S., Schneider, L., & Rigotti, N. A. (2005). Measuring provider adherence to tobacco treatment guidelines: A comparison of electronic medical record review, patient survey, and provider survey. *Nicotine & Tobacco Research*, *7*(Suppl 1), S35–S43. doi:10.1080/14622200500078089

Contrandripoulos, A. P., Denis, J. L., Touati, N., & Rogriguez, C. (2003). *The integration of health care: Dimensions and implementation*. (Working Paper No 4-01). Montréal, Canada: Université de Montréal Groupe deresearche interdisciplinaire en santé.

Department of Health and Human Services. (2001). *HHS pandemic influenza plan supplement 10: Public health communications*. Retrieved May 30, 2010, from http://www.hhs.gov/pandemicflu/plan/sup10.html

Department of Health and Human Services. (2008). *The National Alliance for Health Information Technology report to the Office of the National Coordinator for Health Information Technology on defining key health Information Technology terms*. Retrieved May 30, 2010, from http://healthit.hhs.gov/portal/server.pt/gateway/PTARGS_0_10741_848133_0_0_18/10_2 _hit_terms.pdf

Department of Health and Human Services. (n.d.). *Electronic medical records*. Retrieved May 30, 2010, from http://healthit.hhs.gov/portal/ server.pt?open=512&mode=2&cached=true&objID=1219

Detmer, D. E. (2003). Building the national health information infrastructure for personal health, health care services, public health, and research. *BMC Medical Informatics and Decision Making*, *3*, 1. doi:10.1186/1472-6947-3-1

Dimitropoulos, L., & Rizk, S. (2009). A state-based approach to privacy and security for interoperable health information exchange. *Health Affairs*, *28*(2), 428–434. doi:10.1377/hlthaff.28.2.428

Frohlich, J., Karp, S., Smith, M., & Sujansky, W. (2007). Retrospective: Lessons learned from The Santa Barbara Project and their implications for health information exchange. *Health Affairs*, *26*(5), w589–w591. doi:10.1377/hlthaff.26.5.w589

Galbreth, M., & Shor, M. (2010). (in press). The impact of malicious agents on the enterprise software industry. *Management Information Systems Quarterly*, *34*(3).

Giannangelo, K., & Fenton, S. H. (2008). SNOMED CT survey: An assessment of implementation in EMR/EHR applications. *Perspectives in Health Information Management*, *5*(7), 1–13.

Grimson, J. (2001). Delivering the electronic healthcare record for the 21st century. *International Journal of Medical Informatics*, *64*(2-3), 111–127. doi:10.1016/S1386-5056(01)00205-2

Halamka, J., Overhage, J., Ricciardi, L., Rishel, W., Shirky, C., & Diamond, C. (2005). Exchanging health information: Local distribution, national coordination. *Health Affairs*, *24*(5), 1170–1179. doi:10.1377/hlthaff.24.5.1170

Harlan, G., Srivastava, R., Harrison, L., McBride, G., & Maloney, C. (2009). Pediatric hospitalists and primary care providers: A communication needs assessment. *Journal of Hospital Medicine*, *4*(3), 187–193. doi:10.1002/jhm.456

Haux, R. (2005). Health Information Systems - Past, present, future. *International Journal of Medical Informatics*, *75*(3-4), 268–281. doi:10.1016/j.ijmedinf.2005.08.002

Hersh, W. (2009). A stimulus to define informatics and health Information Technology. *BMC Medical Informatics and Decision Making*, *9*(24). doi:. doi:10.1186/1472-6947-9-24

Hook, J. M., Pan, E., Adler-Milstein, J., Bu, D., & Walker, J. (2006). The value of healthcare information exchange and interoperability in New York State. *AMIA Annual Symposium Proceedings*, (p. 53).

Kaelber, C. D., & Bates, W. D. (2007). Health information exchange and patient safety. *Journal of Biomedical Informatics*, *40*(6), S40–S45. doi:10.1016/j.jbi.2007.08.011

Khoumbati, K., & Themistocleous, M. (2006). Evaluating integration approaches adopted by healthcare organizations. *Journal of Computer Information Systems*, *47*(2), 20–27.

Kokolakis, S., Gritzalis, D., & Katsikas, S. (1999). Generic security policies for healthcare Information Systems. *Health Informatics Journal*, *4*(3), 184–195. doi:10.1177/146045829800400309

Liu, D., Wang, X., Pan, F., Xu, Y., Yang, P., & Rao, K. (2008). Web-based infectious disease reporting using XML forms. *International Journal of Medical Informatics*, *77*(9), 630–640. doi:10.1016/j.ijmedinf.2007.10.011

Lorenzi, N. M., Kouroubali, A., Detmer, D. E., & Bloomrosen, M. (2009). How to successfully select and implement electronic health records (EHR) in small ambulatory practice settings. *BMC Medical Informatics and Decision Making*, *9*, 15. doi:10.1186/1472-6947-9-15

Mandl, K., Simons, W., Crawford, W., & Abbett, J. (2007). Indivo: A personally controlled health record for health information exchange and communication. *BMC Medical Informatics and Decision Making*, *7*, 25. doi:10.1186/1472-6947-7-25

McDonald, C. (2009). Protecting patients in health information exchange: A defense of the HIPAA privacy rule. *Health Affairs*, *28*(2), 447–449. doi:10.1377/hlthaff.28.2.447

McDonald, C. J., Overhage, J. M., Dexter, P., Takesue, B., & Suico, J. G. (1998). What is done, what is needed and what is realistic to expect from medical informatics standards. *International Journal of Medical Informatics*, *48*(1), 5–12. doi:10.1016/S1386-5056(97)00102-0

Mcdonald, C. J., Overhage, J. M., Tierney, W. M., Dexter, P. R., Martin, D. K., & Suico, J. G. (1999). The Regenstrief medical record system: A quarter century experience. *International Journal of Medical Informatics*, *54*(3), 225–253. doi:10.1016/S1386-5056(99)00009-X

McGraw, D., Dempsey, J., Harris, L., & Goldman, J. (2009). Privacy as an enabler, not an impediment: Building trust into health information exchange. *Health Affairs*, *28*(2), 416–427. doi:10.1377/hlthaff.28.2.416

Meinert, D. B. (2005). Resistance to electronic medical records (EMRs): A barrier to improved quality of care. In E. Cohen (Ed.), *Issues in Informing Science and Information Technology, 2*, 493-504. Informing Science Press.

Menon, N. M., Lee, B., & Eldenburg, L. (2000). Productivity of information systems in the healthcare industry. *Information Systems Research*, *11*(1), 83–92. doi:10.1287/isre.11.1.83.11784

Mettler, T., & Vimarlund, V. (2009). Understanding business intelligence in the context of healthcare. *Health Informatics Journal*, *15*(3), 254–264. doi:10.1177/1460458209337446

Moon, T., Fewell, S., & Reynolds, H. (2008). The what, why, when and how of interoperability. *Defense & Security Analysis*, *24*(1), 5–17. doi:10.1080/14751790801903178

Nagarajan, M., & Sosic, G. (2008). Game-theoretic analysis of cooperation among supply chain agents: Review and extensions. *European Journal of Operational Research*, *187*(3), 719–745. doi:10.1016/j.ejor.2006.05.045

Polikandrioti, M., & Stefanou, E. (2009). Obesity disease. *Health Science Journal*, *3*(3), 132–138.

Rahm, E., & Bernstein, A.P. (2001). A survey of approaches to automatic schema matching. *The VLDB Journal — The International Journal on Very Large Data Bases, 10*(4), 334-350.

Raths, D. (2009). *Vetting the vendors- 2009 best in KLAS: Beyond the numbers*. Retrieved May 30, 2010, from http://www.healthcare-informatics.com/ Media/DocumentLibrary/ KLAS_2009_Supplement.pdf

Roberts, S. A. B. (2007). *The impact of Information Technology on small, medium and large hospitals: Quality, safety and financial metrics*. Ph.D. Dissertation, University of Texas at Arlington.

Stiell, A., Forster, A. J., Stiell, I. G., & van Walraven, C. (2003). Prevalence of information gaps in the emergency department and the effect on patient outcomes. *Canadian Medical Association Journal*, *169*, 1023–1028.

The Levin Group, Inc. (2005). *Health Information Technology Leadership Panel final report*. Retrieved May 30, 2010, from http://www.hhs.gov/healthit /HITFinalReport.pdf

Vimarlund, V., Olve, N. G., Scandurra, I., & Koch, S. (2008). Organizational effects of information and communication technology (ICT) in elderly homecare: A case study. *Health Informatics Journal*, *14*(3), 195–210. doi:10.1177/1081180X08092830

Walker, J., Pan, E., Johnston, D., Adler-Milstein, J., Bates, D. W., & Middleton, B. (2005). The value of health care information exchange and interoperability. *Health Affairs*, *24*(5), w10–w18.

Yao, D. Q., Yue, X., & Liu, J. (2006). Vertical cost information sharing in a supply chain with value-adding retailers. *Omega*, *36*(5), 838–851. doi:10.1016/j.omega.2006.04.003

Zafar, A. (2009). *Health information exchange (HIE): Nuts and bolts*. Retrieved June 25, 2010, from http://www.virec.research.va.gov /EducationResources/Seminars/ Informatics071806.PPT

Zhao, X., & Johnson, M. E. (2009). The value of escalation and incentives in managing information access. In Johnson, M. E. (Ed.), *Managing information risk and the economics of security* (pp. 165–177). Springer, US. doi:10.1007/978-0-387-09762-6_8

Section 4
Patient Flow

Chapter 18
Evaluating Patient Flow Based on Waiting Time and Travel Distance for Outpatient Clinic Visits

S. Reza Sajjadi
North Dakota State University, USA

Jing Shi
North Dakota State University, USA

Kambiz Farahmand
North Dakota State University, USA

ABSTRACT

Patient flow greatly affects the quality of service delivered to the patients. Among various performance measures identified for patient flow, this chapter focuses on the analytical modeling of two key measures, namely, patient waiting time and travel distance. Waiting time is analyzed by a promising yet simple analytical tool – queuing theory. Three queuing models, including single station, multiple serial stations, and network systems are presented. Moreover, patient travel distance is investigated by an analytical model to evaluate the patient flow. For both measures, the applicability of models is illustrated with numerical examples.

INTRODUCTION

There are many indices in healthcare delivery by which the quality of service provided to patients can be evaluated. One aspect for evaluation is the smoothness of the patients' movement in their visit to medical facilities, known as patient flow. At the first glance, patient flow is related to the time a patient consumes in a medical facility from arrival to discharge. Any time in which the patient waits to receive the service is considered as waste that might result in the patient's dissatisfaction. As such, patient waiting time is essential to the measurement of patient flow. Combined with

DOI: 10.4018/978-1-60960-872-9.ch018

data collection, analytical modeling approaches can help the management to develop a systematical understanding about operations and make better decisions. Queuing models as a powerful tool have been extensively used in analyzing manufacturing and service systems. Such a tool furnishes mathematical formulas to approximate performance measures in a system. A queuing system can be simply described as customers arriving for service and waiting for service if it is not immediate available, as well as leaving the system after being served. Although the *theory* of queuing requires advanced mathematical background, its *application* side is relatively easier. Being compatible with spreadsheet programs such as Microsoft Excel®, healthcare practitioners can effectively apply the tool. On the other hand, it is also natural to evaluate the patient flow based on the distance a patient travels in a medical facility. In most cases, patients need to travel among multiple places in a visit. Therefore, the total distance traveled during a visit can be considered another key factor for the patient flow. Based on the probability of traveling from one department to another department in a facility, a score can be assigned to each patient route in the facility. The score can be then considered as a performance measure of patient flow.

In this chapter, we focus on the patient flow in outpatient clinics. The second section of this chapter briefly reviews the literature on the general aspects of patient flow. Meanwhile, the management tools and performance measures which have been used in the literature to analyze the patient flow are reviewed. Thereafter, the waiting time is analyzed by queuing models for various healthcare settings in the third section. Queuing principles and applications in healthcare are covered. Three queuing systems known as single station, multiple serial station, and network are then discussed and case studies are provided. In the fourth section, an algorithmic approach is presented by which the patient flow can be measured from the perspective of travel distance. By introducing "from-to" matrix, patient route probability vector, and route accessibility concept, a simple-to-use analytical approach including a case study is furnished to compute the patient flow travel score.

BRIEF LITERATURE REVIEW ON PATIENT FLOW

General Patient Flow

An effective and efficient patient flow is characterized by high patient throughput, low patient waiting time, short length of stay, and low clinic overtime, while maintaining adequate staff utilization rates and low physician idle times(Jun et al., 1999). Potisek et al. (2007) performed a patient flow analysis to identify specific areas of inefficiencies in patient visits and thus improve patient visit efficiency through developing interventions to decrease the mean time of patient visit. It is found that patient flow analysis is an effective method for identifying the inefficiencies and efficiently collecting patient flow data. Generally, patient flow analysis is closely related to three main areas: (i) patient scheduling and admissions, (ii) patient routing and flow schemes, (iii) scheduling and availability of resources (Jun et al., 1999). Patrick et al. (2008) addressed the incorporation of patient priority in a scheduling problem where patients are scheduled to the fixed scheduling slots of a diagnostic resource within the maximum waiting time recommended for each priority. St. John's hospital (Henderson et al., 2004) teamed up with Institute for Healthcare Improvement (IHI) to improve the patient flow in its emergency department. The first approach that they took is to provide a dedicated operating room for the unscheduled and "add-on" cases. By doing so, the number of surgical cases went up by 5 percent and the overall time decreased by 2 percent. Also, the staffing need could be more accurately predicted. Another major approach is to add a standardized fax report form to facilitate the communication between ED nurses and receiving nurses. This way, the time wasted on phone between different departments was significantly reduced. The median time from decision to admit to physical placement in an inpatient bed was reduced by 67%. Garcia et al. (1995) analyzed the effects of using a fast track lane to reduce waiting times of low priority patients in an emergency room. Emergency rooms were prioritized according to the level of patient sickness, hence low priority patients regularly wait for excessively long periods of time. A fast track lane is a lane dedicated to serving a particular type of patient. It was found that a fast track lane that uses a minimal amount of resources could greatly reduce patient waiting times.

Analytical Tools and Performance Measures

One of the most powerful tools for analyzing healthcare systems is to utilize operation management techniques. The kind of tool looks for improvement opportunities in flow of the patients and resources through better usage of resources including man, material, and machine. The operation management techniques reported in the literature include discrete-event simulation, mathematical programming models (e.g., linear, non linear, dynamic, stochastic, and integer programming), Markov chain analysis, queuing, statistical analysis, and Lean. Discrete-event simulation has been more widely used for patient flow analysis than other tools. Compared with the mathematical modeling tools, simulation is featured by its capacity to model complex patient flows and conveniently examine different patient flow rules and policies. Complex patient flows are common in settings such as emergency department, where patients arrive without appointments and require treatment over a large and various set of ailments and conditions. Although the arrival of patients is highly unpredictable, it is still possible to minimize patient waiting time and increase staff utilization by altering patient routing and flow. Blake and Carter (1996) analyzed an emergency department at the Children's Hospital of Eastern Ontario. Based on the simulation results, a fast track lane for treating patients with minor injuries was implemented. Ritondo and Freedman (1993) showed that changing a procedural policy (of ordering tests while in triage) could result in a decrease in patient waiting time in the emergency room and an increase in patient throughput. Goitein (1990) performed Monte Carlo simulation to examine factors such as physician idle time relative to patient waiting time, and he found that patients would experience very long waiting times if the physician overbooked the schedule, even in a slight manner. In two different studies, Holdgate et al. (2007) and Moser et al. (2004) applied simulation models to investigate the accuracy of triage nurses in identifying patients suitable for admission or discharge.

Other modeling tools have also been used for patient flow analysis in literature. Edwards et al. (1994) compared two medical clinics that use different queuing systems: serial processing, where patients wait in a single queue, and quasi-parallel processing, where patients are directed to the shortest queue to maintain flow. It was shown that patient waiting times could be reduced by up to 30% using the quasi-parallel processing. Similarly, Jiang and Giachetti (2008) developed a queuing network to analyze the impact of care parallelization on the patient cycle time in an outpatient clinic. Driven by the need from an urgent care center, the patient flow was required to be improved and the total cycle time was asked to reduce to 3 hours. Note that more literature on the application of queuing systems in healthcare will be discussed in a later section. Moreover, Rohleder et al. (2005) developed a goal programming model to allocate operating room block in an effort to improve patient flow. At the Foothills Medical Centre in Calgary, Alberta, the block schedules derived from the proposed model was compared with actual scheduling practice by running a simulation model built on the actual data. Min and Yih (2010) formulated a stochastic dynamic programming model for a scheduling problem where patients with different priorities are scheduled for elective surgery in a surgical facility of limited capacity. It was found that the consideration of patient priority results in significant differences in surgery schedules from the schedule that ignores the patient priority. As such, different patient scheduling and admission rules and policies can have a significant impact on patient waiting time and provider utilization.

In addition, Kyriacou et al. (1999) studied the patient flow in an emergency department of Los Angeles County Hospital. The purpose was to identify the areas of inefficiency and assess if administrative interventions can improve patient flow and ED efficiency. The major tool used in this study is time study. It was found that time study is an effective tool to identify the inefficiency and also, targeted administrative interventions apparently reduced the total ED LOS and improved overall efficiency. Abdel-Aal (1998) adopted two univariate time-series analysis methods in modeling and forecasting the monthly patient volume at a primary care clinic, where the optimum ARIMA model was determined as an autoregressive model of the fourth order operating on the data after differencing twice at the non seasonal level and once at the seasonal level.

Table 1 lists the typical performance measures found in the literature for evaluating the clinic

Table 1. Performance measures for patient flow

Number	Efficiency Measure
1	Mean total cost (calculated by using relevant combinations of the following factors)
2	Waiting time of patients
3	Cycle time of patients
4	Idle time of doctor(s)
5	Overwork time of provider(s)
6	Idle time of clerks and nurses
7	Overwork time of clerks and nurses
8	Mean, maximum and frequency distribution of the patient's waiting time
9	Mean, variance and frequency distribution of doctor's waiting time
10	Mean, maximum and standard deviation of doctor's overwork time
11	Means and frequency distributions of patient cycle time, process time and lead time
12	Mean, variance and frequency of provider/nurse waiting for information or supplies
13	Percentage of patients seen within the scheduled time
14	Productivity of providers or nurses
15	Utilization of providers or nurses
16	Delays between requests and appointments
17	Percentage of walk in, new and returning patients
18	Equipment utilization
19	Likelihood of patients receiving the slots they requested
20	Mean, variance and frequency distribution of service time for providers or nurses
21	Mean and frequency distribution of number of patients waiting in queue
22	Mean and frequency distribution of number of patients waiting in system

visit efficiency. Waiting time is found to be one of the most important measures for outpatient clinic visit efficiency (Hart, 1995; Cartwright & Windsor, 1992; Evans & Wakeford, 1964; Jones et al., 1987; Clague et al., 1997). Most recently, Bush et al. (2007) included both the waiting times for appointment and in clinic as performance measures for clinic efficiency study. Williams et al. (2009) considered the waiting time of patients and usage of healthcare resources as system performance measures based on their means, variances, and confidence intervals.

WAITING TIME ANALYSIS

Queuing Approach in Healthcare

Queuing theory is an important operations research tool, applicable for various systems where servers (e.g., bank teller, nurses, or providers) provide service to customers. In general, a customer can receive the service immediately once he/she arrives at the system if not all the servers are occupied; otherwise, the customer stays in a queue. Using the rate of customer arrivals and the server process time, it is possible to use queuing models to determine the patient waiting time to receive the service as well as the total time the patient spends in the system. For most healthcare systems, neither the patient arrival rate nor the server processing time is fixed. Even in appointment based systems such as outpatient clinics, there is no guarantee that patients arrive at their exact scheduled times and receive the services exactly as predicted. In such cases, queuing theory which works based on the random process analysis can provide detailed information about the system.

A growing number of researchers use queuing theory in view of its ease of calculation, minimal data requirements, and ability to deliver using spreadsheets (Cochran & Roche, 2009). In contrast to the discrete event simulation methodology that is time consuming and requires skillful modelers, a queuing model can be built in a fraction of time needed for developing a simulation model (Jiang & Giachetti, 2008). Moreover, queuing is easy to use while it does not require dedicated software codes, which may not be affordable for many regular users. Kao and Tung (1981) employed an $M/G/\infty$ model in analyzing the demand for inpatient bed units and allocating beds to minimize overflows, where patient arrival to each unit was estimated and collected from empirical daily admission data. Albin et al. (1990) adopted a queuing network model to investigate the causes of delay in a clinic. The queuing analysis showed that the delays were due to scheduling problems rather than the registration area. It was concluded that although significant differences exist between the real system and the model assumptions, the queuing network model provided insight for the operation of the appointment clinic. Shmueli et al. (2003) modeled the probability distribution of the number of occupied beds in an intensive care unit based on queuing theory. They developed a model for optimizing the admissions so as to maximize its expected incremental number of lives saved. Cochran and Bharti (2006) presented a multi-stage methodology for hospital bed planning, where queuing networks was applied to capacitate areas in the hospital. Su (2003) analyzed several scheduling solutions and found that setting the appropriate arrival time interval for preregistered patients significantly impacts queuing problems in outpatient services. There is a consensus that the efficiency of a system could be improved by combining queues or switching from multiple-queue multiple-server systems to a single-queue multiple server system (Winston, 1993). Meanwhile, some argue that the patient waiting time could not be reduced by adding resources alone and most practitioners would increase their referrals in this case (Hindel, 1972). Worthington (1987) performed a queuing analysis to test this feedback or latent demand phenomenon and concluded that adding resources could not help the wait list problem but improve throughput. However, Martin and Smith

(1999) found that increased resources may reduce waiting time without greatly increasing utilization by investigating the correlation between arrival rates and resource levels.

Queuing Principles

Kendall's Notation

The most common notation for indicating a queuing system is Kendal's notation (Kendall, 1951). A queuing system can be characterized by six terms in order. Such notations can be explained in Table 2. For example, G/M/3/20/100/LIFO represents the queuing system where the customer inter arrival time follows a general distribution, the service time follows an exponential distribution, three parallel servers serve customers, the maximum number of customers allowed in the system is 20, the population of customers is 100, and the last customer is served first. Similarly, an M/M/m system represents a queuing system including m servers while both arrivals and service times follow exponential distributions. Note that the models presented in this chapter only consider queuing systems without any capacity limitation while they take into account FIFO procedure for their queuing lines.

Queuing Formulas Notation

Table 3 shows the symbols that are used in the chapter for the queuing systems. If the rate of patient arriving to the system (λ) is greater than the rate of patient receiving service (μ), the system will eventually explode. Therefore, the fundamental assumption of all queuing systems is to hold the inequality $\lambda/\mu<1$. When parallel servers work at the station m, the condition should be modified to $\lambda/(m\mu)<1$. A queuing system can be evaluated against its performance measures. The common performance measures for evaluating a queuing system are shown in Table 4.

Three useful equations in queuing systems are coefficient of variation (CV), Little's law, and utilization of the station. The CV of a stochastic variable indicates the variation of that variable. CV for customer arrival (CV_a) and server (CV_s) can be calculated as follows,

$$CV_a = \sigma_a/\lambda, \tag{1}$$

Table 2. Kendall's notation for queuing system

Character order	Meaning	Most common notation
1	The statistical distribution of customers' inter arrival times to the system	D: Deterministic
		M: Exponential (Markovian)
		G: General
2	The statistical distribution of servers' processing times	D: Deterministic
		M: Exponential (Markovian)
		G: General
3	Number of parallel servers	A fixed number such as 1, 2, etc.
4	Maximum number of customers allowed in the system	A fixed number such as 1, 2, etc. It also could be assumed infinite.
5	Total population of patient	A fixed number such as 1, 2, etc. It also could be assumed infinite.
6	Queuing discipline	FIFO: First in first out
		LIFO: Last in first out
		SIRO: Service in random order

Table 3. Queuing notations

Symbol	Definition
λ	Rate of patient arrivals to the server per unit of time
$1/\lambda$	Average time between two immediate patient arrivals (inter arrival time)
CV_a	Patient arrival coefficient of variance
σ_a	Standard deviation of customer arrivals
μ	Rate of service per unit of time
$1/\mu$	Average service time
CV_s	Service time coefficient of variance
σ_s	Standard deviation of service time
CV_d	Patient departure coefficient of variance
m	Number of parallel servers at station
ρ	Percentage of time that the server is busy (utilization of station)

Table 4. Performance measures used in the queuing models

Measure	Definition $\rho = \frac{\lambda}{m\mu}$.
L	Expected number of patients in the system
L_q	Expected number of patients in the queue
W	Total time that the patient spends in the system (cycle time)
W_q	Time that the patient spends in the queue

$$CV_s = \sigma_s/\mu. \tag{2}$$

Little's law indicates that the expected number of patients in the system/queue is equal to the total time a customer spends in the system/queue multiplies the rate of customer arrivals. Little's law can be expressed as follows:

$$L=\lambda \cdot W, \tag{3}$$

$$L_q=\lambda \cdot W_q. \tag{4}$$

The next equation is the utilization of the station including m servers,

$$\rho = \frac{\lambda}{m\mu} \tag{5}$$

It is easy to observe that for a single server station,

$$\rho=\lambda/\mu. \tag{6}$$

Poisson and exponential distributions are two important patterns for many queuing systems. In the next section these two distributions are briefly discussed.

Poisson Process

Poisson process is a non-negative stochastic process extensively used in queuing theory. The most important property of a Poisson process is that the occurrences of events are independent. This characteristic is a realistic assumption for many systems such as bank and healthcare in which the arrivals of customers are usually not dependent on each other. There are two types of Poisson processes, namely, homogenous and non-homogenous. Homogenous Poisson process is the focus of this chapter and can be defined as a process in which the number of events occurring in a period of time is fixed. This property may not be true over a long period of time (e.g., a week), but it is appropriate for smaller time intervals. For example, patient arrival in a clinic during working hours (not an entire day) may follow a Poisson process. The non-negative property of the Poisson process is that the process can not handle negative values. For example, the number of patient arrivals to a clinic can not be negative. This characteristic is in contrast to some of other stochastic process such as standard normal process which can cope with negative values. Two useful Poisson processes are Poisson distribution and exponential distribution which are discussed below.

Poisson Distribution

In a homogenous Poisson process, the probability of observing x events from time T to $T+t$ can be calculated from the discrete Poisson distribution as follows,

$$P(x) = \frac{e^{-\lambda t}(\lambda t^{x})}{x!}, \tag{7}$$

where λ is known as the parameter of the Poisson distribution and defined as the rate of occurrences. If $t=1$, the probability distribution function (PDF) of observing x events in one unit of time can be computed by,

$$P(x) = \frac{e^{-\lambda}(\lambda^{x})}{x!}. \tag{8}$$

Values for the cumulative density function (CDF) of Poisson distribution are provided as a table in many statistical books for pre-defined values of λ (Mendenhall & Sincich, 1995). The mean and variance of the Poisson distribution is equal to λ. It is noticeable that Poisson distribution is not limited to events per unit of time. It also can be used to calculate the probability of events per unit of page, distance, etc, which may, for example, include the number of typing error per page, the number of infant mortality per thousand delivery, or the number of defect per batch of production.

Exponential Distribution

While Poisson distributions deal with the number of events per unit of time, the inter arrival times of such events form another statistical distribution known as exponential distribution. Examples include the time between the arrivals of patients, and the service time for the patients in an inpatient clinic. The PDF and CDF of exponential distribution are as follows,

$$P(x) = \frac{1}{\mu}e^{-\frac{1}{\mu}x}\ x \geq 0, \tag{9}$$

$$F(x) = 1 - e^{-\frac{1}{\mu}x}, \tag{10}$$

where μ is the parameter of exponential distribution and defined as the time between two immediate events (i.e., inter arrival time). The mean and standard deviation of exponential distribution are equal to μ.

The parameters of exponential and Poisson distributions have an inverse relation: $\mu=1/\lambda$. One interesting characteristic of exponential distribution is its *memoryless* property. It implies that, the probability of patient arriving after t_1+t_2 provided that the patient arrives after t_1 is equal to the probability of patient arriving in clinic after t_2. This property can be written as Eq. (11). For example, the probability that the next patient arrives after 50 minutes provided that the patient will arrives after 40 minutes is equal to the probability that the patient arrives after 10 minutes.

$$P(T > t_1 + t_2 | T > t_1) = P(T > t_2). \tag{11}$$

Goodness of Fit Tests

One question which is often raised in a queuing system is the statistical distribution of patient arrival and/or server service time. The queuing systems extensively deal with Poisson and exponential distribution. At some point, it is needed to verify the assumption of Poisson or exponential distribution. Since the standard deviation and mean of exponential distribution are the same, one simple method is to collect a sample data and observe if the mean and standard deviation of the data are close to each other. The more robust and reliable technique is, however, the statistical test approach. While there are different statistical approaches to test such hypothesis, Chi-Square (χ^2) and Kolmogrov-Simironov (K-S) tests are two common ones. To illustrate the process of hypothesis test, the Chi-Square test is discussed below using one numerical example. The description of K-S test can be found in many statistical books such as (Law & Kelton, 2003). It is also noticeable that such tests are not limited to exponential and Poisson distributions and they may be open to any type of statistical distribution. The general format of null and claim hypothesis can be written as follows, respectively:

H0: The set of data follows the distribution with function F

H1: The set of data does not follow the distribution with function F

Chi-Square Test

This test can be applied for both discrete and continuous distributions. Poisson, uniform, and Bernoulli are three examples of discrete distribution, while normal, exponential and Weibull are the examples of continuous distribution. To satisfy the accuracy of the χ^2 test, the sample size should be larger than 50. The data should be broken into K adjacent intervals. In some cases, selecting a different K interval may result in a different conclusion. χ^2 goodness of fit test is based on the χ^2 statistics approximation. A value of calculated χ^2 is compared to a value of χ^2 from the χ^2 table in reference books (e.g., Law & Kelton, 2003), and based on that the hypothesis is evaluated.

Suppose k is the data set level, O_i is the observed frequency, E_i is the expected value; and v $(=k\text{-}r+1)$ is the degree of freedom, r is the number of parameters from hypothesized distributions, and α is a threshold value. The χ^2 value can be calculated from the following equation:

$$\chi^2 = \sum_{i=1}^{k} \frac{(O_i - E_i)^2}{E_i} \tag{12}$$

Based on the above data, the rejection criteria would be $\chi^2 > \chi^2\ (v, 1\text{-}\alpha)$. Next, we explain the

Table 5. Number of patients visited and its frequencies

Number of patient seen per hour	Frequency
0	10
1	26
2	12
3	2

procedure of the χ^2 test for case of *discrete* distribution using the following example.

Example: The number of patients seen by provider per hour in a walk-in primary care clinic is obtained from a field observation of 50 hours and the data is shown in Table 5. Is it true that the number of patients seen by the provider follows a Poisson distribution with α=0.05?

First, the null and claim hypothesis can be written as follows:

H0: The number of patient visited follows Poisson distribution

H1: The number of patient visited does not follow Poisson distribution

Then, a table needs to be developed to provide information about the observation number (i), observed data (O_i), and frequency of observed data. Also, we need to approximate the parameter of the candidate distribution using the observed data by calculating the probability of events, P_i, and nP_i where n is sample size. Note that the cells needs to be combined if nP_i is less than or equal to 5. The χ^2 values can be calculated based on Eq. (12). To calculate P_i, the parameter (i.e., λ) of the Poisson distribution should be approximated based on the data collected. Therefore, we have $\lambda = (0 \cdot 10 + 1 \cdot 26 + 2 \cdot 12 + 3 \cdot 2) / 50 = 1.12.$

Thus, the probability function is in the form of $P(x) = 1.12e^{-1.12x} / x!$ Now, the probability for each level of data observed will be computed. For instance,

$$P(x = 0) = P_1 = 1.12e^{-1.12 \times 0} / 0! = 0.33$$

The results are provided in Table 6.

Finally, the calculated χ^2=5.71 should be compared with χ^2 (v, 1-α). In this case, by looking up the χ^2 table, χ^2(v, 1-α)= χ^2 (3-1-1, 0.05)=3.84. Since 5.71>3.84, H0 is rejected. It is concluded that at 95% of confidence level, the number of patients visited does not follow Poisson distribution.

Table 6. χ^2test data

i	Number of patients visited	Frequency (O_i)	P_i	E_i=nP_i	Combined nP_i	χ^2_i
1	0	10	0.33	16.31	16.31	2.44
2	1	26	0.37	18.27	18.27	3.27
3	2	12	0.20	10.23	14.05	0.00
4	3	2	0.08	3.82		
	n=	50			χ^2=	5.71

Figure 1. Single station queuing system

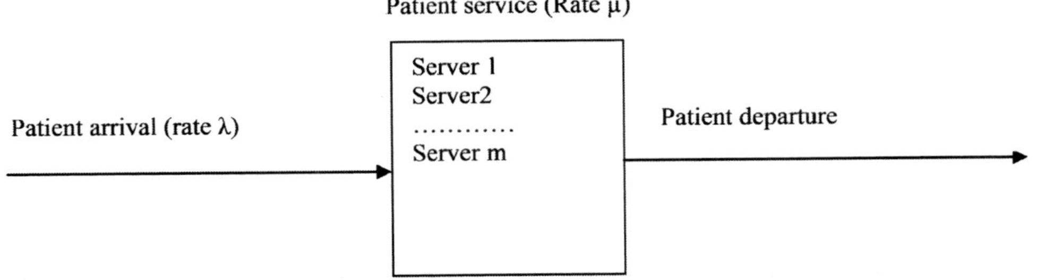

Single Station Queuing System

Figure 1 indicates a single station queuing system, the simplest form of queuing system, where a single server or multiple parallel servers provide service to patients (customers). In such a system, patients wait until a server is available. After being served, they leave the system.

Based on the probability distributions of arrivals and service time, the performance measures are calculated from their corresponding mathematical formulations. Table 7 summarizes these formulations. It should be noted that except the M/M/1 formulas, other queuing systems are calculated using approximation method (Hopp & Spearman, 2008). The exact formulas for queuing systems may be derived based on queuing references such as (Gross & Harris, 2002). However, it requires extensive mathematical manipulations. The first step for using the queuing models is to determine the type of the station and then apply the formulas. This process is shown using a numerical case in the next section. Although some of the formulas may be considered complex, they can be calculated using a spread sheet program such as Microsoft Excel®. For other queuing systems such as M/G/m and G/M/m, it is possible to use G/G/m approximation.

Multiple Serial Station

A sequence of single station systems forms a multiple serial station system where patients sequentially receive service at each station. In

Table 7. Formulations for single station queuing system

Queuing System	Performance measure			
	L	L_q	W	W_q
M/M/1	$\frac{\rho}{1-\rho}$	$\frac{\rho}{1-\rho}$	$\frac{1}{\mu-\lambda}$	$\frac{\rho}{\mu-\rho}$
M/M/m	$(\frac{\rho^{\sqrt{2(m+1)}1}}{1-\rho})+m\rho$	$\frac{\rho^{\sqrt{2(m+1)}}}{1-\rho}$	$\frac{\rho^{\sqrt{2(m+1)}-1}}{m\mu(1-\rho)}+\frac{1}{\mu}$	$\frac{\rho^{\sqrt{2(m+1)}-1}}{m\mu(1-\rho)}$
G/G/1	$(\frac{CV_a^2+CV_s^2}{2})(\frac{\rho\lambda}{\mu-\lambda})+\rho$	$(\frac{CV_a^2+CV_s^2}{2})(\frac{\lambda\rho}{\mu-\lambda})$	$(\frac{CV_a^2+CV_s^2}{2})(\frac{\rho}{\mu-\lambda})+\frac{1}{\mu}$	$(\frac{CV_a^2+CV_s^2}{2})(\frac{\rho}{\mu-\lambda})$
G/G/m	$(\frac{CV_a^2+CV_s^2}{2})(\frac{\rho^{\sqrt{2(m+1)}1}}{1-\rho})+m\rho$	$(\frac{CV_a^2+CV_s^2}{2})(\frac{\rho^{\sqrt{2(m+1)}}}{1-\rho})$	$(\frac{CV_a^2+CV_s^2}{2})(\frac{\rho^{\sqrt{2(m+1)}-1}}{m\mu(1-\rho)})+\frac{1}{\mu}$	$(\frac{CV_a^2+CV_s^2}{2})(\frac{\rho^{\sqrt{2(m+1)}-1}}{m\mu(1-\rho)})$

Figure 2. Multiple stations queuing system

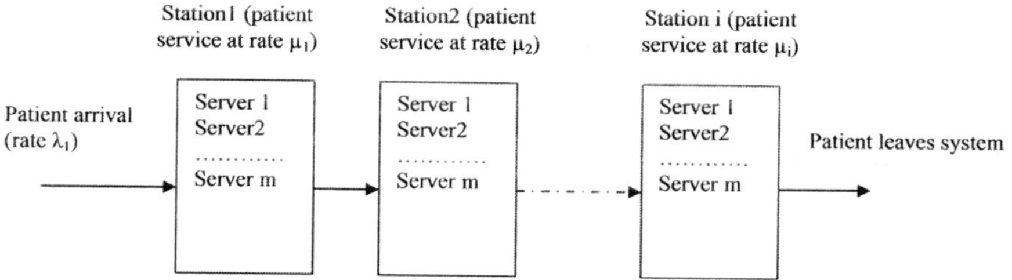

such a system, patients have to wait in multiples queues once they leave a station and arrive to the next station. Figure 2 shows the schematic of such systems. This situation is similar to many situations in healthcare facilities where a patient follows a route within a department or travels among various departments. Each department is like a station in the queuing system.

The concept of single station queuing system can be extended in this section with some further consideration. Suppose that there are *i* single stations in the queuing system. Each station should be analyzed separately to calculate the performance measures at that station. The total waiting time in queue is the summation of individual queues. Similarly, the total cycle time in the system is the summation of individual cycles. However, the waiting time and processing time at one station affects the patient arrivals in the next station. In fact, the departure rate at one station should be the arrival rate to the next station. Buzacott and Shanthikumar (1993) and Hopp and Spearman (2008) estimate the *CV* of departure in Eq. (13). Using Eq. (5) and knowing that $CV_a(i+1)=CV_d(i)$, it is possible to determine the type of queuing model and calculate the performance measures of serial stations.

$$CV_d^2 = 1 + (1-\rho^2)(CV_a^2 - 1) + \frac{\rho^2}{\sqrt{m}}(CV_s^2 - 1) \quad (13)$$

Queuing System: Variability Impact

One interesting application of queuing system is to evaluate the variability of the system. Variability is recognized as one critical source of inefficiency in any system. In the manufacturing industries, the level of process variability is determined by the value of *CV*. Table 8 shows the common definitions. Considering that the same assumption holds for healthcare application, it is possible to perform a variability analysis when the degree of variability is available.

Table 8. Level of variability (Hopp & Spearman, 2008)

Variability level	Coefficient of variance
Low	$CV< 0.75$
Moderate	$0.75<= CV<=1.33$
High	$CV>1.33$

For a serial station system, the variability in patient arrivals and server service time will be combined and this produces higher variability in the patient departure rate. Such phenomenon will be continued throughout the system causing resonance effect in the final station departure. By determining the impact of variability in a queuing system, it is possible to determine the relation between the waiting time and the flow of patients. It is expected to observe an inverse relation between them. The flow of patient can be defined as the percentage of the time the patient receives service when he/she is in the system. Such percentage is calculated as follows,

$$\text{Patient flow\%} = 100 - \frac{W_q}{W}\% \quad (14)$$

It is easy to observe that the best scenario for the patient is to receive the services as soon as he/she enters the system which means that the queuing time is zero and therefore patient flow is 1. It is also possible to define the flow of patient based on the number of patients in queue and in system,

$$\text{Patient flow\%} = 100 - \frac{L_q}{L}\% \quad (15)$$

The impact of variability in a queuing system and patient flow will be further discussed using a case study in the next section.

CASE STUDY 1: A GENERIC PRIMARY CARE SYSTEM

Current Situation

In a primary care clinic, patients follow a set of stations sequentially to receive various services in each station. The patient flow in the primary clinic is illustrated in Figure 3. Basically, once patients arrive in the clinic, they need to check in, and then wait in the waiting area until the nurse call them for the assessment. After assessment, they wait for providers. It can be seen that currently that there are one clerk at check-in station, three nurses at nurse assessment station, and four providers at provider station.

To perform such an analysis, it is needed to identify the type of queuing system for each station first. The current available data on the clinic is provided in Figure 4. It is noticeable that the same arrival rate to check-in station can be assumed for nurse assessment and provider stations.

Now, each station should be individually treated as follows. By indexing clerk, nurse, and provider stations by 1, 2, and 3 respectively; the check-in station is in fact a M/G/1 system because the $CV_a(1)=1$ indicates that the patients inter arrivals in the station follows an exponential distribution. However, $CV_s(1)=2$ indicates a general distribution. By approximating M/G/1 by G/G/1 formulation from Table 7, the performance measures for check-in station are obtained. The departure CV of check-in station is equal to the arrival CV of nurse assessment station, therefore, $CV_a(2)= CV_d(1)=1.17$. As a result, nurse assessment station represents a G/M/3 model, thus, the

Figure 3. A serial queuing system in a primary care clinic

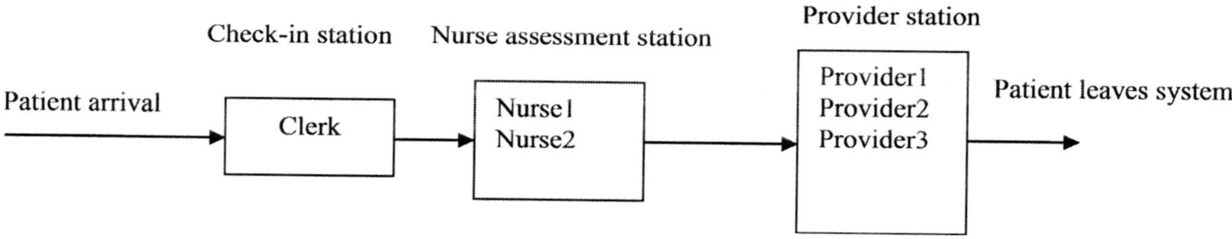

Figure 4. Current operation information for a primary care clinic

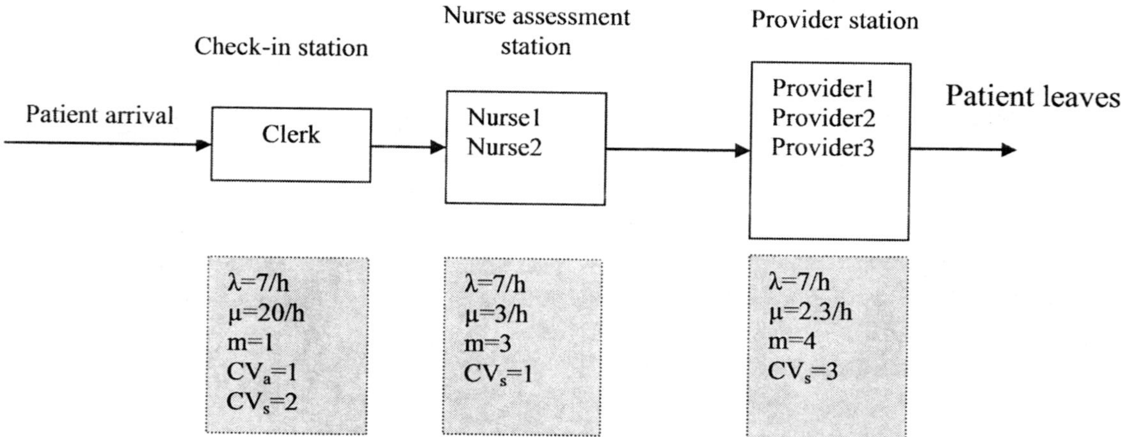

Table 9. Performances of the current system

Station	m	μ	λ	ρ	CV_a	CV_s	CV_d^2	CV_d	Wq	Lq	W	L	Patient Flow
Clerk	1	20	7	0.35	1.00	2.00	1.37	1.17	0.07	0.47	0.12	0.82	0.43
Nurse	3	3	7	0.78	1.17	1.00	1.15	1.07	0.37	2.62	0.71	4.95	0.47
Provider	4	2.3	7	0.76	1.07	3.00	5.69	2.39	1.28	8.94	1.71	11.98	0.25
Total									1.72	12.03	2.54	17.75	0.32

performance measures can be calculated accordingly. The same procedure is followed for the provider station, which is a G/G/4 system. As a result, the performance measures of this clinic are, in fact, the summation of individual station. Table 9 shows the detailed results of calculation for each station, as well as the overall system performances. It reveals that from the time a patient enters the clinic to the time he/she leaves the clinic, it takes 152 minutes which are comprised of 103 minutes for waiting time and 49 minutes for service time.

Spread sheet programs can facilitate the calculation. Figure 5 illustrates how the first case study can be formulated and solved in Microsoft Excel®. In this figure, the input data are plugged into the cells as fixed numbers. Such data include the number of stations, arrival rate, service rate, CVs of all stations, and CV_a of clerk station. Once the input data are plugged in, the queuing formulas are provided accordingly for each cell. For example, in order to calculate $\rho = \lambda/(m\mu)$, the equation, i.e., Eq. (5), is formulated in cells E2 – E4.

Sensitivity Analysis

With the current state in mind, it is also important to know how the system performance will be changed if some variables or conditions are changed. For instance, if the waiting time is deemed to be too long, one intuitive thought is to add more staff. In the following, how the change of staffing level affects the system performance

Figure 5. The spread sheet application of queuing models used in Case Study 1

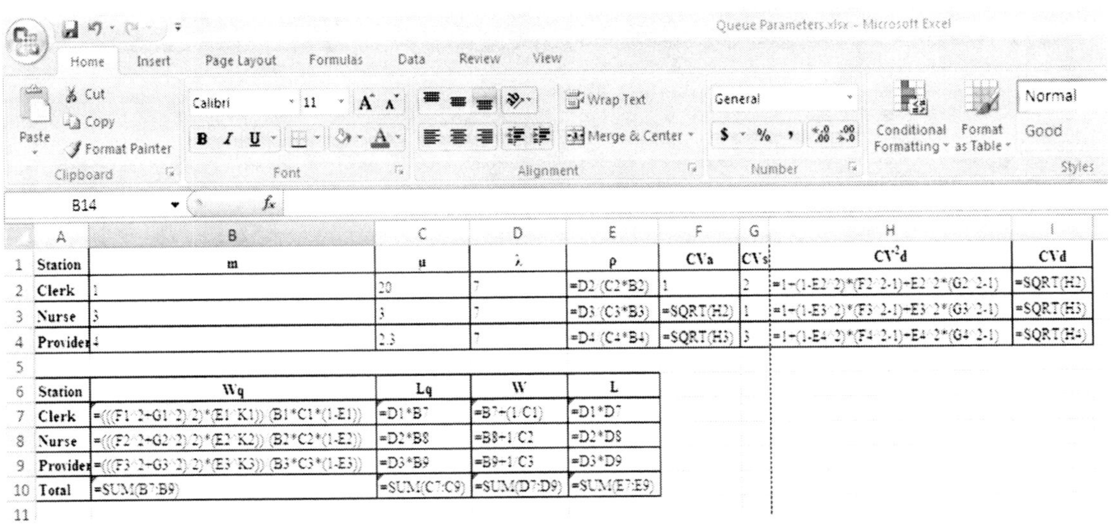

	A	B	C	D	E	F	G	H	I
1	Station	m	μ	λ	ρ	CVa	CVs	CV²d	CVd
2	Clerk	1	20	7	=D2/(C2*B2)	1	2	=1+(1-E2^2)*(F2^2-1)+E2^2*(G2^2-1)	=SQRT(H2)
3	Nurse	3	3	7	=D3/(C3*B3)	=SQRT(H2)	1	=1+(1-E3^2)*(F3^2-1)+E3^2*(G3^2-1)	=SQRT(H3)
4	Provider	4	2.3	7	=D4/(C4*B4)	=SQRT(H3)	3	=1+(1-E4^2)*(F4^2-1)+E4^2*(G4^2-1)	=SQRT(H4)
5									
6	Station	Wq	Lq	W	L				
7	Clerk	=(((F1^2+G1^2)/2)*(E1^K1))/(B1*C1*(1-E1))	=D1*B7	=B7+(1/C1)	=D1*D7				
8	Nurse	=(((F2^2+G2^2)/2)*(E2^K2))/(B2*C2*(1-E2))	=D2*B8	=B8+1/C2	=D2*D8				
9	Provider	=(((F3^2+G3^2)/2)*(E3^K3))/(B3*C3*(1-E3))	=D3*B9	=B9+1/C3	=D3*D9				
10	Total	=SUM(B7:B9)	=SUM(C7:C9)	=SUM(D7:D9)	=SUM(E7:E9)				
11									

is thus briefly investigated. Here, the current system is regarded as the base system. The effect of staffing level at each station is studied separately, and the results are compared with the base system. For the purpose of brevity, the patient flow of the entire clinic is only calculated from Eq. (14). Figure 6 indicates that adding one clerk to check-in station will increase the patient flow from current value 32% to 34%, while adding two clerks or more produces negligible improvement to patient flow coefficient. Similarly, the change of staffing level at nurse station can be revealed in Figure 7. It can be seen that adding one nurse to the base system incurs the improvement of the patient flow by around 4%, but further increase of nurse number alone hardly facilitates the patient flow. On the other hand, Figure 8 shows that the effect of changing provider number is far more significant. In this case, by adding one more provider, the patient flow coefficient increases from 32% to 51%; by adding two more providers, the coefficient reaches about 60%.

Figure 6. Sensitivity analysis on the effect of staffing level at clerk station

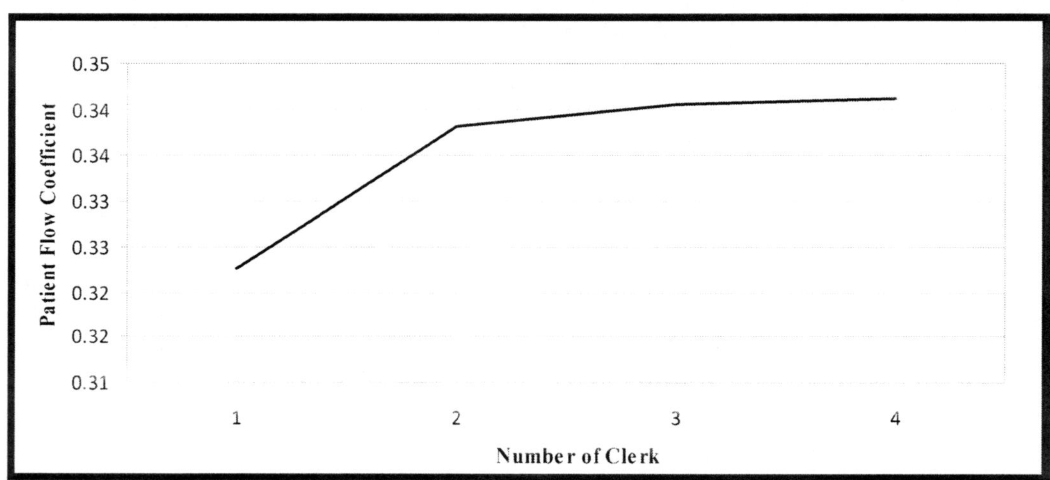

Figure 7. Sensitivity analysis on the effect of staffing level at nurse station

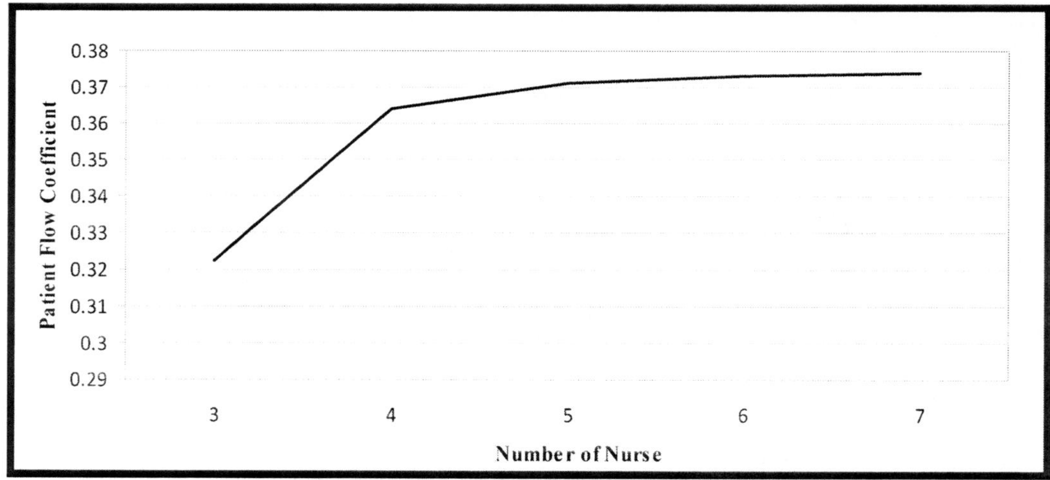

Figure 8. Sensitivity analysis on the effect of staffing level at provider station

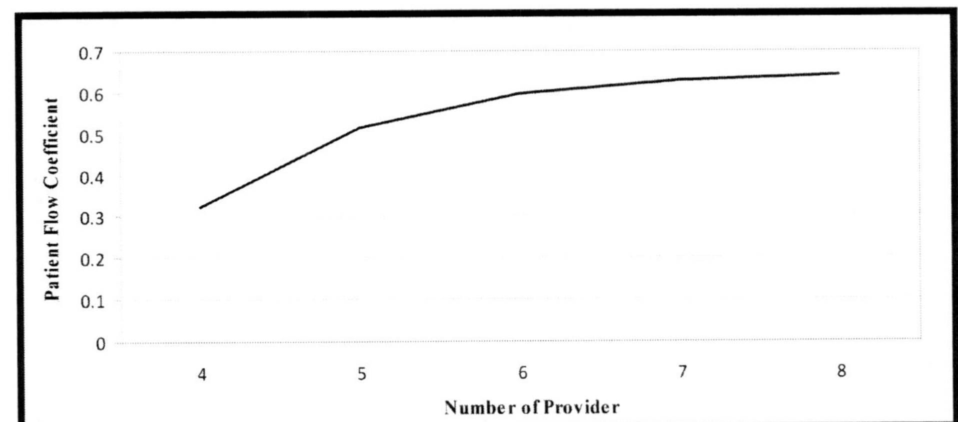

Variability Analysis

It is also interesting to conduct a variability analysis on the performance of the clinic. Basically, a low-variability station generates more standard and reliable output, and the variability at each station depends on the variability of the arrivals and service time. To perform such analysis, different levels of variability can be considered for the arrivals and server service time for each station. Here, three levels of variability, namely, low, moderate, and high, are considered for the patient's arrivals in the check-in station, and for each level of patient arrival variability, three levels of variability for clerk service time are considered as well. As a result, nine scenarios in total are generated, with each representing a unique queuing system. For illustration purpose, the levels of variability are quantified as CV=0.5, 1, 2 for low, medium, and high variability respectively.

Table 10 shows the results of the scenarios. Based on CV_a and CV_s, CV_d is calculated from Eq. (13). Then, the queuing model is determined and performance measures are calculated. The current situation of the system is indicated by scenario 6 in the table. The last column of the table indicates the impact of variability on overall patient flow. The relation between CV_d and patient flow is illustrated in Figure 9. As seen, the trend of the diagram indicates an inverse relation between departure

Table 10. Variability analysis for check-in station

Scenario	CV_a	CV_s	CV_d^2	CV_d	Model	Wq	Lq	W	L	Overall Patient Flow
1	0.5	0.5	0.25	0.50	G/G/1	0.01	0.05	0.06	0.40	0.36
2	0.5	1	0.34	0.58	G/M/1	0.02	0.12	0.07	0.47	0.36
3	0.5	2	0.71	0.84	G/G/1	0.06	0.40	0.11	0.75	0.34
4	1	0.5	0.91	0.95	M/G/1	0.02	0.12	0.07	0.47	0.34
5	1	1	1.00	1.00	M/M/1	0.03	0.19	0.08	0.54	0.34
6	1	2	1.37	1.17	M/G/1	0.07	0.47	0.12	0.82	0.32
7	2	0.5	3.54	1.88	G/G/1	0.06	0.40	0.11	0.75	0.27
8	2	1	3.63	1.91	G/M/1	0.07	0.47	0.12	0.82	0.27
9	2	2	4.00	2.00	G/G/1	0.11	0.75	0.16	1.10	0.26

Figure 9. Relation between departure CV and patient flow

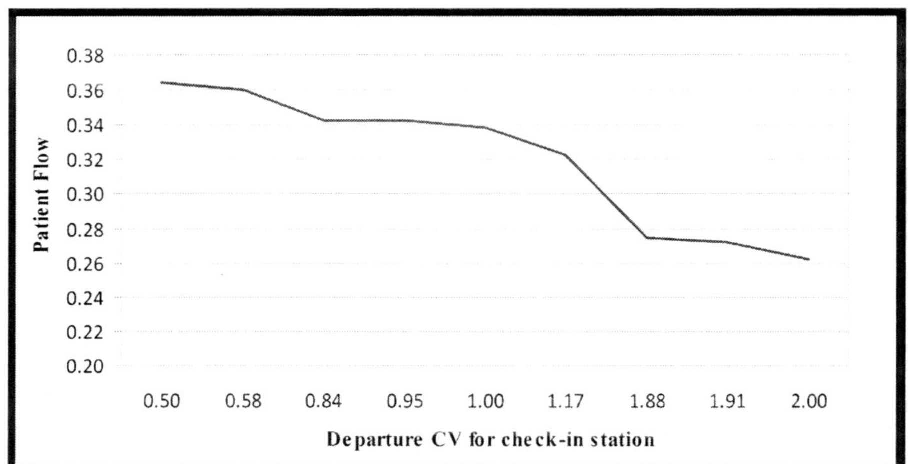

CV and patient flow. This result means that it is expected to observe a larger patient flow when the departure *CV* is small. Note that the departure *CV* value is in fact a combination of two *CV* values, i.e., arrivals and service time. It is seen that the overall patient flow will be optimal at 0.36 when the departure *CV* is minimal at 0.5. As such, the current patient flow will be improved from 0.32 to 0.36 based on the nine scenarios.

Similar analysis can be performed for the nurse assessment and provider stations. Note that the arrivals in these two stations in fact are the departures from their previous stations. For example, if the *CV* of patient arrivals at nurse station is currently 1.17, what if the nurse assessment service variability changes? Considering three levels of nurse variability for nurse service time, the results can be observed in Table 11. The current situation is shown in the second row (CV_a=1.17, and CV_s=1). Therefore, the patient flow coefficient increase from 0.32 to 0.35 when CV_s=0.5. Likewise, the impact of service time variability on the overall patient flow can be identified at provider station. As seen, by changing the provider service variability from 3 to 0.5, the overall patient flow will increase from 0.32 to 0.57.

Clearly, the above analysis shows that if the level of variability becomes lower, more significant improvement can be made on the patient flow. If all stations have the low level of variability, the system performance can be calculated and shown in Table 12. It is interesting to observe that the individual and overall patient flows dramatically improve when low level of variability

Table 11. Impact of service variability at nurse and provider stations on the overall patient flow

Station	CV_a	CV_s	CV_d	Patient Flow
Nurse	1.17	0.5	0.83	0.35
	1.17	1	1.07	0.32
	1.17	2	1.72	0.25
Provider	1.07	0.5	0.79	0.57
	1.07	1	1.03	0.53
	1.07	2	2.39	0.32

Table 12. Patient flow performance with low variability for all stations

Station	m	μ	λ	ρ	CV_a	CV_s	W_q	L_q	W	L	Patient Flow
Check-in	1	20	7	0.35	0.5	0.5	0.01	0.05	0.06	0.40	0.88
Nurse	3	3	7	0.78	0.5	0.5	0.08	0.55	0.41	2.89	0.81
Provider	4	2.3	7	0.76	0.5	0.5	0.06	0.44	0.50	3.48	0.87
							0.15	1.04	0.97	6.77	0.85

is achieved at each station. Under such situation, a patient stays 58 minutes in the clinic in which less than 9 minutes is his/her waiting time. Therefore, it is worth considering the strategies to improve the system through *minimizing the variability*.

Queuing Network

Jackson queuing network is a generalization of queues in series. Many healthcare queuing systems can be represented by the Jackson network. The fundamental assumption is that the patients will arrive from outside at any k station facility according to Poisson process. This is different from the serial network we discussed before where patients have to sequentially follow a single route. In other words, there is only one route in the multiple station system, while in the Jackson network there are multiple routes. The mean arrival rate in station i is considered to be γ_i. All servers (m servers) at station i work with the average service time following an exponential distribution with mean μ_i. Therefore, all servers at a given station are assumed to be identical. The assumption of exponential distribution for the patients inter-arrival times and server service times is reasonable in many cases. For example, the walk-in clinics where the patients arrive randomly are an appropriate fit for such assumption. Even for appointment based clinic, if the sources of variability such as no-shows, walk-ins, new patients, lab results, early arrivals, staff being late or absent, and canceling calls are significant, the assumption of exponential inter arrivals may be a proper fit. Once completing service at station i, the patient joins the queue at station j with probability r_{ij} (i=1, 2, …, k). There is a probability r_{i0} that the patient will leave the network at node i upon completion of service. There is no limit on queue capacity at any station. In this model, performance measures can be calculated using the Jackson's solutions. According to Gross and Harris (2003), the traffic equation is as follows:

$$\lambda_i = \gamma_i + \sum_{j=1}^{k} \lambda_j r_{ji}, \qquad (16)$$

or in the form of vector-matrix,

$$\lambda = \gamma + \lambda R,, \qquad (17)$$

where R is the route matrix and indicates the probability that a patient goes from one station to other stations. The expected number of customers in service can be calculated using,

$$r_i = \frac{\lambda_i}{\mu_i}. \qquad (18)$$

CASE STUDY 2: PRIMARY CARE NETWORK

The primary care case study considered in the previous section represents a single route clinic, in which all patients have to route through sequential stations, namely, check-in, nurse assessment, and

Table 13. Performance measures for a primary care network

Station	m	μ	λ	ρ	CV_a	CV_s	W_q	L_q	W	L	Patient Flow
Clerk	1	20	7	0.35	1	2	0.07	0.47	0.12	0.82	0.43
Nurse	3	3	4.92	0.55	1.17	1	0.10	0.47	0.43	2.11	0.78
Provider	4	2.3	7.23	0.79	1.12	3	1.55	11.18	1.98	14.32	0.22
Total							1.71	12.12	2.53	17.26	0.32

provider. In many cases, however, patients may follow multiple routes rather than a single route. Based on their needs, patients may want to do a nurse-only visit or may need ancillary care after the provider visit. As such, the primary care can form a queuing network. Recall that in the first case study, patients who arrive at the clinic have to check in first. In this case, 95% of patients see the nurse while the rest directly visit the provider. 10% of patients who visit the provider need to see the nurse for ancillary service. Out of patients who visit the nurse, 90% will visit the provider and the rest leave the clinic. The rate of patient arrival is 7 per hour. It is expected that nurse visit time is 20 minutes while provider's is 26 minutes. We evaluate the performance of this queuing system as follows.

Based on the data, route matrix can be formed as,

$$R = \begin{bmatrix} 0 & 0.95 & 0.05 \\ 0 & 0 & 0.90 \\ 0 & 0.10 & 0 \end{bmatrix}.$$

Other data related to the clinic can be summarized in Table 13. Here, the clerk, nurse, and provider stations are considered using M/M/1, M/M/3, and M/M/4 models respectively. It can be observed that the overall system performances are almost the same as those of the serial system; however, the patient flow for nurse assessment station is dramatically increased. This can be attributed to the smaller arrival rate at the station compared to that of the original case. Similarly, it is straightforward to perform a variability analysis on the current network and observe opportunities for improvement – the readers are encouraged to perform this calculation by themselves.

TRAVEL DISTANCE ANALYSIS

Travel distance can be considered as another important patient flow measure. In clinic visits, patients may need to follow a route which normally consists of multiple departments/stations. The distance a patient travels has an immediate effect on the quality of the service. The travel distance also impacts the time a patient spends in the system. The smaller the travel distance, the better the patient flow. As such, practitioners and professionals should also analyze their system in terms of the travel distance. In this section some useful tools are provided to enable users to analytically evaluate the flow of patients from the travel distance perspective.

From-To Matrix

From-To matrix is a tool to show the distance between any two departments/stations in the medical facility. The tool can be represented by a matrix where each array of the matrix indicates the distance between corresponding departments,

$$d = \begin{bmatrix} d_{11} & d_{12} & \cdots & d_{1j} \\ d_{21} & d_{22} & \cdots & \cdots \\ \cdots & \cdots & \cdots & \cdots \\ d_{i1} & \cdots & \cdots & d_{ij} \end{bmatrix}, \qquad (19)$$

where i and j are the indices for rows and columns of the matrix respectively. The distance from department i to j is equal to the distance from department j to i; therefore, $d_{ij}=d_{ji}$. Moreover, $d_{ii}=0$ which means that the distance from each department to itself is zero. Thus, From-To matrix can be shown by a square-triangular matrix where the main diagonal array values are zero:

$$d = \begin{bmatrix} 0 & d_{12} & \cdots & d_{1j} \\ d_{21} & 0 & \cdots & \cdots \\ \cdots & \cdots & \cdots & \cdots \\ d_{j1} & \cdots & \cdots & 0 \end{bmatrix} \quad (20)$$

In order to develop a From-To matrix, a number of factors should be taken into account. Firstly, the unit of all distances should be same. Besides, although the distances can be obtained from engineering drawings, it should be noted that the realistic limitations such as department access, walls, and medical equipment, should be considered. Vertical distance between two departments located in different levels should also be included.

Patient Route Probability Vector

In general, patients follow multiple routes in the clinic based on the service requested. The probability that a patient travel between any two departments can be estimated based on historical data and/or observation. The probabilities can be organized in the following matrix.

$$P = \begin{bmatrix} p_{11} & p_{12} & \cdots & p_{1j} \\ p_{21} & p_{22} & \cdots & \cdots \\ \cdots & \cdots & \cdots & \cdots \\ p_{i1} & \cdots & \cdots & p_{ij} \end{bmatrix}. \quad (21)$$

Note that p_{ij} is not necessarily equal to p_{ji}. From this matrix, the probability vector can be determined for any specific route. This will be a one-row matrix and the number of columns depends on the number of departments to be visited by patient in the route. For a route including j departments visited in ascending order, therefore, the probability vector is,

$$\mathrm{P}(\text{route 1 to } j) = \left[p_{12} \quad p_{23} \quad \cdots \quad p_{j-1,j} \right]. \quad (22)$$

At some clinics, it is expected to observe a steady state of patients flow during the clinic work hours, while other clinics may experience a time dependent patient flow. For example, in a primary care clinic, it is expected to observe that the patients arrive at the clinic in a steady state during the clinic hours (e.g., 8:00 am-5:00pm). This is especially true if the clinic is appointment based in that the patients are scheduled for a specific time slot, which is uniformly spread out over the entire week. However, in some cases such as lab where many patients need to be on fast when taking the test, it is expected that patients flow is higher in the morning than in the afternoon. Therefore, the probability vector can be provided based on the probability matrix type:

i. Time independent probability matrix where the flow of patient is fixed and therefore the probability of travel between any two departments on the route can be approximated by a fixed number, see Eq. (21).
ii. Time dependent probability matrix where the flow of patient is a function of time. In such cases, the probability should be determined by a function. A general form of a time dependent probability matrix can be indicated as follows,

$$P^t = \begin{bmatrix} f_{11}^t & f_{12}^t & \cdots & f_{1j}^t \\ f_{21}^t & f_{22}^t & \cdots & \cdots \\ \cdots & \cdots & \cdots & \cdots \\ f_{i1}^t & \cdots & \cdots & f_{ij}^t \end{bmatrix}. \tag{23}$$

For example, suppose that the lab request from specialty care is high in the morning with the probability of 95% in the first hour of the lab is in operation. However, the requests decrease linearly in the next hours in a way that the probability of observing a patient in the lab at 5pm is 14%. Based on this data, the probability function is $f(t)$=-0.09t+0.95. The probability can be calculated for any time between 8 am to 5 pm. For example, the probability of patient request at 10 am is $f(t)$=0.75.

In contrast to the time independent case, the time dependent probability matrix can not be represented by fixed numbers. In order to represent such a matrix using fixed arrays, the average method can be applied. In this method the time interval t is split into t/n equal sub intervals. For each sub interval a fixed number can be obtained from f_{ij}^t and then taking the average among all fixed numbers results in a fixed number for the probability function.

$$P^t = \begin{bmatrix} \bar{f}_{11}^t & \bar{f}_{12}^t & \cdots & \bar{f}_{1j}^t \\ \bar{f}_{21}^t & \bar{f}_{22}^t & \cdots & \cdots \\ \cdots & \cdots & \cdots & \cdots \\ \bar{f}_{i1}^t & \cdots & \cdots & \bar{f}_{ij}^t \end{bmatrix}. \tag{24}$$

iii. Mixed probability matrix where some arrays in the matrix are indicated with time independent (type i) numbers while others are illustrated by time dependent (type ii) arrays. Such a matrix will be treated using the average method for only time dependent arrays.

Route Accessibility Penalty Function (W_R)

The accessibility of various routes may be different in a medical facility. While some routes are easy to follow, others may be difficult to find. There are various factors that determine the accessibility of a route. For example, if an appropriate signage system is not implemented for a route, patients may not be able to find the route efficiently. Similarly, if a route serving disabled patients and not far from the main entrance clinic door would require many turns or elevators, it is deemed to have low accessibility. One method to determine the accessibility of a route is to assign qualitative levels (e.g., poor, moderate, and good), and then to consider a quantitative score to each level. In this section, three levels of poor, moderate, and good with scores of 1, 3, and 5 respectively are considered.

Patient Flow Traveling Score

The following formula is used to quantify the patient flow traveling score,

Patient flow traveling score (PFTS) =

$$\sum_{i,j \in Routes} \frac{W_R P_{ij}^T d_{ij}}{n-1}, \tag{25}$$

where n is the number of departments on the route, W_R is the route accessibility score, P_{ij}^T is the transpose matrix of probability vector for departments i and j on route R, and d_{ij} is the distance vector between departments i and j. A smaller number of PFTS is more desirable. It is possible to sort all scores to rank the patient flow. In the next section a numerical example is provided to show how PFTS can be applied for an outpatient primary care clinic.

Table 14. Definition of symbols for stations and routes

Station/route symbol	Note
A	Clerk station
B	Nurse station
C	Provider station
D	Lab station
Route 1	ABCD with low level accessibility (5)
Route 2	AB with high level accessibility (1)
Route 3	ABCB with moderate level accessibility (3)
Route 4	DABC with high level accessibility (3)

CASE STUDY 3: MULTIPLE ROUTE PRIMARY CARE

Recall case study 2, and assume that in addition to the 3 stations in the primary case, there is a lab station available where some patients may be directed to the lab after visiting their providers. Besides, there is a possibility that some patients take the lab tests first and then go to the primary care with the lab test results. The stations and routes can be identified as shown in Table 14.

The distance matrix indicating the distance between any two departments is as follows:

$$d = \begin{bmatrix} 0 & 75 & 49 & 52 \\ \ldots & 0 & 64 & 39 \\ \ldots & \ldots & 0 & 49 \\ \ldots & \ldots & \ldots & 0 \end{bmatrix}$$

The probability matrix can be given as,

$$P^t = \begin{bmatrix} - & 0.90 & - & - \\ - & - & -0.05t + 0.45 & - \\ - & 0.1t & - & -0.1t + 0.9 \\ -0.02t + 0.73 & - & - & - \end{bmatrix}$$

With the above information given, the patient flow from distance travel score can be quantified. First, it is seen that the probability matrix is mixed. The very first step is to convert the mixed probability matrix to a fixed one. To do so, the working time from 8 am to 5 pm is split into 9 one-hour intervals and the average of probabilities will be calculated. Thus, the fixed probability matrix can be obtained as,

$$P^t = \begin{bmatrix} - & 0.90 & - & - \\ - & - & 0.225 & - \\ - & 0.45 & - & 0.45 \\ 0.64 & - & - & - \end{bmatrix}$$

Probabilityvectorsforroutesare: *P(ABCD)*=[0.9 0.225 0.45], *P(AB)*=[0.9], *P(ABCD)*=[0.9 0.225 0.45], and P(DABC)=[0.64 0.9 0.225]. Similarly, the corresponding distance vectors become:

$$d^T_{ABCD} = \begin{bmatrix} 75 & 64 & 49 \end{bmatrix},\ d^T_{AB} = \begin{bmatrix} 75 \end{bmatrix},$$

$$d^T_{ABCB} = \begin{bmatrix} 75 & 64 & 64 \end{bmatrix},\ \text{and}$$

$$d^T_{DABC} = \begin{bmatrix} 49 & 75 & 64 \end{bmatrix}.$$

Thus,

$$PFTS(ABDC) = \sum_{i,j \in Route1} \frac{W_R P_{ij} d_{ij}}{n-1} = \frac{5 * \begin{bmatrix} 0.9 & 0.225 & 0.45 \end{bmatrix} * \begin{bmatrix} 75 & 64 & 49 \end{bmatrix}^T}{4-1} = 173.25$$

$$PFTS(AB) = \sum_{i,j \in Route2} \frac{W_R P_{ij} d_{ij}}{n-1} = \frac{1 * [0.9] * [75]^T}{2-1} = 67.5$$

$$PFTS(ABCB) = \sum_{i,j \in Route3} \frac{W_R P_{ij} d_{ij}}{n-1} = \frac{3 * \begin{bmatrix} 0.9 & 0.225 & 0.45 \end{bmatrix} * \begin{bmatrix} 75 & 64 & 64 \end{bmatrix}^T}{4-1} = 110.7$$

$$PFTS(DABC) = \sum_{i,j \in Route4} \frac{W_R P_{ij} d_{ij}}{n-1} = \frac{3 * \begin{bmatrix} 0.64 & 0.9 & 0.225 \end{bmatrix} * \begin{bmatrix} 49 & 75 & 64 \end{bmatrix}^T}{4-1} = 113.26.$$

As a result the rank of routes based on the scores obtained is Route 2, Route 3, Route 4, and Route 1.

Approach Summary

The method provided for identifying the flow of patient based on the distance a patient travels during a visit can be summarized as follows:

- Determine the From-To distance matrix
- Identify the probability matrix
- Determine available routes in the clinic
- Identify the corresponding distance and probability vectors for each route
- Determine the route accessibility
- Calculate patient flow traveling score (PFTS) $= \sum_{i,j \in Routes} \frac{W_R P_{ij}^T d_{ij}}{n-1}$ for each route
- Sort PFTS values to rank the patient flow options.

CONCLUSION

The quality of service giving to the patients is highly dependent on the patient flow in medical facilities. Patient flow can be evaluated using a variety of measures. Waiting time is one of the most important indicators. Researchers have applied various tools from simple time study techniques to complex analytical tools to quantitatively analyze the waiting time. Queuing theory is one of these tools and is discussed in details in this chapter. While there are various health care systems which can be modeled using queuing theory, this chapter presents three queuing systems which are widely used in outpatient clinics (i.e., primary care), namely, single station, multiple serial station, and queuing network. Numerical cases are provided to verify the applicability of the queuing models. Besides, a queuing system approach which considers the system variability is also discussed. It shows how the low variability of patient arrivals and/or service time at the beginning of the patient visit may be propagated and enlarged in the end. Furthermore, the distance traveled by patients can be seen as another measure for patient flow. The functional structure of medical cares forces the patients to travel between departments. This may negatively affect the patient satisfaction. A simple yet useful approach is discussed in this chapter to evaluate the patient flow from distance perspective.

Operation management tools enable practitioners to analyze the health care operations through a systematic and engineering approach. By providing accurate information on the system condition, such tools make the system more understandable for management and other professionals. As such, better decisions can be made, which in turn results in improvement of patient satisfaction, reduction of operation cost, and better usage of resources.

REFERENCES

Abdel-Aal, R. (1998). Modeling and forecasting monthly patient volume at a primary health care clinic using univariate time-series analysis. *Computer Methods and Programs in Biomedicine*, *56*(3), 235–247. doi:10.1016/S0169-2607(98)00032-7

Albin, S. L., Barrett, J., Ito, D., & Mueller, J. E. (1990). A queuing network analysis of a health center. *Queueing Systems*, *7*(1), 51–61. doi:10.1007/BF01158785

Banks, J., & Carson, J. S. (1984). *Discrete-event system simulation*. Prentice-Hall.

Blake, J. T., & Carter, M. W. (1996). An analysis of emergency room wait time issues via computer simulation. *INFOR*, *34*(4), 263–272.

Bush, S. H., Lao, M. R., Simmons, K. L., Goode, J. H., Cunningham, S. A., & Calhoun, B. C. (2007). Patient access and clinical efficiency improvement in a resident hospital-based women's medicine center clinic. *The American Journal of Managed Care*, *13*(12), 686–690.

Buzacott, J. A., & Shnathikumar, J. G. (1993). *Stochastic models of manufacturing systems*. Englewood Ciffs, NJ: Prentice-Hall.

Cartwright, A., & Windsor, J. (1992). *Outpatients and their doctors*. London, UK: HMSO.

Clague, J. E., Reed, P. G., Barlow, J., Rada, R., Clarke, M., & Edwards, R. H. (1997). Improving outpatient clinic efficiency using computer simulation. *International Journal of Health Care Quality Assurance*, *10*, 197–201. doi:10.1108/09526869710174177

Cochran, J. K., & Bharti, A. (2006). A multi-stage methodology for whole hospital bed planning. *International Journal of Industrial and Systems Engineering*, *1*(1), 8–36. doi:10.1504/IJISE.2006.009048

Cochran, J. K., & Roche, K. (2009). A multi-class queuing network analysis methodology for improving hospital emergency department performance. *Computers & Operations Research*, *36*(5), 1497–1512. doi:10.1016/j.cor.2008.02.004

Edwards, R., Clague, J. E., Barlow, J., Clarke, M., Reed, P. G., & Rada, R. (1994). Operations research survey and computer simulation of waiting times in two medical outpatient clinic structures. *Health Care Analysis*, *2*, 164–169. doi:10.1007/BF02249741

Evans, A. M., & Wakeford, J. (1964). Research on hospital outpatients and casualty attendances: A strategy for improvement. *British Medical Journal*, *299*, 722–724.

Garcia, M. L., Centeno, M. A., Rivera, C., & DeCario, N. (1995). Reducing time in an emergency room via a fast-track. In C. Alexopoulos, K. Kang, W. R. Lilegdon, & D. Goldsman (Ed.), *Proceedings of the 1995 Winter Simulation Conference*, (pp. 1048-1053). Washington DC, USA.

Goitein, M. (1990). Waiting patiently. *The New England Journal of Medicine*, *323*, 604–608. doi:10.1056/NEJM199008303230911

Gross, D., & Harris, C. M. (2003). *Fundamentals of queuing theory* (3rd ed.). New York, NY: John Wiley & Sons.

Hart, M. (1995). Improving out-patient clinic waiting times: Methodological and substantive issues. *International Journal of Health Care Quality Assurance*, *8*(6), 14. doi:10.1108/09526869510098813

Henderson, D., Dempsey, C., & Appleby, D. (2004). A case study of successful patient flow methods: St. John's Hospital. *Frontiers of Health Services Management*, *20*(4), 25–30.

Hindel, A. (1972). *Hospital waiting lists – A review*. Internal Report, Department of Operations Research, Lancaster University.

Holdgate, A., Morris, J., Fry, M., & Zecevic, M. (2007). Accuracy of triage nurses in predicting patient disposition. *Emergency Medicine Australasia: EMA*, *19*(4), 341–345. doi:10.1111/j.1742-6723.2007.00996.x

Hopp, W. J., & Spearman, M. L. (2008). *Factory physics* (3rd ed.). New York, NY: McGraw Hill.

Jiang, L., & Giachetti, R. E. (2008). A queuing network model to analyze the impact of parallelization of care on patient cycle time. *Health Care Management Science*, *11*(3), 248–261. doi:10.1007/s10729-007-9040-9

Jones, L., Leneman, L., & MacLean, U. (1987). *Consumer feedback for the NHS: A literature review*. London, UK: King Edward's Hospital Fund.

Jun, J. B., Jacobson, S. H., & Swisher, J. R. (1999). Application of discrete-event simulation in healthcare: A survey. *The Journal of the Operational Research Society*, *50*(2), 109–123.

Kao, E. P. C., & Tung, G. G. (1981). Bed allocation in a public health care delivery system. *Management Science*, *27*(5), 507–520. doi:10.1287/mnsc.27.5.507

Kendall, D. (1951). Some problems in the theory of queues. *Journal of the Royal Statistical Society. Series B. Methodological*, *13*, 151–185.

Kyriacou, D. N., Ricketts, V., Dyne, P. L., McCollough, M. D., & Talan, D. A. (1999). A 5-year time study analysis of emergency department patient care efficiency. *Annals of Emergency Medicine*, *34*(3), 326–335. doi:10.1016/S0196-0644(99)70126-5

Law, A. M., & Kelton, W. D. (2003). *Simulation modeling and analysis* (3rd ed.). New Dehli, India: Tata McGraw-Hill.

Martin, S., & Smith, P. C. (1999). Rationing by waiting lists: an empirical investigation. *Journal of Public Economics*, *71*, 141–164. doi:10.1016/S0047-2727(98)00067-X

Mendenhall, W., & Sincich, T. (1995). *Statistics for engineering and sciences* (4th ed.). Upper Saddle River, NJ: Prentice- Hall.

Min, D., & Yih, Y. (2010). An elective surgery scheduling problem considering patient priority. *Computers & Operations Research*, *37*(6), 1091–1099. doi:10.1016/j.cor.2009.09.016

Moser, M. S., Abu-Laban, R. B., & Van Beek, C. A. (2004). Attitude of emergency department patients with minor problems to being treated by a nurse practitioner. *CJEM: Canadian Journal Of Emergency Medical Care*, *6*(4), 246–252.

Patrick, J., Puterman, M. L., & Queyranne, M. (2008). Dynamic multipriority patient scheduling for a diagnostic resource. *Operations Research*, *56*(6), 1507–1525. doi:10.1287/opre.1080.0590

Potisek, N. M., Malone, R. M., Bryant, B., Ives, T. J., Chelminski, P. R., DeWalt, D. A., & Pignone, M. P. (2007). Use of patient flow analysis to improve patient visit efficiency by decreasing wait time in a primary care-based disease management programs for anticoagulation and chronic pain: A quality improvement study. *BMC Health Services Research*, *7*(8), 1–7.

Ritondo, M., & Freedman, R. W. (1993). The effects of procedure scheduling on emergency room throughput: A simulation study. In Anderson, J. G., & Katzper, M. (Eds.), *SCS Western Multiconference on Simulation: Simulation in the Health Sciences and Services* (pp. 8–11). La Jolla, California, USA: Society for Computer Simulation.

Rohleder, T. R., Sabapathy, D., & Schorn, R. (2005). An operating room block allocation model to improve hospital patient flow. *Clinical and Investigative Medicine. Medecine Clinique et Experimentale*, *28*(6), 353–355.

Shmueli, A., Sprung, C. L., & Kaplan, E. H. (2003). Optimizing admissions to an intensive care unit. *Health Care Management Science*, *6*(3), 131–136. doi:10.1023/A:1024457800682

Su, S. (2003). Managing a mixed-registration-type appointment system in outpatient clinics. *International Journal of Medical Informatics, 70*(1), 31–40. doi:10.1016/S1386-5056(03)00008-X

Williams, P., Tai, G., & Lei, Y. (2009). Simulation based analysis of patient arrival to health care systems and evaluation of an operations improvement scheme. *Annals of Operations Research, 178*(1), 263–279..doi:10.1007/s10479-009-0580-x

Winston, W. L. (1993). *Operations research: Application and algorithms*. International Thomson Publishing.

Worthington, D. (1987). Queuing models for hospital waiting lists. *The Journal of the Operational Research Society, 38*(5), 413–422.

Chapter 19
Using Patient Flow to Examine Hospital Operations

Renata Konrad
Worcester Polytechnic Institute, USA

Beste Kucukyazici
Zaragoza Logistics Center, Spain

Mark Lawley
Purdue University, USA

ABSTRACT

Adopting an admission-to-discharge patient flow perspective has the potential to improve hospital operations. Flow paths provide insight regarding patient care needs, support resource allocation and capacity planning decisions, and improve the operational performance of the hospitals. Studying patient flow through systems engineering tools and applications can help decision makers assess and improve care delivery. This chapter presents current research and techniques used to describe, measure, and model inpatient flow. We formally define patient flow from an operational standpoint and discuss why it is crucial for operational decisions. Systems engineering techniques, which describe and analyze inpatient flow, are introduced. The chapter concludes with a discussion of emerging approaches to capture patient flow.

INTRODUCTION

The coordination and allocation of personnel, physical space, and equipment required to meet patient needs is an important problem for hospitals. Unanticipated waits and delays add tremendous cost and can negatively impact outcomes. For this reason, policy makers advocate the study of patient flow for analyzing operational decisions. (Joint Commission Resources, 2004; Vissers & Beech,2005)

DOI: 10.4018/978-1-60960-872-9.ch019

Compared to sophisticated operations management techniques used in other industries, operations management in hospitals is fairly rudimentary. Most hospitals manage their operations with census snapshot reports along with ad hoc use of multiple data sources to augment their managerial intuition. (Isken, 2002) Since the early 1970s researchers have been advocating a holistic analysis of hospital operations by using a patient flow approach. Although research has illustrated that short term operational decision-making can be refined by adopting a this perspective, implementation rates are scant. As of May 2011, there were approximately 700 article citations in PubMed containing the phrase "patient flow". The vast majority of these studies consider the clinical perspective of patient flow. Of the remaining studies, most take a managerial perspective while a smaller subset considers using patient flow for operational analysis.

The intent of this chapter is to present current research and techniques to describe inpatient flow. The chapter begins with a brief discussion of the advantages of using patient flow and continues with a formal definition of patient flow. Current challenges in measuring patient flow are then presented following by a summary of techniques to describe patient flow. The chapter concludes with an examination of future research areas.

PATIENT FLOW

Patient flow can be described from two perspectives, the clinical and the operational. (Côté, 2000; Marshall et al., 2005) From a clinical point of view, patient flow represents the progression of a patient's health status. Accordingly, understanding patient flow in a clinical sense offers providers, patients, and hospital administration insight about care needs associated with disease progression or recovery status. (Côté, 2000) On the other hand, from an operational point of view, patient flow can be thought of as the movement of patients through a set of events or locations in a health care facility. (Côté, 2000) In the context of this chapter, we focus on patient flow from the operational perspective. This section formally defines patient flow and illustrates why it is important to use this approach when performing operational analysis.

Definition of Patient Flow

Before discussing systems engineering tools and applications used for patient flow, we provide a formal definition of patient flow. Typically flow patterns are defined from the point where the patient first enters, or is admitted to the hospital, and ends at the point of discharge. Between these two points, there is a set of conditions, activities, services, or locations that the patient may encounter. Within these points, the patient requires a variety of health care resources (e.g. beds, examining rooms, operating rooms, physicians, nurses, and/or medical procedures). (Cote, 2000, Marshall et al., 2005, Kucukyazici et al., 2010) Therefore from an operational standpoint, the term patient flow encompasses the following four elements:

- The set of events during a patient's stay,
- The precedence/sequence of events,
- The duration of events, and
- The resources required to perform these events.

In this chapter, we use the term model as an ideal analytical description capable of encompassing the four above concepts. It is important to note that not all existing patient flow models address all four areas of patient flow.

Figure 1 is a simple hypothetical illustration of a patient flow from an operational standpoint. Note that the patient's journey is described in terms of time, resources and events. A patient is registered by a clerk, an event which takes 10 minutes. The patient then waits 45 minutes for a blood draw which requires two resources, a nurse and an exam room (assuming that the materials for drawing blood are negligible). The next event, lab analysis, occurs 200 minutes later and requires a lab technician for 10 minutes. After a 55 minute wait, a physician uses the results from the lab to consult with the patient in an exam room, an event which take 15 minutes. Forty-five minutes later, the patient is discharged, an event which

Figure 1. A sample patient flow path

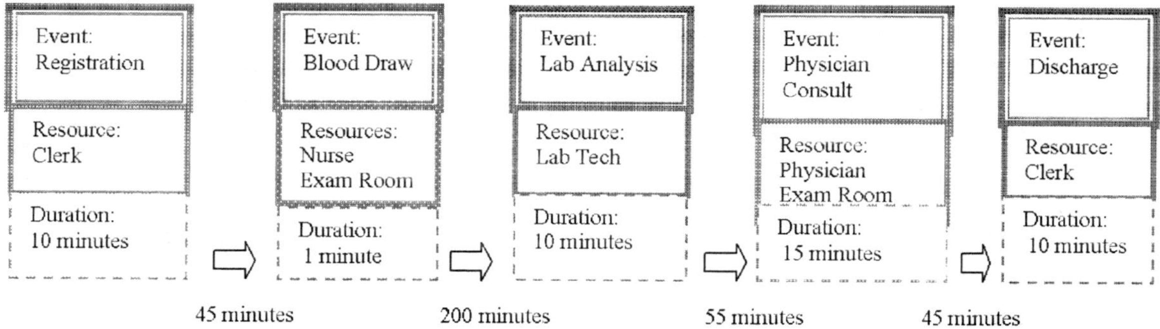

requires 10 minutes of a clerk's time. In reality, a patient's flow through the hospital will be much more complex, would involve a multitude of resources, and several events could happen in parallel. The sequence of events, the timeline, the resources required for these events, and efficiency can fluctuate vastly between patients.

Benefits of Patient Flow Approach

Hospital management tends to focus on the performance of individual departments rather than a holistic portrayal of patient events from admission to discharge. Yet most activities and services required to deliver care are tightly coupled. Hospital departments, such as radiology or the emergency department, do not exist in isolation. Operational decisions regarding resource allocation and usage in one department impacts another. Resources, such as providers or equipment, are often shared across departments. Unfortunately the prevailing localized viewpoint and decision-making leads to inefficient allocation of resources, diminished patient access, and increased costs. Resource allocation, capacity planning, scheduling, and utilization are all affected by patients moving between departments. (Cote, 2000; Kucukyazici et al., 2010) Better management of patient movement requires looking at the whole system of care, exploring the associations between events and services, and recognizing sources of variation in care delivery. One way to achieve this to adopt a patient flow viewpoint.

Patient flow approaches have better matched hospital resources to fluctuating demand levels; reduced ambulance diversions (Cameron, Scown, & Campbell, 2002; Fatovich, Nagree, & Sprivulis, 2005; (Schull, Lazier, Vermeulen, Mawhinney, & Morrison, 2003); reduced periods of under- and overstaffing (Ledersnaider & Channon, 1998), and better managed inpatient bed capacity (Mackay, 2001). Employing a patient flow perspective provides a feedback mechanism for patient quality programs (Wright, Wain, Grillo, Moncure, Macaluso, & Mathisen, 1997); it can explore the effects of changing treatment decisions on resource use and costs (Davies and Davies, 1994), and can be used to structure hospital admission profiles (Clerkin, Fos, & Petry, 1995). In sum improving patient flow through the hospital provides better clinical outcomes, increases patient safety, positively impacts patient and staff satisfaction, and improves a hospital's financial performance. (Haraden and Resar, 2004)

The focus of a patient flow approach is to ensure a smooth progression through a hospital minimizing unnecessary delays for the patient, and ensuring that services are provided at the right time, at the right place by the right provider. In the following section we discuss systems engineering techniques useful for understanding, evaluating, and improving patient flow.

ENGINEERING TOOLS TO MANAGE PATIENT FLOWS

A recently published joint report from the National Academy of Engineering (NAE) and Institute of Medicine (IOM) advocated the widespread application of systems engineering tools to improve health care delivery. (Reid, Compton, Grossman, & Fanjiang, 2005) Systems engineering focuses on the design, control, and orchestration of system activities to meet performance objectives. (Kopach-Konrad, et al., 2007) This is achieved through the application of mathematical modeling and analysis techniques.

There is a growing interest in applying systems engineering techniques to health care. Within the last decade, several universities instituted graduate level degrees Health Systems Engineering. Similarly, a number of health care organizations, such as the Department of Veterans Affairs, created engineering research centers to implement systems engineering solutions in its medical centers.

The use of systems engineering tools has not been lost on patient flow modeling. Among some of the more common techniques are discrete event simulation, Markov processes, queuing theory, Petri nets, and data mining. These techniques are all very useful tools for modeling uncertainty which is inherent in healthcare processes. In this section we briefly describe each approach, provide application examples, and discuss the merits and weaknesses of each technique. We then explore some of the impediments in modeling patient flow.

Current Techniques

Discrete Event Simulation is perhaps the most commonly applied systems engineering tool to model patient flow. In essence, simulation models mimic system behavior in accelerated time. It is the process of designing and creating a model of a real or proposed system for the purpose of conducting numerical experiments to provide a better understanding of the behavior of that system for a given set of conditions.(Law & Kelton, 1999; Kelton, Sadowski, & Sturrock, 2007) It entails building a model of the process to be analyzed, repeatedly running the model with different random inputs under different scenarios, and tabulating the result for different runs to identify process statistics and the likelihood of particular outcomes. Although it cannot be directly used for optimization, it can be combined with optimization techniques or heuristics. Special-purpose simulation languages such as GPSS and SIMAN provide a framework for simulations. More commonly, several high-level software "simulator" products are employed, such as Arena and Automod. These products typically operate through intuitive graphical user interfaces, menus, and dialogs.

Figure 2 is a very simple simulation of a patient arrival process in an Emergency Department built using the software Arena. In this example, there are two types of patient arrivals; either via ambulance or walk-in. Patients are triaged separately and assigned an acuity score. If the triage nurse decides that an ambulance patient requires immediate stabilization, the patient is sent directly to the Emergency Department. Otherwise both types of patients are registered in a central location and, based on their acuity score, the patient is either sent to the Emergency Department or Fast Track. Once the model is simulated over a period of time, statistics can be collected such as the number of patients seen, average wait times, utilization rates of rooms or nurses and so forth.

Simulation enables experimentation without having to make changes in the real world. For example, in this model we can change the number of nurses working in registration to see the effect on patient wait times, or, we could determine nurse utilization rates if all of a sudden the hospital receives three times the amount of ambulance patients. Figure 3 is an example of a more intricate

Figure 2. A screenshot of a simulation model of patients arriving in an emergency department. (The model was built using Arena software).

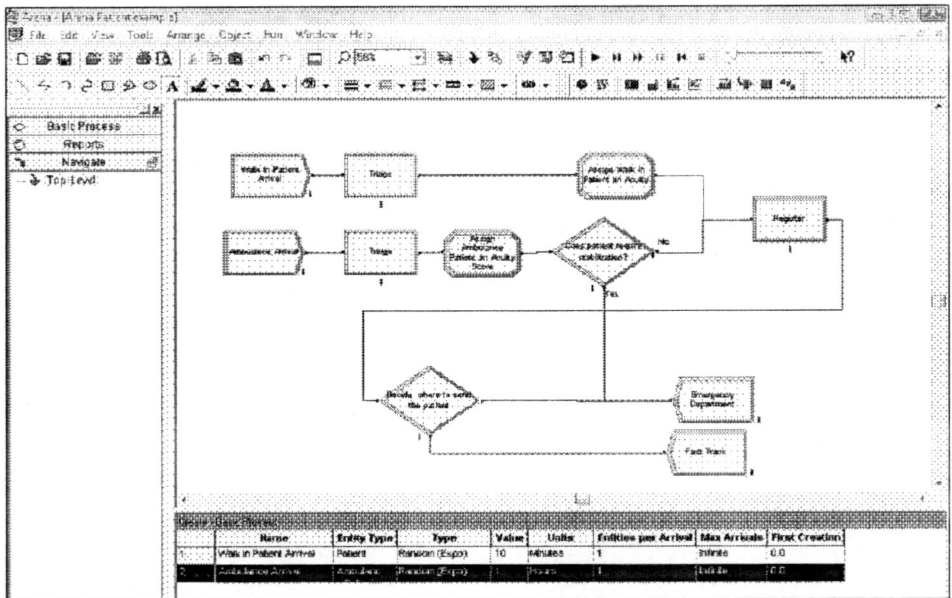

model describing how a patient flows through a hospital's fast track system. This model accounts for events such as bed cleaning, physician visit, laboratory work and so forth.

The main advantage of simulation is its ability model complicated systems making it a versatile and very powerful tool. One of the primary benefits of simulators is that they are able to

Figure 3. A screenshot of a simulation model of patients flow in a fast track department. (The model was built using Arena software).

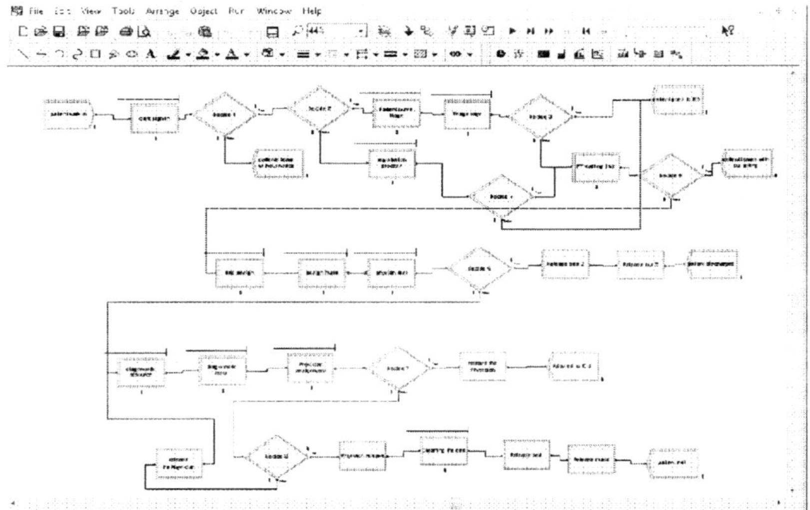

provide users with practical feedback when designing real world systems. This allows the designer to determine the correctness and efficiency of a design (or alternative) before the system is actually implemented. Another benefit of simulators is that they are able to reflect randomness inherent in hospital processes. Third, simulators can be used as an effective means for communicating or demonstrating concepts or the impact of an alternative to end-users. Simulators, like most tools, do have their drawbacks. Simulators use rule-based interactions, and it may not always be possible to full define a set of rules to describe the physical world being modeling. Furthermore, simulations focus on steady state behavior with almost no transient analysis. In reality, transient behavior and its associated variability often contain important information regarding a system.

The use of discrete-event simulation to study patient flow is well documented in the literature. A recent extensive overview of the use of discrete event simulation in healthcare research can be found in (Jacobson, Hall, & Swisher, 2006). Representative examples include (Hoot, et al., 2008) who use simulation to study Emergency Department (ED) congestion by integrating simulation forecasting with ED information systems to obtain short-term projections of wait times, occupancy levels, and boarding time. (Ceglowski, Churilov, & Wasserthiel, 2007) use data mining techniques incorporate core patient treatments into a simulation model, thus identifying bottlenecks between the ED and a hospital ward. (Samaha, Armel, & Starks, 2003) create a simulation model to evaluate operational alternatives, such as the use of a fast track to reduce the length of stay of ED patients. Researchers have also used simulation to address patient flow in observation units (Hung & Kissoon, 2009), specialty clinics (Ramakrishnan, Nagarkar, DeOennaro, Srihari, Courtney, & Emick, 2004), and intensive care (Troy & Rosenberg, 2009).

Another important tool used in modeling patient flow is queuing theory. Queuing theory is the mathematical study of waiting lines, or queues. Figure 4 contains a graphical interpretation of a simple queuing system. For example, assume that we wish to study the system of a nurse taking a patient's vitals. Patients arrive in the system according to some statistical distribution, queue, and then wait to be "served" by a nurse. The patient is then "in service" with a nurse for a given amount of time (also according to a statistical distribution), then leaves the system while the nurse services the next patient. Mathematical expressions calculate system statistics such as: the average time a patient waited; the average number of patients waiting; the average nurse utilization rate, among other measures. For additional discussion of queuing tools, we refer the reader to (Ozcan, 2009).

The majority of queuing applications assess hospital capacity requirements. For example, (de

Figure 4. A graphical representation of a queuing system

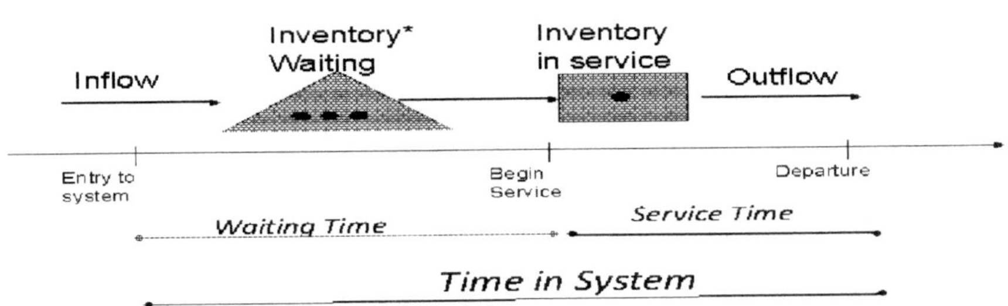

Bruin, Koole, & Visser, 2005), investigate bottlenecks in the emergency care chain of cardiac in-patient flow. The primary goal of their queuing model is to determine the optimal bed allocation over the care chain given a maximum number of refused admissions. Other representative examples include (Xie, Chaussalet, & Rees, 2007) and (Jiang & Giachetti, 2008). Recognizing the connection between limited resource availability and the occurrence of bottlenecks, some queuing models employ blocking (e.g. the waiting space between stations is finite). For example, because of their critical condition, Intensive Care Unit (ICU) patients ready to be transferred from the ICU can wait only in a bed; however a limited number of downstream medical-surgical beds may prevent a unit from accepting ICU patients. (See (McManus, Long, Cooper, & Litvak, 2004) and (Koizumi, Kuno, & Smith, 2005) for examples).

Unfortunately, many queuing models are somewhat restrictive. Queuing models cannot account for the simultaneous allocation of multiple resources which care delivery requires. For example, a patient occupies a bed for the duration of his/her visit. During this visit various resources work intermittently and together to treat the patient. At times, a nurse and a physician may work together; later in the patient's stay, the same nurse may work with a technician. Furthermore, queuing systems are often set up to have a tandem structure in which entities flow in a linear fashion. To circumvent this restriction, queuing systems introduce 'feedback flows' which allow for exogenous input into a server (for example, a patient returning to a server representing physician care). These feedback queuing models could potentially create a deadlock flow problem, a situation in which entities at two or more servers block each other. (Koizumi, Kuno, & Smith, 2005) To the best of our knowledge, all existing queuing models with feedbacks make the simplifying assumption that deadlock is detected and resolved automatically by exchanging the entities between the stations. It should be noted that this portrayal of patient flow is unrealistic. Finally, queuing models assume steady state. In reality, the transient behavior in a hospital and the associated variability in resource availability is the cause of flow bottlenecks.

Markov models are based on well established statistical methodologies and provide a viable approach to measuring and modeling flow. Grounded in probability theory and statistics, Markov models describe time-varying random processes with the property that the next state depends only on the current state. For example, a state of a system could be that all beds on a given unit are assigned to patients. The system state would change if a patient was discharged in which case the new state would be 'one bed available'. Changes in the state of a system are the result of probabilistic rules called transitions. Using the afore mentioned example to construct a Markov model, we would obtain transition data from historical patterns or observations of bed occupancy. For example if we determined that a hospital system is in a "all beds occupied" state, there is a 5% chance that the next state will be "one bed empty", a 1% chance that it is "two beds are empt"y, and 94% chance that the state will remain "all beds occupied". Markov models require that all states of a system be defined.

A number of examples of patient flow Markov models exist. (McClean, Garg, Meenan, & Millard, 2007) use Markov models to identify high probability pathways, groups of patients who incur exceptional high costs and pathways that are very long lasting. Using Markov decision process, (Nunes, de Carvalho, & Rodrigues, 2009) develop patient admission control policies by considering characteristic patient treatment patterns for a hospital. (Côté & Stein, 2000) illustrate and evaluate the applicability and appropriateness of the Erlang model to represent patient flow, but considered the flow of only one group of patients.

To a certain degree Markov models reflect the patient journey and provide insights into transitions between states of a system. However, such models rely on the developer having knowledge of the various states of a system. In a system as large as a hospital, the number of states is exponentially large; thus limiting the use of Markov models to studies that are abstract. Furthermore the patient mix of a hospital requires the introduction of population compartments in a Markov model. This compartmentalization combined with system state enumeration often causes model intractability. Finally while Markov models are useful in deriving steady state utilization rates, these metrics are somewhat limiting for short-term operational analysis.

Petri nets are a graphical and mathematical modeling tool well suited to describe and study patient flow. Petri nets are used to analyze systems characterized as being concurrent, asynchronous, distributed, parallel and/or stochastic (Murata, 1989) and capture how the system state evolves. The main attraction of Petri nets is the way in which system characteristics such as bottlenecks, and resource sharing are captured. Petri Net formalism combines an intuitive graphical notation with a formal mathematical definition, and provides a number of analysis methods. As a mathematical model, it is possible to set up state equations, algebraic equations and other models governing the behavior of the system.

A simple Petri net representing a diagnostic procedure is shown in Figure 5. Petri nets have two kinds of graphical nodes – places and transitions.

Figure 5. An example of a Petri net representing a diagnostic procedure

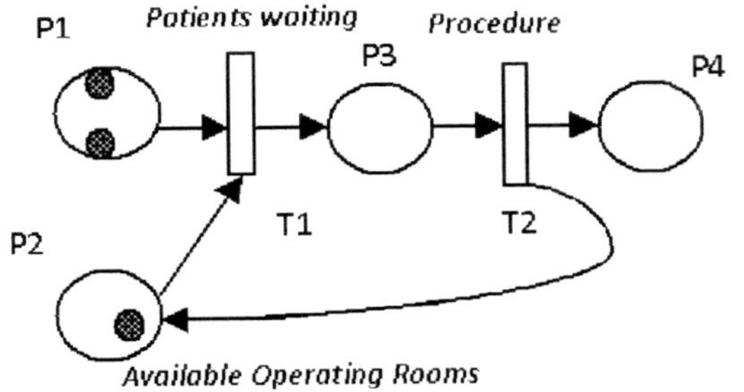

Places are depicted as circles, and transitions are represented as bars. When modeling a system, transitions represent events, and the necessary inputs for the event are modeled as places. In this example the Petri net consists of four places (P1, P2, P3 and P4) and two transitions (T1 and T2). To provide some meaningful interpretations to this net, let

P1: patient ready for the procedure in the Operating Room
P2: available staffed Operating Room
P3: patient in the Operating Room
P4: patient recovery
T1: procedure occurrence in the Operating Room
T2: procedure success

Arcs in a Petri net connect a place to a transition indicating the number input units necessary for an event to occur. For example, in the operating room net of Figure 5, for a procedure to occur, we need a staffed operating room and a patient. The distribution of inputs, known as *tokens*, across the set of places of the Petri net indicates the state of a system. In Figure 5 the current marking indicates that two patients are ready and waiting for a procedure, and one staffed operating room is available. The dynamic behavior of Petri nets can be represented as a set of equations which determine how the system changes over a period of time. Using these equations, a modeler is able to trace the sequence of events which can lead a system, say the Emergency Department, to a bottleneck situation. We refer the reader to (Murata, 1989) for further reading.

Petri nets have long been recognized to be well-suited for workflow modeling including hospital workflowsPetri nets have been studied extensively, resulting in a large body of knowledge and software tools for analysis. As a modeling technique, Petri nets have the following advantages. (1) Flexibility: there are a wide range of Petri net extensions to suit different needs. (2) Visual: Petri nets utilize a graphical modeling notation, making them easy to understand and with which to work. (3) Analytical: Petri nets support formal mathematical analysis of operational properties. The transient behavior of patient flow has been successfully modeled using Petri nets. For example, (Hughes, Carson, Makhlouf, Morgan, & R., 2000) use colored Petri nets to model patient flow between four units in a hospital, and (Maruster, van der Aalst, Weijters, van den Bosch, & Daelemans, 2001) (Konrad & Lawley, 2009) discover workflow Petri nets automatically from hospital process logs. A major weakness of Petri nets is known as the "state-space explosion" problem, that is a Petri net model can become intractably large. Because of this, different approaches have been introduced such as reduction techniques which preserve system properties without loss of generality.

Figure 6 summarizes the four systems engineering techniques which are commonly applied to model patient flow. Other techniques also used include regular expressions (Miró, Sánchez, Espinosa, Coll-Vinent, Bragulat, & Millá, 2003), and systems dynamics (Wolstenholme, 1999). Data mining approaches are often used to describe patient flow patterns. Examples of data mining include the development of clustering techniques to describe inpatient gynecology (Rajagopalan & Isken, 2001), data flow diagrams for radiography (Pohjonen, et al., 1994), and ED "treatment pathways" through process-based self-organizing maps (Ceglowski, Churilov, & Wasserthiel, 2007). The recent establishment of the Unified Modeling Language (UML) for systems analysis and design has led to patient flow studies using UML tools. (Vasilakis, Lecznarowicz, & Lee, 2009)

Figure 6. Systems engineering techniques commonly applied to model patient flow

	Discrete event simulation	Queuing	Markov models	Petri nets
Definition	Imitation of a real-world process or system through software packages	Mathematical analysis of wait times and resource utilization	Depict stochastic processes by defining a set of states which the system may exhibit and probabilistic laws governing movement between these states.	A graphical and mathematical modeling technique which describes and studies systems characterized as being concurrent, asynchronous, distributed, and/or stochastic
Strengths in modeling patient flow	• Able to capture system complexity and develop sophisticated, and detailed models	• Mathematically precise analysis of queue times, utilization rates	• Useful for deriving steady state utilization rates	• Able to analyze transient behavior of a system • Offers both a mathematical and graphical representation of a system
Weaknesses in modeling patient flow	• Focus on steady-state (long run) analysis • Requires software • Building a simulation model is often time-consuming and expensive	• A number of assumptions must be made which may create an unrealistic portrayal of a system • Focus on steady-state analysis	• Requires knowledge of the various states of a system which could be exponentially large • Somewhat limiting for short-term operational analysis.	• Mathematical solutions may be difficult to solve
Additional References	Law, A., & Kelton, W. (1999)	Kleinrock, 1975	Ross, 1996	Murata, 1989

Existing Impediments to Modeling Patient Flow

Although systems engineering tools hold great promise for modeling patient flow, there are significant challenges impeding implementation. Current patient flow models are deficient in four ways. First, these models tend to focus on the analysis of individual units. Most existing patient flow models consider only a single hospital department. Such isolated analysis can be misleading since operations depend on demand from upstream departments and capacity allocation in downstream departments. In reality operational problems in one department can propagate into others. By ignoring the multiple interacting flows of people, materials, and equipment between departments, an operations analysis does not adequately portray a hospital environment (Marshall, Vasilakis, & El-Darzi, 2005) because Not surprisingly, suggested solutions from these incomplete models are problematic. (Harper, 2002; Marshall, Vasilakis, & El-Darzi, 2005; Smith & Goddard, 2002) Vanberkel et al. recently reviewed 88 studies involving two or more hospital departments. All included interactions with downstream departments, while 30 studies explicitly modeled the interaction with upstream departments (i.e. those departments from which patients were referred). Only 13 of the 88 studies consider how diagnostic departments impact patient flow in the hospital. The authors note that "although many patients require blood work, x-rays or other exams in order to be properly treated or diagnosed, very few models include their interactions with the main department under study." (Vanberkel et al., 2009)

In addition to departmental interactions, patient flow models need to aggregate patients into groups, or types, by similarities in flow characteristics. The challenge is to determine the appropriate level of aggregation. Too much aggregation groups patients with dissimilar resource usage, while too little yields an unmanageable number of patient types. Isken and Rajagopalan refer to this as the patient classification problem. Most existing studies consider either a generic patient or only a single patient type. The inherent variability in patient diagnoses has a major impact on analysis of day-to-day hospital operations as it is a primary driver of resource use in hospitals. Appropriate nurse staffing levels are directly affected by the types of patients in a hospital along with the level of care required by each patient. The patient mix also generates demand for a myriad of ancillary services including laboratory, pharmacy, therapy, radiology, housekeeping, and surgical services.

The third limitation faced by patient flow modeling is data requirements. The level of detail required to describe patient flow can be overwhelming with thousands of possible patient paths, and hundreds of procedures with varying durations. Most studies rely on observational and manual data collection (Vanden Bosch & Dietz, 2000), or on a set of electronic databases (Rajagopalan & Isken, 2001). Electronic flow data in healthcare is either non-existent or available only through the integration of multiple, heterogeneous sources, which requires overcoming interoperability and data compatibility and integrity issues (Sanchez, Ferrin, Ogazon, & Sepulveda, 2000). The situation is further exasperated by the problem of amassing and storing vast amounts of data. Some researchers and analysts attempt to address system complexity by sacrificing resolution. (Harper, 2002)

Finally existing flow models typically estimate long-term steady state performance and tend not to address the short term transient behavior with which operational decision making is most concerned. Conventional performance measures, such as bed utilization, do not adequately represent the true situation in the hospital unit (Marshall et al., 2005). Most of these measures focus on the average values in a steady state situation. This is misleading for decision makers. For example perhaps bed capacity is able to satisfy patient demand *on average* (for example over the course of a year); however there may be significant capacity-demand mismatches in shorter intervals (for example in a week). It is essential to consider new models that not only focus on the steady-state measures, but also incorporate short term fluctuations.

DISCUSSION AND RECOMMENDATIONS

Adopting a patient flow perspective promises improved operational performance for hospitals. A number of systems engineering applications have attempted to measure and model patient flow to aid operational decision making. However, as discussed in previous sections efforts to develop comprehensive patient flow models suitable for operational analysis are hampered by a limited representation of the relationships between hospital departments, an incomplete portrayal of the patient population, limited data, and lack of transient behavior descriptions. This section provides direction on how to meet these challenges.

Information Technology

Information is the key element of any patient flow initiative. Representations of patient flow are built from the capture, integration and sharing of information, both within and between departments of the hospitals. (Mahaffey, 2004) Consequently, incorporating recently developed tools in information technology and data processing with patient flow models enables efficient data capture and improves the accuracy and acceptability of these models. Radio Frequency Identification (RFID) technology, sensor networks, and interdepartmental message exchanges can capture the extensive data required to support flow models.

RFID is a technology of identifying unique items using radio waves. (Das, 2004; (Correa, Gil, & Redín, 2005) Hospitals can use RFID systems to capture patient flow pattern with minimal staff involvement in the tracking process. Each RFID implementation is unique; however typically upon arrival or check in a patient will receive a tag. This tag could take on a number of forms including wrist straps or a special badge; and generally are made to be tamperproof to prevent its removal. RFID readers are placed in particular areas of the facility such that a tagged patient's location is read and recorded. Existing technologies such as departmental databases, pagers, or PDAs can be integrated with RFID technology to provide greater details. Depending on the implementation, the RFID system can provide information regarding how much time a patient spent in a particular department or area; different locations visited by the patient; or even which materials and resources a patient used during their stay.

There have been several successful applications of patient tracking systems for managing patient flow. Lancaster General Hospital is often cited as one of the forerunners in using RFIDs to support workflow management. Initially implemented in 1998, this technology is currently operational at three sites, and is on its third generation. Earlier generations enabled the hospital to improve Operating Room (OR) utilization to more than 85% from a previous 50% and reduce OR turnaround time by eliminating an entire step: the patient holding room. Lancaster is using a Radianse active-RFID indoor positioning solution (IPS) which includes small battery-powered ID tags for patients, network ready receivers that plug into the hospital's existing wired/wireless network and location analysis software.

The cost of a RFID implementation varies widely depending on the types of tags, readers, and area covered. Besdies collecting data to describe patient flow patterns, RFID implementations can be used to display current wait and location information for hospital managers, analyze patient and/or provider data, and even be used to track inventory or patients.

In addition to using RFID to model patient flow, hospitals are experimenting with sensor networks. Sensor networks are dense wireless networks of small, low-cost sensors which collect and disseminate physical or environmental data such as motion, sound, or temperatures. (Römer & Friedemann, 2004) Isken et al. (2005) develop a method to automatically characterize outpatient flow from sensor network data. Sensors collected patient location information on various stops visited throughout the outpatient visit: exam room, waiting area, nursing station, and so forth. The study objectives were to propose a data preparation framework capable of analyzing sensor and staff movement data and then to develop data constructs representing patient flow patterns. After data preprocessing and reducing the path by removing consecutive stops, the authors were able to describe the frequency of distinct paths. (Isken, Sugumaran, Ward, Minds, & Ferris, 2005)

Another third approach to capture and model patient flow patterns is to use information from electronic messages passed between hospital information systems. For each patient entering the hospital, information systems generate and communicate with one another through messages regarding procedure orders, lab requests, transfer orders, and so forth. This set of messages represents much of what happens to the patient. Vast amounts of health care information are exchanged on a daily basis in systems prevalent in almost all hospitals, regardless whether the organization uses electronic medical records or not. (Konrad & Lawley, 2009) are developing methods for constructing diagnosis-based patient flow models from these messages. These methods make explicit the expected resource utilization and requirements a patient presents upon admission. By modeling patient flow from the resource consumption perspective, this research provides vital operational information and a method to incorporate these resource requirements into decision support models.

Hybrid Approaches

A second approach to model and measure patient flow is to utilize hybrid methods. Each of the systems engineering methods discussed earlier have their individual strengths and weaknesses. Thus, researchers incorporate the advantages of multiple techniques to create robust hybrids capable of addressing some of the previously mentioned modeling challenges. For example, the integration of simulation in optimization models constitutes a novel and important development and is a good example of hybrid modeling (Swisher et al., 2000). Through their study of a transfusion center of University of Rome, De Angelis et al. (2003) demonstrate the applicability of this framework in the health care domain. As discussed in earlier sections, a simulation model will only allow for scenario analyses; thus limiting analysis to the set of given scenarios. In contrast, simulation-optimization provides a structured approach to determine the *optimal* scenario to maximize the performance. An example managerial concern that can be addressed via simulation-optimization is the optimal staffing ratio to improve the patient flow. While simulation would require testing of alternative scenarios, such as one staff per shift, split shifts, mixing of nursing and ancillary staff, simulation-optimization would search for the most appropriate staffing ratio by running the simulation model iteratively. Another example of such a hybrid approach is Harper (2002). He proposes a framework, where there are various components of analyses combining a preliminary statistical analysis with a further data investigation using methods such as classification and regression tree analysis, and modeling techniques on patient length of stay. This is complemented by a final stage of modeling using simulation techniques.

CONCLUSION AND FUTURE RESEARCH DIRECTIONS

Both researchers and practitioners advocate using a patient flow approach to analyze hospital operations. Patient flow centric approaches better match hospital capacity to demand, improve resource allocation decisions, and enable feedback mechanism for quality programs. A number of systems engineering tools are employed to describe, model, and analyze patient flow. These include discrete event simulation, queuing, Petri nets, Markov models among others. However, these approaches face four key challenges; conducting a multi-departmental analysis, accounting for patient mix, extensive data requirements and identifying appropriate measures. Two emerging directions to meet these challenges are using information technology and developing systems engineering hybrid tools.

REFERENCES

Cameron, P., Scown, P., & Campbell, D. (2002). Managing access block. *Australian Health Review*, *25*, 59–68. doi:10.1071/AH020059

Ceglowski, R., Churilov, L., & Wasserthiel, J. (2007). Combining data mining and discrete event simulation for a value-added view of a hospital emergency department. *The Journal of the Operational Research Society*, *58*(2), 246–254.

Clerkin, D., Fos, P., & Petry, F. (1995). A decision support system for hospital bed assignment. *Hospital & Health Services Administration*, *40*, 386–400.

Correa, F., Gil, M., & Redín, L. (2005). *Benefits of connecting RFID and lean principles in healthcare.* Working Paper 05-44 Business Economics Series 10, Universidad Carlos III de Madrid, Departamento de Economía de la Empresa.

Côté, M., & Stein, W. (2000). An Erlang-based stochastic model for patient flow. *OMEGA: The International Journal of Management Science*, *28*(3), 347–359. doi:10.1016/S0305-0483(99)00045-6

Das, R. (2004). *IDTechEx White Paper: RFID explained.* Retrieved 2009, from www.idii.com/wp/ IDTechExRFID.pdf

de Bruin, A., Koole, G., & Visser, M. (2005). Bottleneck analysis of emergency cardiac inpatient flow in a university setting: An application of queueing theory. *Clinical and Investigative Medicine. Medecine Clinique et Experimentale*, *28*(6), 316–317.

Dempsey, M. (2005). *Intelligent location.* Patient Safety and Quality Healthcare Conference.

Fatovich, D., Nagree, Y., & Sprivulis, P. (2005). Access block causes emergency department overcrowding and ambulance diversion in Perth, Western Australia. *Emergency Medicine Journal*, *22*, 351–354. doi:10.1136/emj.2004.018002

Harper, P. (2002). A framework for operational modelling of hospital resources. *Health Care Management Science*, *5*(3), 165–173. doi:10.1023/A:1019767900627

Hoot, N., LeBlanc, L., Jones, I., Levin, S., Zhou, C., & Gadd, C. (2008). Forecasting emergency department crowding: A discrete event simulation. *Annals of Emergency Medicine*, *52*(2), 116–125. doi:10.1016/j.annemergmed.2007.12.011

Hughes, M., Carson, E. R., Makhlouf, M., Morgan, C. J., & Summers, R. (2000). Modelling a progressive care system using a coloured–timed Petri net. *Transactions of the Institute of Measurement and Control*, *22*(3), 271–283.

Hung, G., & Kissoon, N. (2009). Impact of an observation unit and an emergency department-Admitted patient transfer mandate in decreasing overcrowding in a pediatric emergency department: A discrete event simulation exercise. *Pediatric Emergency Care*, *25*(3), 160–163. doi:10.1097/PEC.0b013e31819a7e20

Isken, M. (2002). Modeling and analysis of occupancy data: A healthcare capacity planning application. *International Journal of Information Technology and Decision Making*, *1*(4), 707–729. doi:10.1142/S0219622002000439

Isken, M., Sugumaran, V., Ward, T., Minds, D., & Ferris, W. (2005). Collection and preparation of sensor network data to support modeling. *Health Care Management Science*, *8*, 87–99. doi:10.1007/s10729-005-0392-8

Jacobson, S., Hall, S., & Swisher, J. R. (2006). Discrete-event simulation of health care systems. In Hall, R. (Ed.), *Reducing delay in healthcare delivery* (pp. 211–252). New York, NY: Springer.

Jiang, L., & Giachetti, R. (2008). A queueing network model to analyze the impact of parallelization of care on patient cycle time. *Health Care Management Science*, *11*(3), 248–261. doi:10.1007/s10729-007-9040-9

Joint Commission Resources. (2004). JCAHO requirement: New leadership standard on managing patient flow for hospitals. *Joint Commission Perspectives*, *24*(2), 13–14.

Jørgensen, J. (2002). Coloured Petri nets in UML-based software development – Designing middleware for pervasive healthcare. In K. Jensen (Ed.), *Proc. of the Fourth International Workshop on Practical Use of Coloured Petri Nets and the CPN.*

Kelton, W., Sadowski, R., & Sturrock, D. (2007). *Simulation with Arena* (4th ed.). McGraw-Hill Science.

Koizumi, N., Kuno, E., & Smith, T. (2005). Modeling patient flows using a queuing network with blocking. *Health Care Management Science*, *8*, 49–60. doi:10.1007/s10729-005-5216-3

Konrad, R., & Lawley, M. (2009). Input modeling for hospital simulaiton models using electronic messages. In M. Rossetti, R. Hill, B. Johansson, A. Dunkin, & A. Ingalls (Eds.), *Winter Simulation Conference*, (pp. 134-147). Austin.

Kopach-Konrad, R., Lawley, M., Criswell, M., Hasan, I., Chakraborty, S., & Pekny, J. (2007). Applying systems engineering principles in improving health. *Journal of General Internal Medicine*, *22*(Suppl 3), 431–437. doi:10.1007/s11606-007-0292-3

Kucukyazici, B., Verter, V., & Mayo, N. E. (2010). (forthcoming). An analytical framework for designing community-based care delivery processes for chronic diseases. *Production and Operations Management.*

Law, A., & Kelton, W. (1999). *Simulation modeling & analysis*. McGraw-Hill Inc.

Ledersnaider, D., & Channon, B. (1998). SDM95—Reducing aggregate care team costs through optimal patient placement. *The Journal of Nursing Administration*, *28*, 48–54. doi:10.1097/00005110-199810000-00010

Mackay, M. (2001). Practical experience with bed occupancy management and planning systems: An Australian view. *Health Care Management Science*, *4*, 47–56. doi:10.1023/A:1009653716457

Marshall, A., Vasilakis, C., & El-Darzi, E. (2005). Length of stay-based patient flow models: Recent developments and future directions. *Health Care Management Science*, *8*(3), 213–220. doi:10.1007/s10729-005-2012-z

Maruster, L., van der Aalst, W., Weijters, A., van den Bosch, A., & Daelemans, W. (2001). Automated discovery of workflow models from hospital data. In B. Krose, M. de Rijke, & G. Schreiber (Eds.), *Proc. 13th Belgium-Netherlands Conference on Artificial Intelligence BNAIC 2001*, (pp. 183-190).

McClean, S., Garg, L., Meenan, B., & Millard, P. (2007). *Using Markov models to find interesting patient pathways*. Twentieth IEEE International Symposium on Computer-Based Medical Systems, 2007. CBMS '07, (pp. 713-718).

McClean, S., McAlea, B., & Millard, P. (1998). Using a Markov reward model to estimate spend-down costs for a geriatric department. *The Journal of the Operational Research Society*, *49*, 1021–1025.

McManus, M., Long, M., Cooper, A., & Litvak, E. (2004). Queueing theory accurately models the need for critical care resources. *Anesthesiology*, *100*, 1271–1276. doi:10.1097/00000542-200405000-00032

Miró, O., Sánchez, M., Espinosa, G., Coll-Vinent, B., Bragulat, E., & Millá, J. (2003). Analysis of patient flow in the emergency department and the effect of an extensive reorganisation. *Emergency Medicine Journal*, *20*(2), 143–148. doi:10.1136/emj.20.2.143

Murata, T. (1989). Petri nets: Properties, analysis and applications. *Proceedings of the IEEE*, *77*(4), 541–580. doi:10.1109/5.24143

Nunes, L., de Carvalho, S., & Rodrigues, R. (2009). Markov decision process applied to the control of hospital elective admissions. *Artificial Intelligence in Medicine*, *47*(2), 159–171. doi:10.1016/j.artmed.2009.07.003

Ozcan, Y. A. (2009). *Quantitative methods in health care management: Techniques and applications*. Wiley, John & Sons, Incorporated.

Pohjonen, H., Bondestam, S., Karp, P., Kinnunen, J., Korhola, O., & Sakari, P. (1994). Quality assurance of the bedside chest radiography process. *Acta Radiologica*, *35*(3), 235–243.

Rajagopalan, B., & Isken, M. (2001). Exploiting data preparation to enhance mining and knowledge discovery. *IEEE T Syst Man Cyb*, *31*(4), 460–471. doi:10.1109/5326.983929

Ramakrishnan, S., Nagarkar, K., DeOennaro, M., Srihari, K., Courtney, A., & Emick, F. (2004). A study of the CT scan area of a healthcare provider. In R. Ingalls, M. Rossetti, J. Smith, & F. Peters (Eds.), *Proc 2004 WSC*, (pp. 2025-2031.).

Reid, P., Compton, W., Grossman, J., & Fanjiang, G. (2005). *Building a better delivery system: A new engineering/healthcare partnership. National Academy of Engineering and Institute of Medicine, Committee on Engineering and the Health Care System*. Washington, DC: National Academy Press.

Römer, K., & Friedemann, M. (2004). The design space of wireless sensor networks. *IEEE Wireless Communications*, *11*(6), 54–61. doi:10.1109/MWC.2004.1368897

Ross, S. M. (1996). *Stochastic processes*. John Wiley&Sons.

Samaha, S., Armel, W., & Starks, D. (2003). The use of simulation to reduce the length of stay in an emergency department. In S. P. Chick (Ed.), *Proc 2003 WSC*, (pp. 1907-1911).

Sanchez, A., Ferrin, D., Ogazon, T., & Sepulveda, J. (2000). Emerging issues in healthcare simulation. In J. Joines, R. Barton, K. Kang, & R. Fishwick (Ed.), *Proc 2000 WSC*, (pp. 1999 – 2003).

Schull, M., Lazier, K., Vermeulen, M., Mawhinney, S., & Morrison, L. (2003). Emergency department contributors to ambulance diverision: A quantitative analysis. *Annals of Emergency Medicine*, *41*, 467–476. doi:10.1067/mem.2003.23

Smith, P., & Goddard, M. (2002). Performance management and operational research: A marriage made in heaven? *The Journal of the Operational Research Society*, *53*, 247–255. doi:10.1057/palgrave.jors.2601279

Troy, P., & Rosenberg, L. (2009). Using simulation to determine the need for ICU beds for surgery patients. *Surgery*, *146*(4), 608–620. doi:10.1016/j.surg.2009.05.021

van der Aalst, W., Weijters, T., & Maruster, L. (2004). Workflow mining: Discovering process models from event logs. *IEEE Transactions on Knowledge and Data Engineering*, *16*(9), 1128–1142. doi:10.1109/TKDE.2004.47

Vanden Bosch, P., & Dietz, D. (2000). Minimizing expected waiting in a medical appointment system. *IIE Transactions*, *32*, 841–848. doi:10.1080/07408170008967443

Vasilakis, C., Lecznarowicz, D., & Lee, C. (2009). Developing model requirements for patient flow simulation studies using the Unified Modelling Language (UML). *J Simul*, *3*(3), 141–149. doi:10.1057/jos.2009.3

Vissers, J., & Beech, R. (2005). *Health operations management: Patient flow logistics in healthcare*. London, UK: Routledge - Taylor and Francis Group.

Wolstenholme, E. (1999). A patient flow perspective of U.K. health services: Exploring the case for new intermediate care initiatives. *System Dynamics Review*, *15*(3), 253–271. doi:10.1002/(SICI)1099-1727(199923)15:3<253::AID-SDR172>3.0.CO;2-P

Wright, C., Wain, J., Grillo, H., Moncure, A., Macaluso, S., & Mathisen, D. (1997). Pulmonary lobectomy patient care pathway: A model to control cost and maintain quality. *The Annals of Thoracic Surgery*, *64*(2), 299–302. doi:10.1016/S0003-4975(97)00548-1

Xie, H., Chaussalet, T., & Rees, M. (2007). A semi-open queueing network approach to the analysis of patient flow in healthcare systems. *Proceedings of the 20th IEEE International Symposium on Computer-Based Medical Systems.*

Young, J. (2005). *RFID applications in the healthcare and pharmaceutical industries: White Paper revolutionizing asset management and the supply chain.* Retrieved 2010, from www.radiantwave.com/whitepapers /healthWP.doc

Section 5
Cost Management

Chapter 20
A New Cost Accounting Model and New Indicators for Hospital Management Based on Personnel Cost

Yoshiaki Nakagawa
Kyoto University, Japan

Hiroyuki Yoshihara
Kyoto University, Japan

Yoshinobu Nakagawa
Kagawa National Children's Hospital, Japan

ABSTRACT

Specified hospital accounting systems in a hospital are necessary for a manager to determine the proper management strategy. We developed a new cost accounting model based on new allocation rules of personnel cost. The model presented in this chapter offers a manager useful tools to calculate the medical cost not only for an individual patient and for each clinical department, but also each DRG system for a specific period.

New financial indicators were developed based on personnel costs which were calculated using this new cost accounting system. Indicator 1: The ratio of the marginal profit after personnel cost per personnel cost (RMP). Indicator 2: The ratio of investment (=indirect cost) per personnel cost (RIP). Operation profit per one dollar of personnel cost (OPP) was demonstrated to be the difference between the RMP and RIP. The break-even point (BEP) and break-even ratio (BER) could be determined by combining the indicators. RMP demonstrates not only the medical efficiency, but also the medical productivity in the case of DPC/DRG groups. OPP can be utilized to compare the medical efficiency of each department in either one hospital or multiple hospitals. It also makes it possible to evaluate the management efficiency of multiple hospitals.

DOI: 10.4018/978-1-60960-872-9.ch020

INTRODUCTION

In order to make suitable management decisions, the hospital manager must analyze the medical revenue and cost of not only the entire hospital, but also individual patient and clinical departments (Cleverley, 2002; Schuhmann, 2008). Even if the medical revenue of a department is apparently high, it is not unusual for the financial balance of the department to be in the red (Nakagawa, 2009). However, it is not easy to recognize the medical efficiency of each department because an adequate and simple medical cost analysis method has not been developed that can determine the financial balance for each patient (as a minimum unit) and/or department. Therefore, it is difficult to compare the efficiency of individual departments in a particular hospital and compare them to the rest of the hospitals in the region. Despite the existence of many kinds of benchmarks or indicators, most of them are not related to efficiency from a medical management point of view (Balicki, 1995; Melony, 1995). The major problem blocking the development of a successful model is how to allocate the indirect costs (depreciation and maintenance cost for a hospital) for each patient and clinical department. The other problem is the allocation rule of personnel cost, which consumes more than 50% of a typical hospital's revenue.

The aim of this chapter is to demonstrate a new allocation rule of personnel cost in a hospital and cost accounting model. The indirect cost is allocated according to the personnel cost computed by the new allocation rule. The new indicators for hospital management based on the personnel cost computed by the new cost accounting model are also presented. These indicators are new tools that can be used as benchmarks or indicators for evaluating the management efficiency and medical productivity of a hospital, as well as of each individual department and DRG (DPC) system.

BACKGROUND

To remain solvent, it is necessary to streamline hospital administration, and it is essential to conduct evaluations at the clinical-department or division level (which can be referred to as evaluations for each sales department) in order to identify areas needing changes. Unfortunately, there are currently no simple and standard evaluation methods that can be used for this purpose (Makie, 2002; Tanaka, 2004). The average length of stay (ALOS) or cost per patient etc. are good benchmarks for a hospital manager to compare his hospital to another hospital, or to compare individual clinical departments within the same hospital. However, there are few indicators that can be used to determine the relationship between the investment and medical productivity or management efficiency of a hospital.

As a cost accounting method, the ratio-cost-to charge (RCC) method and the relative value unit (RVU) method have been widely used (West, 1996). However, the methods were developed primarily in industry and imported into the medical field. The costs in industry are usually divided into two categories; fixed costs and variable costs. The fixed costs, which include the personnel cost, depreciation cost and maintenance cost, were allocated in accordance with machine time and occupancy space. This provides an accurate estimate of efficiency because most of the products are made by a simple production line or process in industry. However, a patient treated in a hospital receives various medical services from different medical sections. One of the major problems preventing the use of these industry-derived methods is how to allocate the depreciation cost and maintenance cost of a hospital to an individual patient (Nakagawa, 2007).

If we calculate the cost of the medical services that each patient receives as a product generated in a factory, we have to consider a large number

Figure 1. Traditional allocation method for calculating medical cost

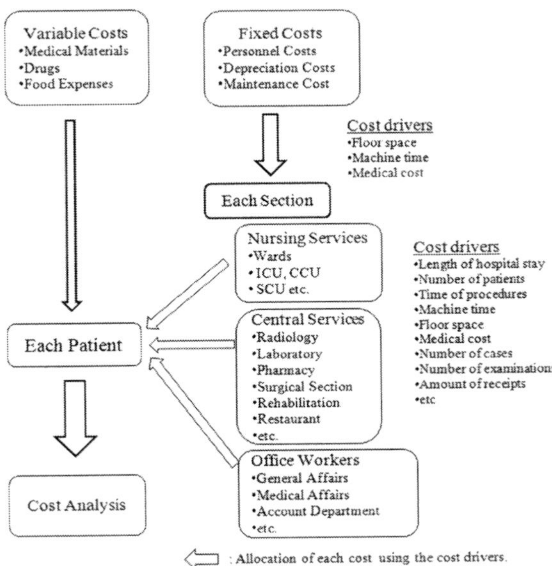

of processes for accounting. Most of the variable costs are directory-allocated to each patient, however, the other part of variable cost and fixed cost is divided into each section, including individual wards, central services, and administrators, according to the floor space, machine time and medical revenue as a cost driver. Thereafter, individual costs, which include personnel cost in each section, are calculated by other cost drivers (Figure 1). Therefore, such accounting systems are complicated and do not provide a reasonable estimate of department cost and revenue. The other problem is the allocation rule of the personnel cost, which accounts for about 50% of the medical revenue in a typical hospital.

Time studies using an activity-based cost (ABC) method been recommended for proportionally dividing the personnel cost (Chan, 1993; Canby, 1995; Player, 1998, Biorn 2003). However, since time studies require extensive time and manpower for a large hospital offering various medical services, their use is not realistic. Furthermore, the physical condition of a patient changes dramatically from day to day, and the number of patients in each clinical department is not uniform throughout the year. Therefore, if the result from a one- or two-day time study are applied to the whole year, the evaluation may prove to be widely different from the actual conditions of a hospital, and may cause incorrect results.

Medical services are provided from multi-product firms composed of highly heterogeneous activities such as cancer centers, heart centers, emergency hospitals or training hospitals. Therefore, in order to evaluate the output of medical service, the allocation rules of medical efficiency or productivity of the health care (clinical outcome or life time etc.) has been discussed. Various methods have so far been established to measure the medical productivity and efficiency. (Cutler and McClellan 2001). One such method is the analysis of the efficiency of medical service based on investment and the level of benefit to the patients. This method makes it possible to directly demonstrate the trend of medical productivity based on the level of benefit provided a given patient. However, there is little correlation between the efficiency and the data such as medical price or output data which are used to evaluate the quality of medical production. The other method is the computation of the price index (PI) using the clinical outcome and medical incidents based on the improvements of health care. However, the price of medical care is usually controlled by the Government, or some other official organization. Medical services are not the same as market services and medical prices do not change depending on the quality of health care, therefore medical prices alone are not suitable for use as deflators to compute the output of productivity. The goal is therefore to measure the output of the medical services by computing the medical productivity, based on such factors as the clinical outcome and life time, etc. However, it is not easy to simplify such indexes because of the wide variations in medical care and the different types of patients. A DRG in the U.S.A and a DPC in Japan were therefore developed to arrange the different aspects of complex medical care and to make a detailed database.

The Diagnosis Related Group (DRG) system was initially applied to Medicare in the United States to control increasing medical costs (Gee, 2006). DRGs or similar grouping systems were progressively introduced into European countries as a tool for hospital reimbursement (Schreyogg, 2006; Bellanger, 2006; Fattore, 2006). In 2003, the modified payment system based on Diagnosis Procedure Combinations (DPC) was introduced as a medical treatment fee system in Japan (Yasunaga, 2005; Yasunaga, 2006; Fushimi, 2007). While the DRG is a "per case payment" system, the DPC based payment system is a "per day payment" system. One of the aims of such a payment system is to standardize the medical care including medical costs. A suitable diagnosis and successful treatment resulted in a shortening of the hospital stay and an increase in medical profit. Both systems were designed for high quality medical care and a better outcome in order to produce a higher medical profit.

In addition to the introduction of this new payment system, dramatic advances in information technology, such as electronic medical records, ordering systems, and new accounting systems have also recently been developed and introduced into hospitals (Tanaka, 2004; Nakagawa 2009). As a result, it has now become easier to compute the direct cost, medical material cost, food expenses and costs of other services in individual sections. Although it might seem that a patient is treated in a single department, however, he/she usually receives different kinds of medical services from the entire hospital, such as nursing services, central crevices, radiation or imaging services, and restaurant and administrative services. Therefore, we developed a new allocation rule of personnel cost and tried to incorporate these medical services with personnel costs according to the total amount of the personnel cost.

A New Cost Accounting Model

The new model consists of three sections as follows:

1. *A medical revenue and cost analysis system.* Medical revenue is computed according to the database of the DPC (DRGs) system, or it can also be calculated using medical receipts or bills from individual patients. The medical direct costs, such as medical materials, and drug and food expenses for each patient are also calculated in the same way.
2. *A system for calculating personnel costs interlinked with the hospital accounting system.* We developed a new allocation rule of personnel cost using simpler cost drives, and proportionally divided depreciation and maintenance costs based on the personnel cost (Figure 2). The personnel cost is allocated for each patient using the cost drivers; number of beds, length of hospital stay, and direct medical cost. The personnel costs in the entire hospital were divided into three groups: Nursing services, Central services and Office/administrative services. Nursing services include the personnel cost of doctors, nurses and other paramedical staff belong to the ward (or department) or ICU. The individual ward usually belongs to each clinical department or two or three minor departments keep one ward together. Then the personnel cost in a ward is allocated according to the cost drivers; number of beds, length of hospital stay, and medical cost. Central services include pharmacy, radiology, laboratory, anesthesiology and operating room, rehabilitation and restaurant costs, etc., which are charged in bills. The personnel cost of central crevice is allocated according to the amount billed for each patient. Office workers who offer indirect services include the administration,

Figure 2. New allocation rule of medical costs

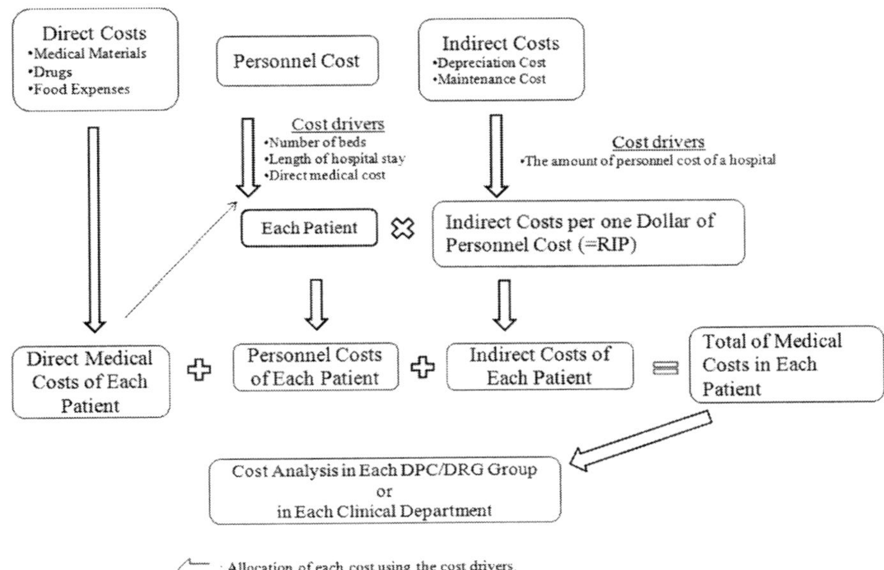

staff for maintenance services, laundry and other indirect services, which are not billed as medical services. The personnel costs of office workers were divided according to the length of hospital stay of all inpatients. The personnel cost of each patient is the total amount of nursing service, central service and the amount paid to office workers based on the individual patients.

3. *Indirect costs for each patient.* The indirect cost consists of depreciation costs and maintenance costs for a hospital. Before allocation of the indirect cost to each patient, the total indirect cost of the hospital is divided by the amount of the personnel cost. This yields the indirect cost per one dollar of personnel cost. The indirect cost of each patient can be calculated by multiplying the personnel cost for each patient and indirect costs per one dollar of personnel cost.

Utilization of a New Cost Accounting Model

The medical cost for each patient can be presented by the amount of the direct medical cost, personnel cost and indirect cost for each patient. It becomes possible to realize the accounting balance not only for each patient, but also for each department and DPC/DRG group (Figure 3).

The data used in this chapter were all obtained from profit and loss statements.

New Indicators for Hospital Management Based on Personnel Cost

A simple and fair benchmarking system or financial indicators for use on the clinical department level that are needed to evaluate the management efficiency and productivity of each clinical department or division of a hospital remains to be established. New indicators have therefore been developed based on personnel costs as follows:

Figure 3. The medical revenue and cost analysis for each department in a hospital

Department	No. of patients	Medical revenue	Personnel cost				Cost of materials			Marginal profit	Indirect cost		Total cost	Net profit
			Doctors	Nurses	Paramedical	Office workers	Medical materials	Drugs	Food expenses		Depreciation cost	Maintenance cost		
General medicine	15,212	6,195,749	899,091	1,421,432	633,359	282,173	141,398	1,243,951	217,536	1,356,810	388,680	942,072	2,933,636	26,058
Respiratology	23,996	9,131,150	952,646	2,799,513	996,758	478,979	176,090	1,052,065	373,510	2,301,589	627,918	1,521,932	3,751,515	151,739
Gastroenterology	14,659	6,006,840	866,590	1,574,203	635,357	291,778	261,627	728,279	161,306	1,487,700	404,519	980,463	2,536,194	102,718
Cardiology	8,151	9,571,757	682,175	1,898,237	412,849	140,449	5,106,566	420,488	129,562	781,431	376,387	912,278	6,945,281	-507,235
Pediatics	2,023	1,051,534	407,860	204,903	46,298	37,470	1,295	91,992	21,914	239,803	83,660	202,772	401,632	-46,629
Generel surgery	64,041	31,957,029	3,808,362	7,898,288	2,724,621	1,230,848	5,686,976	3,536,774	903,827	6,167,334	1,881,164	4,559,518	16,568,258	-273,348
Orthopedic surgery	14,287	7,928,912	1,336,453	2,217,723	559,363	296,544	827,041	535,847	183,789	1,972,152	529,691	1,283,853	3,360,221	158,608
Plastic surgery	634	319,889	61,492	210,072	20,586	13,712	5,454	13,263	9,914	-14,604	36,737	89,042	154,410	-140,383
Neurosurgery	1,320	631,156	77,073	206,679	66,707	26,437	105,193	72,524	19,142	57,402	45,269	109,721	351,849	-97,588
Cardio-vascular surgery	1,973	1,630,365	344,830	851,030	123,403	26,457	495,369	170,946	28,518	-410,188	161,633	391,763	1,248,229	-963,584
Gynecology	3,301	1,398,474	174,794	557,235	143,430	69,867	15,419	261,490	43,578	132,660	113,542	275,201	709,230	-256,083
Opthalmology	2,254	1,294,847	217,622	409,790	155,041	50,703	209,786	24,781	35,251	191,872	100,070	242,547	612,434	-150,744
Otolaryngology	1,936	782,489	207,565	244,321	70,492	39,840	26,776	75,349	26,630	91,515	67,528	163,672	359,955	-139,685
Neurology	2,310	713,298	19,768	241,257	90,923	43,526	22,290	125,119	22,893	147,522	47,500	115,129	332,931	-15,108
Dermatology	182	53,172	101,521	68,242	7,347	3,157	136	5,137	3,104	-135,472	21,652	52,479	82,507	-209,603
Urology	2,625	1,259,833	216,625	340,424	99,895	51,958	47,666	107,565	38,272	357,428	85,146	206,374	485,022	65,908
Total of inpatients	94,863	47,969,464	6,566,107	13,245,062	4,061,808	1,853,050	7,442,106	4,928,794	1,314,918	8,557,621	3,089,931	7,489,298	24,265,047	-2,021,608

RMP: The **r**atio of **m**arginal profit after personnel cost per **p**ersonnel cost.

The RMP is defined as an index which reflects the ratio of marginal profit after personnel cost per one monetary unit (e.g. one dollar or yen) of personnel cost. A new entity "medical marginal profit after personnel cost" was defined to be what remains after the subtraction of direct costs from medical revenues.

The RMP is expressed using the definition in Figure 4 as:

$$RMP = \frac{A - E}{c}$$

Figure 4. Parameters used in this study

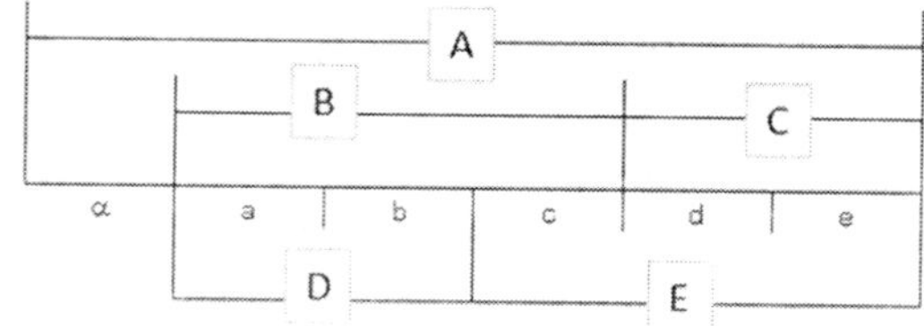

A: (Medical) Revenue, B: Fixed cost, C: Variable cost,
D: Indirect cost, E: Direct cost,
α: Medical profit, a: Depreciation for a hospital,
b: Maintenance cost for a hospital,
c: Personnel costs, d: Cost of medical materials,
e: Food expenses,

The RMP of the hospital is computed using the A, E and c of the whole hospital. However, when the RMP of each department and DPC (DRG) group is computed, the amount of the A, E and c of individual data for each patient calculated by the new accounting model in each department or DPC (DRG) group is used. All components of A, E and c are closely connected and influenced by medical practice revenue, the length of hospital stay, number of patients, length of procedures, etc. which are related to the quality of medical care and the clinical outcome. High personnel costs and the cost of materials resulted in a low RMP. The proper allocation of resources, such as labor and medical materials improves RMP which demonstrates management efficiency of a hospital and clinical department. Equally the change in the RMP reflects how much labor should be invested in individual medical care, thus demonstrating the medical productivity in the DPC/DRG system (Figure 5).

RIP: The **r**atio of **i**nvestment per **p**ersonnel cost

The RIP is defined as an index which reflects the ratio of investment (= indirect cost) per one monetary unit (e.g. one dollar or yen) of personnel cost. The indirect cost of each DPC (DRG) group or department can be computed as the amount of

Figure 5. Medical efficacy demonstrated by RMP, RIP, and OPP in DPC groups ($=US$)

DPC code	Medical revenue/pt/day				MAP	RMP	RIP	OPP
	Blanket portion	FFS	Personnel cost	Materials				
020200XX970X0X	$185.43	$720.00	$200.84	$61.75	$642.84	3.201	0.63	2.571
030350XX97XXXX	$239.82	$776.27	$277.16	$72.69	$666.24	2.404	0.63	1.774
020200XX970X1X	$213.45	$447.90	$203.11	$49.95	$408.29	2.010	0.63	1.380
010030XX01X0XX	$270.98	$790.22	$301.63	$191.88	$567.69	1.882	0.63	1.252
060020XX0100XX	$278.77	$738.51	$333.27	$80.28	$603.73	1.812	0.63	1.182
100260XX97X0XX	$314.19	$548.24	$281.22	$87.54	$493.67	1.755	0.63	1.125
050070XX01X00X	$273.62	$1,754.86	$232.77	$1,415.48	$380.23	1.634	0.63	1.004
050170XX03X1XX	$301.45	$1,347.39	$229.81	$1,045.51	$373.52	1.625	0.63	0.995
050050XX03X2XX	$353.95	$1,508.47	$244.98	$1,221.21	$396.23	1.617	0.63	0.987
060040XX0100XX	$272.07	$582.37	$303.02	$63.00	$488.42	1.612	0.63	0.982
010010XX99X5XX	$415.44	$143.84	$254.84	$245.56	$58.88	0.231	0.63	-0.399
161060XX99X0XX	$171.81	$254.61	$247.00	$125.88	$53.54	0.217	0.63	-0.413
010111XXXXX00X	$171.39	$167.03	$223.26	$68.60	$46.56	0.209	0.63	-0.421
120180XX99XX0X	$130.03	$175.73	$219.38	$47.34	$39.04	0.178	0.63	-0.452
060180XX99X00X	$169.23	$193.71	$225.17	$98.00	$39.77	0.177	0.63	-0.453
060570XX99XXXX	$170.82	$311.66	$323.45	$103.71	$55.32	0.171	0.63	-0.459
130030XX99X30X	$195.56	$252.58	$242.80	$170.28	$35.06	0.144	0.63	-0.486
130030XX97X3XX	$264.19	$242.96	$255.81	$245.06	$6.28	0.025	0.63	-0.605
010110XXXXX4XX	$1,078.42	$137.52	$372.43	$843.55	-$0.04	0.000	0.63	-0.630
120260XX99XXXX	$127.25	$80.70	$216.01	$28.49	-$36.55	-0.169	0.63	-0.799

Materials include cost of medical material,drugs and food expences
FFS: Ferr for service
MAP: marginal profit after personnel cost

indirect cost of individual patient. Therefore, RIP demonstrates the balance between the investment of the whole hospital and the resource of labor.

RIP is expressed using the definition in Figure 1 as:

$$RIP = \frac{D}{c}$$

D is the indirect cost of a whole hospital, and c is the total personnel cost in a hospital. Therefore, each hospital has a single RIP. Therefore, the same value of RIP is used to compute the direct cost for each patient. The indirect cost for each can then be calculated by the following formula:

Indirect cost = RIP $\times$ amount of personnel cost

The medical payment systems such DPC are designed for high quality medical care and outcomes in order to produce higher medical profits. It is thus possible to compare the medical productivity and the management efficiency of clinical departments or DPC (DRGs) groups in a hospital from the point of view of financial management using these two indicators (Figure 6).

If personnel costs are deceased to improve the RMP, the RIP should also increase. To improve the financial balance, a hospital manager tries to improve the RMP in accordance with increasing of the RIP. If the hospital (or department) is in the red, then the RMP should improve more than the RIP, which thus means an improvement in the hospital revenue without increasing personnel costs, and thus indicating an improved medical productivity. If the hospital revenue can improve more than the additional investment which includes personnel costs, then the RMP will increase in opposition to the RIP. As a result, the financial balance changes from being in the red to being in the black.

Figure 6. Sixteen departments of hospital "T" were compared using RMP as a benchmark

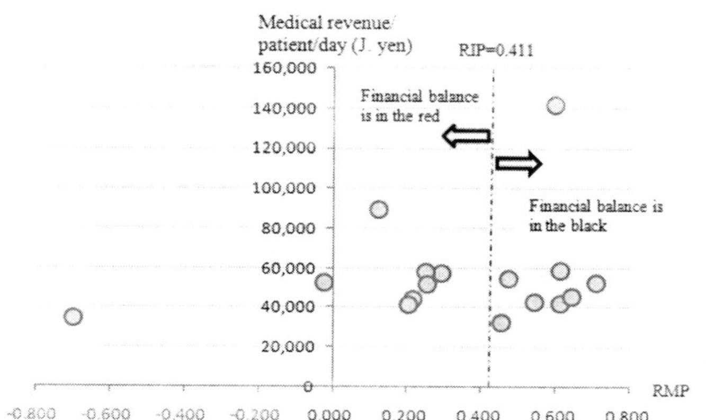

Hospital "T" has 535 beds and 16 clinics. This hospital mainly offers medical services for acute patients. The RIP of the hospital was 0.411, therefore the financial balance of the departments with RMP less than 0.411 was in the red. It was clearly demonstrated that even if the medical revenue/patient/day adequately increases, it does not always demonstrate a better efficiency from the viewpoint of hospital management.

Operation Profit for Personnel Cost (OPP)

The difference after subtracting the RIP from the RMP provides the operation profit per personnel cost (one dollar). The OPP in each department, DRG/DPC system or each hospital demonstrates the financial balance of these factors as well as the management efficiency (Figure 5 and Figure 7). The OPP even for individual patients can be computed. The OPP demonstrate the balance between the medical profit and investment. The comparison of OPP in each medical section becomes able to evaluate the management efficiency.

The net profit can be calculated by the following formula:

Net profit in a hospital (or department) = (RMP - RIP) × amount of personnel cost.

The net profit of an individual department or DPC (DRGs) group can be also calculated the same way.

RMP, RIP and Break-Even Point (BEP)

The BEP can be expressed by the following formula:

$$BEP = \frac{a+b+c}{1-\frac{d+e}{A}} = \frac{A(a+b+c)}{A-(d+e)} = \frac{A(a+b+c)}{\alpha+a+b+c} \tag{1}$$

The RMP is expressed by the following formula:

$$RMP = \frac{A-(c+d+e)}{c} = \frac{a+b+\alpha}{c}$$

Therefore:

$$cRMP = a+b+\alpha \tag{2}$$

RIP is expressed by the following formula:

Figure 7. Comparison of the department of cardiology in two hospitals using RMP, RIP, OPP, and BEP

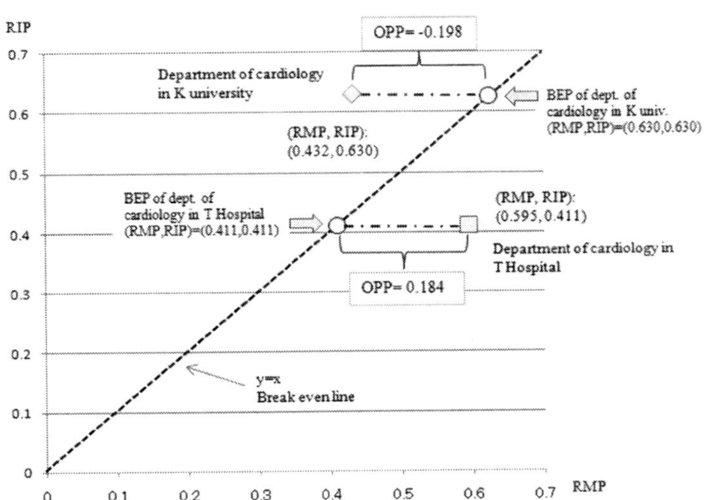

Diamond: Department of Cardiology at K University with (RMP, RIP) = (0.432, 0.630) and financial balance in the red. Square: Department of Cardiology at T Hospital with (PMP, RIP) = (0.595, 0.411) and the financial balance in the black. The line y = x demonstrates the break-even line. The BEP and OPP of each department are demonstrated. The width between RMP of cardiology at K university and the RMP on BEP of the department; 0.432-0.630=-0.198 demonstrates the operating profit per one dollar of personnel cost (OPP) of the department at K University. The width between the RMP of the department of cardiology in T hospital and the RMP on BEP; 0.595-0.411=0.184 demonstrates OPP of the department of the cardiology in hospital T. The value 0.184 demonstrates a better management efficiency than the department at K University.

$$RIP = \frac{D}{c} = \frac{a+b}{c}$$

Therefore:

$$cRIP = a + b \qquad (3)$$

Substituting (2) and (3) into (1) gives

$$BEP = \frac{A(cRIP + c)}{cRMP + c} = \frac{Ac(RIP + 1)}{c(RMP + 1)} = \frac{A(RIP + 1)}{RMP + 1}$$

Therefore, the minimum RMP point for returning to the black is the value of RIP located on the line where y = x (Figure 7). If the RIP and RMP can be estimated in each hospital or department, the turning point in profitability can be demonstrated on the break even line (y=x).

RMP, RIP and Break-Even Ratio (BER)

The break-even ratio (BER) is expressed by the following formula:

$$BER = BEP \times \frac{1}{A} = \frac{A(RIP + 1)}{RMP + 1} \times \frac{1}{A} = \frac{RIP + 1}{RMP + 1}$$

Therefore:

$$BER(RMP + 1) = RIP + 1$$
$$RIP = BER(RMP + 1) - 1$$

A turning point in profitability similar to the break-even point (BEP) and break-even ratio

(BER) could be also defined by combining the RMP and RIP. The merits of these two indicators are not only the ability to indicate the relationship between the medical profit and the investments in the hospital, but also the capability to demonstrate such indicators as BEP, BER and OPP on a single graph (Figure 7). The total medical revenue of the department of cardiology in Hospital T was 881,054/year (US dollars). OPP was demonstrated as the width between RMP of the department of cardiology in Hospital T and BEP of the department; 0.595- 0.411 = 0.184. The total medical revenue of the department of cardiology at University K was 1,668,738/year (US dollars). However, OPP of the department of cardiology at the university was -0.198 (=0.432 - 0.630). The amount of medical revenue of the department of cardiology in University K was much higher than that of Hospital T. However, the value 0.184 (OPP in hospital T) was much better than that of University K, and had better medical efficiency from a hospital management viewpoint.

Application of the Indicators to the Hospitals of the NHO

The two indicators were applied to the hospitals in the National Hospital Organization (NHO). Using these two indicators, it was possible to evaluate the management efficiency and medical activity not only of the whole hospital, but also in each department and DPC/DRG group. This will be of use to a manager of a hospital for evaluating the management efficiency of his/her hospital, and will be useful despite the variations among hospitals, departments and divisions.

The data for each hospital reported by the administration of the 144 NHO hospitals in 2008 was analyzed. Seventy three out of the 144 hospitals offer mainly acute-phase medical care services. The other 71 hospitals offer medical services mainly for chronic patients (chronic hospitals). They have wards for handicapped children (or adults), wards for patients with severe neurological diseases such as muscular dystrophy and amyotrophic lateral sclerosis, wards for patients with tuberculosis, or wards for psychiatric patients. The 144 hospitals that were used in the investigation are all organized and operated under the same rules and have the same payroll system. The new financial indicators, RMP and RIP, were applied to evaluate the management efficiency and medical activity for each hospital.

Forty-three out of the 73 hospitals were in the black (OPP>0). The other 30 hospitals were in the red (OPP<0). Only 3 hospitals out of the 12 hospitals that had an RIP value of greater than 0.6 were in the black (Figure 8). Sixty-eight hospitals out of the 71 chronic hospitals were in the black. However, both RMP and RIP were smaller for these institutions than for the acute-phase hospitals. These findings indicated that the investment in chronic hospitals is smaller than in acute-phase hospitals which normally have a larger number of staff members.

Characteristic Changes of the Indicators at Four Hospitals from 2004-2008

The characteristic changes of the two indicators at four hospitals are shown in Figure 9. The four hospitals offering acute-phase medical care services have 580 beds in hospital A, 500 beds in B, 600 beds in C, and 580 beds in D. After comparing both indicators and the financial balance for the 5 year period, the management efficiency and activities of each hospital became clear. Hospital A had very high RMP and RIP in 2004, thus suggesting that it was well-managed, however, the data indicated that there were an insufficient number of staff and that the staff were over-worked. The hospital increased the hospital staff and tried to improve the efficiency. As a result, both RMP and RIP decreased in 2008, however, OPP markedly improved. The hospital was on the 90% BER line, which indicated that the financial balance of hospital A was improved and was holding a

Figure 8. The relationship among the RMP, RIP, and the financial balance in 73 NHO hospitals

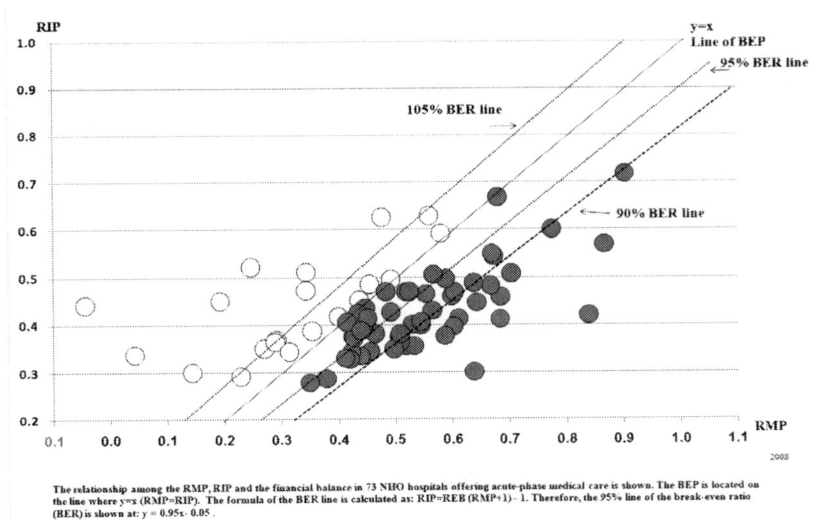

steady state. Hospital B had very high investment, which was indicated by the high RIP. A gradual increase in the RMP in the last 5 years without any marked changes in the RIP revealed good balanced changes between the depreciation cost and personnel cost. The hospital tried to improve medical efficiency, thus resulting in a continuous increase in the OPP, and the financial balance returned to the black in 2008. Hospital C had a high RIP and a large deficit in the financial balance in

Figure 9. Changes in the financial balance demonstrated by RMP and RIP during a 5 year period and the characteristics of 3 hospitals

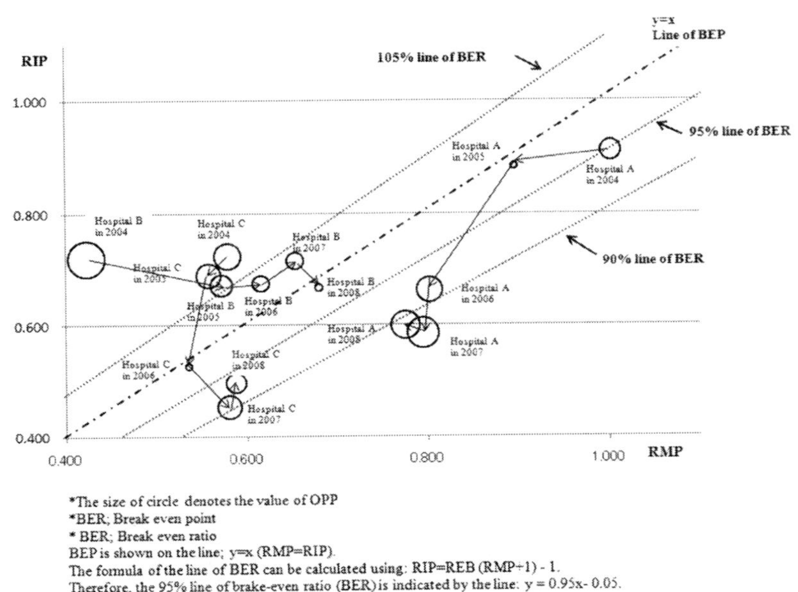

2004. Thanks to the continuous decrease in their depreciation costs and increasing number of staff members with minimum additional investment, there was a continuous decrease in the RIP. The OPP demonstrates the medical efficiency of the hospital to have improved, as demonstrated by the increase in RMP in 2007. The financial balance was in the black in 2007, and additional investment was therefore likely in 2008.

DISCUSSION

In order to appreciate the medical efficiency and activity in a hospital, the manager analyzes the medical revenue and costs of not only the hospital but also each clinical department. Managers predominantly use a traditional method, such as the ratio-cost-to charge (RCC) method, or the relative value unit (RVU) method (West 1996). However, it is well-known that there are problems regarding how to allocate the indirect costs (the depreciation and maintenance cost for a hospital and personnel cost). Peden and Baker (2002) tried to allocate physician overhead costs to activities using the ABC method, and reported that if overhead costs are to be allocated on the basis of work (pay multiplied by hours), and if physician and nonphysician work are somewhat substitutable, then (overhead) costs may be allocated on the basis of physician and nonphysician work combined, which is fairly closely related to the sum of physician work and direct costs. The depreciation cost is influenced by past investments, and the maintenance cost reflects the size and structure of the hospital which directly reflects the hospitalization and medical status. While it might appear that a patient is treated in a specific department, he/she actually receives always medical care or services from the entire hospital, including nursing services, central services, and service from office workers. When a hospital is considered as an aggregate of various departments and sections, it might be better to proportionally allocate the total indirect cost to individual patients according to the amount of the medical service that they receive (Nakagawa, 2009). The transaction of the cost in a hospital is different from that in industry on the balance sheet. The cost in industry is usually classified into two categories; fixed cost and variable cost. Depreciation cost, maintenance cost and personnel costs are usually classified into the fixed cost. On the other hand, the depreciation cost and maintenance cost for a hospital are classified as indirect costs in the medical field. The personnel cost, cost of medical materials, and food expenses are classified as direct costs. The personnel cost of an entire hospital is almost fixed, however, the personnel cost for individual patients are variable.

On the other hand, the medical revenue is basically composed of two parts; one is basic hospital fees, including nursing services in a ward and administrative services. The basic hospital fee is demanded in accordance with the length of hospital stay. The other is a medical fee, which reflects the direct medical services for each patient (Central cervices). Therefore, the personnel costs in the entire hospital can be divided into three groups: nursing services, central services, and services from office workers. Nursing services include the personnel cost of doctors, nurses and other paramedical staff belong to the ward (or department) or ICU. Therefore, the personnel cost of nursing services is allocated to an individual patient in accordance with the number of beds, the length of hospital stay, and direct medical costs. Central services include pharmacy, radiology, laboratory, surgery (anesthesiology and operation room), rehabilitation and restaurant services, etc., which are considered to be direct services and are charged by bills (direct cost). Therefore, the personnel cost of the central services is allocated to each patient according to the total amount of their bills. The cost of central services includes the costs of doctors who belong to each section, such as a radiologist in radiology, a pathologist in the laboratory, an anesthesiologist in the surgical section, and a doctor in rehabilitation. Office workers who offer indirect services, include the administrative staff, staff for maintenance services, laundry, and other indirect services, which are not billed as medical services. The cost for office workers is allocated to each patient according to the length of their hospital stay of all patients. As a result, the personnel cost of each patient is computed as the amount of personnel costs in nursing service, central service and service from office workers.

The new allocation rule of personnel cost revealed that the hospital services can be substituted for personnel cost. Therefore, the indirect costs were allocated to each patient in accordance with the total amount of the personnel cost computed under the new allocation rule of personnel cost. It should be noted that the personnel cost of an entire hospital is fixed, but the personnel cost for individual patients is variable. These factors prompted us to define the new indicators RMP and RIP.

The RIP is defined as the ratio of investment (=indirect cost) per one momentary unit of personnel cost which means the balance between investment of the whole hospital and the resource of labor. Therefore, the RIP is fixed and single value, not only in a hospital, but also in every department and all DPC (DRG) groups and even each patient. On the other hand, the RMP is defined as an index which reflects the ratio of marginal profit after calculating the personnel cost per one monetary unit (e.g. one dollar or yen) of personnel cost. All the components, such as medical revenue, personnel cost and medical materials are composed of data as pertaining to each individual patient. Therefore, the RMP demonstrates the ratio of marginal profit after personnel cost per one monetary unit (e.g. one dollar or yen) of personnel cost not only in an entire hospital, but also for individual patients, each department and DPC (DRG) system. As a result it was revealed that the indicators can be used as a benchmark to compare the medical efficiency of the individual departments, the DPC (DRG) system in a hospital and productivity. On the other hand, RIP reveals that the ratio of investment (indirect cost; depreciation cost and maintenance cost for a hospital) per personnel cost is a fixed indicator in a hospital. Therefore, the difference after subtracting the RIP from RMP indicates that the operating income per personnel cost (OPP) in both the entire hospital, and also in each clinical department and DPC/DRGs group. OPP may therefore yield useful data for hospital managers. Fortunately, it is not difficult to compute the personnel cost per patient or personnel cost per DPC/DRG group. This can be done not only on a yearly basis, but also every week or month using the previously reported accounting system. When the personnel cost per patient or DPC/DRG group is computed, the RMP, RIP and OPP will be automatically calculated.

The break-even point (BEP) and OPP are simple and intelligible methods to evaluate the management efficiency and are practically used in industry. Both concepts were well known, however, it was not usually used in the medical field. Despite the fact that industrial businesses are somewhat standardized and uniform, the variety of products (disease and diagnosis, inpatient and outpatient) has not been standardized in health care systems. Therefore, in order to use the break-even point as an indicator in a hospital, there are prerequisite conditions for standardization or unification (Gandjour, 2001). Both the RMP and the RIP are based on personnel costs, which is the largest expenditure item in hospital management. The RIP is invariable in a hospital or department while the RMP is changed in proportion to the number of patients. BER is the relationship between the RIP and the RMP. Therefore, the prerequisite condition in order to use the BEP as an indicator in a hospital may be fulfilled.

The theoretical break-even point (BEP) and break-even ratio (BER) can be directly expressed by using the new indicators and can be plotted on a single graph. Only by comparing the RMP and RIP does the correlation between the revenue from treatment and the amount invested (fixed costs) become clear. Using the BEP and BER as criteria indicates that the value of the RMP needs to be greater than that of the RIP or BER in order to maintain a surplus or stability in the current account. Furthermore, because the RIP indicates the ratio of investment (=indirect cost) per one monetary unit (e.g. one dollar or yen) of personnel cost, this value can indicate not only the BEP of the hospital, but also the BEP in each medical department and DPC group. Therefore, the ideal values for stabilized hospital management would be values in which the RMP of each medical department exceeds the RIP (Nakagawa, 2009).

In order to improve hospital management, the hospital manager will need to increase the RMP or to decrease the RIP. The conditions for increasing the RMP include reducing the personnel costs by reducing the number of staff members, or to relatively reduce the personnel costs per person by securing a larger number of patients and increasing the income for treatment, thus resulting in an improved medical efficiency and product. On the other hand, the RIP does not change unless reductions in the indirect expenses or in the personnel costs can be effectively implemented. If only the personnel costs are reduced, then the RIP should increase. In other words, the closure of a department or section to improve the financial balance has little effect on the depreciation cost, which will be transferred to other departments, thereby causing an increase in the RIP. It is therefore important to consider the balance between the RMP and the RIP when making future management plans, and new investments should also be considered.

CONCLUSION

The new cost accounting model presented in this chapter provides an accountant with useful tools to calculate the medical cost of not only an individual patient, but also of each DRG group for a specific period of time. It brought a lot of useful information and also allows for the financial balance in each clinical department and DPC group in the hospital to be calculated every week or month.

The new indicators should provide good benchmarking, not only for comparisons between hospitals, but also for evaluations of the medical productivity per department or DPC (DRG group and the management efficiency from a management perspective.

REFERENCES

Balicki, B., Kelly, W. P., & Miller, H. (1995). Establishing benchmarks for ambulatory surgery costs. *Healthcare Financial Management*, *49*(9), 40–46.

Bellanger, M. M., & Tardif, L. (2006). Accounting and reimbursement schemes for inpatient care in France. *Health Care Management Science*, *9*, 295–305. doi:10.1007/s10729-006-9097-x

Biorn, E., Hagen, T., Iversen, T., & Magnussen, J. (2003). The effect of activity-based financing on hospital efficiency: A panel data analysys of DEA efficiency scores 1992-2000. *Health Care Management Science*, *6*, 271–283. doi:10.1023/A:1026212820367

Canby, J. B. IV. (1995). Applying activity-based costing to healthcare settings. *Healthcare Financial Management*, *49*(2), 50–52, 54–56.

Chan, Y. C. L. (1993). Improving hospital cost accounting with activity-based costing. *Health Care Management Review*, *18*(1), 71–77.

Cleverley, W. O. (2002). The hospital cost index: A new way to assess relative cost-efficiency. *Healthcare Financial Management*, *56*(7), 36–42.

Cutler, D. M., & McClellan, M. (2001). Productivity change in health care. *The American Economic Review*, *91*(2), 281–286. doi:10.1257/aer.91.2.281

Fattore, G., & Torbica, A. (2006). Inpatient reimbursement system in Italy: How do tariffs relate to cost? *Health Care Management Science*, *9*, 251–258. doi:10.1007/s10729-006-9092-2

Fushimi, K., Hashimoto, H., Imanaka, Y., Kuwabara, K., Horiguchi, H., Ishikawa, K., & Masuda, S. (2007). Functional mapping of hospitals by diagnosis-dominant case-mix analysis. *BMC Health Services Research*, *7*(50). Retrieved from http://www.biomedicentral.com/1472-6963/7/50.

Gandjour, A., & Lauterbach, K. W. (2001). A method for assessing the cost-effectiveness and the break-even point of clinical practice guidelines. *International Journal of Technology Assessment in Health Care*, *17*(4), 503–516.

Gee, P. (2006). DRG do over the need for a service-line strategy. *Financial Management*, *60*(8), 52–55.

Makie, T., Miyazaki, M., Kobayashi, S., Yamanaka, T., Kinukawa, N., Hanada, E., & Nose, Y. (2002). A simple method for calculating the financial balance of hospital based on proportional dividing. *Journal of Medical Systems*, *26*(2), 105–112. doi:10.1023/A:1014801808798

Melony, W. (1995). Benchmarking to improve financial performance. *Health Management Technology*, *16*(2), 10–12.

Nakagawa, Y., Noguchi, M., Takemura, T., & Yoshihara, H. (2009). Change of the management strategy before and after DPC introduction: Influence on the hospital profit caused by improvement of sickbed turnover ratio. *The Journal of Japan Society for Health Care Management*, *9*(4), 511–518.

Nakagawa, Y., Noguchi, M., Takemura, T., & Yoshihara, H. (2009). New accounting system for financial balance based on personnel cost after the introduction of a DPC/DRG system. *Journal of Medical Systems*, *35*(2), 251–264..doi:10.1007/s10916-009-9361-y

Nakagawa, Y., Takemura, T., Shirakami, G., & Yoshihara, H. (2007). The cost analysis and problems of day surgery unit in the university hospital- Second report: Study of the performance improvement. *Journal of the Japanese Society on Hospital Administration*, *44*(3), 263–272.

Peden, A., & Baker, J. J. (2002). Allocation physicians' overhead costs to service: An econometric/accounting-activity based-approach. *Journal of Health Care Finance*, *29*, 57–75.

Player, S. (1998). Activity-based analyses lead to better decision making. *Healthcare Financial Management*, *52*(8), 66–70.

Schreyogg, J., Stargardt, T., Tiemann, O., & Busse, R. (2006). Methods to determine reimbursement rates for diagnosis related groups (DRG)-A comparison of nine European countries. *Health Care Management Science*, *9*, 215–223. doi:10.1007/s10729-006-9040-1

Schuhmann, T. M. (2008). Hospital financial performance trends to watch. *Healthcare Financial Management*, *62*(7), 59–66.

Tanaka, K., Sato, J., Guo, J., Takada, A., & Yoshihara, H. (2004). A simulation model of hospital management based on cost accounting analysis according to disease. *Journal of Medical Systems*, *28*(6), 689–710. doi:10.1023/B:JOMS.0000044970.82170.ae

West, T. D., Balas, E. A., & West, D. A. (1996). Contrasting RCC, RVU, and ABC for managed care decisions. *Healthcare Financial Management*, *50*(8), 54–61.

Yasunaga, H., Ide, H., Imamura, T., & Ohe, K. (2005). Impact of the Japanese diagnosis procedure combination-based payment system on cardiovascular medicine-related costs. *International Heart Journal*, *46*(5), 855–866. doi:10.1536/ihj.46.855

Yasunaga, H., Ide, H., Imamura, T., & Ohe, K. (2006). Influence of Japan's new diagnosis procedure combination-based payment system on the surgical sector: Does it really shorten the hospital stay? *Surgery Today*, *36*(7), 577–585. doi:10.1007/s00595-006-3203-z

KEY TERMS AND DEFINITIONS

Break-Even Point: a turning point in profitability

Break-Even Ratio: Demonstrate the level of stability of the finance

DPC: Diagnosis Procedure Combinations, Medical treatment fee system of Japan

DRG: Diagnosis Related Group, Medical treatment fee system introduced in the United States.

Financial Indicator: indicator to evaluate the financial status

Hospital Cost Accounting: Accounting for the cost of the medical service in a hospital

Management Efficiency: the quality and affectivity of the management from a hospital management viewpoint

OPP: The difference after subtracting the RIP from the RMP provides the **o**peration **p**rofit per **p**ersonnel cost (one dollar). The OPP in each department, DRG/DPC system or each hospital demonstrates the financial balance of these factors and management efficiency. A comparison of OPP in each group also becomes able to compare management efficiency.

RIP: The RIP is defined as an index which reflects the **r**atio of **i**nvestment (= indirect cost) per one monetary unit (e.g. one dollar or yen) of **p**ersonnel cost. RIP demonstrates the balance between the investment of the whole hospital and resource of labor.

RMP: The **r**atio of **m**arginal profit after personnel cost per **p**ersonnel cost. The RMP is defined as an index which reflects the ratio of marginal profit after personnel cost per one monetary unit (e.g. one dollar or yen) of personnel cost. A new entity "medical marginal profit after personnel cost" was defined to be what remains after subtracting the direct costs from medical revenues. High personnel costs and the cost of materials resulted in a low RMP. The proper allocation of resources, such as labor and medical materials improves RMP which demonstrates management efficiency. On the other hand RMP also demonstrates how much resources of labor should be invested in individual medical care that demonstrates medical productivity especially in DPC/DRG system.

Compilation of References

Abdel-Aal, R. (1998). Modeling and forecasting monthly patient volume at a primary health care clinic using univariate time-series analysis. *Computer Methods and Programs in Biomedicine*, *56*(3), 235–247. doi:10.1016/S0169-2607(98)00032-7

Adan, I., Bekkers, J., Dellaert, N., Vissers, J., & Yu, X. (2009). Patient mix optimisation and stochastic resource requirements: A case study in cardiothoracic surgery planning. *Health Care Management Science*, *12*(2), 129. doi:10.1007/s10729-008-9080-9

Adler-Milstein, D., Bates, D. W., & Jha, K. J. (2009). U.S. regional health information organizations: Progress and challenges. *Health Affairs*, *28*(2), 483–492. doi:10.1377/hlthaff.28.2.483

Agarwal, S., Joshi, A., Finin, T., Yesha, Y., & Ganous, T. (2007, March). A pervasive computing system for the operating room of the future. *Mobile Networks and Applications*, *12*(2-3), 215–228. doi:10.1007/s11036-007-0010-8

Agency for Health Research and Quality. (2004). Literacy and health outcomes. Retrieved from http://www.ahrq.gov/ downloads/ pub/ evidence/ pdf/ literacy/ literacy.pdf

Agency for Healthcare Research and Quality. (2002). *Healthcare costs fact sheet.* (AHRQ Publication No. 02-P033). Rockville, MD: Author. Retrieved from http://www.ahrq.gov/ news/ costsfact.htm

AHRQ. (2010). Electronic medical record systems. Retrieved July 12, 2010, from http://wci-pubcontent/publish/communities/k_o/knowledge_library/key_topics/health_briefing_01232006114616/electronic_medical_record_systems.html

Aiken, A. (2008). *Lean: Concepts and realities*. Lanner Corporation Publication.

Akao, Y. (1990). *History of quality function deployment in Japan* (vol. 3, pp. 183-196). International Academy for Quality: IAQ Book Series.

Albin, S. L., Barrett, J., Ito, D., & Mueller, J. E. (1990). A queuing network analysis of a health center. *Queueing Systems*, *7*(1), 51–61. doi:10.1007/BF01158785

Allenbach, R. L., & Huffman, J. E. (1998). Improving simulation engineering practices I - A capability maturity model for simulation processes improvement. *International Journal of Industrial Engineering: Theory Applications and Practice*, *5*(2), 150–156.

Almborg, A. H., Ulander, K., Thulin, A., & Berg, S. (2008). Patients` perceptions of their participation in discharge planning after acute stroke. *Journal of Clinical Nursing*, *18*, 199–209. doi:10.1111/j.1365-2702.2008.02321.x

Alshawi, S., Missi, F., & Eldabi, T. (2003). Healthcare information management: The integration of patient's data. *Logistics Information Management*, *16*(3/4), 286–295. doi:10.1108/09576050310483772

American Medical Association. (1999). Ad hoc committee on health literacy for the council on scientific affairs. *Journal of the American Medical Association*, *281*, 552–557. doi:10.1001/jama.281.6.552

American Recovery and Reinvestment Act of 2009.P.L. 111-5. Washington, DC: GPO, 2009.

American Telemedicine Association. (2010). *Telemedicine in U.S. healthcare reform*. Retrieved from http://www.americantelemed.org/ files/ public/ policy/ Telemedicine%20in% 20National%20Health% 20Reform.pdf

Analytics, H. I. M. S. S. (2010). *EMR adoption model*. Retrieved July 20, 2010, from http://www.himssanalytics.org/ hc_providers/emr_adoption.asp

Anand, P. (2003). The integration of claims to healthcare: A programming approach. *Journal of Health Economics*, *22*(5), 731–745. doi:10.1016/S0167-6296(03)00024-9

Anand, S. G., Adams, W. G., & Zuckerman, B. S. (2010). Specialized care of overweight children in community health centers. *Health Affairs*, *29*(4), 712–717. doi:10.1377/hlthaff.2009.1113

Anderson, P., Lingaard, A.-M., Prgomet, M., Creswick, N., & Westbrook, J. I. (2009). Mobile and fixed computer use by doctors and nurses on hospital wards: Multi-method study on relationships between clinician role, clinical task and device choice. *Journal of Medical Internet Research*, *11*(3), 32. doi:.doi:10.2196/jmir.1221

Annichiarico, R., Cortés, U., & Urdiales, C. (Eds.). (2008). *Agent technology and e-health*. Basel, Switzerland: Birkhuser Verlag. doi:10.1007/978-3-7643-8547-7

Armstrong, W., & Taege, A. (2007). HIV screening for all: The new standard of care. *Cleveland Clinic Journal of Medicine*, *74*(4), 297–301. doi:10.3949/ccjm.74.4.297

Asaro, P. V., & Boxerman, S. B. (2008). Effects of computerized provider order entry and nursing documentation on Work ow. *Academic Emergency Medicine*, *15*, 908–915. doi:10.1111/j.1553-2712.2008.00235.x

Ash, J. S., Berg, M., & Coiera, E. (2004). Some unintended consequences of Information Technology in healthcare: The nature of patient care Information System-related errors. *Journal of the American Medical Informatics Association*, *11*, 104–112. doi:10.1197/jamia.M1471

Association of American Medical Colleges. (2008). *The complexities of physician supply and demand: Projections through 2025*. Retrieved from http://www.tht.org/ education/ resources/ AAMC.pdf

Atzeni, P., Cappellari, P., & Gianforme, G. (2007). MIDST: Model independent schema and data translation. In *Proc. ACM SIGMOD '07*, (pp. 1134-1136).

Australia's Health. (2010). *Australian Institute of Health and Welfare*. Retrieved from http://www.aihw.gov.au/ publications/aus/ah10/11374-c07.pdf

Bacheldor, B. (2006, December 11). RFID tag built to survive gamma rays. *RFID Journal*. Retrieved October 29, 2010, from http://www.rfidjournal.com/ article/print/2884

Bagust, A., Place, M., & Posnett, J. W. (1999). Dynamics of bed use in accommodating emergency admissions: Stochastic simulation model. *British Medical Journal*, *319*(7203), 158.

Bailey, N. (1952). A study of queues and appointment systems in hospital outpatient departments, with special reference to waiting-times. *Journal of the Royal Statistical Society. Series A (General)*, *14*, 185–189.

Baker, D. R., Pronovost, P. J., Morlock, L. L., Geocadin, R. G., & Holzmueller, C. G. (2009). Patient flow variability and unplanned readmissions to an intensive care unit. *Critical Care Medicine*, *37*(11), 2882–2887. doi:10.1097/ CCM.0b013e3181b01caf

Balestra, G., Gaetano, L., & Puppato, D. (2008). *A model for simulation of clinical engineering department activities* (pp. 5109–5112). Vancouver, Canada: In EMBC.

Balestra, G., Gaetano, L., Puppato, D., Prato, G., Freda, P., Morena, F., et al. Lombardo, M. (2009). Modeling a regional network of clinical engineering departments. In *Proceeding ORAHS 2009*, Leuven, Belgium July 12-17, 2009.

Balicki, B., Kelly, W. P., & Miller, H. (1995). Establishing benchmarks for ambulatory surgery costs. *Healthcare Financial Management*, *49*(9), 40–46.

Banks, J., & Carson, J. S. II. (1984). *Discrete events smulation*. Englewoods Cliffs, NJ: Prentice Hall, Inc.

Banning, P. (2009). Economic-recovery plan to include health info. *MLO: Medical Laboratory Observer*, *41*(2), 48.

Barach, P., & Dickerman, K. N. (2009). Patient safety: We shape our buildings, then they kill us. *World Health Design*. Retrieved from http://www.worldhealthdesign.com/science.aspx

Bargren, M., & Lu, D.-F. (2009). An evaluation process for an electronic bar code medication administration Information System in an acute care unit. *Urologic Nursing*, *29*(5), 355–368.

Barth, T., & Algee, J. (1996). *Proving and improving your processes with simulation.* Paper presented at the International Industrial Engineering Conference, Minneapolis, MN, USA.

Bates, D. W. (2010). Getting in step: Electronic health records and their role in care coordination. *Journal of General Internal Medicine, 25*(3), 174–176. doi:10.1007/s11606-010-1252-x

Bauer, D. T., Guerlain, S., & Brown, P. J. (2010). The design and evaluation of a graphical display for laboratory data. *Journal of the American Medical Informatics Association, 17*, 416–424. doi:10.1136/jamia.2009.000505

Bean, A. G., & Talaga, J. (1995). Predicting appointment breaking. *Journal of Health Care Marketing, 15*(1), 29–34.

Becker, E., Metsis, V., Arora, R., Vinjumur, J., Xu, Y., & Makedon, F. (2009, June). SmartDrawer: RFID-based smart medicine drawer for assistive environments. *Proceedings of the 2nd International Conference on Pervasive Technologies Related To Assistive Environments* (PETRA '09), (pp. 1-9). New York, NY: ACM. DOI= http://doi.acm.org/10.1145/ 1579114.1579163

Bekker, R., & de Bruin, A. M. (2010). Time-dependent analysis for refused admissions in clinical wards. *Annals of Operations Research, 178*(1), 45–65. doi:10.1007/s10479-009-0570-z

Belien, J., Demeulemeester, E., & Cardoen, B. (2009). A decision support system for cyclic mater surgery scheduling with multiple objectives. *Journal of Scheduling, 12*, 147–161. doi:10.1007/s10951-008-0086-4

Beliën, J. (2007). Exact and heuristic methodologies for scheduling in hospitals: Problems, formulations and algorithms. *4OR: A Quarterly Journal of Operations Research, 5*(2), 157-160.

Bellanger, M. M., & Tardif, L. (2006). Accounting and reimbursement schemes for inpatient care in France. *Health Care Management Science, 9*, 295–305. doi:10.1007/s10729-006-9097-x

Bennett, R. E., Tuttle, M., May, K., Harvell, J., & Coleman, E. A. (2007). *Health information exchange in post-acute and long-term care case study findings: Final report.* submitted to the U.S. Department of Health and Human Services Assistant Secretary for Planning and Evaluation Office of Disability, Aging and Long-Term Care Policy.

Bernstein, S. L., Aronsky, D., Duseja, R., Epstein, S., Handel, D., Hwang, U., & Asplin, B. A. (2009). The effect of emergency department crowding on clinically oriented outcomes. *Academic Emergency Medicine, 16*(1), 1–10. doi:10.1111/j.1553-2712.2008.00295.x

Bertsimas, D., & De Boer, S. (2005). Simulation-based booking limits for airline revenue management. *Operations Research, 53*(1), 90–106. doi:10.1287/opre.1040.0164

Berwick, D. M. (2002). A user's manual for the IOM's "quality chasm" report. *Health Affairs, 21*(3), 80–90. doi:10.1377/hlthaff.21.3.80

Biorn, E., Hagen, T., Iversen, T., & Magnussen, J. (2003). The effect of activity-based financing on hospital efficiency: A panel data analysys of DEA efficiency scores 1992-2000. *Health Care Management Science, 6*, 271–283. doi:10.1023/A:1026212820367

Blake, J. T., Carter, M. W., & Richardson, S. (1996). An analysis of emergency room wait time issues via computer simulation. *INFOR, 34*(4), 263–272.

Blake, J. T., Dexter, F., & Donald, J. (2002). Operating room manager's use of integer programming for assigning block time to surgical groups: A case study. *Anesthesia and Analgesia, 94*, 143–148.

Blanco, W. M. J., & Pike, M. C. (1964). Appointment systems in out-patients' clinics and the effect of patients' unpunctuality. *Medical Care, 2*(3), 133–145. doi:10.1097/00005650-196407000-00002

Blendon, R. J., DesRoches, C. M., Brodie, M., Benson, J. M., Rosen, A. B., & Schneider, E. (2002). Views of practicing physicians and the public on medical errors. *The New England Journal of Medicine, 347*(24), 1933–1940. doi:10.1056/NEJMsa022151

Blumenthal, D. (2009). Stimulating the adoption of health information technology. *The New England Journal of Medicine, 360*(15), 1477–1479. doi:10.1056/NEJMp0901592

Blumenthal, D., & Tavernner, M. (2010). The meaningful use regulation for electronic health records. *The New England Journal of Medicine, 363*(6). Retrieved on July 13, 2010, from http://www.nejm.org/doi/full/ 10.1056/NEJMp1006114

Booth, A., & Falzon, L. (2001). Evaluating information service innovations in the health service: If I was planning on going there I wouldn't start from here. *Health Informatics Journal*, *7*(1), 13–19. doi:10.1177/146045820100700104

Bouhaddou, O., Warnekar, P., Parrish, F., Do, N., Mandel, J., Kilbourne, J., & Lincoln, M. J. (2008). Exchange of computable patient data between the Department of Veterans Affairs (VA) and the Department of Defense (DoD): Terminology mediation strategy. *Journal of the American Medical Informatics Association*, *15*(2), 174–183. doi:10.1197/jamia.M2498

Bourne, L. M., & Walker, D. H. T. (2005). Visualising and mapping stakeholder influence. *Management Decision*, *43*(5), 649–660. doi:10.1108/00251740510597680

Boyd, A. D., Funk, E. A., Schwartz, S. M., Kaplan, B., & Keenan, G. M. (2010). Top EHR challenges in light of the stimulus. Enabling effective interdisciplinary, intradisciplinary and cross-setting communication. *Journal of Healthcare Information Management*, *24*(1), 18–24.

Bozzette, S. (2005). Routine screening for HIV infection-timely and cost effective. *The New England Journal of Medicine*, *352*, 620–621. doi:10.1056/NEJMe048347

Bracco, D., Favre, J. B., Bissonnette, B., Wasserfallen, J. B., Revelly, J. P., & Ravussin, P. (2001). Human errors in a multidisciplinary intensive care unit: A 1-year prospective study. *Intensive Care Medicine*, *27*(1), 137–145. doi:10.1007/s001340000751

Braglia, M., Carmignani, G., & Zammori, F. (2006, September 15). A new value stream mapping approach for complex production systems. *International Journal of Production Research*, *44*(18/19), 3929–3952. doi:10.1080/00207540600690545

Brailsford, S. (2005). Overcoming the barriers to implementation of operations research simulation models in healthcare. *Clinical and Investigative Medicine. Medecine Clinique et Experimentale*, *28*(6), 312–315.

Brailsford, S. C., Harper, P. R., Patel, B., & Pitt, M. (2009). An analysis of the academic literature on simulation and modelling in health care. *Journal of Simulation*, *3*(3), 130–140. doi:10.1057/jos200910

Brailsford, S. C., & Hilton, N. A. (2001). A comparison of discrete event simulation and system dynamics for modelling health care systems. In Riley, J. (Ed.), *Planning for the future: Health service quality and emergency accessibility. Operational research applied to health services (ORAHS)*. Glasgow Caledonian University.

Brailsford, S. C. (2007). Tutorial: Advances and challenges in healthcare simulation modelling. *Proceeding of the 2007 Winter Simulation Conference* (pp. 1436-1448).

Brandeau, M. L., Sainfort, F., & Pierskalla, W. P. (2004). *Operations reserach and health care-A handbook of methods and applications*. Springer.

Brennan, T. A., Leape, L. L., Laird, N. M., Hebert, L., Localio, A. R., & Lawthers, A. G. (1991). Incidence of adverse events and negligence in hospitalized patients. Results of the Harvard medical practice study I. *The New England Journal of Medicine*, *324*(6). doi:10.1056/NEJM199102073240604

Brokel, J. M. (2009). Redesigning care processes using an electronic health record: A system's experience. *Joint Commission Journal on Quality and Patient Safety*, *35*(2), 82–92.

Brown, G. E. (2004). *Clinical trials' EDC endgame. Forrester helping business thrive on technology change*. Retrieved from http://www.oracle.com/corporate/analyst-portal/insider/forrester_clinical_trials_edc_endgame.pdf

Bundy, D. G. (2005). Open access in primary care: results of a North Carolina pilot project. *Pediatrics*, *116*(1), 82–87. doi:10.1542/peds.2004-2573

Bureau of Infrastructure. Transport and Regional Economics. (2009). *Cost of road crashes in Australia 2006*. Report 118 Australian Government. Retrieved from http://www.bitre.gov.au/publications/48/Files/Cost_of_road_crashes_in_Australia.pdf

Bush, S. H., Lao, M. R., Simmons, K. L., Goode, J. H., Cunningham, S. A., & Calhoun, B. C. (2007). Patient access and clinical efficiency improvement in a resident hospital-based women's medicine center clinic. *The American Journal of Managed Care*, *13*(12), 686–690.

Butler, T. (1995). Management science/Operations research projects in healthcare: Administrator's perspective. *Health Care Management Review*, *20*(1), 19–25.

Buttell Crane, A. (2007). Management engineers. *Hospitals & Health Networks (H&HN), April*, 50. Retrieved from http://www.hhnmag.com/hhnmag_app/jsp/

Buzacott, J. A., & Shnathikumar, J. G. (1993). *Stochastic models of manufacturing systems*. Englewood Ciffs, NJ: Prentice-Hall.

Cahill, W., & Render, M. (1999). Dynamic simulation modelling of ICU bed availability. *Proceedings of the 1999 Winter Simulation Conference, 2*, (pp. 1573-1576).

Callen, J. L., Braithwaite, J., & Westbrook, J. I. (2008). Contextual implementation model: A framework for assisting clinical information system implementations. *Journal of the American Medical Informatics Association, 15*(2), 255–262. doi:10.1197/jamia.M2468

Cameron, P., Scown, P., & Campbell, D. (2002). Managing access block. *Australian Health Review, 25*, 59–68. doi:10.1071/AH020059

Campbell, E. M., Sittig, D. F., Ash, J. S., Guappone, K. P., & Dykstra, R. H. (2006). Types of unintended consequences related to computerized provider order entry. *Journal of the American Medical Informatics Association, 13*, 547–556. doi:10.1197/jamia.M2042

Canby, J. B. IV. (1995). Applying activity-based costing to healthcare settings. *Healthcare Financial Management, 49*(2), 50–52, 54–56.

Cangialosi, A., Monaly, J. E., & Yang, S. C. (2007, September). Leveraging RFID in hospitals: Patient life cycle and mobility perspectives. *IEEE Communications Magazine, 45*(9), 18–23. doi:10.1109/MCOM.2007.4342874

Card, S., Moran, T., & Newell, A. (1983). *The psychology of human-computer interaction*. Hillsdale, NJ: Lawrence Erlbaum Associates.

Cardoen, B., Demeulemeester, E., & Beliën, J. (2010). Operating room planning and scheduling: A literature review. *European Journal of Operational Research, 201*(3), 921–932. doi:10.1016/j.ejor.2009.04.011

Carter, M. (2002). Healthcare management-Diagnosis: Mismanagement of resources. *Operation Research/Management Science (OR/MS). Today, 29*(2), 26–32.

Cartwright, A., & Windsor, J. (1992). *Outpatients and their doctors*. London, UK: HMSO.

Casey, R. G., Quinlan, M. R., Flynn, R., Grainger, R., McDermott, T. E., & Thornhill, J. A. (2007). Urology out-patient non-attenders: Are we wasting our time? *Irish Journal of Medical Science, 176*(4), 305–308. doi:10.1007/s11845-007-0028-8

Cates, G. R., & Mollaghasemi, M. (2005). *Supporting the vision for space with discrete event simulation.* Paper presented at the Winter Simulation Conference.

Cayirli, T., Veral, E., & Rosen, H. (2006). Designing appointment scheduling systems for ambulatory care services. *Health Care Management Science, 9*, 47–58. doi:10.1007/s10729-006-6279-5

Cayirli, T., & Veral, E. (2003). Outpatient scheduling in health care: A review of literature. *Production and Operations Management Society, 12*(4), 519–549. doi:10.1111/j.1937-5956.2003.tb00218.x

Cayirli, T., Veral, E., & Rosen, H. (2004). *Assessment of patient classification in appointment systems*, 1st Conference of the POMS College of Service Operations.

CDC. (2008). HIV prevalence estimates-USA, 2006. *MMWR Weekly, 57*(39), 1073–1076.

Ceglowski, R., Churilov, L., & Wasserthiel, J. (2007). Combining data mining and discrete event simulation for a value-added view of a hospital emergency department. *The Journal of the Operational Research Society, 58*(2), 246–254.

Center for Medicare and Medicaid Services, Office of the Actuaries. (2010). *Estimated financial effects of the Patient Protection and Affordable Care Act as amended.* Washington, DC: U.S. Government Printing Office. Retrieved from https://www.cms.gov/ ActuarialStudies/ Downloads/ PPACA_2010-04-22.pdf

Center for Telemedicine Law. (2003). *Telemedicine reimbursement report*. Prepared for the Office of Advancement of Telehealth, Health Resources and Services Administration. Washington, DC: Center for Telemedicine Law. Retrieved from ftp://ftp.hrsa.gov/ telehealth/ licen.pdf

Chahal, K., & Eldabi, T. (2010). A multi-perspective comparison for selection between system dynamics and discrete event simulation. *International Journal of Business Information Systems, 6*(1), 4–17.

Chan, Y. C. L. (1993). Improving hospital cost accounting with activity-based costing. *Health Care Management Review*, *18*(1), 71–77.

Chand, S., Moskowitz, H., Norris, J. B., Shade, S., & Willis, D. R. (2009). Improving patient flow at an outpatient clinic: Study of sources of variability and improvement factors. *Health Care Management Science*, *12*(3), 325–340. doi:10.1007/s10729-008-9094-3

Chang, I. C., Hwang, H. G., Hung, M. C., Lin, M. H., & Yen, D. C. (2007). Factors affecting the adoption of electronic signature: Executives' perspective of hospital information department. *Decision Support Systems*, *44*, 350–359. doi:10.1016/j.dss.2007.04.006

Chantler, C. (1999). The role and education of doctors in the delivery of health care. *Lancet*, *353*(9159), 1178–1181. doi:10.1016/S0140-6736(99)01075-2

Checkland, P. (1981). *Systems thinking, systems practice*. Chichester, UK: Wiley.

Chen, M., Gonzalez, S., Leung, V., Zhang, Q., & Li, M. (2010). A 2G-RFID-based e-healthcare system. *IEEE Wireless Communications*, *17*(1), 37–43. doi:10.1109/MWC.2010.5416348

Chen, C., Garrido, T., Chock, D., Okawa, G., & Liang, L. (2009). The Kaiser Permanente electronic health record: Transforming and streamlining modalities of care. *Health Affairs*, *28*(2), 323–333. doi:10.1377/hlthaff.28.2.323

Chen, P. (2010). Doctors and patients, lost in paperwork. *New York Times*, pp. 1-3.

Chisolm, C. D. (2008). A comparison of observed versus documented physician assessment and treatment of pain: The physician record does not reflect the reality. *Annals of Emergency Medicine*, *52*(4), 383–389. doi:10.1016/j.annemergmed.2008.01.004

Christoffel, T. (2008). Thinking outside the box. *Biomedical Instrumentation & Technology*, *3*(42), 173.

Chu, W. H. J., & Lee, C. C. (2006). Strategic information sharing in a supply chain. *European Journal of Operational Research*, *174*(3), 1567–1579. doi:10.1016/j.ejor.2005.02.053

Civelek, A. C. (2009). Patient safety and privacy in the electronic health information era: Medical and beyond. *Clinical Biochemistry*, *42*(4-5), 298–299. doi:10.1016/j.clinbiochem.2008.09.018

Clague, J. E., Reed, P. G., Barlow, J., Rada, R., Clarke, M., & Edwards, R. H. (1997). Improving outpatient clinic efficiency using computer simulation. *International Journal of Health Care Quality Assurance*, *10*, 197–201. doi:10.1108/09526869710174177

Clancy, T. R., Delaney, C. W., Segre, A., Carley, K., Kuziak, A., & Yu, H. (2007). Predicting the impact of an electronic health record on practice patterns using computational modeling and simulation. *AMIA Annual Symposium Proceedings*, (pp. 145-9).

Clerkin, D., Fos, P., & Petry, F. (1995). A decision support system for hospital bed assignment. *Hospital & Health Services Administration*, *40*, 386–400.

Cleverley, W. O. (2002). The hospital cost index: A new way to assess relative cost-efficiency. *Healthcare Financial Management*, *56*(7), 36–42.

Cochran, J. K., & Bharti, A. (2006). A multi-stage methodology for whole hospital bed planning. *International Journal of Industrial and Systems Engineering*, *1*(1), 8–36. doi:10.1504/IJISE.2006.009048

Cochran, J. K., & Roche, K. (2009). A multi-class queuing network analysis methodology for improving hospital emergency department performance. *Computers & Operations Research*, *36*(5), 1497–1512. doi:10.1016/j.cor.2008.02.004

Cole, D. N. (comp). (2005). *Computer simulation modeling of recreation use: Current status, case studies, and future directions*. (Gen. Tech. Rep. RMRS-GTR-143). Fort Collins, CO: US Department of Agriculture, Forest Service, Rocky Mountain Research Station.

Commonwealth of Australia. (2009). *A healthier future for all Australians*. Final report of the National Health and Hospitals Reform Commission.

Conforti, D., Guerriero, F., & Guido, R. (2008). Optimization models for radiotherapy patient scheduling. *4OR: A Quarterly Journal of Operations Research*, *6*(3), 263-278.

Congressional Budget Office. (2009). *The long-term budget outlook.* (Publication No. 3216). Washington DC: Author. Retrieved from http://www.cbo.gov/ ftpdocs/ 102xx/ doc10297/ 06-25-LTBO.pdf

Congressional Budget Office. H.R. 4872, Reconciliation Act of 2010. Washington, DC. March 18, 2010. Retrieved from http://www.cbo.gov/ ftpdocs/ 113xx/ doc11355/ hr4872.pdf

Connelly, L. G., & Bair, A. E. (2004). Discrete event simulation of emergency department activity: A platform for system-level operations research. *Academic Emergency Medicine*, *11*(11), 1177–1185. doi:10.1111/j.1553-2712.2004.tb00702.x

Conroy, M., Majchrzak, N., Silverman, C., Chang, Y., Regan, S., Schneider, L., & Rigotti, N. A. (2005). Measuring provider adherence to tobacco treatment guidelines: A comparison of electronic medical record review, patient survey, and provider survey. *Nicotine & Tobacco Research*, *7*(Suppl 1), S35–S43. doi:10.1080/14622200500078089

Contrandripoulos, A. P., Denis, J. L., Touati, N., & Rogriguez, C. (2003). *The integration of health care: Dimensions and implementation.* (Working Paper No 4-01). Montréal, Canada: Université de Montréal Groupe deresearche interdisciplinaire en santé.

Cook, R. I., & Woods, D. (1994). Operating at the sharp end: The complexity of human error. In Bogner, M. (Ed.), *Human errors in medicine*. Hillsdale, NJ: Erlbaum.

Cook, C., & Perez, R. (2003). A management engineering approach to improving throughput and shortening overall LOS: A unique model for efficiency and time studies. *Collaborative Case Management – The Official Publication of the American Case Management Association. 1*(4).

Corbin, A. (2007). The 360-degree approach. EHRs are only a first step in what should be an effort to integrate clinical and financial applications. *Healthcare Informatics*, *24*(5), 42.

Corfield, L., Schizas, A., Noorani, A., & Williams, A. (2008). Non-attendance at the colorectal clinic: A prospective audit. *Annals of the Royal College of Surgeons of England*, *90*(5), 377–380. doi:10.1308/003588408X301172

Correa, F., Gil, M., & Redín, L. (2005). *Benefits of connecting RFID and lean principles in healthcare.* Working Paper 05-44 Business Economics Series 10, Universidad Carlos III de Madrid, Departamento de Economía de la Empresa.

Costa, A., Ridley, S., Shahani, A., Harper, P., De Senna, V., & Nielsen, M. (2003). Mathematical modeling and simulation for planning critical care capacity. *Anesthesia*, *58*, 320–327. doi:10.1046/j.1365-2044.2003.03042.x

Costa, A. X., Ridely, S. A., Shahani, A. K., Harper, P. R., De Senna, V., & Nielsen, M. S. (2003). Mathematical modeling and simulation for planning critical care capacity. *Anesthesiology*, *58*, 320–327.

Côté, M., & Stein, W. (2000). An Erlang-based stochastic model for patient flow. *OMEGA: The International Journal of Management Science*, *28*(3), 347–359. doi:10.1016/S0305-0483(99)00045-6

Cox, T. F., Birchall, J. F., & Wong, H. (1985). Optimizing the queuing system for an ear, nose and throat outpatient clinic. *Journal of Applied Statistics*, *12*(2), 113–126. doi:10.1080/02664768500000017

Cross, H. M. (2009). The EHR in our emerging future. *Behavioral Healthcare*, *29*(8), 40.

Cutler, D. M., & McClellan, M. (2001). Productivity change in health care. *The American Economic Review*, *91*(2), 281–286. doi:10.1257/aer.91.2.281

Das, R. (2004). *IDTechEx White Paper: RFID explained.* Retrieved 2009, from www.idii.com/wp/ IDTechExRFID.pdf

David, Y., & Jahnke, E. G. (2004). Planning hospital medical technology management. *IEEE Engineering in Medicine and Biology Magazine*, *23*(3), 73–79. doi:10.1109/MEMB.2004.1317985

Davies, R. (1994). Simulation for planning services for patients with coronary artery disease. *European Journal of Operational Research*, *72*(2), 323–332. doi:10.1016/0377-2217(94)90313-1

D'Avolio, L. W. (2009). Electronic medical records at a crossroads: Impetus for change or missed opportunity? *Journal of the American Medical Association*, *302*(10), 1109–1111. doi:10.1001/jama.2009.1319

Dawes, K. S. (1972). Survey of general practice records. *British Medical Journal*, *3*, 219–223. doi:10.1136/bmj.3.5820.219

de Bruin, A., Koole, G., & Visser, M. (2005). Bottleneck analysis of emergency cardiac in-patient flow in a university setting: An application of queueing theory. *Clinical and Investigative Medicine. Medecine Clinique et Experimentale*, *28*(6), 316–317.

De Bruin, A., van Rossum, A., Visser, M., & Koole, G. (2007). Modeling the emergency cardiac in-patient flow: An application of queuing theory. *Health Care Management Science*, *10*, 125–137. doi:10.1007/s10729-007-9009-8

Dean, A., & Voss, D. (1999). *Design and analysis of experiments*. New York, NY: Springer-Verlag, Inc. doi:10.1007/b97673

Dean, B. B., Lam, J., Natoli, J. L., Butler, Q., Aguilar, D., & Nordyke, R. J. (2008). Toward a model of successful electronic health record adoption. *Healthcare Quarterly (Toronto, Ont.)*, *11*(3), 84–91.

Dellinger, R. P., Carlet, J. M., Masur, H., Gerlach, H., Calandra, T., & Cohen, J. (2004). Surviving sepsis campaign guidelines for management of severe sepsis and septic shock. *Critical Care Medicine*, *32*(3), 858–873. doi:10.1097/01.CCM.0000117317.18092.E4

Dempsey, M. (2005). *Intelligent location*. Patient Safety and Quality Healthcare Conference.

Denton, B., Viapiano, J., & Vogl, A. (2007). Optimization of surgery sequencing and scheduling decisions under uncertainty. *Health Care Management Science*, *10*, 13–24. doi:10.1007/s10729-006-9005-4

Department of Finance and Deregulation. Australian Government. (2010). *Best practice regulation: Value of a statistical life*. Retrieved from http://www.finance.gov.au/obpr/docs/ValuingStatisticalLife.rtf

Department of Health and Human Services. (2001). *HHS pandemic influenza plan supplement 10: Public health communications*. Retrieved May 30, 2010, from http://www.hhs.gov/pandemicflu /plan/sup10.html

Department of Health and Human Services. (2008). *The National Alliance for Health Information Technology report to the Office of the National Coordinator for Health Information Technology on defining key health Information Technology terms*. Retrieved May 30, 2010, from http://healthit.hhs.gov/portal/ server.pt/gateway/PTARGS_0_10741_848133_0_0_18/10_2_hit_terms.pdf

Department of Health and Human Services. (n.d.). *Electronic medical records*. Retrieved May 30, 2010, from http://healthit.hhs.gov/portal/ server.pt?open=512&mode=2 &cached=true&objID=1219

Dervin, J. V., Stone, D. L., & Beck, C. H. (1978). The no-show patient in the model family practice unit. *The Journal of Family Practice*, *7*(6), 1177–1180.

DesRoches, C. M., Campbell, E. G., & Rao, S. R. (2008). Electronic health records in ambulatory care: A national survey for physicians. *The New England Journal of Medicine*, *359*, 50–60. doi:10.1056/NEJMsa0802005

Detmer, D. E. (2003). Building the national health information infrastructure for personal health, health care services, public health, and research. *BMC Medical Informatics and Decision Making*, *3*, 1. doi:10.1186/1472-6947-3-1

Detty, R., & Yingling, J. (2000, January 20). Quantifying benefits of conversion to lean manufacturing with discrete event simulation: A case study. *International Journal of Production Research*, *38*(2), 429–445. doi:10.1080/002075400189509

Deyo, R. A., & Inui, T. S. (1980). Dropouts and broken appointments: A literature review and agenda for future research. *Medical Care*, *18*(11), 1146–1157. doi:10.1097/00005650-198011000-00006

Dimitropoulos, L., & Rizk, S. (2009). A state-based approach to privacy and security for interoperable health information exchange. *Health Affairs*, *28*(2), 428–434. doi:10.1377/hlthaff.28.2.428

Dittus, R. S., Klein, R. W., DeBrota, D. J., Dame, M. A., & Fitzgerald, J. F. (1996). Medical resident work schedules: Design and evaluation by simulation modeling. *Management Science*, *42*(6), 891–906. doi:10.1287/mnsc.42.6.891

Dittus, R. S. (2001). Discrete-event simulation modeling of the content, processes and structures of healthcare. In Institute of Medicine Committee on Quality of Healthcare in America (Eds.), *Crossing the quality chasm: A new health system for the 21st century.*

Doebbeling, B. N., & Pekny, J. (2008). The role of systems factors in implementing health information technology. *Journal of General Internal Medicine*, *23*(4), 500–501. doi:10.1007/s11606-008-0559-3

Does, R., Vermaat, T., Verver, J., Bisgaard, S., & Van Den Heuvel, J. (2009). Reducing start time delays in operating rooms. *Journal of Quality Technology*, *41*(1), 95–109.

Donchin, Y., Gopher, D., Olin, M., Badihi, Y., Biesky, M., & Sprung, C. L. (2003). A look into the nature and causes of human errors in the intensive care unit. *Quality & Safety in Health Care*, *12*(2), 143–147. doi:10.1136/qhc.12.2.143

Dong, Y., Lu, H., Rotz, J., Schieffer, C., Kashyap, R., & Pickering, B. W. (2009). Simulation modeling of healthcare delivery during sepsis resuscitation. *Critical Care Medicine*, *37*(Suppl S), 686.

Dong, Y., Suri, H. S., Cook, D. A., Kashani, K. B., Mullon, J. J., & Enders, F. T. (2010). Simulation-based objective assessment discerns clinical proficiency in central line placement: A construct validation. *Chest*, *137*(5). doi:10.1378/chest.09-1451

Dubin, R. (1976). Organizational effectiveness: Some dilemmas of perspective. In Lee, S. (Ed.), *Organizational effectiveness: Theory-research-utilization* (p. 7). Kent, OH: Kent State University Press.

Duggan, J. (2008). Using system dynamics and multiple objective optimization to support policy analysis for complex systems. In Qudrat-Ullah, H., Spector, J. M., & Davidsen, P. I. (Eds.), *Complex decision making: Theory and practice* (pp. 59–81). Cambridge, MA: Springer.

Dyer, J. S., Fishburn, R. E., Wallenius, J., & Zionts, S. (1992). Multiple criteria decision making, multiattribute utility theory: The next ten years. *Management Science*, *38*(5), 645–654. doi:10.1287/mnsc.38.5.645

Edwards, R., Clague, J. E., Barlow, J., Clarke, M., Reed, P. G., & Rada, R. (1994). Operations research survey and computer simulation of waiting times in two medical outpatient clinic structures. *Health Care Analysis*, *2*, 164–169. doi:10.1007/BF02249741

Ehsani, J. P., Jackson, T., & Duckett, S. J. (2006). The incidence and cost of adverse events in Victorian hospitals 2003–04. *The Medical Journal of Australia*, *184*(11), 551–555.

Eldabi, T., Irani, Z., & Paul, R. J. (2002). A proposed approach for modelling health-care systems for understanding. *Journal of Management in Medicine*, *16*(2-3), 170–187. doi:10.1108/02689230210434916

Eldabi, T., Paul, R. J., & Young, T. (2007). Simulation modelling in healthcare: Reviewing legacies and investigating futures. *The Journal of the Operational Research Society*, *58*(2), 262–270.

EPCglobal. (2007). *Tag data standards version 1.3.1.* EPCglobal Inc

Eriksson, H. (2000). *Medical research and its impact on healthcare design.* International Academy for Design and Health. Retrieved from http://www.designandhealth.com/uploaded/documents/Publications/Papers/Hakan-Eriksson-WCDH2000.pdf

Etzioni, A. (1964). *Modern organizations.* Englewood Cliffs, NJ: Prentice-Hall.

Evans, A. M., & Wakeford, J. (1964). Research on hospital outpatients and casualty attendances: A strategy for improvement. *British Medical Journal*, *299*, 722–724.

Fabri, P. (2008). Can healthcare engineering fix healthcare? *American Medical Association Journal of Ethics*, *10*(5), 317–319.

Fatovich, D., Nagree, Y., & Sprivulis, P. (2005). Access block causes emergency department overcrowding and ambulance diversion in Perth, Western Australia. *Emergency Medicine Journal*, *22*, 351–354. doi:10.1136/emj.2004.018002

Fattore, G., & Torbica, A. (2006). Inpatient reimbursement system in Italy: How do tariffs relate to cost? *Health Care Management Science*, *9*, 251–258. doi:10.1007/s10729-006-9092-2

Fei, H., Chu, C., & Meskens, N. (2009). Solving a tactical operating room planning problem by a column-generation based heuristic procedure with four criteria. *Annals of Operations Research*, *166*, 91–108. doi:10.1007/s10479-008-0413-3

Fei, H., Meskens, N., & Chu, C. (2010). A planning and scheduling problem for an operating theatre using an open scheduling strategy. *Computers & Industrial Engineering*, *58*(2), 221. doi:10.1016/j.cie.2009.02.012

Ferrer, R., Artigas, A., Levy, M. M., Blanco, J., Gonzalez-Diaz, G., & Garnacho-Montero, J. (2008). Improvement in process of care and outcome after a multicenter severe sepsis educational program in Spain. *Journal of the American Medical Association*, *299*(19), 2294–2303. doi:10.1001/jama.299.19.2294

Fetter, R., & Thompson, J. (1966). Patients' waiting time and doctors' idle time in the outpatient setting. *Health Services Research*, *1*, 66–90.

Fischman, D. (2010). Applying lean six sigma methodologies to improve efficiency, timeliness of care, and quality of care in an internal medicine residency clinic. *Quality Management in Health Care*, *19*(3), 201–210.

Fletcher, A., & Worthington, D. (2009). What is a generic hospital model?—A comparison of generic and specific hospital models of emergency patient flows. *Health Care Management Science*, *12*(4), 374–391. doi:10.1007/s10729-009-9108-9

Fomundam, S., & Herrmann, J. (2007). *A survey of queuing theory applications in healthcare. The Institute of Systems Research, A. James Clarke School of Engineering*. University of Maryland.

Fone, D., Hollinghurst, S., Temple, M., Round, A., Lester, N., & Weightman, A. (2003). Systematic review of the use and value of computer simulation modelling in population health and health care delivery. *Journal of Public Health Medicine*, *25*(4), 325–335. doi:10.1093/pubmed/fdg075

Forrester, J. W. (1961). *Industrial dynamics*. Productivity Press.

Forster, A. J., Stiell, I., & Wells, G. (2003). The effect of hospital occupancy on emergency department length of stay and patient disposition. *Academic Emergency Medicine*, *10*, 127–133. doi:10.1111/j.1553-2712.2003.tb00029.x

Fries, B., & Marathe, V. (1981). Determination of optimal variable-sized multiple-block appointment systems. *Operations Research*, *29*(2), 324–345. doi:10.1287/opre.29.2.324

Fries, J. F. (1974). Alternatives in medical record formats. *Medical Care*, *12*, 871–881. doi:10.1097/00005650-197410000-00006

Frohlich, J., Karp, S., Smith, M., & Sujansky, W. (2007). Retrospective: Lessons learned from The Santa Barbara Project and their implications for health information exchange. *Health Affairs*, *26*(5), w589–w591. doi:10.1377/hlthaff.26.5.w589

Fushimi, K., Hashimoto, H., Imanaka, Y., Kuwabara, K., Horiguchi, H., Ishikawa, K., & Masuda, S. (2007). Functional mapping of hospitals by diagnosis-dominant case-mix analysis. *BMC Health Services Research*, *7*(50). Retrieved from http://www.biomedicentral.com/1472-6963/7/50.

Galbreth, M., & Shor, M. (2010). (in press). The impact of malicious agents on the enterprise software industry. *Management Information Systems Quarterly*, *34*(3).

Gallucci, G., Swartz, W., & Hackerman, F. (2005). Brief reports: Impact of the wait for an initial appointment on the rate of kept appointments at a mental health center. *Psychiatric Services (Washington, D.C.)*, *56*(3), 344–346. doi:10.1176/appi.ps.56.3.344

Gandjour, A., & Lauterbach, K. W. (2001). A method for assessing the cost-effectiveness and the break-even point of clinical practice guidelines. *International Journal of Technology Assessment in Health Care*, *17*(4), 503–516.

Garcia, M. L., Centeno, M. A., Rivera, C., & DeCario, N. (1995). Reducing time in an emergency room via a fast-track. In C. Alexopoulos, K. Kang, W. R. Lilegdon, & D. Goldsman (Ed.), *Proceedings of the 1995 Winter Simulation Conference*, (pp. 1048-1053). Washington DC, USA.

Garfinkel, S. L., Juels, A., & Pappu, R. (2005, May-June). RFID privacy: An overview of problems and proposed solutions. *IEEE Security & Privacy*, *3*(3), 34–43. doi:10.1109/MSP.2005.78

Garrett, D. (2010). Tapping into the value of health data through secondary use. *Healthcare Financial Management*, *64*(2), 76–83.

Garrouste-Orgeas, M., Timsit, J. F., Vesin, A., Schwebel, C., Arnodo, P., & Lefrant, J. Y. (2010). Selected medical errors in the intensive care unit: Results of the IATROREF study: Parts I and II. *American Journal of Respiratory and Critical Care Medicine*, *181*(2), 134–142. doi:10.1164/rccm.200812-1820OC

Gawande, A. (2007, December 10). The checklist If something so simple can transform intensive care, what else can it do? *New Yorker (New York, N.Y.)*, 86–101.

Gee, P. (2006). DRG do over the need for a service-line strategy. *Financial Management*, *60*(8), 52–55.

Ghaferi, A. A., Birkmeyer, J. D., & Dimick, J. B. (2009). Variation in hospital mortality associated with inpatient surgery. *The New England Journal of Medicine*, *361*, 1368–1375. doi:10.1056/NEJMsa0903048

Giachetti, R. E., Centeno, E. A., Centeno, M. A., & Sundaram, R. (2005). Assessing the viability of an open access policy in an outpatient clinic: A discrete-event and continuous simulation modeling approach. *Proceedings of the 2005 Winter Simulation Conference*.

Giannangelo, K., & Fenton, S. H. (2008). SNOMED CT survey: An assessment of implementation in EMR/EHR applications. *Perspectives in Health Information Management*, *5*(7), 1–13.

Gilmer, T. P., & Kronick, R. G. (2010). Hard times and health insurance: How many Americans will be uninsured by 2010? *Health Affairs*, *28*(4), w573–w577. doi:10.1377/hlthaff.28.4.w573

Glantz, S., & Slinker, B. (2001). *Applied regression & analysis of variance* (2nd ed.). McGraw-Hill, Inc.

Glaser, J. (2009). Implementing electronic health records: 10 factors for success. *Healthcare Financial Management*, *63*(1), 50–52, 54.

Glowacka, K., Henry, R., & May, J. (2009). A hybird data mining/simulation approach for modelling outpatient no-shows in clinic scheduling. *The Journal of the Operational Research Society*, *60*(8), 1056–1068. doi:10.1057/jors.2008.177

Goitein, M. (1990). Waiting patiently. *The New England Journal of Medicine*, *323*, 604–608. doi:10.1056/NEJM199008303230911

Goldman, L., Freidin, R., Cook, E. F., Eigner, J., & Grich, P. (1982). A multivariate approach to the prediction of no-show behavior in a primary care center. *Archives of Internal Medicine*, *142*(3), 563–567. doi:10.1001/archinte.142.3.563

Goldratt, E., & Cox, J. (2004). *The goal* (3rd ed., p. 384). Great Barrington, MA: North River Press.

Goldschmidt-Clermont, P. J., Dong, C., Rhodes, N. M., McNeill, D. B., Adams, M. B., & Gilliss, C. L. (2009). Autonomic care systems for hospitalized patients. *Academic Medicine*, *84*, 1727–1731. doi:10.1097/ACM.0b013e3181bf9bfd

Goodman, C. S. (2004). *HTA 101: Introduction to health technology assessment.* Retrieved August 2010, from http://www.nlm.nih.gov/ nichsr/ outreach.html

Gordon, T., Lyles, A. P. S., & Fountain, J. (1988). Surgical unit time review: Resource utilization and management implications. *Journal of Medical Systems*, *12*, 169–179. doi:10.1007/BF00996639

Graham, R. L. (1969). Bounds on multiprocessing timing anomalies. *SIAM Journal on Applied Mathematics*, *17*, 263–269. doi:10.1137/0117039

Green, L. V., & Savin, S. (2008). Reducing delays for medical appointments: A queueing approach. *Operations Research*, *56*(6), 1526–1538. doi:10.1287/opre.1080.0575

Green, L. (2006). Queuing analysis in healthcare. In Hall, R. (Ed.), *Patient flow: Reducing delay in healthcare delivery* (pp. 281–307). New York, NY: Springer.

Griffiths, J. D., Jones, M., Read, M. S., & Williams, J. E. (2010). A simulation model of bed-occupancy in a critical care unit. *Journal of Simulation*, *4*(1), 52–59. doi:10.1057/jos.2009.22

Grimes, S. L. (2003). The future of clinical engineering: The challenge of change. *IEEE Engineering in Medicine and Biology Magazine*, *22*(2), 91–99. doi:10.1109/MEMB.2003.1195702

Grimson, J. (2001). Delivering the electronic healthcare record for the 21st century. *International Journal of Medical Informatics*, *64*(2-3), 111–127. doi:10.1016/S1386-5056(01)00205-2

Grol, R., & Grimshaw, J. (2003). From best evidence to best practice: Effective implementation of change in patients' care. *Lancet*, *362*(9391), 1225–1230. doi:10.1016/S0140-6736(03)14546-1

Gross, D., & Harris, C. M. (2003). *Fundamentals of queuing theory* (3rd ed.). New York, NY: John Wiley & Sons.

Gruber, J. (2009). Getting the facts straight on healthcare reform. *The New England Journal of Medicine*, *361*, 2497–2499. doi:10.1056/NEJMp0911715

Grunebaum, M., Luber, P., Callahan, M., & Leon, A. C. (1996). Predictors of missed appointments for psychiatric consultations in a primary care clinic. *Psychiatric Services (Washington, D.C.)*, *47*(8), 848–852.

Gruzd, D. C., Shear, C. L., & Rodney, M. (1986). Determinants of no-show appointment behavior: The utility of multivariate analysis. *Family Medicine*, *18*(4), 217–220.

Guo, M., Wagner, M., & West, C. (2003). Outpatient clinic scheduling – A simulation approach. *Proceedings of the 2004 Winter Simulation Conference*.

Gupta, D., & Denton, B. (2008). Appointment scheduling in health care: Challenges and opportunities. *IIE Transactions*, *40*(9), 800–819. doi:10.1080/07408170802165880

Gupta, D., & Denton, B. (2008). Appointment scheduling in health care: Challenges and opportunities. *IIE Transactions*, *40*, 800–819. doi:10.1080/07408170802165880

Hagland, M. (2009). A glass slipper? For cash-strapped organizations with EMR dreams, open-source software may be a perfect fit. *Healthcare Informatics*, *26*(8), 32–36.

Halamka, J., Overhage, J., Ricciardi, L., Rishel, W., Shirky, C., & Diamond, C. (2005). Exchanging health information: Local distribution, national coordination. *Health Affairs*, *24*(5), 1170–1179. doi:10.1377/hlthaff.24.5.1170

Hall, R. W. (Ed.). (2006). *Patient flow: Reducing delay in healthcare delivery*. Los Angeles, CA: Springer.

Halpern, N. A., & Pastores, S. M. (2010). Critical care medicine in the United States 2000-2005: An analysis of bed numbers, occupancy rates, payer mix, and costs. *Critical Care Medicine*, *38*(1), 65–71. doi:10.1097/CCM.0b013e3181b090d0

Handler, T. (2008). Gartner 2008 North American enterprise CPR generation evaluation: Nearly half the products evaluated have finally reached generation 3. *Gartner*, 1-9.

Hannan, T. (1999). Variation in health care – The roles of the electronic medical record. *International Journal of Medical Informatics*, *54*, 127–136. doi:10.1016/S1386-5056(98)00175-0

Hanser, F., Gruenerbl, A., Rodegast, C., & Lukowicz, P. (2008, February). *Design and real life deployment of a pervasive monitoring system for dementia patients*. Second International Conference on Pervasive Computing Technologies for Healthcare, (pp. 279-280).

Haraden, C., Nolan, T., & Litvak, E. (2003). *Optimizing patient flow: Moving patients smoothly through acute care setting*. Cambridge, MA: Institute for Healthcare Improvement Innovation.

Haraden, C., & Resar, R. (2004). Patient flow in hospitals. *Frontiers of Health Services Management*, *20*(4), 3–15.

Harlan, G., Srivastava, R., Harrison, L., McBride, G., & Maloney, C. (2009). Pediatric hospitalists and primary care providers: A communication needs assessment. *Journal of Hospital Medicine*, *4*(3), 187–193. doi:10.1002/jhm.456

Harper, P. R., & Gamlin, H. M. (2003). Reduced outpatient waiting times with improved appointment scheduling: A simulation modelling approach. *OR-Spektrum*, *25*(2), 207–222. doi:10.1007/s00291-003-0122-x

Harper, P. (2002). A framework for operational modelling of hospital resources. *Health Care Management Science*, *5*(3), 165–173. doi:10.1023/A:1019767900627

Hart, M. (1995). Improving out-patient clinic waiting times: Methodological and substantive issues. *International Journal of Health Care Quality Assurance*, *8*(6), 14. doi:10.1108/09526869510098813

Haut, E. R., Chang, D. C., Hayanga, A. J., Efron, D. T., Haider, A. H., & Cornwell Iii, E. E. (2009). Surgeon- and system-based influences on trauma mortality. *Archives of Surgery*, *144*(8), 759–764. doi:10.1001/archsurg.2009.100

Haux, R. (2005). Health Information Systems - Past, present, future. *International Journal of Medical Informatics*, *75*(3-4), 268–281. doi:10.1016/j.ijmedinf.2005.08.002

Hawrylak, P. J., Cain, J. T., & Mickle, M. H. (2007). Analytic modeling methodology for analysis of energy consumption for ISO 18000-7 RFID networks. *International Journal of Radio Frequency Identification Technology and Applications, 1*(4), 371–400. doi:10.1504/IJRFITA.2007.017748

Hawrylak, P. J., Mats, L., Cain, J. T., Jones, A. K., Tung, S., & Mickle, M. H. (2006, July). Ultra low-power computing systems for wireless devices. *International Review on Computers and Software, 1*(1), 1–10.

Hawrylak, P. J., Cain, J. T., & Mickle, M. H. (2008). RFID tags. In Yan, L., Zhang, Y., Yang, L. T., & Ning, H. (Eds.), *The Internet of things: From RFID to pervasive networked systems*. Boca Raton, FL: Auerbach Publications, Taylor & Francis Group. doi:10.1201/9781420052824.ch1

Hawrylak, P. J., & Mickle, M. H. (2009). EPC Gen-2 standard for RFID. In Y. Zhang, L. T. Yang & J. Chen (Eds.), *RFID and sensor networks: Architectures, protocols, security and integrations* (pp. 97-124), Boca Raton, FL: Taylor & Francis Group, CRC Press.

Haynes, A. B., Weiser, T. G., Berry, W. R., Lipsitz, S. R., Breizat, A. H. S., & Dellinger, E. P. (2009). A surgical safety checklist to reduce morbidity and mortality in a global population. *The New England Journal of Medicine, 360*(5), 491–499. doi:10.1056/NEJMsa0810119

Health Care Advisory Board. (n.d.). *HHS release meaningful use rule, shaping HER adoption*. Retrieved on July 14, 2010, from http://www.advisory.com/login/ login.aspx?URL=/members/ new_layout/default.asp?contentid =92039&program=1&collect

Healthcare and Education Reconciliation Act of 2010. P.L. 111-152. Washington, DC: GPO, 2010.

Healthcare at the Crossroads. (2008). *Guiding principles for the development of the hospital of the future.* The Joint Commission. Retrieved from http://www.jointcommission.org/NR/rdonlyres/1C9A7079-7A29-4658-B80D-A7DF8771309B/0/Hosptal_Future.pdf

Henderson, D., Dempsey, C., & Appleby, D. (2004). A case study of successful patient flow methods: St. John's Hospital. *Frontiers of Health Services Management, 20*(4), 25–30.

Hennessy-Fiske, M. (2010). UCLA is fined $95,000 for violating patient privacy. Retrieved June 30, 2010 from http://latimesblogs.latimes.com /lanow/2010/06/ucla-fined --for-violating-patient-privacy.html

Herasevich, V., Pickering, B. W., Dong, Y., Peters, S. G., & Gajic, O. (2010). Informatics infrastructure for syndrome surveillance, decision support, reporting, and modeling of critical illness. *Mayo Clinic Proceedings, 85*(3), 247–254. doi:10.4065/mcp.2009.0479

Herman, T., Pemmaraju, S. V., Segre, A. M., Polgreen, P. M., Curtis, D. E., & Fries, J. … Severson, M. (2009, May). Wireless applications for hospital epidemiology. In *Proceedings of the 1st ACM International Workshop on Medical-Grade Wireless Networks*, (pp. 45-50). New York, NY: ACM.

Hersh, W. (2007). Adding value to the electronic health record through secondary use of data for quality assurance, research, and surveillance. *The American Journal of Managed Care, 13*(6 Part 1), 277–278.

Hersh, W. (2009). A stimulus to define informatics and health Information Technology. *BMC Medical Informatics and Decision Making, 9*(24). doi:.doi:10.1186/1472-6947-9-24

Hiatt, J. (2006). *Awareness desire knowledge ability reinforcement: How to implement successful change in our personal lives and professional careers*. Loveland, CO: Prosci.

Hill, D. L., Marchant, R. J., & Gant, P. D. (2007). *Reported road crashes in Western Australia 2005*. Perth, Western Australia: Road Safety Council of Western Australia.

Hillier, F. S., & Lieberman, G. J. (Eds.). (2000). *Introduction to operation research.* New York, NY: McGraw-Hill Companies, Inc.

Hindel, A. (1972). *Hospital waiting lists – A review.* Internal Report, Department of Operations Research, Lancaster University.

Hixon, A. L., Chapman, R. W., & Nuovo, J. (1999). Failure to keep clinic appointments: Implications for residency education and productivity. *Family Medicine, 31*(9), 627–630.

Ho, C., & Lau, H. (1992). Minimizing total cost in scheduling outpatient appointments. *Management Science, 38*(12), 1750–1764. doi:10.1287/mnsc.38.12.1750

Ho, C., & Lau, H. (1999). Evaluating the impact of operating conditions on the performance of appointment scheduling rules in service systems. *European Journal of Operational Research, 112*, 542–553. doi:10.1016/S0377-2217(97)00393-7

Ho, C., Lau, H., & Li, J. (1995). Introducing variable-interval appointment scheduling rules in service systems. *International Journal of Operations & Production Management, 15*(6), 59–68. doi:10.1108/01443579510090345

Holdgate, A., Morris, J., Fry, M., & Zecevic, M. (2007). Accuracy of triage nurses in predicting patient disposition. *Emergency Medicine Australasia: EMA, 19*(4), 341–345. doi:10.1111/j.1742-6723.2007.00996.x

Holpp, L. (1993). Eight definitions of quality in healthcare. *Journal for Quality and Participation, 16*(3), 18–26.

Hook, J. M., Pan, E., Adler-Milstein, J., Bu, D., & Walker, J. (2006). The value of healthcare information exchange and interoperability in New York State. *AMIA Annual Symposium Proceedings*, (p. 53).

Hoot, N., LeBlanc, L., Jones, I., Levin, S., Zhou, C., & Gadd, C. (2008). Forecasting emergency department crowding: A discrete event simulation. *Annals of Emergency Medicine, 52*(2), 116–125. doi:10.1016/j.annemergmed.2007.12.011

Hopp, W. J., & Spearman, M. L. (2008). *Factory physics* (3rd ed.). New York, NY: McGraw Hill.

Hripcsak, G., Senqupta, S., Wilcox, A., & Green, R. A. (2007). Emergency department access to a longitudinal medical record. *Journal of the American Medical Informatics Association, 14*(2), 235–238. doi:10.1197/jamia.M2206

Hrúz, B., & Zhou, M. (2007). *Modeling and control of discrete-event dynamic systems: With Petri nets and other tools* (1st ed.). Springer.

Huang, X. (1994). Patient attitude towards waiting in an outpatient clinic and its applications. *Health Services Management Research, 7*(1), 2–8.

Huang, Y. L. (2009). *An alternative outpatient scheduling system*. Germany: VDM Publishing House Ltd.

Hufnagel, S. P. (2009). Interoperability. *Military Medicine, 174*(5), 43–50.

Hughes, M., Carson, E. R., Makhlouf, M., Morgan, C. J., & Summers, R. (2000). Modelling a progressive care system using a coloured–timed Petri net. *Transactions of the Institute of Measurement and Control, 22*(3), 271–283.

Hung, G., & Kissoon, N. (2009). Impact of an observation unit and an emergency department-Admitted patient transfer mandate in decreasing overcrowding in a pediatric emergency department: A discrete event simulation exercise. *Pediatric Emergency Care, 25*(3), 160–163. doi:10.1097/PEC.0b013e31819a7e20

Huschka, T. R., Denton, B. T., Narr, B. J., & Thompson, A. C. (2008). Using simulation in the implementation of an outpatient procedure center. *Proceedings of the 2008 Winter Simulation Conference*, (pp. 1547-1552).

Huschka, T., Denton, B., Gul, S., & Fowler, J. (2007). Bi-criteria evaluation of an outpatient procedure center via simulation. *Proceedings of the 2007 Winter Simulation Conference*, (pp. 1510-1518).

Hutzschenreuter, A. (2004). *Waiting patiently: An analysis of the performance aspects of outpatient scheduling in health care institutes. BMI Paper*. Amsterdam, The Netherlands: Vrije Universiteit.

Indiana University School of Medicine. (2010, February 26). The most frequent error in medicine. ScienceDaily. Retrieved July 12, 2010, from http://www.sciencedaily.com /releases/2010/02/ 100226101330.htm

Institute for Healthcare Improvement (IHI). (2005). *Office practices*. Retrieved from http://www.ihi.org/IHI/Topics/OfficePractices/SpecialtyCareAccess/EmergingContent/Appointment+Sequence+Simulation.htm

Institute of Medicine. (2001). *Crossing the quality chasm: A new health system for the 21st century*. Committee on Quality of Healthcare in America.

Isken, M. (2002). Modeling and analysis of occupancy data: A healthcare capacity planning application. *International Journal of Information Technology and Decision Making, 1*(4), 707–729. doi:10.1142/S0219622002000439

Isken, M., Sugumaran, V., Ward, T., Minds, D., & Ferris, W. (2005). Collection and preparation of sensor network data to support modeling. *Health Care Management Science, 8*, 87–99. doi:10.1007/s10729-005-0392-8

ISO/IEC DTR 9126-4. (2001). *Software engineering-Product quality – Part 4: Quality in use metrics*. International Standards Organization.

Jack, B., Greenwald, J., Forsythe, S., O'Donnell, J., Johnson, A., & Schipelliti, L. ... Chetty, V. K. (2009). Developing the tools to administer a comprehensive hospital dischargep: The reengineered discharge (RED) program. Retrieved from http://innovations.ahrq.gov/content.aspx?id=1777

Jacobson, S., Hall, S., & Swisher, J. R. (2006). Discrete-event simulation of health care systems. In Hall, R. (Ed.), *Reducing delay in healthcare delivery* (pp. 211–252). New York, NY: Springer.

Jarvis, C. W. (2009). Investigate funding alternatives to support successful EHR implementation. *The Journal of Medical Practice Management, 24*(6), 335–338.

Jebali, A., Hadi Alouane, A. B., & Ladet, P. (2006). Operating rooms scheduling. *International Journal of Production Economics, 99*, 52–62. doi:10.1016/j.ijpe.2004.12.006

Jensen, K. (1996). *Coloured Petri nets. Basic concepts, analysis methods and practical use*. Berlin, Germany: Springer-Verlag EATCS Monographs on Theoretical Computer Science.

Jha, A. K., DesRoches, C. M., Campbell, E. G., Donelan, K., Rao, S. R., & Ferris, T. G. (2009). Use of electronic health records in U.S. hospitals. *The New England Journal of Medicine, 360*, 1628–1638. doi:10.1056/NEJMsa0900592

Ji, Y., Ying, H., Yen, J., Zhu, S., Barth-Jones, D. C., Miller, R. E., & Massanari, R. M. (2007). A distributed adverse drug reaction detection system using intelligent agents with a fuzzy recognition-primed decision model. *International Journal of Intelligent Systems, 22*, 827–845. doi:10.1002/int.20230

Jiang, L., & Giachetti, R. E. (2008). A queuing network model to analyze the impact of parallelization of care on patient cycle time. *Health Care Management Science, 11*(3), 248–261. doi:10.1007/s10729-007-9040-9

Jiang, L., & Giachetti, R. (2008). A queueing network model to analyze the impact of parallelization of care on patient cycle time. *Health Care Management Science, 11*(3), 248–261. doi:10.1007/s10729-007-9040-9

Jobson, J. D. (1992). *Applied multivariate data analysis, vol. 2: Categorical and multivariate methods*. New-York, NY: Springer-Verlag, LLC.

Johnson, S. M. (1954). Optimal two- and three-stage production schedules with setup times included. *Naval Research Logistics Quarterly, 1*(1), 61–68. doi:10.1002/nav.3800010110

Joint Commission Resources. (2004). JCAHO requirement: New leadership standard on managing patient flow for hospitals. *Joint Commission Perspectives, 24*(2), 13–14.

Jones, L., Leneman, L., & MacLean, U. (1987). *Consumer feedback for the NHS: A literature review*. London, UK: King Edward's Hospital Fund.

Jørgensen, J. (2002). Coloured Petri nets in UML-based software development – Designing middleware for pervasive healthcare. In K. Jensen (Ed.), *Proc. of the Fourth International Workshop on Practical Use of Coloured Petri Nets and the CPN*.

Journal, R. F. I. D. (2010a, April 29). RFID news roundup –April 29, 2010. *RFID Journal*. Retrieved April 30, 2010, from http://www.rfidjournal.com/ article/view/7564

Journal, R. F. I. D. (2010b, July 8). RFID news roundup – July 8, 2010. *RFID Journal*. Retrieved October 29, 2010, form http://www.rfidjournal.com/article/view/7712

Joustra, P., van der Sluis, E., & van Dijk, N. (2010). To pool or not to pool in hospitals: A theoretical and practical comparison for a radiotherapy outpatient department. *Annals of Operations Research, 178*, 77–89. doi:10.1007/s10479-009-0559-7

Juels, A. (2006, February). RFID security and privacy: A research survey. *IEEE Journal on Selected Areas in Communications, 24*(2). doi:10.1109/JSAC.2005.861395

Jun, G. T., Ward, J., Morris, Z., & Clarkson, J. (2009). Health care process modelling: Which method when? *International Journal for Quality in Health Care, 21*(3), 214–224. doi:10.1093/intqhc/mzp016

Jun, J. B., Jacobson, S. H., & Swisher, J. R. (1999). Applications of discrete-event simulation in health care clinics: A survey. *The Journal of the Operational Research Society*, *50*(2), 109–123.

Kaandorp, G., & Koole, G. (2007). Optimal outpatient appointment scheduling. *Health Care Management Science*, *10*(3), 217–229. doi:10.1007/s10729-007-9015-x

Kaelber, C. D., & Bates, W. D. (2007). Health information exchange and patient safety. *Journal of Biomedical Informatics*, *40*(6), S40–S45. doi:10.1016/j.jbi.2007.08.011

Kahn, J. M., & Bates, D. W. (2008). Improving sepsis care: The road ahead. *JAMA -. Journal of the American Medical Association*, *299*(19), 2322–2323. doi:10.1001/jama.299.19.2322

Kahn, J. M., & Rubenfeld, G. D. (2005). Translating evidence into practice in the intensive care unit: The need for a systems-based approach. *Journal of Critical Care*, *20*(3), 204–206. doi:10.1016/j.jcrc.2005.06.001

Kaiser Family Foundation. (2009). *The uninsured and the difference health insurance makes*. Retrieved from http://www.kff.org/ uninsured/ upload/ 1420-11-2.pdf

Kano, N. (1984, April). Attractive quality and must-be quality. *Journal of the Japanese Society for Quality Control*, *14*(2), 39–48.

Kao, E. P. C., & Tung, G. G. (1981). Bed allocation in a public health care delivery system. *Management Science*, *27*(5), 507–520. doi:10.1287/mnsc.27.5.507

Karnas, J., & Robles, J. (2007). Implementing the electronic medical record: Big Bang or phased rollout? *Creative Nursing*, *13*(2), 13–14.

Keller, T. F., & Laughhunn, D. J. (1973). An application of queuing theory to a congestion problem in an outpatient clinic. *Decision Sciences*, *4*(3), 379–394. doi:10.1111/j.1540-5915.1973.tb00563.x

Kelley, R. (2009). *Where can $700 billion in waste be cut annually from the U.S. healthcare system?* Retrieved July 27, 2010, from http://thomsonreuters.com/content/corporate/articles/healthcare_reform

Kelton, W., Sadowski, R., & Sturrock, D. (2007). *Simulation with Arena* (4th ed.). McGraw-Hill Science.

Kendall, D. (1951). Some problems in the theory of queues. *Journal of the Royal Statistical Society. Series B. Methodological*, *13*, 151–185.

Khoumbati, K., & Themistocleous, M. (2006). Evaluating integration approaches adopted by healthcare organizations. *Journal of Computer Information Systems*, *47*(2), 20–27.

Kim, S. C., Horowitz, I., Young, K. K., & Buckley, T. A. (1999). Analysis of capacity management of the intensive care unit in a hospital. *European Journal of Operational Research*, *115*, 36–46. doi:10.1016/S0377-2217(98)00135-0

Kim, S., & Giachetti, R. E. (2006). A stochastic mathematical appointment overbooking model for healthcare providers to improve profits. *IEEE Transactions on Systems, Man, and Cybernetics*, *36*(6), 1211–1219. doi:10.1109/TSMCA.2006.878970

Kim, Y., & Jo, H. (2009, August). Patient information display system in hospital using RFID. In *Proceedings of the 2009 International Conference on Hybrid Information Technology*, (pp. 397-400). New York, NY: ACM. Aug. 27 - 29, 2009.

Kirsch, I., Jungeblut, A., Jenkins, L., & Kolstad, A. (2002). *Adult literacy in America: A first look at the findings of the national adult literacy survey*, 3rd edition, vol. 201. Washington, DC: National Center for Education, U.S. Department of Education, 2002.

Klassen, K. J., & Rohleder, T. R. (1996). Scheduling outpatient appointment in a dynamic environment. *Journal of Operations Management*, *14*, 83–101. doi:10.1016/0272-6963(95)00044-5

Klassen, K. J., & Rohleder, T. R. (2004). Outpatient appointment scheduling with urgent clients in a dynamic, multi-period environment. *International Journal of Service Industry Management*, *15*(2), 167–186. doi:10.1108/09564230410532493

Kluger, J. (2009, March 25). Electronic health records: What's taking so long? Time Online.

Knaup, P., Garde, S., & Haux, R. (2007). Systematic planning of patient records for cooperative care and multicenter research. *International Journal of Medical Informatics*, *76*(2-3), 109–117. doi:10.1016/j.ijmedinf.2006.08.002

Kohn, L. T., Corrigan, J. M., & Donaldson, M. S. (Eds.). (2000). *To err is human: Building a safer health system. Committee on Quality of Healthcare in America*. Institute of Medicine.

Koizumi, N., Kuno, E., & Smith, T. (2005). Modeling patient flows using a queuing network with blocking. *Health Care Management Science*, *8*, 49–60. doi:10.1007/s10729-005-5216-3

Kokolakis, S., Gritzalis, D., & Katsikas, S. (1999). Generic security policies for healthcare Information Systems. *Health Informatics Journal*, *4*(3), 184–195. doi:10.1177/146045829800400309

Kolb, E. M. W., Schoening, S., Peck, J., & Lee, T. (2008). Reducing emergency department overcrowding: Five patient buffer concepts in comparison. *Proceedings of the 40th Conference on Winter Simulation*, December 07-10, 2008, Miami, Florida.

Kolker, A. (2008). Process modeling of emergency department patient flow: Effect of patient length of stay on ED diversion. *Journal of Medical Systems*, *32*(5), 389–401. doi:10.1007/s10916-008-9144-x

Kolker, A. (2009). Process modeling of ICU patient flow: Effect of daily load leveling on elective surgeries on ICU diversions. *Journal of Medical Systems*, *33*(1). doi:10.1007/s10916-008-9161-9

Kolker, A. (2010a). Queuing theory and discrete events simulation for healthcare: From basic processes to complex systems with interdependencies. In Abu-Taieh, E., & El Sheik, A. (Eds.), *Handbook of research on discrete event simulation technologies and applications* (pp. 443–483). Hershey, PA: IGI Global.

Kolker, A. (2010b). System engineering and management science for healthcare: Examples and fundamental principles. *Proceedings of the SHS/ASQ Conference and Expo*. Atlanta, GA, February 26, 2010.

Konrad, R., & Lawley, M. (2009). Input modeling for hospital simulaiton models using electronic messages. In M. Rossetti, R. Hill, B. Johansson, A. Dunkin, & A. Ingalls (Eds.), *Winter Simulation Conference*, (pp. 134-147). Austin.

Kopach, R., DeLaurentis, P.-C., Lawley, M., Muthuraman, K., Ozsen, L., & Rardin, R. (2007). Effects of clinical characteristics on successful open access scheduling. *Health Care Management Science*, *10*(2), 111–124. doi:10.1007/s10729-007-9008-9

Kopach-Konrad, R., Lawley, M., Criswell, M., Hasan, I., Chakraborty, S., & Pekny, J. (2007). Applying systems engineering principles in improving health. *Journal of General Internal Medicine*, *22*(Suppl 3), 431–437. doi:10.1007/s11606-007-0292-3

Koppel, R., Metlay, J. P., Cohen, A., Abaluck, B., Localio, A. R., Kimmel, S. E., & Strom, B. L. (2005). Role of computerized physician order entry systems in facilitating medication errors. *Journal of the American Medical Association*, *293*(10), 1197–1203. doi:10.1001/jama.293.10.1197

Koppel, R., Wetterneck, T., Telles, J. L., & Karsh, B. (2008). Workarounds to barcode medication administration systems: their occurrences, causes, and threats to patient safety. *Journal of the American Medical Informatics Association*, *15*(4), 408–423. doi:10.1197/jamia.M2616

Kreke, J. E., Schaefer, A. J., & Roberts, M. S. (2004). Simulation and critical modeling. *Current Opinion in Critical Care*, *10*(5), 395–398. doi:10.1097/01.ccx.0000139361.30327.20

Kros, J., Dellana, S., & West, D. (2009). Overbooking increases patient access at East Carolina University's student health services clinic. *Interfaces*, *39*(3), 271–291. doi:10.1287/inte.1090.0437

Kruse, G. R. (2002). Factors associated with attendance at a first appointment after discharge from a psychiatric hospital. *Psychiatric Services (Washington, D.C.)*, *53*(4), 473–476. doi:10.1176/appi.ps.53.4.473

Ku, L., & Waidmann, T. (2003). *How race/ethnicity, immigration status and language affect health insurance coverage, access to care and quality of care among the low-income population*. Prepared for the Kaiser Commission on Medicaid and the Uninsured, August 2003.

Kucukyazici, B., Verter, V., & Mayo, N. E. (2010). (forthcoming). An analytical framework for designing community-based care delivery processes for chronic diseases. *Production and Operations Management*.

Kujala, J., Lillrank, P., Kronstrom, V., & Peltokorpi, A. (2006). Time-based management of patient processes. *Journal of Health Organization and Management*, *20*(6), 512–524. doi:10.1108/14777260610702262

Kuljis, J., Paul, R. J., & Stergioulas, L. K. (2007). *Can health care benefit from modeling and simulation methods in the same way as business and manufacturing has?* Paper presented at the Winter Simulation Conference.

Kumar, K., Zarychanski, R., Bell, D. D., Manji, R., Zivot, J., & Menkis, A. H. (2009). Impact of 24-hour in-house intensivists on a dedicated cardiac surgery intensive care unit. *The Annals of Thoracic Surgery*, *88*(4), 1153–1161. doi:10.1016/j.athoracsur.2009.04.070

Kyriacou, D. N., Ricketts, V., Dyne, P. L., McCollough, M. D., & Talan, D. A. (1999). A 5-year time study analysis of emergency department patient care efficiency. *Annals of Emergency Medicine*, *34*(3), 326–335. doi:10.1016/S0196-0644(99)70126-5

LaGanga, L. R., & Lawrence, S. R. (2007). Clinic overbooking to improve patient access and increase provider productivity. *Decision Sciences*, *38*(3), 251–276. doi:10.1111/j.1540-5915.2007.00158.x

Lahtela, A. (2009, September) *A short overview of the RFID technology in healthcare*. Paper presented at the Fourth International Conference on Systems and Networks Communications, (pp. 165-169). Sept. 20-25, 2009.

Lai, C.-H., Chien, S.-W., Chang, L.-H., Chen, S.-C., & Fang, K. (2007, August). *Enhancing medication safety and healthcare for inpatients using RFID*. Paper presented at Portland International Center for Management of Engineering and Technology, (pp. 2783-2790). August 5-9, 2007.

Lane, D. C., Monefeldt, C., & Husemann, E. (2003). Client involvement in simulation model building: Hints and insights from a case study in a London hospital. *Health Care Management Science*, *6*(2), 105–116. doi:10.1023/A:1023385019514

Lane, D. C., Monefeldt, C., & Rosenhead, J. V. (2000). Looking in the wrong place for healthcare improvements: A system dynamics study of an accident and emergency department. *The Journal of the Operational Research Society*, *51*, 518–531.

Langabeer, J. R. (2007). *Health care operations management* (p. 438). Sudbury, MA: Jones and Bartlett Publishers.

Larsen, A., Madsen, O. B. G., & Solomon, M. M. (2008). Recent developments in dynamic vehicle routing systems. In Golden, B., Raghavan, S., & Wasil, E. (Eds.), *The vehicle routing problem: Latest advances and new challenges* (*Vol. 43*, pp. 199–218). Operations Research/Computer Science Interfaces Series. doi:10.1007/978-0-387-77778-8_9

Lau, H., & Lau, A. H. (2000). A fast procedure for computing the total system cost of an appointment schedule for medical and kindred facilities. *IIE Transactions*, *32*(9), 833–839. doi:10.1080/07408170008967442

Lavine, G. (2008, August). RFID technology may improve contrast agent safety. *American Journal of Health-System Pharmacy*, *65*(15), 1400–1403. doi:10.2146/news080064

Law, A., & Kelton, W. D. (1999). *Simulation modeling and analysis* (3rd ed.). McGraw-Hill Science/Engineering/Math.

Lawrence, D. (2005). Bridging the quality chasm. In Reid, P. P., Compton, W. D., Grossman, J. H., & Fanjiang, G. (Eds.), *Building a better delivery system: A new engineering/healthcare partnership* (p. 99). Committee on Engineering and the Health Care System, Institute of Medicine and National Academy of Engineering.

Lawrie, G. J. G., & Cobbold, I. C. (2004). Third-generation balanced scorecard: Evolution of an effective strategic control tool. *International Journal of Productivity and Performance Management*, *5*(7), 611–623. doi:10.1108/17410400410561231

Ledersnaider, D., & Channon, B. (1998). SDM95—Reducing aggregate care team costs through optimal patient placement. *The Journal of Nursing Administration*, *28*, 48–54. doi:10.1097/00005110-199810000-00010

Lee, C., & Matzo, G. A. D. (1998). An evaluation of process capability for a fuel injector process using Monte Carlo simulation. In R. Peck, L. D. Haugh, & A. Goodman (Eds.), *Statistical case studies: A collaboration between academe and industry*. Philadelphia, PA: Society for Industrial and Applied Mathematics/ Virginia: American Statistical Association.

Lee, S.-Y., & Cho, G.-S. (2007, September). *A simulation study for the operations analysis of dynamic planning in container terminals considering RTLS.* Paper presented at Second International Conference on Innovative Computing, Information and Control (ICICIC '07), (p. 116).

Leonard, T. (2007). Paving the way for the second wave of EHR adoption. *Health Management Technology, 28*(2), 24, 26, 28.

Levy, M. M., Dellinger, R. P., Townsend, S. R., Linde-Zwirble, W. T., Marshall, J. C., & Bion, J. (2010). The surviving sepsis campaign: Results of an international guideline-based performance improvement program targeting severe sepsis. *Critical Care Medicine, 38*(2), 367–374. doi:10.1097/CCM.0b013e3181cb0cdc

Lewin Group and Ingeinx Consulting. (2010). *Brave new world: Healthcare reform - An update on the impact on government and commercial payers and providers.* April 1, 2010. Retrieved from http://www.lewin.com/healthreformwebinars/

Lian, Y., & Van Landeghem, H. (2007, July). Analyzing the effects of Lean manufacturing using a value stream mapping-based simulation generator. *International Journal of Production Research, 45*(13), 3037–3058. doi:10.1080/00207540600791590

Liang, B. A. (2000). Risks of reporting sentinel events. *Health Affairs, 19*(5). doi:10.1377/hlthaff.19.5.112

Lin, C. P., Payne, T. H., Nichol, W. P., Hoey, P. J., Anderson, C. L., & Gennari, J. H. (2008). Evaluating clinical decision support systems: Monitoring CPOE order check override rates in the Department of Veterans Affairs' Computerized Patient Record System. *Journal of the American Medical Informatics Association, 15*(5), 620–626. doi:10.1197/jamia.M2453

Litvak, E., & Long, M. (2000). Cost and quality under managed care: Irreconcilable difference? *The American Journal of Managed Care, 6*(3), 305–312.

Liu, C.-M., Wang, K.-M., & Guh, Y.-Y. (1991). A Markov chain model for medical record analysis. *The Journal of the Operational Research Society, 42*(5), 357–364.

Liu, L., & Liu, X. (1998). Block appointment systems for outpatient clinics with multiple doctors. *The Journal of the Operational Research Society, 49*(12), 1254–1259.

Liu, D., Wang, X., Pan, F., Xu, Y., Yang, P., & Rao, K. (2008). Web-based infectious disease reporting using XML forms. *International Journal of Medical Informatics, 77*(9), 630–640. doi:10.1016/j.ijmedinf.2007.10.011

Liu, A. X., & Bailey, L. A. (2008). RFID authentication and privacy. In Yan, L., Zhang, Y., Yang, L. T., & Ning, H. (Eds.), *The Internet of things: From RFID to pervasive networked systems.* Boca Raton, FL: Auerbach Publications, Taylor & Francis Group.

Liu, N., Ziya, S., & Kulkarni, V. G. (2009). Dynamic scheduling of outpatient appointments under patient no-shows and cancellations. *Manufacturing & Service Operations Management,* Articles in Advance. DOI: 10.1287/ msom.1090.0272

Lombardo, M., Vajo, F., Balestra, G., Freda, P., Knaflitz, M., Prato, G., & Puppato, D. (2007). *Studio di un Modello Sostenibile di Rete Regionale di Servizi di Ingegneria Clinica: I presupposti metodologici.* AReSS report. Retrieved August 2010, from http://www.aress.piemonte.it/ Documenti.aspx

Lorenzi, N. M., Kouroubali, A., Detmer, D. E., & Bloomrosen, M. (2009). How to successfully select and implement electronic health records (EHR) in small ambulatory practice settings. *BMC Medical Informatics and Decision Making, 9,* 15. doi:10.1186/1472-6947-9-15

Ludwick, D. A., & Doucette, J. (2009). Adopting electronic medical records in primary care: Lessons learned from health information systems implementation experience in seven countries. *International Journal of Medical Informatics, 78*(1), 22–31. doi:10.1016/j.ijmedinf.2008.06.005

Mackay, M. (2001). Practical experience with bed occupancy management and planning systems: An Australian view. *Health Care Management Science, 4,* 47–56. doi:10.1023/A:1009653716457

Maillart, L. M., Kamrani, A., Norman, B. A., Rajgopal, J., & Hawrylak, P. J. (2010). Optimizing RFID tag-inventorying algorithms. *IIE Transactions, 42*(9), 690–702. doi:10.1080/07408171003705714

Maio, V., & Manzoli, L. (2002). The Italian health care system: W.H.O. ranking versus public perception. *Pharmacy & Therapeutics, 6*(27), 301–308.

Makie, T., Miyazaki, M., Kobayashi, S., Yamanaka, T., Kinukawa, N., Hanada, E., & Nose, Y. (2002). A simple method for calculating the financial balance of hospital based on proportional dividing. *Journal of Medical Systems*, *26*(2), 105–112. doi:10.1023/A:1014801808798

Mandl, K., Simons, W., Crawford, W., & Abbett, J. (2007). Indivo: A personally controlled health record for health information exchange and communication. *BMC Medical Informatics and Decision Making*, *7*, 25. doi:10.1186/1472-6947-7-25

Manton, K. G., Gu, X. L., Ullian, A., Tolley, H. D., Headen, A. E. Jr, & Lowrimore, G. (2009). Long-term economic growth stimulus of human capital preservation in the elderly. *Proceedings of the National Academy of Sciences of the United States of America*, *106*(50), 21080–21085. doi:10.1073/pnas.0911626106

Marcon, E., & Kharraja, S. (2002). *Etude exploratoire sur la strategie de dimensionnement d'une SSPI*. Actes de la 2 Conference Internationale Francophone d'Aitomatique, Nantes, France.

Marjamaa, R. A., Torkki, P. M., Hirvensalo, E. J., & Kirvelä, O. A. (2009). What is the best workflow for an operating room? A simulation study of five scenarios. *Health Care Management Science*, *12*(2), 142–147. doi:10.1007/s10729-008-9073-8

Marshall, A., Vasilakis, C., & El-Darzi, E. (2005). Length of stay-based patient flow models: Recent developments and future directions. *Health Care Management Science*, *8*, 213–220. doi:10.1007/s10729-005-2012-z

Martin, S., & Smith, P. C. (1999). Rationing by waiting lists: an empirical investigation. *Journal of Public Economics*, *71*, 141–164. doi:10.1016/S0047-2727(98)00067-X

Martinez, E. A., Marsteller, J. A., Thompson, D. A., Gurses, A. P., Goeschel, C. A., & Lubomski, L. H. (2010). The society of cardiovascular anesthesiologists' FOCUS initiative: Locating errors through networked surveillance (LENS) project vision. *Anesthesia and Analgesia*, *110*(2), 307–311. doi:10.1213/ANE.0b013e3181c92b9c

Maruster, L., van der Aalst, W., Weijters, A., van den Bosch, A., & Daelemans, W. (2001). Automated discovery of workflow models from hospital data. In B. Krose, M. de Rijke, & G. Schreiber (Eds.), *Proc. 13th Belgium-Netherlands Conference on Artificial Intelligence BNAIC 2001*, (pp. 183-190).

Matthews, C. H. (2005). Using Linear programming to minimize the cost of nurse personnel. *Journal of Health Care Finance*, *32*(1), 37–49.

McCarthy, K., McGee, H. M., & O'Boyle, C. A. (2000). Outpatient clinic waiting times and non-attendance as indicators of quality. *Psychology Health and Medicine*, *5*(3), 287–293. doi:10.1080/713690194

McClean, S., McAlea, B., & Millard, P. (1998). Using a Markov reward model to estimate spend-down costs for a geriatric department. *The Journal of the Operational Research Society*, *49*, 1021–1025.

McClean, S., Garg, L., Meenan, B., & Millard, P. (2007). *Using Markov models to find interesting patient pathways*. Twentieth IEEE International Symposium on Computer-Based Medical Systems, 2007. CBMS '07, (pp. 713-718).

McClellan, M. (2010). *Reforming provider payment to promote models of integrated delivery.* Presented at National Health Policy Conference. Washington, DC. February 8, 2010.

Mcdonald, C. J., Overhage, J. M., Tierney, W. M., Dexter, P. R., Martin, D. K., & Suico, J. G. (1999). The Regenstrief medical record system: A quarter century experience. *International Journal of Medical Informatics*, *54*(3), 225–253. doi:10.1016/S1386-5056(99)00009-X

McDonald, T., Van Aken, E., & Rentes, A. (2002, July). Utilizing simulation to enhance value stream mapping: A manufacturing case application. *International Journal of Logistics: Research & Applications*, *5*(2), 213–232. doi:10.1080/13675560210148696

McDonald, C. (2009). Protecting patients in health information exchange: A defense of the HIPAA privacy rule. *Health Affairs*, *28*(2), 447–449. doi:10.1377/hlthaff.28.2.447

McDonald, C. J., Overhage, J. M., Dexter, P., Takesue, B., & Suico, J. G. (1998). What is done, what is needed and what is realistic to expect from medical informatics standards. *International Journal of Medical Informatics*, *48*(1), 5–12. doi:10.1016/S1386-5056(97)00102-0

McGowan, J. J., Cusack, C. M., & Poon, E. G. (2008). Formative evaluation: A critical component in EHR implementation. *Journal of the American Medical Informatics Association*, *15*(3), 297–301. doi:10.1197/jamia.M2584

McGraw, D., Dempsey, J., Harris, L., & Goldman, J. (2009). Privacy as an enabler, not an impediment: Building trust into health information exchange. *Health Affairs*, *28*(2), 416–427. doi:10.1377/hlthaff.28.2.416

McManus, M., Long, M., Cooper, A., & Litvak, E. (2004). Queuing theory accurately models the need for critical care resources. *Anesthesiology*, *100*(5), 1271–1276. doi:10.1097/00000542-200405000-00032

McManus, M., Long, M., Cooper, A., Mandell, J., Berwick, D., Pagano, M., & Litvak, E. (2003). Variability in surgical caseload and access to intensive care services. *Anesthesiology*, *98*(6), 1491–1496. doi:10.1097/00000542-200306000-00029

Medved, C. K. (1994, February). *Staffing and labor cost analysis using structured estimating techniques.* Paper presented at the Health Information Management Systems Society, Phoenix, Arizona.

Mehrotra, A., Keehl-Markowitz, L., & Ayanian, J. Z. (2008). Implementing open-access scheduling of visits in primary care practices: A cautionary tale. *Annals of Internal Medicine*, *148*(12), 915–922.

Meinert, D. B. (2005). Resistance to electronic medical records (EMRs): A barrier to improved quality of care. In E. Cohen (Ed.), *Issues in Informing Science and Information Technology, 2*, 493-504. Informing Science Press.

Mello, M. M., & Brennan, T. A. (2002). Deterrence of medical errors: Theory and evidence for malpractice reform. *Texas Law Review*, 80.

Melony, W. (1995). Benchmarking to improve financial performance. *Health Management Technology*, *16*(2), 10–12.

Mendenhall, W., & Sincich, T. (1995). *Statistics for engineering and sciences* (4th ed.). Upper Saddle River, NJ: Prentice- Hall.

Menon, N. M., Lee, B., & Eldenburg, L. (2000). Productivity of information systems in the healthcare industry. *Information Systems Research*, *11*(1), 83–92. doi:10.1287/isre.11.1.83.11784

Merkle, J. F. (2002). Computer simulation: A methodology to improve the efficiency in the Brooke Army Medical Center Family Care Clinic. *Journal of Healthcare Management*, *47*(1), 58–67.

Mettler, T., & Vimarlund, V. (2009). Understanding business intelligence in the context of healthcare. *Health Informatics Journal*, *15*(3), 254–264. doi:10.1177/1460458209337446

Meza, J. (1998). Patient waiting times in a physician's office. *The American Journal of Managed Care*, *4*(5), 703–712.

Mickle, M. H., Mats, L., & Hawrylak, P. J. (2008). Resolution and integration of HF and UHF. In Miles, S. B., Sarma, S. E., & Williams, J. R. (Eds.), *RFID technology and applications* (pp. 47–60). New York, NY: Cambridge University Press. doi:10.1017/CBO9780511541155.005

Miller, D. W., Jr. (2008). The transition from paper to digital: Lessons for medical specialty societies. *AMIA Annual Symposium Proceedings,* (pp. 475-9).

Min, D., & Yih, Y. (2010). An elective surgery scheduling problem considering patient priority. *Computers & Operations Research*, *37*(6), 1091–1099. doi:10.1016/j.cor.2009.09.016

Miró, O., Sánchez, M., Espinosa, G., Coll-Vinent, B., Bragulat, E., & Millá, J. (2003). Analysis of patient flow in the emergency department and the effect of an extensive reorganisation. *Emergency Medicine Journal*, *20*(2), 143–148. doi:10.1136/emj.20.2.143

Mitchell, R. K., Agle, B. R., & Wood, D. (1997). Toward a theory of stakeholder identification and salience: Defining the principle of who and what really counts. *Academy of Management Review*, *22*(4), 853–888.

Moon, T., Fewell, S., & Reynolds, H. (2008). The what, why, when and how of interoperability. *Defense & Security Analysis*, *24*(1), 5–17. doi:10.1080/14751790801903178

Moreno, A., & Nealon, J. (Eds.). (2003). *Applications of software agents technology in the health care domain*. Basel, Switzerland: Birkhuser Verlag Whitestein series in software agent technology

Moser, M. S., Abu-Laban, R. B., & Van Beek, C. A. (2004). Attitude of emergency department patients with minor problems to being treated by a nurse practitioner. *CJEM: Canadian Journal Of Emergency Medical Care*, *6*(4), 246–252.

Motwani, J., Klein, D., & Harowitz, R. (1996). The theory of constraints in services: Part 2-Examples from healthcare. *Managing Service Quality*, *6*(2), 30–34. doi:10.1108/09604529610109738

Murata, T. (1989). Petri nets: Properties, analysis and applications. *Proceedings of the IEEE*, *77*(4), 541–580. doi:10.1109/5.24143

Murer, C. G. (2007). EHRs: Issues preventing widespread adoption. *Rehab Management*, *20*(5), 38–39.

Murray, M., & Tantau, C. (1999). Redefining open access to primary care. *Managed Care Quarterly*, *7*(3), 45–55.

Mustain, J. M., Lowry, L. W., & Wilhoit, K. W. (2008). Change readiness assessment for conversion to electronic medical records. *The Journal of Nursing Administration*, *38*(9), 379–385. doi:10.1097/01.NNA.0000323956.06673.bf

Muthuraman, K., & Lawley, M. (2008). A stochastic overbooking model for outpatient clinical scheduling with no-shows. *IIE Transactions*, *40*(9), 820–837. doi:10.1080/07408170802165823

Nagarajan, M., & Sosic, G. (2008). Game-theoretic analysis of cooperation among supply chain agents: Review and extensions. *European Journal of Operational Research*, *187*(3), 719–745. doi:10.1016/j.ejor.2006.05.045

Nagle, L. M., & Catford, P. (2008). Toward a model of successful electronic health record adoption. *Healthcare Quarterly (Toronto, Ont.)*, *11*(3), 84–91.

Nakagawa, Y., Noguchi, M., Takemura, T., & Yoshihara, H. (2009). Change of the management strategy before and after DPC introduction: Influence on the hospital profit caused by improvement of sickbed turnover ratio. *The Journal of Japan Society for Health Care Management*, *9*(4), 511–518.

Nakagawa, Y., Noguchi, M., Takemura, T., & Yoshihara, H. (2009). New accounting system for financial balance based on personnel cost after the introduction of a DPC/DRG system. *Journal of Medical Systems*, *35*(2), 251–264..doi:10.1007/s10916-009-9361-y

Nakagawa, Y., Takemura, T., Shirakami, G., & Yoshihara, H. (2007). The cost analysis and problems of day surgery unit in the university hospital- Second report: Study of the performance improvement. *Journal of the Japanese Society on Hospital Administration*, *44*(3), 263–272.

Narasimhan, J., Parthasarathy, L., & Narayan, P. S. (2007). Increasing the effectiveness of value stream mapping using simulation tools in engine test operations. *Proceedings of 18th IASTED International Conference '07: Modeling and Simulation*. Montreal, Quebec, Canada

Nason, E., & Roberts, G. (2009). *Taming the queue VI-Improving patient flow*. Canadian Policy Research Networks.

National Academy of Engineering. (2005). Building a better delivery system: A new engineering/health care partnership, (p. 64).

National Patient Safety Foundation. (2010). *Unmet needs: Teaching physicians to provide safe patient care*. Report of the Lucian Leape Institute Roundtable On Reforming Medical Education.

Noon, C. E., Hankins, C. T., & Cote, M. J. (2003). Understanding the impact of variation in the delivery of healthcare services. *Journal of Healthcare Management*, *48*(2), 82–98.

Nordman, E., Cermak, D., & McDaniel, K. (2004). *Medical malpractice insurance report: A study of market conditions and potential solutions to the recent crisis*. Kansas City, MO: National Association of Insurance Commissioners.

Nunes, L., de Carvalho, S., & Rodrigues, R. (2009). Markov decision process applied to the control of hospital elective admissions. *Artificial Intelligence in Medicine*, *47*(2), 159–171. doi:10.1016/j.artmed.2009.07.003

Nursing. (2006, December). Replacing bar coding: Radio frequency identification. *Nursing*, *36*(12), 30.

O'Connor, M. E., Matthews, B. S., & Gao, D. (2006). Effect of open access scheduling on missed appointments, immunizations, and continuity of care for infant well-child care visits. *Archives of Pediatrics & Adolescent Medicine*, *160*(9), 889–893. doi:10.1001/archpedi.160.9.889

O'Hare, C. D., & Corlett, J. (2004). The outcomes of open access scheduling. *Family Practice Medicine*, *11*(2), 35–38.

O'Connor, M. C. (2006). Insurer running VeriChip trial. *RFID Journal*. Retrieved April 22, 2010, from http://www.rfidjournal.com/ article/articleview/2496/1/1/

Oden, J. T., Belytschko, T., Fish, J., Hughes, T. J. R., Johnson, C., Keyes, D., … Yip, S. (2006). *Revolutionizing engineering science through simulation*. Report of the National Science Foundation Blue Ribbon Panel on Simulation-Based Engineering Science.

Office of Road Safety. (2006). *Metropolitan area, road crash and injury summaries including vehicle factors*. Perth, Western Australia: Office of Road Safety. Retrieved from http://www.ors.wa.gov.au/ResearchFactsStats/YearCrashStats/Pages/MetropolitanArea.aspx

Organization of Economic Cooperation and Development. (2010). *OECD health data 2010*. Retrieved from http://www.oecd.org/ document/ 16/ 0,3343,en_2649_34631_2085200_1_1 _1_37407,00.html

Ozcan, Y. A. (2009). *Quantitative methods in health care management: Techniques and applications*. Wiley, John & Sons, Incorporated.

Padgham, L., & Winikoff, M. (2004). *Developing intelligent agent systems*. Wiley & Sons Ltd. doi:10.1002/0470861223

Page, D. (2009). Taking the guesswork out of scheduling surgeries. *Hospitals & Health Networks*, *83*(6), 12.

Pamuk, E., Makuc, D., Heck, K., Reuben, C., & Lochner, K. (1998). *Socioeconomic status and health chartbook: United States, 1998*. Hyattsville, MD: National Center for Health Statistics.

Pang, Z., Chen, Q., & Zheng, L. (2009, November). *A pervasive and preventive healthcare solution for medication noncompliance and daily monitoring*. Paper presented at the 2nd International Symposium on Applied Sciences in Biomedical and Communication Technologies (pp. 1-6). November 24-27, 2009.

Pappas, G., Queen, S., Hadden, W., & Fisher, G. (1993). The increasing disparity between socioeconomic groups in the United States, 1990 and 1996. *The New England Journal of Medicine*, *329*, 103–109. doi:10.1056/NEJM199307083290207

Parasher, A. K., Tien, J. M., & Goldschmidt-Clermont, P. J. (2010a). *Healthcare delivery as a service system: The barriers to co-production*. Manuscript Submitted for Publication.

Parasher, A. K., Tien, J. M., & Goldschmidt-Clermont, P. J. (2010b). *The Patient Protection and Affordable Care Act: The implications for healthcare reform for service co-production*. Manuscript Submitted for Publication.

Patient Protection and Affordable Care Act. P.L. 111-148. Washington, DC: GPO, 2010.

Patrick, J., Puterman, M. L., & Queyranne, M. (2008). Dynamic multipriority patient scheduling for a diagnostic resource. *Operations Research*, *56*(6), 1507–1525. doi:10.1287/opre.1080.0590

Patterson, E. S., Cook, R. I., & Render, M. L. (2002). Improving patient safety by identifying side effects from introducing bar coding in medication administration. *Journal of the American Medical Informatics Association*, *9*, 540–553. doi:10.1197/jamia.M1061

Peden, A., & Baker, J. J. (2002). Allocation physicians' overhead costs to service: An econometric/accounting-activity based-approach. *Journal of Health Care Finance*, *29*, 57–75.

Pennsylvania Patient Safety Authority. (2008). Care at discharge—A critical juncture for transition to posthospital care. Pennsylvania Patient Safety Authority, 5(2), 39-43. Retrieved June 20, 2010, from http://patientsafetyauthority.org /ADVISORIES/AdvisoryLibrary /2008/Jun5%282%29/Pages/39.aspx

Pentecost, R. (2009). *Standpoint: Shaping the future.* Retrieved from http://www.worldhealthdesign.com/Standpoint-Shaping-the-future.aspx

Phan, K., & Brown, S. (2009). Decreased continuity in a residency clinic: A consequence of open access scheduling. *Family Medicine Journal*, *41*(1), 46–50.

PHLO. (2008). *Creating and running proactive hospital operations website*. Retrieved from http://phlo.typepad.com/phlo/2008/01/the-worst-thing.html

Pickering, B., Herasevich, V., Ahmed, A., & Gajic, O. (2010). Novel representation of clinical information in the ICU: Developing user interfaces which reduce information overload. *Applied Clinical Informatic*, *1*(2), 116–131. doi:10.4338/ACI-2009-12-CR-0027

Pidd, M. (1999). *Tools for thinking: Modelling in management science*. Wiley and Son.

Pinedo, M. (1995). *Scheduling theory, algorithms and systems*. Prentice Hall.

Pinedo, M. (1995). *Scheduling: Theory, algorithms, and systems*. New Jersey: Prentice Hall, Inc.

Pinedo, M. L. (2009). *Planning and scheduling in manufacturing and services*. New York, NY: Springer. doi:10.1007/978-1-4419-0910-7

Pitt, M. (1997). A generalised simulation system to support strategic resource planning in healthcare. In S. Andradóttir, K. J. Healy, D. H. Withers, & B. L. Nelson (Eds.), *Proceedings of the 1997 Winter Simulation Conference*.

Pitts, S. R., Niska, R. W., Xu, J., & Burt, C. W. (2008). *National hospital ambulatory medical care survey: 2006 emergency department summary. National health statistics reports no. 7*. Hyattsville, MD: National Center for Health Statistics.

Player, S. (1998). Activity-based analyses lead to better decision making. *Healthcare Financial Management*, *52*(8), 66–70.

Pohjonen, H., Bondestam, S., Karp, P., Kinnunen, J., Korhola, O., & Sakari, P. (1994). Quality assurance of the bedside chest radiography process. *Acta Radiologica*, *35*(3), 235–243.

Polikandrioti, M., & Stefanou, E. (2009). Obesity disease. *Health Science Journal*, *3*(3), 132–138.

Poon, E. G., Wright, A., Simon, S. R., Jenter, C. A., Kaushal, R., & Volk, L. A. (2010). Relationship between use of electronic health record features and health care quality: Results of a statewide survey. *Medical Care*, *48*(3), 203–209. doi:10.1097/MLR.0b013e3181c16203

Porter, M. E. (2009). A strategy for health care reform - Toward a value-based system. *The New England Journal of Medicine*, *361*(2), 109–112. doi:10.1056/NEJMp0904131

Potisek, N. M., Malone, R. M., Bryant, B., Ives, T. J., Chelminski, P. R., DeWalt, D. A., & Pignone, M. P. (2007). Use of patient flow analysis to improve patient visit efficiency by decreasing wait time in a primary care-based disease management programs for anticoagulation and chronic pain: A quality improvement study. *BMC Health Services Research*, *7*(8), 1–7.

Press, W., Flannery, B., Teukolsky, S., & Vetterling, W. (1988). *Numerical recipes in C: The art of scientific computing* (p. 735). New York, NY: Cambridge University Press.

Pronovost, P., & Vohr, E. (2010). *Safe patients, smart hospitals: How one doctor's checklist can help us change health care from the inside out* (1st ed.). Hudson Street Press.

Pyzdek, T. (2003). *Quality engineering handbook*. Tucson, AZ: Quality Publishing.

Rahimi, B., Moberg, A., Timpka, T., & Vimarlund, V. (2008). Implementing an integrated computerized patient record system: Towards an evidence-based information system implementation practice in healthcare. *AMIA Annual Symposium Proceedings*, (pp. 616-20).

Rahm, E., & Bernstein, A.P. (2001). A survey of approaches to automatic schema matching. *The VLDB Journal — The International Journal on Very Large Data Bases*, *10*(4), 334-350.

Rajagopalan, B., & Isken, M. (2001). Exploiting data preparation to enhance mining and knowledge discovery. *IEEE T Syst Man Cyb*, *31*(4), 460–471. doi:10.1109/5326.983929

Ramakrishnan, S., Nagarkar, K., DeOennaro, M., Srihari, K., Courtney, A., & Emick, F. (2004). A study of the CT scan area of a healthcare provider. In R. Ingalls, M. Rossetti, J. Smith, & F. Peters (Eds.), *Proc 2004 WSC*, (pp. 2025-2031.).

Raths, D. (2009). *Vetting the vendors- 2009 best in KLAS: Beyond the numbers*. Retrieved May 30, 2010, from http:// www.healthcare-informatics.com/ Media/DocumentLibrary/ KLAS_2009_Supplement.pdf

Reason, J. (2000). Human errors: Models and management. *British Medical Journal*, *320*, 768. doi:10.1136/ bmj.320.7237.768

Regione Piemonte. (2010). Determina Dir. Sanità Regione Piemonte n. 41 del 27.01.2010. *Linea guida per l'applicazione di un modello organizzativo regionale di servizi di ingegneria clinica.*

Reid, P., Compton, W., Grossman, J., & Fanjiang, G. (Eds.). (2005). *Building a better delivery system: A new engineering / healthcare partnership. National Academy of Engineering and Institute of Medicine*. Washington, DC: The National Academy Press.

Reiner, J., & Sullivan, M. (2005, June). RFID in healthcare: A panacea for the regulations and issues affecting the industry? *Healthcare Purchasing News*, *29*(6), 74–76.

Research, C. f. H. S. (2009). *Federal funding for health services research. Nominal spending increase does not compensate for years of real declines.* Retrieved March 10, 2010, from http://www.chsr.org/ coalitionfunding2008.pdf

Revere, L., Black, K., & Zalila, F. (2010). RFIDs can improve the patient care supply chain. *Hospital Topics*, *88*(1), 26–31. doi:10.1080/00185860903534315

Ridge, J. C., Jones, S. K., Nielson, M. S., & Shahani, A. K. (1998). Capacity planning for intensive care units. *European Journal of Operational Research*, *105*, 346–355. doi:10.1016/S0377-2217(97)00240-3

Rising, E. J., Baron, R., & Averill, B. (1973). A system analysis of a university health service outpatient clinic. *Operations Research*, *21*(5), 1030–1047. doi:10.1287/ opre.21.5.1030

Ritondo, M., & Freedman, R. W. (1993). The effects of procedure scheduling on emergency room throughput: A simulation study. In Anderson, J. G., & Katzper, M. (Eds.), *SCS Western Multiconference on Simulation: Simulation in the Health Sciences and Services* (pp. 8–11). La Jolla, California, USA: Society for Computer Simulation.

Roark, D. C., & Miguel, K. (2006, February). RFID: Bar coding's replacement? *Nursing Management*, *37*(2), 28–31. doi:10.1097/00006247-200602000-00009

Roberts, S. A. B. (2007). *The impact of Information Technology on small, medium and large hospitals: Quality, safety and financial metrics*. Ph.D. Dissertation, University of Texas at Arlington.

Robinson, J. C. (2001). Theory and practice in the design of physician payment incentives. *The Milbank Quarterly*, *79*(2). doi:10.1111/1468-0009.00202

Robinson, L. W., & Chen, R. R. (2009). *The effects of patient no-shows on traditional and open-access appointment scheduling policies*. (UC Davis Graduate School of Management Research No. 16-09 / Johnson School Research Paper Series No. 43-09). Retrieved June 1, 2010, from http://papers.ssrn.com/ sol3/ papers.cfm? abstract_id= 1478736

Robinson, L., & Chen, R. (2009). A comparison of traditional and open-access policies for appointment scheduling. *Manufacturing & Service Operations Management*, Articles in Advance. DOI: 10.1287/msom.1090.0270

Rohleder, T. R., Sabapathy, D., & Schorn, R. (2005). An operating room block allocation model to improve hospital patient flow. *Clinical and Investigative Medicine. Medecine Clinique et Experimentale*, *28*(6), 353–355.

Roland, B., Di Martinelly, C., Riane, F., & Pochet, Y. (2010). Scheduling an operating theatre under human resource constraints. *Computers & Industrial Engineering*, *58*(2), 212. doi:10.1016/j.cie.2009.01.005

Römer, K., & Friedemann, M. (2004). The design space of wireless sensor networks. *IEEE Wireless Communications*, *11*(6), 54–61. doi:10.1109/MWC.2004.1368897

Ross, J. (2009). Electronic medical records: The promises and challenges. *Journal of Perianesthesia Nursing*, *24*(5), 327–329. doi:10.1016/j.jopan.2009.08.002

Ross, S. M. (1996). *Stochastic processes*. John Wiley&Sons.

Roth, C. P., Lim, Y. W., Pevnick, J. M., Asch, S. M., & McGlynn, E. A. (2009). The challenge of measuring quality of care from the electronic health record. *American Journal of Medical Quality*, *24*(5), 385–394. doi:10.1177/1062860609336627

Rothchild, J. M., & Keohane, C. (2008). *The role of barcoding and smart pump safety: Perspective*. Agency for Healthcare Research and Quality Web Morbility and Mortality Rounds. Retrieved on July 19, 2010, from http://www.webmm.ahrq.gov/ perspective.aspx? perspectiveID=64

Rouse, W. (2007). Health care as a complex adaptive system: Implications for design and management.

Rowland, D., Hoffman, C., & McGinn-Shapiro, M. (2009). *Healthcare and the middle class: More costs and less coverage*. Washington, DC: Kaiser Family Foundation.

Rudin, R. S., Simon, S. R., Volk, L. A., Tripathi, M., & Bates, D. (2009). Understanding the decisions and values of stakeholders in health information exchanges: Experiences from Massachusetts. *American Journal of Public Health*, *99*(5), 950–955. doi:10.2105/AJPH.2008.144873

Rust, C. T., Callups, N. H., Clark, W. S., Jones, D. S., & Wilcox, W. E. (1995). Patient appointment failures in pediatric resident continuity clinics. *Archives of Pediatrics & Adolescent Medicine*, *149*(6), 693–695.

Rutherford, R. (2007). TimeLine: Visualizing integrated patient records. *IEEE Transactions on Information Technology in Biomedicine*, *11*(4), 462–473. doi:10.1109/TITB.2006.884365

Ryan, T. P. (2007). *Modern engineering statistics*. Hoboken, NJ: John Wiley and Sons, Inc. doi:10.1002/9780470128442

Ryckman, F., Yelton, P., Anneken, A., Kissling, P., Schoettker, P., & Kotagal, U. (2009). Redesigning intensive care unit flow using variability management to improve access and safety. *Joint Commission Journal on Quality and Patient Safety*, *35*(11), 535–543.

Sage, W. (2003). Medical liability and patient safety. *Health Affairs*, *22*(4), 26–36. doi:10.1377/hlthaff.22.4.26

Saleem, J. J., Russ, A. L., Justice, C. F., Hagg, H., Ebright, P. R., Woodbridge, P. A., & Doebbeling, B. N. (2009). Exploring the persistence of paper with the electronic health record. *International Journal of Medical Informatics*, *78*(9), 618–628. doi:10.1016/j.ijmedinf.2009.04.001

Samaha, S., Armel, W., & Starks, D. (2003). The use of simulation to reduce the length of stay in an emergency department. In S. P. Chick (Ed.), *Proc 2003 WSC*, (pp. 1907-1911).

Samaras, E. A., & Samaras, G. M. (2010). Using Human-Centered Systems Engineering to Reduce Nurse Stakeholder Dissonance. *Biomedical Instrumentation & Technology*, *44*(s1), 25–32. doi:10.2345/0899-8205-44.s1.25

Samaras, G. M. (2006). An approach to human factors validation. *Journal of Validation Technology*, *12*(3), 190–201.

Samaras, G. M. (2010a). The use, misuse, and abuse of design controls. *IEEE Engineering in Medicine and Biology Magazine*, *29*(3), 12–18. doi:10.1109/MEMB.2010.936551

Samaras, G. M., & Horst, R. L. (2005). A systems engineering perspective on the human-centered design of health information systems. *Journal of Biomedical Informatics*, *38*(1), 61–74. doi:10.1016/j.jbi.2004.11.013

Samaras, G. M., & Samaras, E. A. (2009). Feasibility of an e-health initiative: Information NWDs of cancer survivor stakeholders. *Proceedings of IEA 2009*. Beijing. *China*, (August): 9–14.

Samaras, G. M. (2010b). Human-centered systems engineering: Building products, processes, and services. *Proc. 2010 SHS/ASQ Joint Conference*. February 25-28. Atlanta, Georgia USA.

Sanchez, A., Ferrin, D., Ogazon, T., & Sepulveda, J. (2000). Emerging issues in healthcare simulation. In J. Joines, R. Barton, K. Kang, & R. Fishwick (Ed.), *Proc 2000 WSC*, (pp. 1999 – 2003).

Sanders, D., Mukhi, S., Laskowski, M., Khan, M., Podaima, B. W., & McLeod, R. D. (2008, August). *A network-enabled platform for reducing hospital emergency department waiting times using an RFID proximity location system*. Paper presented at International Conference on Systems Engineering, 2008 (ICSENG '08), (pp. 538-543).

Santibanez, P., Begen, M., & Atkins, D. (2007). Surgical block scheduling in a system of hospitals: An application to resource and wait list management in a British Columbia health authority. *Health Care Management Science, 10*, 269–282. doi:10.1007/s10729-007-9019-6

Santibáñez, P., Chow, V. S., French, J., Puterman, M. L., & Tyldesley, S. (2009). Reducing patient wait times and improving resource utilization at British Columbia Cancer Agency's ambulatory care unit through simulation. *Health Care Management Science, 12*(4), 392–407. doi:10.1007/s10729-009-9103-1

Saraniti, B. (2006). Optimal pooled testing. *Health Care Management Science, 9*, 143–149. doi:10.1007/s10729-006-7662-y

Savage, S. (2009). *The flaw of averages* (p. 392). Hoboken, NJ: John Wiley & Sons, Inc.

Savage, G. T., Nix, T. W., Whitehead, C., & Blair, J. (1991). Strategies for assessing and managing organizational stakeholders. *The Academy of Management Executive, 5*(2), 61–76.

Schmidt, J. W., & Taylor, R. E. (1970). *Simulation and analysis of industrial systems*. Homewood, IL: R. D. Irwin.

Schneiderman, A. M. (2006). *The first Balanced Scorecard*. Retrieved on July 19, 2010, from www.Schneiderman.com/ Concepts/ The_First_Balanced_Scorecard/ BSC_INTRO AND CONTENTS.htm

Schrage, M. (1999). Measure prototyping paybacks. In Schrage, M. (Ed.), *Serious play: How the world's best companies simulate to innovate*. Harvard Business School Press.

Schreyogg, J., Stargardt, T., Tiemann, O., & Busse, R. (2006). Methods to determine reimbursement rates for diagnosis related groups (DRG)-A comparison of nine European countries. *Health Care Management Science, 9*, 215–223. doi:10.1007/s10729-006-9040-1

Schuhmann, T. M. (2008). Hospital financial performance trends to watch. *Healthcare Financial Management, 62*(7), 59–66.

Schull, M., Lazier, K., Vermeulen, M., Mawhinney, S., & Morrison, L. (2003). Emergency department contributors to ambulance diverision: A quantitative analysis. *Annals of Emergency Medicine, 41*, 467–476. doi:10.1067/mem.2003.23

Schuster, H. G. (1998). *Deterministic chaos: Introduction*. Weinheim, Germany: Physik Verlag.

Sen, A. K. (1999). *Development as freedom*. New York, NY: Alfred A. Knopf.

Shachak, A., & Jadad, A. R. (2010). Electronic health records in the age of social networks and global telecommunications. *Journal of the American Medical Association, 303*(5), 452–453. doi:10.1001/jama.2010.63

Sharp, D. J. (2001). Non-attendance at general practices and outpatient clinics: Local systems are needed to address local problems. *British Medical Journal, 323*(7321), 1081–1082. doi:10.1136/bmj.323.7321.1081

Sheth, R. S., Ramly, E., & Brennan, P. F. (2010). *Industrial and systems engineering and health care: Critical areas of research*.

Shmueli, A., Sprung, C. L., & Kaplan, E. H. (2003). Optimizing admissions to an intensive care unit. *Health Care Management Science, 6*(3), 131–136. doi:10.1023/A:1024457800682

Shonick, W., & Klein, B. W. (1977). An approach to reducing the adverse effects of broken appointments in primary care systems: Developing a decision rule based on estimated conditional probabilities. *Medical Care, 15*(5), 419–429. doi:10.1097/00005650-197705000-00008

Silver, E. A., Pyke, D., & Peterson, R. (1998). *Decision systems for inventory management and production planning and control* (3rd ed.). New York, NY: Wiley.

Simon, H. A. (1957). *Models of man: Social and rational*. New York, NY: Wiley.

Simul8 Corporation. (2008). *Simul8 user manual*. Simul8 Corporation.

Sinreich, D., & Marmor, Y. (2005). Emergency department operations: The basis for developing a simulation tool. *IIE Transactions, 37*(3), 233–245. doi:10.1080/07408170590899625

Sittig, D. F., & Classen, D. C. (2010). Safe electronic health record use requires a comprehensive monitoring and evaluation framework. *Journal of the American Medical Association, 303*(5), 450–451. doi:10.1001/jama.2010.61

SK&A. (2009). *Physician office acceptance of government insurance programs report*. October 2009.

Sloane, E. B., & Carey, C. C. (2007). Using standards to automate electronic health records (EHRs) and to create integrated healthcare enterprises. *Proceedings of the Annual International Conference of the IEEE Engineering in Medicine & Biology Society*, *2007*, 6178–6179.

Smalley, H. (1982). Hospital management engineering: A guide to the improvement of hospital management systems.

Smith, W. E. (1956). Various optimizers for single-stage production. *Naval Reserach Logistic Quarterly*, *3*(1-2), 59–66. doi:10.1002/nav.3800030106

Smith, P., & Goddard, M. (2002). Performance management and operational research: A marriage made in heaven? *The Journal of the Operational Research Society*, *53*, 247–255. doi:10.1057/palgrave.jors.2601279

Soliman, F. (1998). Optimum level of process mapping and least cost business process re-engineering. *International Journal of Operations & Production Management*, *18*(9-10), 810–816. doi:10.1108/01443579810225469

Soriano, A. (1966). Comparison of two scheduling systems. *Operations Research*, *14*, 388–397. doi:10.1287/opre.14.3.388

Sprivulis, P. C., Da Silva, J.-A., Jacobs, I. G., Frazer, A. R. L., & Jelinek, G. A. (2006). The association between hospital overcrowding and mortality among patients admitted via Western Australian emergency departments. *The Medical Journal of Australia*, *184*(5), 208–212.

State Government of Victoria. (2010). *Capital development guidelines, functional benchmarks*. Retrieved from http://www.capital.dhs.vic.gov.au/Assets/Files/Functional_Benchmarks[1].doc

Steele, C. (2002). *An introduction to clinical risk management* (pp. 24-27). Retrieved August 2010, from http://www www.optometry. co.uk

Stiell, A., Forster, A. J., Stiell, I. G., & van Walraven, C. (2003). Prevalence of information gaps in the emergency department and the effect on patient outcomes. *Canadian Medical Association Journal*, *169*, 1023–1028.

Story, P. (2010). *Dynamic capacity management for healthcare: Advanced methods and tools for optimization*. Productivity Press/Taylor and Francis Publishing. doi:10.1201/b10393

Story, P. (2009). *Are we thinking systems yet?* American Society for Quality (ASQ), January, 2009. Retrieved from http://www.asq.org/pdf/healthcare/are-we-thinking-systems-yet.pdf

Studdert, D. M., Mello, M. M., Gawande, A. A., Gandhi, T. K., Kachalia, A., & Yoon, C. (2006). Claims, errors, and compensation payments in medical malpractice litigation. *The New England Journal of Medicine*, *354*, 2024–2033. doi:10.1056/NEJMsa054479

Sturdevant, M. (2009, November 19). 1.5 million medical files at risk in health net data breach. The Hartford Courant. Retrieved June 20, 2010, from http://articles.courant.com/ 2009-11-19/news/ hc-healthbreach1119.artnov 19_1_health-net-data-breach-theft-or-health-united-bank-customer-information

Su, S., & Shih, C. L. (2003a). Modeling an emergency medical services system using computer simulation. *International Journal of Medical Informatics*, *72*, 57–72. doi:10.1016/j.ijmedinf.2003.08.003

Su, S., & Shih, C. L. (2003b). Managing a mixed-registration-type appointment system in outpatient clinics. *International Journal of Medical Informatics*, *70*(1), 31–40. doi:10.1016/S1386-5056(03)00008-X

Suneja, A., & Suneja, C. (2010). *Lean doctors*. Milwaukee, WI: ASQ Quality Press.

Swedberg, C. (2010a). Byrne Group automates asset management, orders. *RFID Journal*. Retrieved April 2, 2010, from http://www.rfidjournal.com/ article/articleview/7508

Swedberg, C. (2010b). San Jose Medical Center installs ZigBee-based RTLS across 10 buildings. *RFID Journal*. Retrieved April 1, 2010, form http://www.rfidjournal.com/ article/view/7470

Swedberg, C. (2010c). Trident health system boosts patient throughput, asset utilization. *RFID Journal*. Retrieved April 22, 2010, from http://www.rfidjournal.com/ article/view/7547

Swedberg, C. (2010d). Wright University researchers test RFID and ultrasound for 3-D RTLS. *RFID Journa*l. Retrieved April 23, 2010, from http://www.rfidjournal.com/ article/view/7546

Swedberg, C. (2010e). Zimmer Ohio to use RFID to manage orthopedic products. *RFID Journal*. Retrieved May 13, 2010, from http://www.rfidjournal.com/ article/view/7588

Swedberg, C. (2010f). U.S. customs' bonded warehouse deploys virtual perimeter. *RFID Journal*. Retrieved May 13, 2010, from http://www.rfidjournal.com/ article/view/7591

Swedberg, C. (2010g). Israelita Albert Einstein hospital uses RFID to track temperatures, assets. *RFID Journal*. Retrieved June 2, 2010, from http://www.rfidjournal.com/ article/view/7639

Swedberg, C. (2010h). RFID to take the chill out of frozen plasma tracking. *RFID Journal*. Retrieved June 2, 2010, from http://www.rfidjournal.com/ article/view/7632

Swedberg, C. (2010i). Nyack Hospital tracks medication compliance. *RFID Journal*. Retrieved June 2, 2010, from http://www.rfidjournal.com/ article/view/7631

Swedberg, C. (2010j). RFID-based hand-hygiene system prevents health-care acquired infections. *RFID Journal*. Retrieved June 11, 2010, from http://www.rfidjournal.com/ article/view/7660

Swedberg, C. (2010k). Mobile RTLS tracks health-care efficiency. *RFID Journal*. Retrieved June 16, 2010, from http://www.rfidjournal.com/ article/view/7668

Swedberg, C. (2010l). New Oregon hospital adopts IR-RFID hybrid system. *RFID Journal*. Retrieved June 16, 2010, from http://www.rfidjournal.com/ article/view/4846

Swisher, J. R., Jacobson, S. H., Jun, J. B., & Balci, O. (2001). Modeling and analyzing a physician clinic environment using discrete-event (visual) simulation. *Computers & Operations Research*, *28*(2), 105–125. doi:10.1016/S0305-0548(99)00093-3

Tanaka, K., Sato, J., Guo, J., Takada, A., & Yoshihara, H. (2004). A simulation model of hospital management based on cost accounting analysis according to disease. *Journal of Medical Systems*, *28*(6), 689–710. doi:10.1023/B:JOMS.0000044970.82170.ae

Tarrant, C., Stokes, T., & Colman, A. M. (2004). Models of the medical consultation: Opportunities and limitations of a game theory perspective. *Quality Safety in Health Care Journal*, *13*, 461–466. doi:10.1136/qshc.2003.008417

Teow, K. L. (2009). Practical operations research applications for healthcare managers. *Annals of the Academy of Medicine, Singapore*, *38*(6), 564–566.

Testi, A., & Tànfani, E. (2009). Tactical and operational decisions for operating room planning: Efficiency and welfare implications. *Health Care Management Science*, *12*(4), 363. doi:10.1007/s10729-008-9093-4

Testi, A., Tanfani, E., & Torre, G. (2007). A three-phase approach for operating theatre schedules. *Health Care Management Science*, *10*, 163–172. doi:10.1007/s10729-007-9011-1

The Economist. (September 4, 2010). Poison pills. *The Economist*.

The Levin Group, Inc. (2005). *Health Information Technology Leadership Panel final report*. Retrieved May 30, 2010, from http://www.hhs.gov/healthit /HIT-FinalReport.pdf

Thomas, E. J., Studdert, D. M., Burstin, H. R., Orav, E. J., Zeena, T., & Williams, E. J. (n.d.). … Brennan, T. A. Incidence and types of adverse events and negligent care in Utah and Colorado. *Medical Care*, *38*(3).

Thompson, C. W., & Thompson, D. R. (2007, May-June). Identity management. *Internet IEEE Computing*, *11*(3), 82–85. doi:10.1109/MIC.2007.60

Tien, J. M. (2003). Towards a decision informatics paradigm: A real-time, information-based approach to decision making. *IEEE Transactions on Systems, Man, and Cybernetics, Special Issue*, *33*(1), 102–113. doi:10.1109/TSMCC.2003.809345

Tien, J. M., & Berg, D. (2003). A case for service systems engineering. *Journal of Systems Science and Systems Engineering*, *12*(1), 13–38. doi:10.1007/s11518-006-0118-6

Tien, J. M., & Goldschmidt-Clermont, P. J. (2009). Healthcare: A complex service system. *Journal of Systems Science and Systems Engineering*, *18*(4), 285–310.

Tierney, W. M., Miller, M. E., Overhage, J. M., & McDonald, C. J. (1993). Physician inpatient order writing on microcomputer workstations. Effects on resource utilization. *Journal of the American Medical Association*, *269*(3), 379–383. doi:10.1001/jama.269.3.379

Trček, D., & Jäppinen, P. (2008). RFID security. In Yan, L., Zhang, Y., Yang, L. T., & Ning, H. (Eds.), *The Internet of things: From RFID to pervasive networked systems*. Boca Raton, FL: Auerbach Publications, Taylor & Francis Group.

Troy, P., & Rosenberg, L. (2009). Using simulation to determine the need for ICU beds for surgery patients. *Surgery, 146*(4), 608–620. doi:10.1016/j.surg.2009.05.021

Tufo, H. M., & Speidel, J. J. (1971). Problems with medical records. *Medical Care, 9*(6), 509–517. doi:10.1097/00005650-197111000-00007

Tufte, E. (1983). *The visual display of quantitative information*. Cheshire, CT: Graphics Press.

Turner, B. J., Weiner, M., Yang, C., & TenHave, T. (2004). Predicting adherence to colonoscopy or flexible sigmoidoscopy on the basis of physician appointment–keeping behavior. *Annals of Internal Medicine, 140*(7), 528–532.

U. S. Department of Health and Human Services. (2009). *Shortage designation: HPSAs, MUAs & MUPs*. Washington, DC. Retrieved from http://bhpr.hrsa.gov/ shortage/ index.htm

U.S. Bureau of Labor Statistics. (2006). *Employment statistics*. Retrieved from http://www.bls.gov/ bls/ employment.htm

U.S. Census Bureau. (2006). *Survey of income and program participation, October 2001–January 2002*. Retrieved from http://www.census.gov/ prod/ 006pubs/ p70-106.pdf

Ulgen, O. M., & Williams, E. J. (2001). Simulation modeling and analysis. In Zandin, K. B. (Ed.), *Maynard's industrial engineering handbook*. New York, NY: McGraw-Hill Companies, Inc.

Urban Institute. (2005). *Analysis of the 2005 annual and social economic supplement to the current population survey for the Kaiser Commission on Medicaid and the uninsured*. Washington, DC: Kaiser Family Foundation.

van der Aalst, W., Weijters, T., & Maruster, L. (2004). Workflow mining: Discovering process models from event logs. *IEEE Transactions on Knowledge and Data Engineering, 16*(9), 1128–1142. doi:10.1109/TKDE.2004.47

van der Aalst, W. M. P. (1996). Three good reasons for using a Petri-net-based workflow management system. In S. Navathe & T. Wakayama, (Eds.), *Proceedings of the International Working Conference on Information and Process Integration in Enterprises (IPIC'96)*, (pp. 179–201) Cambridge, Massachusetts, Nov 1996.

van der Aalst, W., & van Hee, K. (2004). *Workflow management: Models, methods, and systems*. The MIT Press, paperback edition.

van Sambeek, J. R. C., Cornelissen, F. A., Bakker, P. J. M., & Krabbendam, J. J. (2010). Models as instruments for optimizing hospital processes: A systematic review. *International Journal of Health Care Quality Assurance, 23*(4), 356–377. doi:10.1108/09526861011037434

VanBerkel, P. T., & Blake, J. T. (2007). A comprehensive simulation for wait time reduction and capacity planning applied in general surgery. *Health Care Management Science, 10*(4), 373–385. doi:10.1007/s10729-007-9035-6

Vanden Bosch, P. M., Dietz, C. D., & Sumeoni, J. R. (1999). Scheduling customer arrivals to a stochastic service system. *Naval Research Logistics, 46*, 549–559. doi:10.1002/(SICI)1520-6750(199908)46:5<549::AID-NAV6>3.0.CO;2-Y

Vanden Bosch, P. M., & Dietz, D. C. (2000). Minimizing expected waiting in a medical appointment system. *IIE Transactions, 32*(9), 841–848. doi:10.1080/07408170008967443

Vankipuram, M., Kahol, K., Cohen, T., & Patel, V. L. (2010). Toward automated workflow analysis and visualization in clinical environments. *Journal of Biomedical Informatics*.

Vasilakis, C., Lecznarowicz, D., & Lee, C. (2009). Developing model requirements for patient flow simulation studies using the Unified Modelling Language (UML). *J Simul, 3*(3), 141–149. doi:10.1057/jos.2009.3

Villegas, E. L. (1967). Outpatient appointment system saves time for patients and doctors. *Hospitals, 41*(8), 52–57.

Vimarlund, V., Olve, N. G., Scandurra, I., & Koch, S. (2008). Organizational effects of information and communication technology (ICT) in elderly homecare: A case study. *Health Informatics Journal, 14*(3), 195–210. doi:10.1177/1081180X08092830

Vincent, C., Moorthy, K., Sarker, S. K., Chang, A., & Darzi, A. W. (2004). Systems approaches to surgical quality and safety: From concept to measurement. *Annals of Surgery*, *239*(4), 475–482. doi:10.1097/01.sla.0000118753.22830.41

Vinjumur, J. K., Becker, E., Ferdous, S., Galatas, G., & Makedon, F. (2010). Web based medicine intake tracking application. In *Proceedings of the 3rd International Conference on Pervasive Technologies Related To Assistive Environments*. June 23 - 25, 2010.

Viscusi, W. K. (Ed.). (2002). *Regulation through litigation*. Washington, DC: AEI-Brookings Joint Center for Regulatory Studies.

Visser, J. M. H. (1998). Patient flow-based allocation of inpatient resources: A case study. *European Journal of Operational Research*, *105*, 356–370. doi:10.1016/S0377-2217(97)00242-7

Vissers, J. M. H., Adan, I. J. B. F., & Bekkers, J. A. (2005). Patinet mix optimization in cardiothoracic surgery planning: A case study. *IMA Journal of Management Math*, *16*, 281–304. doi:10.1093/imaman/dpi023

Vissers, J. (1979). Selecting a suitable appointment system in an outpatient setting. *Medical Care*, *17*(12), 1207–1220. doi:10.1097/00005650-197912000-00004

Vissers, J., & Beech, R. (2005). *Health operations management: Patient flow logistics in healthcare*. London, UK: Routledge - Taylor and Francis Group.

Vladeck, B. C. (2010). Fixing Medicare's physician payment system. *New England Journal of Medicine*. Retrieved from http://content.nejm.org/ cgi/ content/ short/ NEJMp1004709v1? rss=1&query=current

Wainer, G. A. (Ed.). (2009). *Discrete-event modeling and simulation: A practitioner approach*. Boca Raton, FL: CRC Press, Taylor and Francis Group.

Wakefield, D. S., Halbesleben, J. R., Ward, M. M., Qiu, Q., Brokel, J., & Crandall, D. (2007). Development of a measure of clinical information systems expectations and experiences. *Medical Care*, *45*(9), 884–890. doi:10.1097/MLR.0b013e3180653625

Walker, D. H. T., Bourne, L. M., & Shelley, A. (2008). Influence, stakeholder mapping and visualization. *Construction Management and Economics*, *26*(6), 645–658. doi:10.1080/01446190701882390

Walker, J., Pan, E., Johnston, D., Adler-Milstein, J., Bates, D. W., & Middleton, B. (2005). The value of health care information exchange and interoperability. *Health Affairs*, *24*(5), w10–w18.

Wang, P. P. (1993). Static and dynamic scheduling of customer arrivals to a single-server system. *Naval Research Logistics*, *40*, 345–360. doi:10.1002/1520-6750(199304)40:3<345::AID-NAV3220400305>3.0.CO;2-N

Wang, S.-W., Chen, W.-H., Ong, C.-S., Liu, L., & Chuang, Y.-W. (2006, January). RFID application in hospitals: A case study on a demonstration RFID project in a Taiwan hospital. In the *Proceedings of the 39th Annual Hawaii International Conference on System Sciences* (vol. 8, p. 184a).

Warden, J. (1995). 4.5-million outpatients miss appointments. *British Medical Journal*, *310*(6988), 1158–1158.

Washington Hospital Center. (n.d.). Electronic medical records help physicians and boost revenues while saving millions. Retrieved June 20, 2010, from http://download.microsoft.com /documents/australia/healthcare /washington.doc

Weiss, E. N. (1990). Models for determining estimated start times and case orderings in hospital operating rooms. *IIE Transactions*, *22*(2), 143–150. doi:10.1080/07408179008964166

Welch, J. D. (1964). Appointment systems in hospital outpatient departments. *Operational Research Quarterly*, *15*(3), 224–237. doi:10.1057/jors.1964.43

Welch, J. D., & Bailey, N. (1952). Appointment systems in hospital outpatient departments. *Lancet*, *259*, 1105–1108. doi:10.1016/S0140-6736(52)90763-0

West, T. D., Balas, E. A., & West, D. A. (1996). Contrasting RCC, RVU, and ABC for managed care decisions. *Healthcare Financial Management*, *50*(8), 54–61.

Westfall, J. M., Mold, J., & Fagnan, L. (2007). Practice-based research-"Blue highways" on the NIH roadmap. *Journal of the American Medical Association*, *297*(4), 403–406. doi:10.1001/jama.297.4.403

Wetterneck, T. B., Skibinski, K. A., Roberts, T. L., Kleppin, S. M., Schroeder, M. E., & Enloe, M. (2006). Using failure mode and effects analysis to plan implementation of smart i.v. pump technology. *American Journal of Health-System Pharmacy*, *63*, 1528–1538. doi:10.2146/ajhp050515

White, C. R., Best, J. B., & Sage, C. K. (1992). Simulation of emergency medical service scheduling. *Hospital Topics*, *70*, 34–37.

White, M. J. B., & Pike, M. C. (1964). Appointment systems in outpatients' clinics and the effect on patients' unpunctuality. *Medical Care*, *2*(3), 133–145. doi:10.1097/00005650-196407000-00002

Wicks, A. M., Visich, J. K., & Li, S. (2006). Radio frequency identification applications in hospital environments. *Hospital Topics*, *84*(3), 3–8. doi:10.3200/HTPS.84.3.3-9

Wijewickrama, A. (2006). Simulation analysis for reducing queues in mixed-patients' outpatient department. *International Journal of Simulation Modelling*, *5*(2), 56–68. doi:10.2507/IJSIMM05(2)2.055

Wijewickrama, A., & Takakuwa, S. (2005). Simulation analysis of appointment scheduling in an outpatient department of internal medicine. *Proceedings of the 2005 Winter Simulation Conference*.

Williams, P., Tai, G., & Lei, Y. (2009). Simulation based analysis of patient arrival to health care systems and evaluation of an operations improvement scheme. *Annals of Operations Research*, *178*(1), 263–279..doi:10.1007/s10479-009-0580-x

Winston, W. L. (1993). *Operations research: Application and algorithms*. International Thomson Publishing.

Woehrle, S., & Abu-Shady, L. (2010). Using dynamic value stream mapping and lean accounting box scores to support lean implementation. *2010 EABR & ETLC Conference Proceedings,* (pp. 839-840).

Wolfson, M., Kaplan, G., Lynch, J., Ross, N., & Backlund, E. (1999). Relation between income inequality and mortality: Empirical demonstration. *British Medical Journal*, *319*, 953–957.

Wolstenholme, E. (1999). A patient flow perspective of U.K. health services: Exploring the case for new intermediate care initiatives. *System Dynamics Review*, *15*(3), 253–271. doi:10.1002/(SICI)1099-1727(199923)15:3<253::AID-SDR172>3.0.CO;2-P

Womack, J. P., Jones, D. T., & Roos, D. (1990). *The machine that changed the world: The story of lean production-- Toyota's secret weapon in the global car wars that is now revolutionizing world industry*. New York, NY: Free Press.

Worthington, D. (1987). Queuing models for hospital waiting lists. *The Journal of the Operational Research Society*, *38*(5), 413–422.

Wright, C., Wain, J., Grillo, H., Moncure, A., Macaluso, S., & Mathisen, D. (1997). Pulmonary lobectomy patient care pathway: A model to control cost and maintain quality. *The Annals of Thoracic Surgery*, *64*(2), 299–302. doi:10.1016/S0003-4975(97)00548-1

Wullink, G., Van Houdenhoven, M., Hans, E., van Oostrum, J., van der Lans, M., & Kazemier, G. (2007). Closing emergency operating rooms improves efficiency. *Journal of Medical Systems*, *31*, 543–546. doi:10.1007/s10916-007-9096-6

Xiao, Y., Shen, X., Sun, B., & Cai, L. (2006, April). Security and privacy in RFID and applications in telemedicine. *IEEE Communications Magazine*, *44*(4), 64–72. doi:10.1109/MCOM.2006.1632651

Xie, H., Chaussalet, T., & Rees, M. (2007). A semi-open queueing network approach to the analysis of patient flow in healthcare systems. *Proceedings of the 20th IEEE International Symposium on Computer-Based Medical Systems.*

Xiong, J., Seet, B.-C., & Symonds, J. (2009, July). *Human activity inference for ubiquitous RFID-based applications*. Paper presented at the 2009 Symposia and Workshops on Ubiquitous, Autonomic and Trusted Computing, (pp. 304-309). July 7-9, 2009.

Yackanicz, L., Kerr, R., & Levick, D. (2010). Physician buy-in for EMRs. *Journal of Healthcare Information Management*, *24*(2), 41–44.

Yang, K. K., Lau, M. L., & Quek, S. A. (1998). A new appointment rule for a single-server, multiple-customer service system. *Naval Research Logistics*, *45*(3), 313–326. doi:10.1002/(SICI)1520-6750(199804)45:3<313::AID-NAV5>3.0.CO;2-A

Yao, D. Q., Yue, X., & Liu, J. (2006). Vertical cost information sharing in a supply chain with value-adding retailers. *Omega*, *36*(5), 838–851. doi:10.1016/j.omega.2006.04.003

Yasunaga, H., Ide, H., Imamura, T., & Ohe, K. (2005). Impact of the Japanese diagnosis procedure combination-based payment system on cardiovascular medicine-related costs. *International Heart Journal*, *46*(5), 855–866. doi:10.1536/ihj.46.855

Yasunaga, H., Ide, H., Imamura, T., & Ohe, K. (2006). Influence of Japan's new diagnosis procedure combination-based payment system on the surgical sector: Does it really shorten the hospital stay? *Surgery Today*, *36*(7), 577–585. doi:10.1007/s00595-006-3203-z

Yellowlees, P. M., Marks, S. L., Hogarth, M., & Turner, S. (2008). Standards-based, open-source electronic health record systems: A desirable future for the U.S. health industry. *Telemedicine Journal and e-Health*, *14*(3), 284–288. doi:10.1089/tmj.2007.0052

Yoon-Flannery, K., Zandieh, S. O., Kuperman, G. J., Langsam, D. J., Hyman, D., & Kaushal, R. (2008). A qualitative analysis of an electronic health record (EHR) implementation in an academic ambulatory setting. *Informatics in Primary Care*, *16*(4), 277–284.

Young, T. (2005). An agenda for healthcare and information simulation. *Health Care Management Science*, *8*(3), 189–196. doi:10.1007/s10729-005-2008-8

Young, T., Brailsford, S., Connell, C., Davies, R., Harper, P., & Klein, J. H. (2004). Using industrial processes to improve patient care. *British Medical Journal*, *328*(7432), 162–164. doi:10.1136/bmj.328.7432.162

Young, J. (2005). *RFID applications in the healthcare and pharmaceutical industries: White Paper revolutionizing asset management and the supply chain.* Retrieved 2010, from www.radiantwave.com/whitepapers /healthWP.doc

Young, T., Eatock, J., Jahangirian, M., Naseer, A., & Lilford, R. (2009). *Three critical challenges for modeling and simulation in healthcare.* Paper presented at the Winter Simulation Conference.

Zafar, A. (2009). *Health information exchange (HIE): Nuts and bolts*. Retrieved June 25, 2010, from http://www.virec.research.va.gov /EducationResources/Seminars/Informatics071806.PPT

Zandin, K. B. (Ed.). (2001). *Maynard's industrial engineering handbook*. New York, NY: McGraw-Hill Companies, Inc.

Zeleny, M. (1998). Multiple criteria decision making: Eight concepts of optimality. *Human Systems Management*, *17*, 97–107.

Zelman, W.N., Glick, N. D., & Blackmore, C. C. (2001). Animated-simulation modeling facilitates clinical-process costing - Healthcare organizations finance department use new software. *Healthcare Financial Management, September*.

Zhang, J., & Butler, K. A. (2007). *UFuRT: A work-centered framework and process for design and evaluation of information systems*. HCI International Proceedings.

Zhao, X., & Johnson, M. E. (2009). The value of escalation and incentives in managing information access. In Johnson, M. E. (Ed.), *Managing information risk and the economics of security* (pp. 165–177). Springer, US. doi:10.1007/978-0-387-09762-6_8

Zheng, K., Padman, R., Johnson, M. P., & Diamond, H. S. (2009). An interface-driven analysis of user interactions with an electronic health records system. *Journal of the American Medical Informatics Association*, *16*(2), 228–237. doi:10.1197/jamia.M2852

Zhou, J., & Dexter, F. (1998). Methods to assist in the scheduling of add-on surgical cases: Upper prediction bounds for surgical case durations based on log-normal distribution. *Anesthesiology*, *89*(5). doi:10.1097/00000542-199811000-00024

Zhu, Z. C., Heng, B. H., & Teow, K. L. (2009). Simulation study of the optimal appointment number for outpatient clinics. *International Journal of Simulation Modelling*, *3*, 156–165. doi:10.2507/IJSIMM08(3)3.132

About the Contributors

Alexander Kolker is currently an Outcomes Operations Project Manager in Children's Hospital and Health System, Wisconsin, USA. He has extensive practical expertise in quantitative methods for healthcare management, such as hospital capacity expansion planning, system-wide patient flow optimization, staffing planning, forecasting trends, and market expansion analysis. He widely applies process simulation and other advanced analytical and computer methodologies to analyze different scenarios for allocation resources that result in the most efficient operational hospital management solutions. He actively publishes in peer-reviewed journals, edits books, and speaks at the national conferences in the area of management engineering and system and process improvement in healthcare settings. He serves on the review boards of *Healthcare Management Science* and *Journal of Medical Systems.* Previously he has worked for Froedtert Memorial Lutheran Hospital, and for General Electric Co, GE Healthcare, as a simulation specialist, and reliability engineer. He can be reached at alexanderkolker@yahoo.com

Pierce Story is a Senior Consulting Manager for the Care Design group, part of GE Healthcare's Performance Solutions division. He works with a team of clinical experts, process and systems engineers, and simulationists to provide dynamic facility and operations optimization, capacity analysis, and staffing algorithms to new and existing facilities. Pierce has been engaged in healthcare process simulation development and deployment for over eleven years, and has worked in the healthcare industry for over twenty. Pierce is a Diplomate-level member and Past President of the Society for Health Systems (SHS), a current Board member for the Healthcare Division of the American Society for Quality (ASQ), and a member of HIMSS and IIE. His is author of the new book, Dynamic Capacity Management for Hospitals, (to be published in Oct. 2010 by Productivity Press) and is co-author of the book *Management Engineering for Effective Healthcare Delivery: Principles and Applications*. He has written numerous articles for healthcare and engineering journals including Quality Progress and the Journal of Industrial Engineering. He has also spoken at over twenty healthcare conferences, including the ACHE Annual Congress. Pierce earned a Master's Degree in Health Policy and Management from the University of Southern Maine. His passions include bringing engineering principles, tools, and concepts to the everyday management of hospital capacity and care delivery, and developing viable solutions to the challenges of reducing the total cost of the provision of American healthcare. Pierce understands the issues facing the future of the US healthcare systems, and believes strongly that GE is in a unique position to help make it financially viable, clinically safe, and openly accessible. Pierce currently resides in Wells, ME, where he is an active member of his local Baptist church, and enjoys fly-fishing, riding his 1988 Harley Davidson, and growing championship roses.

* * *

Arben Asllani is a UC Foundation Professor of Management at the University of Tennessee at Chattanooga. He has published over 24 journal articles and presented and published over twenty conference proceedings. His most recent research has been published in such journals as *Omega*, *European Journal of Operational Research*, *Knowledge Management*, and *Computers & Industrial Engineering*. Dr. Asllani is a member of the Decision Sciences Institute, the Academy of Information and Management Sciences, and the Academy of Marketing Research. He has consulted with a number of businesses in the field of healthcare scheduling, open source software, database design, and computer simulations.

Gabriella Balestra received the Laurea degree in Computer Science from Università degli Studi di Torino and the Ph.D. degree from Politecnico di Torino. Since 1993 she is Research Assistant Professor at Politecnico di Torino teaching classes on medical informatics, biomedical data interpretation and decision support systems, and clinical engineering. Her research interests include biomedical data interpretation, decision support systems, medical informatics and telemedicine, healthcare technology management. She has developed several support systems based on fuzzy logic, genetic algorithms, neural networks, multicriteria methods, et cetera. She has authored and coauthored over 15 papers and book chapters, and 50 conference papers. She is a member of several scientific societies (IEEE, ORAHS, AAMI, AIRO, HTAi).

David Ben-Arieh is a Professor of Industrial Engineering at Kansas State University. Prior to joining Kansas State University, Dr. Ben-Arieh taught at the Department of Industrial Engineering and Management, Ben-Gurion University in Beer Sheva, Israel. His industrial experience includes working for AT&T Bell Laboratories, and consulting for the aerospace industry and NASA. Dr. Ben- Arieh holds a PhD in Industrial Engineering from Purdue University. Dr. Ben-Arieh concentrates mainly on applications systems design and modeling and holds one patent in this area. In recent years Dr. Ben-Arieh has focused on applications in health care systems management, including patients flow, Information Systems integration, and patient quality and safety improvements.

Brian Denton is an Associate Professor at North Carolina State University in the Edward P. Fitts Department of Industrial & Systems Engineering. Previously he has been a Senior Associate Consultant at Mayo Clinic in the College of Medicine, and a Senior Engineer at IBM. He is currently a Fellow at the Cecil Sheps Center for Health Services Research at University of North Carolina. His primary research interests are in optimization under uncertainty and applications to health care delivery and medical decision making. He completed his Ph.D. in Management Science at McMaster University, his M.Sc. in Physics at York University, and his B.Sc. in Chemistry and Physics at McMaster University in Hamilton, Ontario, Canada.

Amerett L. Donahoe-Anshus is a Unit Head in Systems and Procedures, the internal consulting group at Mayo Clinic. She began her career at Mayo in 1983 in the Department of Physical Medicine and Rehabilitation. After 15 years in clinical outpatient, hospital, and home health care settings, she joined the Division of Systems & Procedures. Amy has led and assisted with the implementation of multiple hospital and clinic-based electronic applications and quality initiatives. Amy's current leadership and consulting roles include the S&P Quality Initiatives Support Unit, Mayo's electronic environment, practice convergence, curriculum development, and instruction for Mayo's Change Management and S&P Decision Support & Data Analysis courses and other collaborations with administrative and physician leaders to support Mayo Clinic's strategic priorities. Amy received a Master's in Human and Health Service Administration from St. Mary's College of Minnesota; a Bachelor's in Physical Therapy from the University of Health Sciences/Chicago Medical School; and a Bachelor's in Psychology from the College of St. Benedict.

Yue Dong trained as an anesthesiologist in China and finished research fellowship of anesthesiology and physiology in Mayo Clinic. He is currently a patient safety researcher at Multidisciplinary Simulation Center Simulation Center and METRIC group at Mayo Clinic. With collaboration with a multidisciplinary team of clinicians, researchers, and engineers, his research interest is to apply application of modeling and simulation to the study of healthcare delivery factors which improve patient safety and in acute care settings. Three main themes emerge from this interest: 1) Using a systems engineering/operation research approaches to study system performance and provide re-designed alternatives to improve safety and efficiency of healthcare delivery; 2) Study the effectiveness of simulation based medical education (SBME) by developing valid outcome measurements which stretch measurement endpoints from the simulation lab into clinical practice, and in the process provide highly reliable data for decision support and high-stakes testing; 3) Using simulation as a tool to study human performance variation under different "stress conditions" (fatigue, cognition, workload, etc.) and to conduct usability testing of devices and processes.

Ergin Erdem obtained his B.S. and M.Sc. degrees from Middle East Technical University, Ankara, Turkey in the field of Industrial Engineering. He served as an instructor at Atilim University, where he taught various courses such as Ergonomics and Heuristic Methods for Optimization. He is a Ph.D. candidate in the Department of Industrial & Manufacturing Engineering at North Dakota State University. At NDSU, he has served in different academic positions such as Graduate Teaching Assistant, Instructor, and Graduate Research Assistant. Currently, he actively participates in the improvement and system redesign projects conducted at Veteran Affairs Healthcare Centers at local and national levels. His research interests include RFID applications in food and pharmaceutical distribution networks, wind energy engineering, healthcare Information Systems, metaheuristic methods for optimization, and mathematical modeling for healthcare applications.

Kambiz Farahmens is a Professor and department head in the Department of Industrial and Manufacturing Engineering at North Dakota State University. He is an internationally recognized expert in Productivity Improvement. He has published over 50 refereed papers, has over $3.5 million in research, and is a recipient of numerous awards. Dr. Farahmand has over 30 years of experience as an engineer, manager, and educator. His primary teaching and research activities are in the areas of manufacturing systems, lean manufacturing and implementation, ergonomics, safety and human factors engineering, human exposure and physiology simulation, simulation and modeling, facilities and production layout planning, operations & materials management and strategic planning, ISO and QS 9000 standards, and healthcare management. He has been involved in joint research and consulting with DOE, ARMY, NAVY, NASA, VHA, and industry. He is a registered professional engineer in the states of Texas and North Dakota.